Tending Animals in the Global Village

D0871066

A Guide to International Veterinary Medicine

About the Author

Dr. David M. Sherman is a graduate of Antioch College. He received his veterinary degree from the Ohio State University in 1977 and a Masters of Science degree in veterinary medicine from the University of Minnesota in 1979. He became board certified in Veterinary Internal Medicine in 1990. He has taught large animal clinical medicine at the University of Minnesota and at Tufts University School of Veterinary Medicine (TUSVM). He is coauthor of the veterinary textbook *Goat Medicine*, published in 1994. Dr. Sherman joined the Section of International Veterinary Medicine at TUSVM in 1990 and was appointed head of section in 1995. He also participated in the creation of the Center for Conservation Medicine at TUSVM and was appointed director of the center in 1997. Currently, Dr. Sherman is the chief of the Bureau of Animal Health for the Commonwealth of Massachusetts. He is the president of Farm Africa USA and the editor-in-chief of *Small Ruminant Research*, the journal of the International Goat Association.

Dr. Sherman's first international experience was in 1969 as an exchange student at University College, Nairobi, Kenya, where he studied zoology. As a veterinarian, he has been actively involved in international work. Dr. Sherman has performed international consultancies for a variety of organizations including the private voluntary organizations Mercy Corps International, Heifer Project International, and Farm Africa UK. He has worked for the United Nations Development Programme and has consulted for the Food and Agricultural Organization of the United Nations, the International Livestock Centre for Africa, and the Pan African Rinderpest Campaign of the Organization of African Unity. These consultancies have focused on a variety of issues, including transboundary animal disease control, community-based animal health service delivery, dairy goat health and production, livestock disease investigation, and veterinary education. Dr. Sherman has worked in Afghanistan, Barbados, China, Egypt, Ethiopia, Israel, Kenya, Mongolia, Pakistan, Rwanda, Tanzania, Uganda, and Zimbabwe. He has also lectured in Brazil, Colombia, France, India, and Indonesia.

Tending Animals in the Global Village

A Guide to International Veterinary Medicine

David M. Sherman, DVM, MS, Diplomate, ACVIM

LIBRARY
FRANKLIN PIERCE COLLEGE
RINDGE, NH 03461

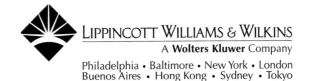

LIPPINCOTT WILLIAMS & WILKINS
A **Wolters Kluwer** Company

Philadelphia • Baltimore • New York • London
Buenos Aires • Hong Kong • Sydney • Tokyo

Editor: David Troy
Managing Editor: Dana Battaglia
Marketing Manager: Paul Jarecha
Production Editor: Paula C. Williams
Designer: Armen Kojoyian
Printer: Maple Press

Copyright © 2002 Lippincott Williams & Wilkins

351 West Camden Street
Baltimore, Maryland 21201-2436 USA

530 Walnut Street
Philadelphia, Pennsylvania 19106-3621 USA

All rights reserved. This book is protected by copyright. No part of this book may be reproduced in any form or by any means, including photocopying, or utilized by any information storage and retrieval system without written permission from the copyright owner.

The publisher is not responsible (as a matter of product liability, negligence, or otherwise) for any injury resulting from any material contained herein. This publication contains information relating to general principles of medical care which should not be construed as specific instructions for individual patients. Manufacturers' product information and package inserts should be reviewed for current information, including contraindications, dosages, and precautions.

Printed in the United States of America

Library of Congress Cataloging-in-Publication Data
Sherman, David M.
   Tending animals in the global village : a guide to international veterinary medicine /
David M. Sherman.
      p. ; cm.
   Includes bibliographical references and index.
   ISBN 0-683-18051-7
    1. Veterinary medicine. I. Title.
   [DNLM: 1. Veterinary medicine—trends. 2. International Cooperation. 3.
   Socioeconomic Factors SF 745 S553t 2002]
   SF745 .S45 2002
   636.089--dc21

pen underlining pg 4+5 noted 1\2020

200201620

The publishers have made every effort to trace the copyright holders for borrowed material. If they have inadvertently overlooked any, they will be pleased to make the necessary arrangements at the first opportunity.

To purchase additional copies of this book call our customer service department at **(800) 638-3030** or fax orders to **(301) 824-7390**. International customers should call **(301) 714-2324.**

Visit Lippincott Williams & Wilkins on the Internet: **http://www.lww.com.** Lippincott Williams & Wilkins customer service representatives are available from 8:30 am to 6:00 pm, EST, Monday through Friday, for telephone access.

02 03 04
1 2 3 4 5 6 7 8 9 10

This work is dedicated to

my father,

Harvey W. Sherman

(1924–2000)

who gave me his love and a moral compass,

to

my friend and mentor,

Martin F. Fuhrer, D.V.M.

(1922–1999)

who set me on the path of veterinary medicine.

and to

Leonard R. Faulkner

(1929–2002)

dairy farmer and neighbor,

who gave me the gift of community.

I dearly miss you all.

Preface

The science and practice of veterinary medicine continue to grow increasingly more sophisticated, with tremendous technological advances in clinical care and preventive medicine. Veterinarians generally do an excellent job of keeping up with the technical advances in their profession through continuing education efforts and by their general willingness to change and adapt. However, a great many trends and influences are at work outside the technical realm of veterinary science that exert profound effects on how the veterinary profession serves society and how veterinarians themselves will define their role as health professionals in a rapidly changing world. These trends and influences are rarely discussed in textbooks aimed at the veterinary community, though their importance to the veterinary profession is constantly growing. This book represents an effort to address that deficiency. It attempts to provide veterinary students, veterinarians, and other interested readers with an introduction to the global trends and international issues that are shaping the future of veterinary medicine in this era of globalization.

The goal of this text is to provide a framework for understanding the diverse potentialities of veterinary medicine in a global context. It offers an overview of the social, economic and environmental forces that influence the relationship of animals and society and which thereby create new challenges and opportunities for veterinary medicine in an increasingly interconnected world. The text is presented in ten chapters, briefly described as follows.

Chapter 1, *The Global Society and Veterinary Medicine*, presents an introductory summary of the major social, economic, and technological trends that are shaping contemporary global society and suggests how these trends are affecting veterinary medicine. Such trends include increased travel and improved communication; advances in science and technology; human population growth and its impact on the global food supply; increasing affluence and heightened consumer demand; the explosive growth in international trade; the spread of democracy; increasing pressure on natural resources; growing concerns about global environmental health; the degradation of natural habitats and the loss of biodiversity; and the global resurgence of infectious diseases.

Chapter 2, *Animal Domestication and Human Society*, provides a historical perspective on the origins and evolving relationship of domestic animals and human society. The various domestications are discussed in the context of the ecological, geographical, social, and economic conditions that surrounded the domestication process at different points and places in human social development. The chapter emphasizes that domestication is an ongoing process and points to the need for veterinarians to participate actively in the selection and domestication of new species to address evolving societal needs.

Chapter 3, *Cultural Attitudes Concerning the Use of Animals*, identifies some key cultural differences among various peoples and regions of the world regarding the use of particular animals and animal products and discusses the factors that have led to the emergence of these cultural differences. The general topics include food preferences and prohibitions; keeping animals as pets; and the influences of economic development and social transformation on societal attitudes toward the human use of animals. Perceptual differences between economically developed and developing countries are emphasized.

Chapter 4, *Animal Agriculture and Food Production Worldwide*, considers the important roles that animals play in global food production. The chapter begins with a discussion of the factors that influence the use of animals in agriculture and then presents information on the current distribution and use of various livestock species around the world. This is followed by a review of the different functions that animals perform in agriculture and daily life and a summary of the major systems of animal management found in different regions of the world. The geographical, cultural, and economic conditions that influence the selection of various animal management systems are emphasized. In closing, the role of animals in promoting sustainable agricultural practices is discussed, and various approaches to improving animal productivity are presented. Challenges and opportunities for veterinarians to enhance the sustainable contribution of livestock to the global food supply are identified.

Chapter 5, *Animals, Food Security, and Socioeconomic Development*, explores the pressing global problems of rural poverty and undernutrition and discusses the role that livestock can play in improving the health, welfare, and quality of life for subsistence farmers, pastoralists, and the landless poor in developing countries. The global situation relative to hunger is reviewed, and the factors that contribute to the persistence of poverty are examined. Then, the subject of international development assistance is discussed, including an overview of the organizations and mechanisms involved in providing such assistance. The role of veterinarians in socioeconomic development is emphasized, and examples of veterinary participation in international development are presented.

Chapter 6, *Animals and the Environment*, addresses growing global concern about environmental degradation. These concerns are examined from two perspectives: first, the role that animals and animal agriculture may play in the various forms of environmental degradation and, second, the impact that such degradations may have on the health and productivity of animals and humans. Topics considered include issues of land transformation such as land degradation, desertification, and deforestation; issues of climate change including global warming, the El Niño phenomenon, and ozone depletion; and issues of environmental contamination, including chemical pollutants associated with endocrine disruption, radiation hazards, and pollutants associated with livestock production. Challenges and opportunities for veterinary researchers, practitioners, and policymakers to address by the various forms of environmental degradation are presented throughout the chapter.

Chapter 7, *Preservation of Biodiversity, Wildlife, and Conservation Medicine*, examines the threats of accelerating biodiversity loss and wildlife extinctions and their implications for human society. Numerous causes are identified and reviewed including habitat loss, overexploitation of wildlife resources, competition from invasive species, and, of particular concern to veterinarians, disease. Efforts to preserve biodiversity, promote wildlife conservation, and protect endangered species are described from a global perspective, and the opportunities for veterinary participation in these *in situ* and *ex situ* efforts are discussed. Finally, the emerging field of conservation medicine is described, wherein veterinarians, physicians, conservation biologists, and other scientists can apply their skills and training to the promotion and integration of animal, human, and environmental health through interdisciplinary cooperation.

Chapter 8, *Delivery of Animal Health Care Services Worldwide*, describes the various services that organized veterinary medicine provides to society, both in the public and private sectors, using the United States structure of veterinary service delivery as a frame of reference. This is followed by a discussion of the constraints on veterinary service delivery in developing countries where, paradoxically, people depend most crucially on animals for their livelihood, yet often have the least reliable access to animal health care. In the final section of the chapter, opportunities to improve veterinary service delivery in developing countries are identified and discussed, including cost recovery; privatization of clinical veterinary services; development of community-based paraprofessional animal health care delivery; an expanded role for ethnoveterinary medicine; and curricular changes in veterinary education tailored to national or regional animal health care situations. Opportunities for involvement of veterinarians from developed countries in these efforts are presented in the discussion.

Chapter 9, *International Trade, Food Safety, and Animal Disease Control*, examines the impact that globalization and the expansion of free trade are having on the international trade of livestock and livestock products, particularly with regard to matters concerning food safety and the control of foreign animal diseases. The chapter begins with an overview of the process of globalization and the movement toward free trade, with special reference to agriculture in general and animal agriculture in particular. This is followed by consideration of the current challenges that veterinarians face in implementing effective animal disease control worldwide, along with a review of some of the

newer tools available to better understand, track, and control the spread of animal disease. Contemporary issues in food safety are then examined. A global overview of food-borne illness is first provided, followed by a review of various food safety concerns including food-borne pathogens, drug residues and antibiotic resistance, genetically modified foods, the welfare of animals raised for food, and the relationship of international trade to food safety. New tools available for managing food safety are also discussed. The chapter closes with a consideration of foreign animal disease control in the United States, emphasizing the role of veterinary practitioners as a critical element of the overall national disease control effort.

Chapter 10, *Career Opportunities in International Veterinary Medicine*, is intended as a practical guide for readers interested in adding an international dimension to their careers in veterinary medicine. The chapter begins with guidelines for conducting a self-assessment to determine both the reader's own suitability for international work and the type of international work that might best reflect the reader's personality and interests. This is followed by a discussion of how the reader can acquire relevant skills, training, and experience during different stages of his or her professional development. Suggestions are provided for readers at the undergraduate, veterinary school, and postgraduate level. Next, there is a presentation of the various types of organizations that might employ veterinarians for international work. The activities of various categories of agencies are described, and specific examples of organizations in each category are provided. The chapter closes with a discussion of how to go about finding work that matches the reader's interests, skills, and experience.

At the end, the book has an appendix that provides contact information for various organizations relevant to the subject of international veterinary medicine. These are divided into several categories, including biodiversity, wildlife, and environmental groups; donor and lending institutions; international development and aid agencies; international technical organizations; nongovernmental organizations involved in general relief and development; nongovernmental organizations focused on veterinary relief and development; pharmaceutical and animal nutrition firms; private consulting firms; professional veterinary and related organizations; research and policy institutions; training, fellowship, and grant opportunities; and United States government agencies.

Numerous, dramatic events in 2001 have made it indisputably clear that veterinarians live and work in a global village. The spread of bovine spongiform encephalopathy throughout Europe and into Japan, the emergence of that same disease as a deadly zoonotic pathogen, the devastating outbreak of foot and mouth disease in the United Kingdom, the specter of that same disease entering the United States, the rapid spread of West Nile virus through the eastern half of the United States, the horrific terrorist attacks of September 11 in New York and Washington, D.C., and the subsequent fear of bioterrorism, including agricultural terrorism, all serve to underscore the global dimension of contemporary veterinary medicine and illustrate that all veterinary medicine is becoming international veterinary medicine. It is the author's hope that this text will serve as an informative and helpful guidebook that veterinarians can use to navigate through the complex landscape of international veterinary medicine, develop a greater knowledge of the terrain, and better appreciate the expanded role they can play in creating a safer, healthier, and more equitable world.

David M. Sherman
Newton, Massachusetts
January, 2002

If you see your neighbor's ox or sheep gone astray, do not ignore it ... you must not remain indifferent.

Deuteronomy 22:1–3

Acknowledgments

First and foremost, I must thank my wonderful wife and best friend, Laurie Miller, for the love, patience, understanding, and support, both emotional and material, that she steadily provided during my seemingly interminable effort to write this book. I also thank her for her willingness to endure numerous and extended separations over the years as I pursued various opportunities in veterinary medicine around the globe. Next, I want to thank my mother, Blossom Sherman, who, against her better judgment and her strong maternal instincts, opened the world to me by consenting to allow me to do a year of undergraduate study in zoology at the University College, Nairobi, in 1969 when I was nineteen years old. I thank Dr. Robert Pelant of Heifer Project International for offering me my first international consultancy in 1985, evaluating an HPI dairy goat development project in Taiwan. I also want to thank Dr. Al Sollod and Dr. Chip Stem for inviting me to join them in the International Program at Tufts University School of Veterinary Medicine in 1990 and for demonstrating, through their innovative efforts, the feasibility, importance, and value of cultivating a global perspective among veterinary students during their period of professional training.

Many individuals provided assistance during the preparation of this book by reviewing draft chapters, offering technical criticism and editorial advice, or by providing general encouragement and support. I want to thank them all for their help and acknowledge their contribution. These individuals included Dr. Nick A. Beresford, Dr. Robert H. Dunlop, Dr. Anthony W. English, Dr. Deana Fritcher, Mr. John K. Greifer, Dr. Michael R. Goe, Dr. Borje K. Gustafsson, Dr. Pierre H. Y. Hierneaux, Dr. Sylvia Kaneko, Dr. Ellen Messner Rogers, Mr. Brad Mitchell, Dr. Mary Pearl, Dr. William G. Smith, Dr. Marilyn J. Wolfe, and Dr. Michael Woodford. These individuals provided excellent counsel and any errors in the book are solely my own responsibility. Dr. Ellen Messner Rogers also provided considerable assistance in the preparation of the appendix of this text, for which I thank her.

In addition, numerous individuals, including some listed in the preceding paragraph, were kind enough to provide photographs for use in this text. Their contribution is hereby acknowledged with appreciation. Photographs supplied by Farm Africa UK were made available through the efforts of Mr. Richard Turner. Other individuals who provided photographs are identified in the captions associated with the photographs they provided. Also, I wish to thank Robert and Betty Kaufman of Silver Visions, Newton, MA, for creative and technical assistance with the photographs used on the cover and in the book.

Finally, I wish to thank my managing editor at Lippincott Williams & Wilkins, Ms. Dana Battaglia, who proved to be a most able shepherdess, leading me gently but firmly to the end of this project despite my incessant bleating and my tendency to stray from the path.

Contents

Chapter 1
The Global Society and Veterinary Medicine

OBJECTIVES FOR THIS CHAPTER:

After completing this chapter, the reader should be able to

- Identify the major global trends that are redefining how people and animals will live on Earth in the coming years
- Recognize the effects that human transformation of the Earth has on the global ecosystem and the implications for human, animal, and environmental health
- Begin to identify new challenges and opportunities for veterinarians to contribute meaningfully as health professionals and as world citizens to the well-being of humans, animals, and Earth itself

Introduction

Some of the most powerful visual images in history are the photographs of Earth taken from space by moon-bound astronauts on the Apollo missions of the late 1960s and early 1970s (Fig. 1-1). These photos of Earth, cradled in a thin wisp of cottony atmosphere and suspended in limitless space, have forever changed the way we look at life on our planet. The unity of the global ecosystem is an undeniable reality when Earth is viewed from space. The interdependence of humans, animals, the land, the sea, and the air is readily apparent. The fragility and beauty of the biosphere are made plain. The need for balance, sharing, and peaceful coexistence is clear. Our own, unique, earthly paradise is revealed to us, as is our responsibility for its stewardship.

Alas, back here on the ground, it is difficult to maintain this perspective of unity. Daily life seems punctuated as much by conflict as by consensus. In fact, we live in a time of great contradiction and contrast. Consider, for example, the following:

- Remarkable advances have been made in recent years in medicine and biotechnology, yet at the same time, the threat of infectious disease has increased, with the emergence of new infections and the resurgence of old infections in more virulent forms. Large segments of the earth's population still have little or no access to reliable health care services for themselves or their animals.

- Population growth rates in the most affluent countries have stabilized or even declined, while population growth rates in the poorest countries are among the highest in the world.

- Globalization of the free market economy has created economic opportunity for millions of people around the world, but millions more remain on the margins, with little prospect of climbing out of abject poverty.

- Science and technology have facilitated enormous increases in agricultural productivity, yet as many as 800 million of the world's people experience hunger or malnutrition daily.

- Citizens in developed countries are cutting back on their meat consumption for medical and ethical reasons while per capita meat consumption in the developing world is skyrocketing.

- The risk of war between nations has diminished as former enemies sign arms limitation and peace agreements and become trading partners. At the same time, armed conflict within nations has increased, as more civil wars are fought over issues of ethnicity, religion, lack of representation, or localized claims to natural resources.

- A love of, and fascination with, wild animals has emerged as a major cultural force in developed countries, yet worldwide, animal extinctions and associated habitat destruction are accelerating at an alarming rate.

Every day, the poorest among us struggle to survive, the comfortable among us, to be more comfortable, and the wealthy among us, to be wealthier. These aspirations all represent a daily competition for increased access to, and exploitation of, the finite resource base that is Earth. The collective strivings and competing interests of human society reverberate through the planet in many forms-civil war, deforestation, desertification, urbanization, emerging disease, air pollution, animal extinctions, and loss of biodiversity. As the human population continues to increase, our own collective human needs-for food, water, shelter, transportation, jobs, entertainment-are placing additional stresses on our global ecosystem and displacing its other, nonhuman inhabitants. Human beings, through the power of science and technology, have, in our time, achieved hegemony over Earth and control over its destiny.

The long-term impact of our collective, cumulative, daily human activity on the viability of Earth itself is only imperfectly understood. As the influence of human society expands, new questions emerge, more quickly it seems than answers:

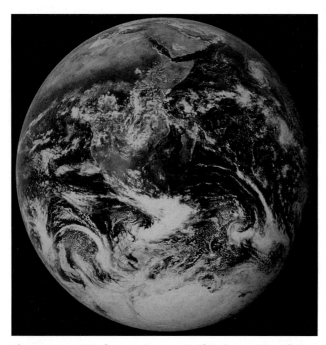

Figure 1-1. This famous photograph of Earth, now identified as the "Blue Marble," was taken by the astronauts aboard the Apollo 17 spacecraft on their way to the moon in 1972. The Horn of Africa and the Arabian Peninsula are clearly visible. NASA believes this to be the most widely distributed image in human history. (Used with permission from the National Space Science Data Center, National Aeronautics and Space Administration.)

- As an ecosystem, does the Earth have enough resiliency and regenerative capacity to withstand the relentless assault of human exploitation on its forests, oceans, and atmosphere?

- Can human population growth exceed the carrying capacity of Earth?

- Will advances in biotechnology and agricultural science help us to succeed in feeding a human population that doubles every 40 years?

- What effect will inexorable population growth have on patterns of human and animal disease?

- What are the implications of dwindling biodiversity on human society and on Earth itself?

- Is the inevitable consequence of the global market economy that people of all nations will enjoy the same standard of living currently enjoyed by people in the prosperous nations of the West? If so, can the Earth tolerate such a level of individual consumption on a worldwide basis?

- What effects will it have on the world if most of the world's population owns automobiles at the rate that people in the industrialized nations currently own them?

- What will be the impact on food production if most of the world's population consumes meat at a rate equivalent to the current rate in industrialized nations?

These questions are not simply rhetorical. They need to be addressed to ensure that Earth can continue to sustain the increasing material desires of an expanding human population without damage to its own viability. Human society has demonstrated an awesome ability to transform the Earth to suit its own needs. However, it remains to be seen whether human beings, having established de facto ownership of the Earth, can demonstrate proper stewardship of the planet.

The fact is that human beings do not have much experience in managing a planet. Earth itself is 5 billion years old. Vertebrate life on the planet emerged about 450 million years ago. The hominid ancestors of human beings evolved just 4.5 million years ago. Agricultural society emerged only about 10,000 years ago, while industrialized society and the germ theory of disease developed only within the last 200 years. Modern communication and transportation technology are about 100 years old, and our modern experiment in cooperative world governance, the United Nations, is just 50 years old.

We still have a lot to learn about our stewardship of the Earth. As the noted biologist Dr. E. O. Wilson observed, at a recent lecture on the loss of biodiversity, "We have no clue where we are going, but we have incredible tools to get there." We do indeed require a clearer idea of where we are going and must begin

to chart that course for the future, taking into account the interdependency that defines life on Earth, which is so eloquently represented in the Apollo mission photographs.

Veterinarians have much to contribute to the health management of our planet and its animal and human inhabitants. Veterinary medicine, at its core, focuses on the interdependent relationships of people, animals, and the environment and how to maintain these components in a healthful equilibrium. Whether at the kennel, the dairy barn, or the zoo, the veterinarian, as diagnostician and healer, must assess and manage numerous aspects of the environment at hand. Ventilation, water quality, general hygiene, food supply, and living space are some of the factors that are routinely considered to manage disease effectively and promote health and productivity. There is a tremendous need and opportunity for veterinarians to expand their environmental frame of reference beyond man-made structures and to apply their solid training, skills, and perspective to managing the health and sustainability of natural environments such as forests, savannas, rivers, and wetlands and their inhabitants. Ultimately, the health and well-being of all creatures depends on a greater understanding of, and respect for Earth—the global ecosystem we call home.

Important Global Trends for Veterinary Medicine

Today, as in the past, the human use of animals and human concern for animals remain as fundamental themes in human society. However the human-animal relationship is a dynamic relationship. It is being constantly redefined by the powerful forces of rapid change that characterize modern, global society. In the following sections of this chapter, key, contemporary, global trends that are reshaping the practice and perspective of modern veterinary medicine are presented, with reference to the opportunities and challenges that these global trends present for veterinarians and the animals and people who rely on them.

Increased Travel and Improved Communication

Clearly, nothing has caused our world to "shrink" or accelerated the pace of life more than modern developments in transportation and telecommunications. Nowadays, virtually everywhere and everyone on the planet is potentially accessible on short notice (see sidebar "Doing Business in Asia: Then and Now"). Those of the world's citizens who can afford it have taken exuberantly to traveling for business or simply for pleasure. Tourism has become the fastest growing sector of the global economy, currently providing over 100 million jobs worldwide. In 2000, almost 700 million people left their own countries to visit other countries as tourists and then return home. The World Tourism Organization projects that international tourism arrivals will exceed 1 billion by the year 2010 and reach 1.5 billion by 2020. Millions more people travel on business. In the United States alone, annual arrivals of international air passengers more than quintupled in the last quarter of the 20th century, from 10.9 million in 1975 to 56.2 million in 1998, according to data reported by the United States Department of Transportation.

This globe-trotting fervor has serious implications for veterinary medicine. A key responsibility of veterinarians is to protect a nation's animals from the introduction of diseases that do not already occur within its borders. The speed, frequency, and volume of modern jet travel make this an increasingly challenging task. Travelers carry with them an astounding array of souvenirs and artifacts when returning from trips abroad, including many products of vegetable and animal origin that may harbor infectious agents or pests that threaten vulnerable plant and animal life at home.

For instance, meat-based products, such as sausages, may contain viable organisms capable of producing African swine fever, classical swine fever, or foot and mouth disease. The introduction of such organisms into countries presently free of these agents could wreak economic havoc on indigenous livestock industries, as such diseases may produce high mor-

Doing Business in Asia: Then and Now

One of the dominant features of modern economic life is the robust trade that flourishes between Asia and the West. While this trade did not always exist, its putative beginnings, over 700 years ago, are known. In the 13th century, Venice was the mercantile capital of the world and embodied the entrepreneurial spirit of the time. Venetian businessmen sought new business and trade opportunities wherever they might arise. Around AD 1260, Nicolo and Maffeo Polo, two brothers and merchants of Venice, set out eastward on a trading expedition to the Crimea and beyond. Early in their travels, they met an ambassador of Kublai Khan, the emperor of the eastern Tartar Empire, who proposed that the Polos visit the court of the Great Khan near what is today Beijing, China. Curious about the business opportunities that might develop, the brothers agreed to travel further east. Kublai Khan warmly welcomed the Polo brothers, and after hearing their tales of life in Europe, the Great Khan expressed interest in bringing Christian teachings to his eastern empire. He asked the two Venetians to serve as his emissaries and return to Europe to request that the pope send 100 religious teachers to his kingdom. Thus, the linkage of commerce with cultural exchange was clearly established.

It took Nicolo and Maffeo 3 years of grueling overland travel with horse, donkey, and camel caravans to get back to Europe from Beijing, only to discover that Pope Clement IV had died a year before their arrival. They waited in Venice for two more years while the College of Cardinals wrangled over the election of a new pope. Finally, they left again for China, accompanied by two friars of questionable knowledge and talent, hastily assigned to their mission by the new pope, Gregory X. Both friars, terrified by the perils and hardships of the overland journey, fled back to Europe, while Nicolo and Maffeo, accompanied now by Nicolo's son, Marco, continued slowly onward to China. Finally, after 31/2 years of return travel, including a year's stay in the mountains of northern Afghanistan to allow young Marco to recover from fever, they once again reached the court of the Great Khan, sans friars, but with some sacred oil from the Holy Land, and a letter of greeting from the pope.

While trade between Europe and Asia has continued to increase following the return of the Polos to Venice, history tells us that Christianity never did make very significant inroads into China. The trials and tribulations experienced by Nicolo, Maffeo, and Marco Polo on their long and arduous journey help to explain why. The window of opportunity opened by Kublai Khan was shut by delays in travel and communication. Clearly, modern travel has profoundly altered the way the world conducts business across long distances, and modern telecommunication has virtually erased time as a constraint on human interaction.

Today, things might have turned out differently. A modern family Polo responding to the Great Khan's proposal would have scheduled an audience at the Vatican by cellular phone while still in Beijing, hopped a flight from Beijing to Rome, arranged for a program of religious instruction for the Tartar Empire via satellite teleconferencing using friars based in Italy, air freighted the sacred oil of the Holy Land to Beijing by overnight express, emailed the Pope's letter back to the Great Khan as an attachment, and had the whole deal wrapped up in less than a week-in which case the communists' Great Hall of the People in Beijing might today be listed in tourist guide books instead as the Great Cathedral of China.

bidity and mortality in immunologically naive animal populations and require the slaughter of large numbers of exposed or at-risk animals to control further spread of the disease. This was the case in the United Kingdom in 2001 when foot and mouth disease was introduced into the country and close to 4.0 million cattle, sheep, goats, and swine were destroyed before the infection was stamped out. The risk of rapid spread of introduced diseases may be exacerbated in countries where intensive animal production is practiced and large numbers of animals are concentrated in close proximity. This is a major concern in the United States, where feedlot cattle, swine, and poultry are routinely raised under intensive management conditions.

In the United States, the Animal and Plant Health Inspection Service (APHIS) of the United States Department of Agriculture (USDA) is the agency officially charged with excluding foreign diseases and pests from the nation. Through its Plant Protection and Quarantine Division, APHIS employs about 1300 inspectors, stationed at ports of entry into the United States, including international airports, to screen passengers and their baggage for potentially dangerous plant and animal products. In the last decade, these inspectors have been joined in their efforts by over 60 Beagle dogs at 21 ports of entry around the country. These dogs are trained to sniff out various meat and vegetable odors. In 2001, following the outbreak of foot and mouth disease in the United Kingdom and elsewhere, the U.S. secretary of Agriculture authorized $32 million in spending to hire 350 new inspection personnel and double the size of the USDA Beagle Brigade. This additional help will be welcome, as APHIS inspectors (and their canine colleagues) face a formidable challenge, given the ever increasing flow of air traffic into the United States. In addition to tourism, the expanding international trade in animals and animal products is increasing the risk of new, foreign animal-disease introductions, which pose potential threats to animal and, sometimes, human health. A more detailed discussion of issues in international disease control and international trade is provided in Chapter 9.

Ecotourism, whereby travelers specifically seek out holiday experiences in natural settings to view fauna and flora in their relatively undisturbed state, is one of the fastest growing segments of the tourist economy. Ecotourism results in increased contacts between people and animals throughout the world, with important implications for both human and animal health. In some instances, ecotourism has been embraced as a mechanism for promoting the conservation of threatened and endangered species. The income generated by visiting tourists is offered as an economic justification for preserving the threatened or endangered species in its natural habitat. However, this rationale for ecotourism is a two-edged sword. The pursuit of income puts pressure on site managers to allow increased tourist numbers, which in turn can lead to degradation of the habitat and expose the animals to increased health risks, an outcome contrary to the original intent. This is particularly true of endangered primates, who are susceptible to many of the same disease organisms as humans. More infor-

mation on ecotourism and the opportunities and challenges it poses for veterinarians is presented in Chapter 8.

Modern satellite communication and the internet have turned the world into a "global village," a term coined in the 1960s by communications theorist and educator Marshall MacLuhan to describe the transforming effects of electronic media on human society. In his book *Understanding Media: The Extensions of Man,* MacLuhan[9] proposed that, "In the electric age, when our central nervous system is technologically extended to involve us in the whole of mankind and to incorporate the whole of mankind in us, we necessarily participate, in depth, in the consequences of our every action." MacLuhan's observation was prophetic. Today, modern communication allows us to experience world events directly as they take place, while modern jet travel allows us to participate directly in such events almost immediately. For example, when man-made or natural disasters strike, veterinarians are increasingly becoming involved in providing support to victims, both animal and human at distant locations around the globe, sometimes within a matter of hours.

In the United States, veterinarians have formed the American Academy of Veterinary Disaster Medicine to promote the welfare of animals during and after disasters. In addition, the organization provides consultative services and professional advice to agencies responsible for developing emergency response procedures and tries to foster the inclusion in emergency management plans of protocols specifically addressing the rescue and care of animals at risk. The World Society for the Protection of Animals, in the United Kingdom, is a nonprofit agency that fields teams worldwide to rescue livestock and pets following natural disasters around the world (see http://www.wspa.org.uk/). Another nonprofit organization, Veterinaires Sans Frontieres-France (VSF), or Veterinarians Without Borders, provides veterinary services and training in difficult environments and situations in which people who depend on animals for their livelihood are threatened by war, drought, or other major calamities. VSF is currently working in 16 developing countries around the world (see http://www.vsf-france.org/). Delivery of animal health care services worldwide is discussed in more detail in Chapter 8, and the role of veterinary assistance in developing countries is discussed further in Chapter 5.

Advances in Science and Technology

Science and technology have reshaped our modern world in such profound ways that a discussion of their total impact on contemporary society is well beyond the scope of this book. However, some specific scientific and technological developments bear directly on the future of veterinary medicine and merit at least a brief introduction here. These developments include biotechnology, satellite sensing, and computer modeling.

Biotechnology

At the same time that space exploration has provided us with metaphorical imagery for the unity of life, advances in molecular biology and genetics have provided the scientific evidence for that unity. We now know that at the molecular level the structure and function of all forms of life are defined by their genetic code and that there is remarkable uniformity and homology to the molecular composition of genes, from single-celled organisms through complex mammalian organisms, including humans. This basic knowledge and the techniques developed to obtain this knowledge are now being regularly applied throughout the rapidly expanding biotechnology industry, to develop new products and services in a variety of areas of human activity. Many of these applications have direct and indirect implications for veterinarians in a global context.

Background on Biotechnology   It was in 1953 that James Watson and Francis Crick deduced the structure of deoxyribonucleic acid (DNA), the fundamental molecule of genetic expression. The structure they described is both simple and elegant. Simple in that it consists of only four basic nucleotides linked in a double-stranded chain. Elegant in that the repeating structure of the chain allows for enormous variation in the genetic expression of different proteins. The basic building blocks of genes are the same for bacteria as they are for mammals, but the sequence of nucleotides within genes permits them to express different proteins and thereby regulate the growth and differentiation of organisms, each according to its own particular genetic blueprint. In this manner, bacteria are destined to become more bacteria and mammals are destined to beget mammals.

In 1967, Har Gobind Khorana and Marshall Nirenberg unlocked the genetic code. They determined which specific sequence of three nucleotides (a codon) or set of codons in a DNA molecule were responsible for expressing each of the 20 amino acids that serve as the basic constituents of all proteins. With this knowledge, if the structure of a protein were known, then it would be possible, with appropriate technology and skill, to work backward to identify the gene responsible for the production of that protein, study it, and even, perhaps, manipulate it. Therein lies the basis for modern genetic engineering and applied biotechnology.

Scientists now have taken advantage of this knowledge and have developed techniques to manipulate genes in extraordinarily ingenious ways. Early recombinant DNA techniques allowed, for example, a mammalian gene to be introduced into a bacterium so that a culture of bacteria would produce the mammalian protein, say insulin, coded for by that gene. These recombinant DNA techniques have become sufficiently advanced that now, transgenic mammals are being produced routinely. For example, human genes are being introduced into the DNA of goat or sheep embryos, and their expression manipulated so that when the transgenic sheep or goat matures, it will produce the desired human protein, but only in the cells of the sheep or goat's mammary tissue. In this way, the protein can be harvested from the animal's milk as a pharmaceutical product, while the gene and its product exert no apparent direct effect on the sheep or goat itself, outside of the mammary gland.

Techniques for genetic manipulation have become so sophisticated that the cloning of mammals, including sheep and cattle, has been accomplished by transferring somatic cell nuclei from an adult animal into unfertilized ova whose own nuclear material has been removed. In this process, a cow muscle cell, for example, with a full complement of cow genes but only expressing those genes required for it to function as muscle, reverts to full expression of all its genes. The manipulated ovum is transferred to the uterus of a recipient cow that carries the developing embryo through to term pregnancy. The embryonic maturation of the manipulated ova containing the muscle cell nucleus leads to the development of a fully differentiated, functioning calf. This calf is an identical clone of the cow from which the muscle cell was taken.

Genetic engineering and biotechnology already have, and will continue to have, much influence on the art, science, and practice of veterinary medicine. Three key areas can be identified in which that influence will be felt, namely clinical medicine, animal agriculture, and the environment. In all of these areas, there are challenges and opportunities of a global nature for interested veterinarians.

Biotechnology and Clinical Medicine   In clinical medicine, biotechnology is offering new prospects for the diagnosis, treatment, and prevention of animal disease. In the area of diagnosis, monoclonal antibodies, produced by hybridoma technology are greatly improving the specificity and sensitivity of diagnostic tests, such as the enzyme-linked immunosorbant assay (ELISA), for the identification of antibody or antigen associated with infectious agents. DNA amplification techniques, such as the polymerase chain reaction (PCR), are being used to identify minute quantities of DNA associated with infectious agents so that early or latent infections are more readily detectable. Such advances are providing better opportunities to manage individual cases in clinical practice, identify and control diseases in livestock herds, improve surveillance in regulatory disease control programs, and even improve opportunities for international trade of livestock (see sidebar "Goat Disease, Polymerase Chain Reactions, and International Relations").

Biotechnology is opening the door to new therapies and therapeutic applications for animal disease as well. For example, the tools of genetic engineering, in conjunction with advances in computer science, are enabling researchers to identify the specific, three-dimensional structure of microbial proteins and their related receptor sites in host cells. Based on this knowledge, antimicrobial drugs can be rationally designed to specifically block entry, adherence, or metabolic expression of important pathogens.

Perhaps the greatest potential of biotechnology in veterinary medicine is in the area of disease prevention and disease resistance. Recombinant DNA technology is facilitating novel approaches to immunization, with the potential to increase immunogenicity, reduce the risk of reversion to virulence, minimize vaccination stress on animals, permit new routes of administration, allow discrimination of antibody responses due to vaccination from responses due to natural infection, and improve stability and ease of handling of vaccines in the field.

Improved stability and ease of handling in the field are particularly significant issues in the developing world, where livestock are important to local economies, but infectious disease control through vaccination is difficult to achieve. In many such places, rural infrastructure, in terms of roads, electricity, and refrigeration, is not available to keep live vaccines cold for extended periods of time under field conditions. With these constraints in mind, some of the early vaccine development efforts by veterinary researchers focused on the creation of effective, genetically engineered vaccines with suitable characteristics for use in the field under adverse conditions. Rinderpest, peste des petits ruminants, foot and mouth disease, and East Coast fever are some of the tropical diseases of livestock targeted in these efforts.

Manipulation of natural disease resistance in animals, is another opportunity facilitated by advances in biotechnology. It is known that certain breeds of livestock in different locations around the world show resistance to specific diseases. Sometimes this is the result of acquired immunity, but in other cases, the disease resistance may have a genetic basis. One new approach to manipulating disease resistance is to identify breeds or families of animals that demonstrate natural resistance to infection by certain pathogens, attempt to identify a genetic basis for the resistance, isolate the responsible genes, and introduce them into the germ cell line of nonresistant breeds of animals that might have other superior production characteristics but lack the disease resistance. Such investigations are already ongoing with regard to livestock diseases of international significance, for example, the assessment of the local N'Dama breed of cattle in west Africa for genetically based resistance to the protozoal disease trypanosomiasis.

Another approach to promoting disease resistance is the introduction into animals of nonmammalian genes that may produce enzymes deleterious to parasites, but which are innocuous to the host animal. For example, blowfly strike is an important disease of sheep in which blowflies lay eggs in skin wounds of sheep and the larvae develop by feeding on sheep tissues. Blowfly larvae have a structural polysaccharide called chitin in their outer cover, but mammals, including sheep, do not possess chitin. Some plants, however, produce an enzyme, chitinase, that breaks down chitin, as a defense against insect predators. Currently, veterinary scientists in the animal production branch of the Commonwealth Scientific and Industrial Research Organization (CSIRO) in Australia are working on the introduction of a plant gene coded for the production of chitinase into sheep, which would be expressed in the animal's sweat glands. The hope is that sweat containing chitinase, secreted onto the sheep's skin, will inhibit the development of blowfly larvae.

Biotechnology and Animal Agriculture In the realm of animal agriculture, biotechnology offers tools to improve the productivity of livestock in various ways. One opportunity is to improve adaptability of animals to adverse environments by improving, for example, heat tolerance in the tropics or, as just described above, disease resistance through the use of transgenic animals. Another approach is to improve growth rates of animals through the use of growth promoters, including somatotropin. The growth hormones may be produced exogenously for parenteral administration to animals, or genes regulating increased production of growth hormones may be introduced into germ cell lines to produce transgenic animals. This has already been done with genetically engineered, farm-fished Atlantic salmon.[11] The genetically modified salmon can reach market weight in 18 months compared with 24 to 30 months for conventional fish.

The quantity or quality of a product produced by animals may also be manipulated, as has already been done with bovine somatotropin, or BST, to increase milk production in dairy cows. Other applications under consideration or development include manipulation of carcass characteristics in pigs and poultry to increase muscle mass and reduce fat, reduction of the fat content of cow's milk, transgenic alteration of fiber quality in sheep and goats to produce finer grades of wool and cashmere, and reduction of cholesterol content of eggs, to name but a few. Using biotechnology, it might someday be possible to carry out mass cultivation of animal muscle cells *in vitro* to produce a meat-type, animal protein product that could be harvested, processed, and then packaged much like sausage is today, without the exploitation of live animals.

Plants used as feed for animals may also be genetically altered to improve animal production by increasing overall protein content, altering the production ratios of essential amino acids, or including immunizing antigens against animal diseases into plants so that animals eating those plants have their enteric mucosal immunity stimulated continuously against specific infections.

Biotechnology and the Environment Bioremediation is the branch of biotechnology that addresses the reduction of environmental pollution through the use of plants and microorganisms with the ability to capture or degrade toxins and pollutants and thereby remove them from the environment. Genetic engineering offers the opportunity to improve the efficiency and broaden the spectrum of microorganisms and plants that can be used in bioremediation. Bioremediation is already finding application in the cleanup of oil spills by use of oil-digesting bacteria, the clearance of heavy metals such as lead from contaminated soils by use of plants of the mustard family, and the removal of uranium from water by pumping it through filters containing uranium-binding bacteria bound to polymer beads.

There is increasing awareness of the potential adverse impacts that modern agricultural practices can have on the environment. This includes management practices in animal agriculture. Bioremediation offers opportunities to alleviate the environmental stresses of farming. For example, intensification of animal production in large-scale confinement units has led to the concentration and storage of vast quantities of animal

Goat Disease, Polymerase Chain Reactions (PCR), and International Relations

In 1982, I attended the Third International Conference on Goat Production and Disease, held in Tucson, Arizona. At one session, a Kenyan official in attendance stood up and angrily accused the U.S. government of trying to undermine the well-being and development of his country by willfully and knowingly encouraging the exportation to Kenya of American purebred dairy goats infected with the virus that causes CAE, thus putting millions of Kenyan goats at risk for a disease which previously did not occur in that country. The goats in question had been sent as part of a USAID-funded livestock development project. More than a few eyebrows were raised by this spontaneous and public accusation at a scientific meeting.

In truth, it is quite likely that dairy goats exported from the United States prior to 1982 may have been infected with CAE virus. However, the Kenyan's position that the export of infected goats was the purposefully malevolent act of a hostile government had no merit. The problem had less to do with politics and international intrigue than with the state of our knowledge about CAE and the tools available to detect infection at that point in time. Nevertheless, the story does serve to emphasize how international livestock trade can become a contentious matter and how important animal health and disease issues are in maintaining harmonious international trading relations. Since that conference, biotechnological applications in veterinary medicine have led to a better understanding of the pathogenesis of CAE infection and resulted in the development of new diagnostic approaches that would have effectively detected infected goats well before they were shipped to Kenya.

CAE is caused by a retrovirus. The disease affects primarily goats and has a neurological and an arthritic form. The neurological form was first recognized in 1974, and the virus was first isolated from the arthritic form of the disease in 1980, so at the time of the Tucson conference, CAE was still a relatively new and incompletely understood disease. It is now known, thanks to modern

manure, leading to associated problems of waste disposal, as discussed further in Chapter 6. In the United States, concerns about the contamination of water supplies, adverse impacts on wildlife, and possible effects on human health from animal manure in the environment led the Environmental Protection Agency (EPA) to introduce stricter regulations on animal manure treatment and disposal in 1998. New approaches to the problems of animal waste management and new opportunities for waste utilization must be developed. Bioremediation is likely to provide useful methods to reduce harmful chemical and microbial constituents in animal waste, speed the process of waste degradation, and increase the production of byproducts from animal manure usable, for example, as fuel, fertilizer, or feed. Transgenic science may also offer solutions to waste management. In 1999, scientists at the University of Guelph, in Canada, developed the "Enviropig," a genetically engineered hog that contains a mouse/*Escherichia coli* transgene that promotes secretion of salivary phytase. This enables the pig to absorb the phosphorus in cereal feeds more efficiently, which thus reduces the amount of phosphorus in manure. Contamination of groundwater with phosphorus from livestock manure runoff is recognized as a significant contributor to reduced water quality.

Public Concerns about Biotechnology The preceding discussion highlights some of the opportunities that scientific advances in molecular biology and genetic engineering offer to improve animal health, food production and human nutrition, and environmental quality. It reflects the enormous sense of scientific power and potential that the biotechnology industry itself promotes to society at large. There are considerable segments of society, however, that voice a healthy skepticism concerning the power and promise of biotechnology and who see it, rather, as a potentially dangerous and disruptive force threatening our future well-being. Eric Grace,[8] in his informative book *Biotechnology Unzipped*, offers a useful summary of the main concerns commonly expressed about biotechnology and discusses their significance. He identifies the issues as follows:

- Altering genes is unnatural.
- Swapping genes between species is unnatural.
- Genetic engineering breaches fundamental species boundaries.
- New combinations of genes in microbes are likely to produce dangerous and uncontrollable mutant germs.
- We are altering evolution by creating new combinations of genes.

techniques of molecular biology, that the causative retrovirus has a predilection for host cells of the monocyte-macrophage line. In the infected goat, the virus enters host mononuclear cells, and the viral genome is integrated into the host cell DNA where it may reside in latent form for extended periods of time.

In 1982, the only diagnostic test routinely available for the detection of CAE infection was the agar gel immunodiffusion (AGID) test, which identified the presence of circulating antibody to the CAE virus in the serum of infected goats. However, antibody tests are actually indirect tests of infection, identifying not the infection itself, but only the host's reaction to it. Unknown in 1982, but known now, is the fact that there may be a considerable lag time between the introduction of the CAE virus into the host's mononuclear cells and the subsequent development of an antibody response by the infected host. One study reported this delay to be as long as 8 months. That means that serum taken from an infected goat might give false-negative responses on an AGID test for as long as 8 months following infection. So even if the goats shipped to Kenya had been tested and found negative on the AGID test and identified, in good faith, as disease free, they might still in fact have been infected, with the virus present in the host cell genome, but not yet stimulating an antibody response.

Advances in biotechnology have now enabled veterinary scientists to eliminate these false-negative test results by direct identification of the viral DNA. Polymerase chain reaction (PCR) is a technique, first developed in 1985, that allows minute quantities of DNA to be amplified from small samples. Using PCR, DNA from the CAE virus could be directly identified from cells of an infected goat, and by 1993, PCR was being applied to the diagnosis of CAE infection. A blood sample is taken from the goat. Peripheral blood mononuclear cells are separated from whole blood and disrupted, and the PCR procedure is applied to the prepared sample. The amplified quantity of DNA fragments are separated by gel electrophoresis and then transferred by blotting to nitrocellulose paper. Then, CAE-specific DNA probes are applied to detect the presence of proviral DNA from the monocyte samples to confirm retroviral infection. Unlike the situation in 1982, countries importing goats today can avoid the risk of accepting CAE-infected goats with false-negative diagnostic test results by requiring a negative PCR test result as a condition of shipment.

- Biotechnology brings unprecedented new power to humanity, with new ethical dilemmas.

Some of the skepticism concerning biotechnology is a direct reaction to the assertive optimism of the biotechnology industry itself in promoting the development and application of biotechnology. Many critics perceive that the industry is driven essentially by the goal of corporate profit, not social progress, and therefore, believe that industry makes claims about the promise of biotechnology that overstate its benefits and understate its risks. This perception has led to a variety of societal responses including organized protests against individual biotechnology firms, academic forums on the role of biotechnology in society, the creation of independent oversight groups to monitor industry developments, and increasing calls for government regulation of the biotechnology industry, particularly with regard to safety testing of new products before they are released for market.

It is probably fair to say that biotechnology is neither a total panacea nor a total pariah. The situation today with regard to biotechnology is analogous to the situation presented to society in the 1940s with the discovery of organochlorine pesticides. When DDT was first introduced in 1942, it was heralded as a gift from God, revolutionizing public health efforts to control vector-borne diseases.[7] In the early 1940s, malaria was still present in the American South, the Caribbean, and Europe and killed over 800,000 people a year in India alone. DDT appeared miraculously effective in eliminating the vectors for this and other dreaded diseases such as typhus. Yet, it was not until two decades later, with the publication of *Silent Spring* by Rachel Carson[4] that the profound, adverse environmental effects of widespread organochlorine pesticide application were recognized. As a result, the use of organochlorine pesticides today has been severely restricted and has become heavily regulated.

Again, with biotechnology, as with organochlorine pesticides, society is being offered new and powerful technology that promises new benefits, but which also may carry new risks. It is reasonable for society to expect that the risks will be vigorously identified and evaluated at the same time that the opportunities are being pursued and that the general public safety is not being compromised. It is also reasonable to expect that the products developed by the biotechnology industry truly reflect the goals, needs, and values of the societies and cultures in which the products are to be marketed. Vigorous, informed debate is essential to this exercise, as is responsible leadership.

Biotechnology Challenges for Veterinarians Veterinarians have a tremendous potential to assume a leadership role in guiding the socially responsible development and application of biotechnology. Veterinarians receive training in comparative medicine, animal agriculture, food safety, and public health and increasingly in ethics, animal welfare, and environmental science. Furthermore, veterinary medicine has always been a service profession, receptive to, and responsive to, public need and expectation. This unique mix of training and experience is most relevant in the biotechnology arena. It enables veterinarians to understand the science of biotechnology, grasp the potential scope of its application, evaluate its safety and utility, and assess the social and economic implications of many new products and processes.

Veterinarians interested in biotechnology and its role in society can become engaged in many important ways. They can be directly involved in basic genetic research, product identification and development, design and implementation of field trials, safety and efficacy testing, regulatory oversight and as responsible, informed critics. Whether veterinarians work in industry, government, or academia or with public interest groups, the voice of veterinary medicine needs to be heard more clearly in the biotechnology arena.

This is particularly true in the international context. Considerable differences in public attitude about biotechnology exist around the globe. European nations were much quicker to impose regulatory constraints on the biotechnology industry than was the United States, and some developing nations have shown a high degree of suspicion about biotechnology, leading to outright refusal to allow genetically engineered agricultural and medical products into their countries. Yet, the biotechnology industry has consistently identified the developing world as a major potential beneficiary of the promise of biotechnology, particularly in the areas of human health and agricultural productivity. Veterinarians with first-hand experience working in the developing world on issues of health and food production can help to resolve misunderstandings about the promise and the reality of biotechnology and can help to bridge the communications gap between government, industry, and the public in numerous ways: Veterinarians can carry out needs assessments, help to set product priorities, anticipate or identify adverse consequences, establish guidelines for cooperation and regulation, and help to develop marketing, educational, and outreach campaigns to gain acceptance for safe and worthwhile products that are eventually produced.

Nevertheless, the complexity of issues that will require consideration when introducing biotechnology into the developing world should not be underestimated. Biotechnology is a powerful tool of transformation. Applying it wisely and appropriately will require great sensitivity, insight, patience, trust, mutual respect, open lines of communication, and, most of all, a strong sense of the interdependence of all things.

Other Relevant Technologies

Two other powerful technologies merit brief discussion in terms of their impact on global veterinary medicine. These are remote sensing and computer modeling. Space-based satellite photography and computer-based geographic information systems (GIS) allow the integration of animal population and disease data with mapping data on terrain, vegetation, temperature, and other agricultural and environmental parameters that can affect animal disease patterns and animal productivity around the globe. Veterinary epidemiologists are increasingly using these tools to analyze complex animal-environmental interactions so as monitor disease outbreaks and to model improved disease control strategies.

For instance, the optimal timing of vaccinations or anthelmintic treatments, the adjustment of animal stocking rates, or the manipulation of reproductive schedules can be modeled on the basis of historical climate and vegetation patterns recorded by satellite and be subsequently stored and analyzed by computer. The distribution of disease vectors, such as mosquitoes, tsetse flies, or snails, may be correlated with satellite-derived geographic and climatic data to help model disease outbreaks and plan disease control efforts.[1,12,13] During contagious disease outbreaks, such as foot and mouth disease, satellite data are now being used to map farm locations in conjunction with topographic features and water source information. This allows a more accurate and rational determination of the shape and size of effective quarantine zones and also, when large-scale carcass disposal is necessary, reduces the risk of potential environmental contamination. Such tools also have application in wildlife conservation to map and monitor patterns of habitat transformation that could adversely affect resident endangered species. These tools can also help wildlife conservationists to identify and protect contiguous habitat on wildlife corridor routes, to ensure the undisrupted movement of migratory animals to distant feeding and nesting sites, as discussed further in Chapter 7.

Human Population Growth and Food Needs

About 10,000 years ago, humans began the transition from food procurement to food production, switching their survival strategy from gathering and hunting to the cultivation of crops and domestication of animals. The advance of agriculture allowed people to adopt sedentary living patterns and produce and store surpluses of food. In turn, reliable food stores facilitated an acceleration of human population growth that has continued unabated to the present day. Increases in agricultural productivity have historically kept ahead of human population growth, thus allowing, through access to adequate food, further increases in human population. Whether or not agricultural productivity can continue to outpace population growth in contemporary society to provide an adequate food supply for all the world's citizens is perhaps the most critical question of our time.

Various estimates put the total human population of Earth at the time of the development of agriculture in the Neolithic era at about 10 million people. Today the human population of Earth is very close to 6 billion people. Each and every day, there is a net increase of 230,000 human beings added to the world's population, or 84 million more people per year. The rate of population growth has accelerated over time as well. In the Neolithic era, when the population growth rate was estimated to be less than 0.5% per year, a doubling of the total human population required 140 or more years. Today, with population growth rates in some parts of the world reaching as high as 3.0%, a doubling of the world population may take only 35 to 45 years. By 2050, within the lifetime of many readers of this book, the United Nations projects that the human population will reach 11 billion people. Just like you and me, each of these people will expect to eat sufficient food to maintain a healthy and productive life every single day of their lives.

The amount of land available on Earth for production of food is more or less fixed. While there has been replacement of forest by farmland and the use of otherwise unusable land through irrigation or terracing, the major increases in food production that have supported human population growth have come primarily by increasing the productivity of land, not by increasing the quantity of land itself. This increased productivity has come primarily through periodic technological advances in agriculture. Major advances include: improved labor efficiency through the use of animals and machinery; soil conservation and enrichment practices including manuring and fertilization; improved plant and animal genetics for increased growth and yield and adaptation to harsh environment; chemical control of weeds and pests; and, improved techniques for food storage and preservation.

However, the technological advances of agriculture have been neither universally available nor universally applied. Agricultural inputs in the form of machinery, fuel, chemicals, irrigation pumps, and improved seeds cost money and require a well-developed supporting infrastructure. As such, the greatest gains in agricultural productivity have occurred in the developed, industrialized nations of Europe and North America. With some notable exceptions, such as India and China, gains in the developing world have been less substantial, and recently there have been actual losses in per capita agricultural production among the least developed nations, particularly in Africa, as discussed in Chapter 5.

This is not to say that all the technological advances developed primarily for temperate zone agriculture are necessarily appropriate for, or transferable to, tropical agricultural systems. Nevertheless, efforts to improve agricultural output in the tropics have never received the level of economic and scientific investment that has been afforded agriculture in the temperate regions. Today, largely as a result of mechanization and intensification, countries such as the United States, with less than 3% of the workforce directly engaged in agriculture, produce consistent food surpluses, while many of the least developed countries, where more than 50% of the workforce may be directly involved in agriculture are unable to maintain self sufficiency in food production.

The disparity in food production is exacerbated by parallel disparities in population growth. The highest rates of population growth (>2.0% per annum) in the world occur among the least developed nations of Central America, Africa, and South Asia, where increases in agricultural productivity have been limited. Thus, even if agricultural output remains stable in these countries, per capita food production may decrease. In contrast, the United States, Canada, Japan, and most of Europe have population growth rates less than 0.9% per annum. Several European countries are actually experiencing population loss.

Continued population growth in poor countries coupled with inadequate production of food will have dire consequences. Food insecurity constrains economic growth and is politically destabilizing. Chronic undernutrition undermines physical and intellectual growth and predisposes to disease. Low agricultural productivity coupled with expanding population puts additional pressure on natural resources, leading to environmental degradation and habitat destruction. Countries that could be active participants in the global economy instead are sidelined because of inadequate food production or distribution. The relationship of food security and population growth is discussed further in Chapter 5.

Animals continue to play diverse and vital roles in agriculture and daily life in much of the developing world. They are an integral part of small farming systems, providing fertilizer, agricultural power, food, income, transportation, and risk diversification, as discussed further in Chapter 4. There is much still to be learned about how to improve the health and productivity of animals in developing countries and how to integrate them more efficiently, profitably, and sustainably into traditional farming systems. As discussed in Chapter 5, effective interventions in rural development require experience with, and an understanding of, local conditions and constraints. Local experience increases the likelihood that appropriate technologies will be developed and applied to strengthen and sustain productive agricultural systems around the world. Feeding the world's people will be one of the major challenges of the next century. Given the continued importance of animals in agriculture, it is clear that veterinarians have an important role to play, at home and abroad (see sidebar "Trypanosomiasis Control in Africa: A Debate Among the Well-Meaning").

Increasing Affluence and Consumer Demand

The last two decades have been characterized by a dramatic transformation of the global economy. Expansion of international trade and the movement of foreign capital investment into developing countries, especially in Asia and South America, have stimulated substantial economic and social development. Major outcomes include increased industrialization, increased urbanization, and an improved standard of living for countless millions of people. Modern India, for example, with its burgeoning economy, now has a largely urban middle class numbering about 250 million people, a number approaching the entire population of the United States.

Trypanosomiasis Control in Africa: A Debate Among the Well-Meaning

Africa is a continent of great beauty and diversity, with tremendous human, animal, and natural resources. However, the continent faces many challenges. Africa has had more than its fair share of political instability and military conflict in recent years. Economic development in general lags behind that of other world regions. Population growth rates are among the highest in the world, exceeding 2.5% per year in most countries on the continent, while the world mean is 1.4%. Food production, per capita, in Africa has been decreasing, with a 16% drop recorded between 1980 and 1993. As many as 35% of Africa's people experience chronic malnourishment. Improving the prospects for future food production in Africa is a major priority. One important constraint to such improvement is the disease trypanosomiasis.

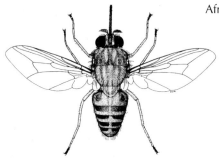

African trypanosomiasis is a hemoparasitic infection of humans, domestic mammals, and wild mammals caused by various flagellated protozoa of the genus *Trypanosoma*. Trypanosomes are transmitted to susceptible hosts by blood-feeding tsetse fly vectors of the genus *Glossina*, for example, *G. morsitans*. Infection is usually subclinical in wild mammals. In humans, the disease produced is known as sleeping sickness, and in domestic animals, Nagana. It is characterized by fever, cyclic parasitemia, anemia, enlarged lymph nodes, loss of body condition, lethargy, and high mortality. Acute and chronic forms of the disease occur. Though all types of domesticated mammals are susceptible to varying degrees, cattle are most commonly and most severely affected.

Glossina morsitans, one of the several *Glossina* species of blood-sucking tsetse fly vectors of Africa responsible for transmitting trypanosomiasis in humans and animals. (Reproduced with permission from Soulsby EJL. Helminths, Arthropods and Protozoa of Domesticated Animals, 7th Ed. Philadelphia: Lea & Febiger, 1982.)

As such, trypanosomiasis is a major constraint on ruminant livestock production in Africa. The distribution and intensity of animal trypanosomiasis in sub-Saharan Africa follows the distribution and intensity of the various species of the tsetse fly vectors, as shown on the accompanying map. An estimated 10 million km^2, or 37% of the African continent, is tsetse infested, much of it savanna and forest. This area includes at least 37 countries, covering most of West and Central Africa and parts of East Africa and listed in the accompanying table. Various estimates suggest that the livestock-carrying capacity of tsetse-infested areas of sub-Saharan Africa could be increased five- to sevenfold by eliminating or controlling animal trypanosomiasis.

Efforts to control trypanosomiasis began in 1910, and significant progress was made over the following 50 or so years, largely through the control of tsetse fly populations through heavy application of insecticides and destruction of known tsetse fly habitats. Though effective, these approaches had negative environmental and ecological impacts.[10] Following the African independence movement of the 1960s, trypanosomiasis control efforts declined. Newly independent governments lacked the economic resources or management experience to maintain existing control programs, or wars and civil unrest disrupted these activities. As a result, there has been a dramatic resurgence of clinical trypanosomiasis in people and animals in recent times. Currently, however, improved knowledge has created new opportunities for control. There is greater understanding of the natural history of the disease and the bi-

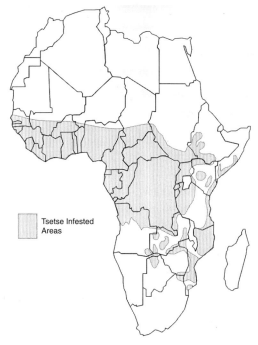

Tsetse Infested Areas

General distribution of tsetse flies in Africa.

Middle-class status implies that families and individuals have disposable income beyond that necessary for subsistence and are able to enter the marketplace to purchase goods and services that enhance their own quality of life. In addition to India, increased purchasing power has become a reality for many cit-izens in a variety of countries in recent years, notably China, Taiwan, South Korea, Hong Kong, Singapore, Malaysia, and Indonesia in Asia and Chile and Brazil in South America. Collectively, this represents enormous new global consumer demand.

ology of trypanosomes and tsetse flies. There have also been advances in integrated pest management, epidemiological monitoring, and the prospect of new approaches to control made possible through biotechnology, such as the development of novel vaccines or the possibility of developing transgenic livestock resistant to trypanosome infection. Thus, interest in trypanosomiasis control efforts in Africa has been revived in recent years. This new interest, however, has stimulated significant debate.

African Countries with Animal Trypanosomiasis	
• Epidemic	Equatorial Guinea
Angola	Kenya
Democratic Republic of Congo	Malawi
	Mali
Uganda	Niger
Sudan	Togo
• Highly Endemic	Zambia
Cameroon	Zimbabwe
Chad	**• Sporadic, At Risk, or**
Congo	**Status Poorly Defined**
Central African Republic	Burundi
Guinea	Botswana
Ivory Coast	Ethiopia
Mozambique	Gambia
Tanzania	Liberia
• Endemic	Namibia
Benin	Rwanda
Burkina Faso	Senegal
Eritrea	Sierra Leone
Gabon	Somalia
Ghana	South Africa

Advocates of vigorously renewed control efforts view the control of animal trypanosomiasis as an opportunity to expand cattle production in savanna regions, to make greater use of the grasslands for the production of animal protein that will help to improve the food supply and nutritional standard of millions of Africans. Others, however, see the expansion of extensive cattle raising as ill advised, claiming it will produce poor economic returns and improve the food situation only minimally. Conservationists raise concerns that it will accelerate the degradation of grasslands, lead to the displacement and destruction of indigenous flora and fauna, and further contribute to the general loss of biodiversity. It is further argued that the attraction of the famous African savannas to ecotourists will be diminished, thus damaging national economies dependent on tourism.

Encompassed within these points of view are the seeds of a healthy debate, which must be informed by solid scientific research and which must lead to a thorough, critical analysis by policymakers in each affected country before aggressive trypanosomiasis control is undertaken. Clearly, veterinarians, through research, informed advocacy, technical consultation, and innovative thinking, have a critical role to play in guiding the debate on the issue of trypanosomiasis control in Africa.

In our complex, fast-moving world, even the noblest impulses can create conflict. What right-minded person would oppose feeding the hungry? And what right-minded person would oppose protecting the great treasure that is African wildlife? Not many on either count. Yet, how many right-minded people want to feed the hungry at the expense of wildlife? And how many right-minded people want to protect wildlife at the expense of the hungry? Now the answer is not so clear, as these choices carry unwanted consequences. Veterinarians, with professional credibility in the areas of livestock health and production, wildlife medicine, public health, and, increasingly, environmental health, can serve as bridge builders between the different constituencies in this debate and provide an important leadership role in developing solutions that yield the maximum of intended benefits and the fewest undesired consequences.

A wide range of organizations will be involved in the ongoing debate and decision-making process concerning policies for trypanosomiasis control in Africa. Many of these organizations already employ veterinarians in some capacity and could use veterinary expertise to address the issue of trypanosomiasis control. Examples of relevant organizations include multinational agencies such as the World Bank and the Food and Agriculture Organization of the United Nations, research institutions such as the International Livestock Research Institute, government development agencies such as USAID, conservation groups such as the World Wildlife Fund, and private voluntary organizations involved in agricultural and rural development, such as FARM Africa. Opportunities for veterinarians to work with these and other organizations in different areas of international veterinary medicine are discussed in Chapter 10.

For most people climbing out of poverty, the first choice they make with increased income is to diversify their diet and eat higher on the food chain. This usually means the addition of animal products to a previously monotonous cereal-based diet augmented with fruits and vegetables. The choice of animal protein will vary according to cultural preferences and proscriptions as discussed in Chapter 3. Most Indians, for example, as Hindus, will not eat beef, but prize dairy products. Muslims will not eat pork, but eat considerable amounts of lamb and goat. Religious preferences notwithstanding, the overall demand for meat, fish, dairy products, and eggs around the world has increased dramatically. Over the 20-year period from 1977 to 1997, world meat production increased from 117 million tons to 206 million tons, representing a global per capita increase from 27.6 to 35.7 kg per person. The International Food Policy Research Institute (IFPRI) estimates that for the period 1993 to 2020, global meat demand will increase in developing countries at a rate of between 2.8 and 3.3% per year. This means that by 2020, these countries will consume 100 million metric tons more meat and 223 million metric tons more milk than in 1993.[6]

In some countries, notably in Asia, economic development has already led to tremendous increases in meat consumption. In China, for example, per capita meat consumption, which was 10.3 kg per person in 1977, reached 41.2 kg per person by 1996, a 400% increase. As China is a nation of 1.25 billion people, this increase in demand for meat, mainly in the form of pork and poultry products, is enormous. It has created major new opportunities for increased international trade in livestock and livestock products and is challenging China's capacity to be self-sufficient in food production.

The skyrocketing global demand for animal protein presents some serious challenges. If increased demand for poultry and pork continues at present rates, demand will be met mainly by further intensification of the swine and poultry industries, both of which are based on the feeding of grain. Some analysts are deeply concerned that the expanding world demand for meat, milk, and eggs will result in more grain being produced specifically to feed animals, with less grain, at higher prices, being available for direct consumption by humans. Some expect demand for cereal grains for use as animal feed in developing countries to double between now and 2020. Other observers express concern about animal welfare, as increased numbers of animals are raised in confinement under intensively managed conditions in countries without adequate animal welfare legislation or enforcement.

In response to the increasing world demand for animal products in the human diet, veterinarians have many roles to play as researchers, practitioners, industry consultants, and international development workers. They must actively participate to improve production efficiency of livestock, reduce losses through stress and disease, help to develop production systems that are sustainable and appropriate to local conditions, and work to promote the welfare of food-producing animals.

Another result of increased affluence is growth in the number of companion animals worldwide. The emergence of the middle class, coupled with urbanization in many newly prosperous nations, has led to an increase in the keeping of dogs and cats. Even in the poorest countries, the urban elite in the capital cities maintain dogs either as companion animals or for household security and are willing to pay for veterinary services when such services are available. The direct provision of companion animal veterinary services or the provision of continuing education services for indigenous veterinarians on cur-

rent developments in companion animal practice are potential opportunities for international veterinary work.

While pet ownership has increased worldwide, there are still many less-fortunate, uncared-for dogs and cats frequently observed in developing countries. These animals are often malnourished and diseased, act as a dangerous reservoir for human rabies and other zoonotic diseases, and often have no one to advocate for their care (Fig. 1-2). There is tremendous need and opportunity for humane societies in developed countries to assume a greater active role in providing technical and financial support for the establishment or expansion of humane services in the developing world. This is clearly an area of international activity in which veterinarians can play a leadership role. The Massachusetts Society for the Prevention of Cruelty to Animals, for example, has supported a veterinary clinic, the American Fondouk, in Fez, Morocco, for decades to provide clinical and preventive care for animals whose owners would otherwise not be able to afford veterinary services (see http://www.mspca.org/).

Growth in International Trade

The widespread economic growth and increased global prosperity of the last two decades has been fueled in large part by a tremendous expansion in international trade. According to statistics available from the World Trade Organization (WTO), the total value of merchandise and commercial services exported globally more than tripled between 1980 and 2000, from US$2.40 trillion to US$7.77 trillion. The United States remains the world's leading importer and exporter. In 2000, the U.S. share of the world's imported goods and services was 18.1% and valued at US$1.46 trillion. The same year, the U.S. generated 13.6% of global exports, valued at US$1.06 trillion.

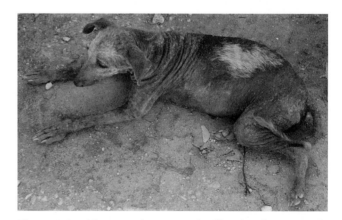

Figure 1-2. This street dog is severely affected with mange and, probably, gastrointestinal parasites, judging by the distended belly. This particular dog was photographed in Trinidad, though sadly, the world is full of such neglected animals. While working in Pakistan, the author literally peeled a half-dead puppy about this size off the top of a rotting trash heap in an empty lot. The puppy responded well to subcutaneous fluids, anthelmintics, and a new home, only to die 2 months later from complications of postdistemper encephalitis. (Photo by Dr. David M. Sherman)

This growth in trade has been spurred by cooperative efforts between nations to encourage and facilitate nonrestrictive, or free, trade. The General Agreement on Tariffs and Trade (GATT), agreed upon by 92 nations, calls for lowering a variety of tariffs on a wide spectrum of commodities and manufactured goods, eliminating import quotas, and protecting copyrights and patents. The GATT agreement, signed in 1994, also established the WTO, a permanent institution based in Geneva, Switzerland, that has the power, backed by international law, to monitor trade agreements, enforce trade rules, and settle disputes. By the middle of 2001, 142 countries had become members of the WTO, thereby agreeing to abide by its trade rules and arbitration decisions (see http://www.wto.org/).

In addition to GATT, many regional trading partnerships have been created in recent years to stimulate fair and free trade among neighbors. Most notable among these are the European Union (EU) and the North American Free Trade Agreement (NAFTA). Other, similar regional trade agreements exist for South American nations (MERCO-SUR), Central American nations (CACM), Caribbean nations (CARICOM), African nations (ECOWAS, COMESA), and Asian nations (APEC, ASEAN) (see Table 1-1).

Trade in agricultural commodities and food products has been stimulated by free trade agreements and facilitated by advances in modern transportation. A leg of lamb purchased in Boston is just as likely to come from Australia as from Colorado, and a chicken wing consumed in Beijing is just as likely to come from Arkansas as from Sichuan. The increased world trade in livestock and livestock products and the new rules that regulate it have important consequences for veterinary medicine and present a wide range of new opportunities for veterinarians.

Outbreaks of animal disease, or even the perceived threat of animal disease, can adversely affect world markets in livestock products and even affect diplomatic relations. If zoonotic diseases are involved, posing a risk to human health, the effects on trade can be catastrophic. There have been a number of instances in recent years in which animal disease has significantly disrupted trade:

- In Japan, food-borne E. coli outbreaks in school children in 1996 resulted in a sharp reduction in beef imports.

- An outbreak of avian influenza in Hong Kong in 1997, with the suggestion that the disease might be transmissible to humans, resulted in destruction of the entire national poultry flock and a loss of consumer confidence in the wholesomeness of poultry products throughout Asia.

- An extensive outbreak of foot and mouth disease in the swine industry in Taiwan in 1997 led to an overall 20% drop in production in that major pork-exporting nation and resulted in the loss of a significant share of Taiwan's lucrative Japanese pork export market to other international competitors.

- Classical swine fever outbreaks in the Netherlands in 1997 reduced swine inventories in that country and created a boon in swine exports for nearby Denmark. Disease eradication costs alone exceeded US$2 billion.

- The association of human variant Creutzfeldt-Jakob disease (vCJD) with bovine spongiform encephalopathy (BSE) in the United Kingdom in 1994 added a horrible new dimension to a cattle disease that had already devastated the cattle industry in that country through mass destruction of

Table 1-1 Major Regional Trading Groups Around the World		
Acronym	**Full Name**	**Membership**
EU	European Union	16 European nations
NAFTA	North American Free Trade Association	3 North American nations
COMESA	Common Market for Eastern and Southern Africa	20 East and South African nations
ECOWAS	Economic Community of West Africa	16 West African nations
APEC	Asia Pacific Economic Cooperation	19 Nations bordering the Pacific Ocean
ASEAN	Association of South East Asian Nations	9 South East Asian nations
MERCO-SUR	Mercado Comun del Cono Sur (Southern Cone Common Market)	4 South American nations
CACM	Central American Common Market	5 Central American nations
CARICOM	Caribbean Community and Common Market	14 Caribbean nations

cattle and loss of export markets. When BSE was diagnosed in a native-born cow in Germany in November, 2000, beef consumption among Germans dropped as much as 75% according to some media reports, largely due to consumer fears of contracting vCJD.

Clearly, competitiveness in the world marketplace for livestock and livestock products will depend increasingly on improving and maintaining animal health, a critical responsibility and vigorous challenge for veterinarians worldwide. The impact of livestock disease on international trade is discussed further in Chapter 9.

There is a growing concern that animal health issues will themselves be used to block international trade in livestock and livestock products. As tariffs and quotas disappear as a result of GATT, some countries, whose own livestock industries feel threatened by competing imports, may seek to exploit health regulations as nontariff barriers to trade. In such cases alleged concerns about animal health and safety are used as a smoke-screen for trade protectionism. A relevant example of this surfaced in 1996 when Russia banned the import of U.S. poultry meat, ostensibly because of the risk of salmonellosis. In reality, there was no more risk of salmonellosis from imported U.S. poultry than from domestic Russian poultry, and the ban was imposed primarily to protect the domestic Russian poultry industry, fragile from reorganization into the private sector. In the year preceding the ban, U.S. poultry exports to Russia were worth US $500 million, so the ban was not a trivial matter to U.S. poultry producers.

The WTO is alert to issues such as protectionism and nontariff barriers to trade. The WTO also recognizes the real need to protect animal health and ensure food safety. In response, the WTO has developed, through consultation with member nations, a set of standardized sanitary and phytosanitary (SPS) measures to ensure that importing and exporting nations are reasonably and rightfully protected from disease risks associated with agricultural products. Members of the WTO agree to abide by these SPS measures. The WTO has assigned responsibility for international SPS animal health standards to the Office International des Epizooties (OIE) in Paris, France. The OIE is a cooperative international body that provides technical support and disease-reporting services to the national veterinary services of member nations. This important organization is described further in Chapter 9.

In support of the WTO initiative, the OIE identifies specific diagnostic tests and test protocols acceptable as official screening tests and sets standards for disease surveillance and monitoring within countries to ensure disease-free status for countries and regions with regard to specific diseases. As there is tremendous variation around the world in the technical capacity of different countries to carry out diagnostic testing and disease monitoring, the establishment of international testing and monitoring standards is essential. This variability offers significant challenges and opportunities for well-trained veterinary diagnosticians and epidemiologists to assist in establishing world-class diagnostic and surveillance capabilities in many countries around the world.

The Spread of Democracy

Over the last 20 years there has been enormous and significant movement toward democratic government for nations in many parts of the world. The most notable event in this regard was the demise of the Soviet Union and its client states in Eastern Europe. This effectively ended the Cold War and, at the same time, created a host of newly independent states in central Asia and Eastern Europe. Most of these new nations are experimenting, with varying degrees of success, with democratic government. In addition, there have also been many important political changes in nations of Latin America and Asia, where military dictatorships or despotic oligarchies have been replaced by democratically elected governments with new constitutions. Brazil, Chile, Argentina, Taiwan, and South Korea are good examples.

This positive trend is encouraged and assisted by the power and pervasiveness of modern telecommunications, which helps bring to light social inequities and injustice anywhere in the world and exposes the perpetrators to international scrutiny and potential sanction. Arbitrary arrests and torture, the exploitation of child labor, the lack of equal rights for women, and genocidal activities in warfare are examples of unacceptable behavior that are being increasingly subjected to the spotlight of public opinion and being more vigorously addressed by United Nations agencies, public advocacy groups such as Amnesty International, and ordinary citizens who express their disapproval through economic boycotts and other forms of political activism.

Participatory, democratic government changes the landscape of human society. It empowers ordinary citizens, gives them a voice in their own future, keeps government accountable to the people, facilitates change, and tends to redistribute wealth, resources, and opportunity more equitably. Yet people who have lived in fear of authority, who have been consistently deprived of freedom of expression, and who have not had the opportunity to define their own goals and ambitions do not, overnight, create thriving, fully actualized democratic societies. There are growing pains, as the present economic and political turmoil in Russia makes clear. There is a need, indeed an obligation, for experienced democracies to provide education, encouragement, and material support.

One healthy and vigorous response to this need has been the emergence of a new generation of international and national private voluntary organizations with the mission of providing direct support to the citizens of newly democratic nations at the grassroots level. These private voluntary organizations (PVOs), also known as nongovernmental organizations (NGOs), vary in their stated goals or areas of interest but share a common goal of working "people-to-people," rather than "top-down" through government bureaucracies. Areas of focus for different NGOs include strengthening democratic institutions, monitoring and improving human rights, encouraging community organization, stimulating local economic development, implementing the appropriate transfer of technology, fostering private initiative and enterprise, and establishing lending schemes geared toward individual, small-scale entrepreneurs at the village level, a process known as microcredit.

A number of NGOs focus primarily on issues of agriculture and food production. While these are fundamental matters in any country regardless of the type of government, agricultural issues are particularly important in emerging democracies, because the democratizing process has frequently resulted in major transformations in agricultural production. For example, collectivized farms in the former Soviet Union have largely been divided and privatized, and there is considerable need for advice and guidance on the technical and financial management of smaller, privately owned farms to keep them both productive and competitive in the global marketplace for agricultural products. This applies to livestock enterprises as well as crop enterprises. Similarly, as changes in governance and economic structure are instituted, many veterinarians, especially in developing countries, have been released from government service and encouraged to enter the private sector. Yet these veterinarians may have little experience with, or understanding of how to succeed in, private clinical practice. As such, there are increased opportunities for veterinarians from developed countries with experience in livestock health and production to serve as consultants and/or volunteers with NGOs working in agricultural development and veterinary service delivery as discussed further in Chapter 5. In addition, corporations and businesses in the private sector that are seeking agricultural investment opportunities and partnerships in the new democracies sometimes require the services of veterinarians and other agricultural specialists.

The governments of established democracies, such as the United States and various western European countries, have recognized the importance of strengthening fledgling democracies around the world and ensuring that they remain capable of feeding themselves. These western governments are increasingly providing financial support to NGOs as a way of carrying out their foreign aid goals. The United States Agency for International Development (USAID), for example, provides funds for the American farmers' cooperative Land O' Lakes to provide technical and marketing assistance, including veterinary expertise, to newly privatized dairy farmers in former Soviet republics. Similarly the USAID supports international programs of the NGO known as ACDI/VOCA, which places volunteers with expertise in all phases of agriculture, including livestock disease control, in developing countries and emerging democracies (see http://www.acdivoca.org/).

Ownership of their own land is a dream of poor farmers everywhere, and the process of democratization has made this dream a reality for many, since democratically elected governments are much more likely to respond to calls for land reform than are dictatorships. However, land reform is not always carried out in ideal ways. Politicians may find themselves hav-

ing to please several competing constituencies and may come up with compromise plans that contain undesirable outcomes. In a number of Latin American countries, for example, government land reform policies have addressed the desire for land among the landless and poor largely by opening up the rainforests to agricultural exploitation rather than by redistributing large tracts of existing agricultural land held by relatively few, but influential landholders. Thus, to fulfill the aspirations of their disenfranchised citizens, without alienating the well-to-do, these governments risk trading away their unique ecological heritage and abundant biodiversity.

Veterinarians interested in environmental issues, wildlife conservation, and livestock health and production all can find professional challenges and opportunities in such situations. They can work in the areas of research and policy to document the impacts of habitat destruction; assist in the protection of endangered species; develop animal production systems that integrate with, rather than replace, forests; or help to improve agricultural productivity of subsistence farmers and herders so that existing land resources are used as efficiently and wisely as possible.

Increasing Pressure on Natural Resources

Lester R. Brown[2] of the Worldwatch Institute has characterized the period of 1950 to 1990 as the *economic* era in modern development. In contrast, he describes the period from 1991 through 2030 as the *environmental* era. He suggests by this characterization that during the economic era, social growth and development were constrained only by human ambition and imagination, technological innovation and adaptation, the exercise of political will, and the investment of capital. Opportunities for growth seemed limitless. Relatively little attention was paid to Earth's ability to accommodate or withstand the accelerating transformation of natural landscapes and the consumption of natural resources that has come to characterize the contemporary advance of human civilization.

However, in the current environmental era, ambition, imagination, technology, political will, and capital investment may not suffice to ensure further growth and prosperity. Brown believes that human society is on a "collision course" between economic growth and Earth's many natural limits. The growth of population and human aspirations for a better material life may be exceeding Earth's carrying capacity.

The challenge of expanding food production illustrates the limits imposed by natural resources in the environmental era. Nothing is more fundamental to the ongoing growth, development, and prosperity of human society than an adequate and nutritious food supply. Today, however, there are growing concerns about an adequate resource base to support agriculture. The best farmland on the planet has long been under cultivation, and as food production requirements increase, marginal lands are increasingly being brought under cultivation. Making marginal land productive often requires irrigation. Presently, over 80% of the water consumed annually in the world is consumed by agricultural use, and demand continues to increase. As a result, the expanded use of deep-well irrigation is depleting aquifers, lowering water tables, and overall straining water supplies. Even irrigation itself can, over time, reduce the usefulness of land for agricultural purposes by salinizing topsoil and waterlogging subsoils. Expansion of livestock production in response to increased world demand for meat may further exacerbate the water supply problem. It can take 100 times more water to produce 1 kg of animal protein than 1 kg of vegetable protein.

Pressure for agricultural land also encourages deforestation. In turn, the loss of trees reduces the water retention capacity of the land. The resultant increase in water runoff contributes to flooding in regions of heavy rainfall and leads to excessive soil erosion and further degradation of farmland. This is only one of the many adverse consequences of widespread deforestation. It also results in the acceleration of global warming, as discussed in Chapter 6, and the loss of biodiversity, as discussed in Chapter 7.

Paradoxically, even as new, suboptimal farmland is created and brought under cultivation at the expense of forests and grasslands, some of the world's finest farmland is disappearing as a result of industrialization, urbanization, and the development of transportation infrastructure. In the United States, for example, during the 30 years following the end of World War II, an area of prime agricultural land, approximately equal in size to the state of Ohio was lost, just as a result of blacktopping for roads, driveways, and parking lots. In Japan, the total area of land available for grain production decreased by half between 1955 and 1995 because of the industrialization and urbanization that occurred during Japan's extraordinary rise as a global economic power.

Currently, in China, cropland is being lost at the rate of 1.4% a year, equal to the rate of loss in Japan over the last 40 years. As was the case earlier in Japan, the cropland loss in China is associated with rapid industrialization and urbanization. If the Chinese population continues to grow and become more affluent, with expectations of a more diverse diet containing increased amounts of meat derived from grain-fed livestock, there is serious question as to whether China will be able to continue to feed itself in the coming decades. This prospect of food scarcity in China and its implications for world agriculture and food supplies are discussed in the book *Who Will Feed China?* by Lester Brown.[2] Though not everyone agrees about the inevitability of the food scarcity scenario in China, Brown's book nonetheless makes compelling reading and underscores the potential limits on economic growth imposed by such basic resources as land and water in the so-called environmental era.

Of course, it is not only in the realm of agriculture that natural resource constraints may impose limits on future economic growth. Our major transportation systems, power-generating stations, and many of our key industries, including mechanized agriculture, are fueled largely with fossil fuel derivatives, which are essentially nonrenewable resources. Experts differ on the total world reserve of crude oil. However, disagreements

about when projected world demand for oil is likely to exceed known world supplies are now being debated not in terms of millennia or even centuries, but rather in decades; in other words, possibly within our lifetimes.

Despite active exploration, some 80% of the oil produced today comes from oil fields identified before 1973, and many of these older fields are experiencing decline. It is hard to imagine the full adverse impact that severe oil shortages will have on the current structure of world trade, transportation, economic growth, and agricultural productivity. It is equally hard to imagine why the development of alternative energy sources did not become a higher priority in the advanced industrialized nations following the oil shortage dress rehearsal of the 1970s. A generous explanation is the unwillingness of the human spirit to accept limits, but less generous explanations abound.

The most confident advocates of continued industrial growth and broader prosperity suggest that science and technology will continue to find ways to meet the future needs and challenges of continued human population growth and the increased demand for material comforts. Recent advances in the life sciences do encourage this perspective, and indeed, biotechnology will likely help to improve agricultural outputs. Yet biotechnology is unlikely to produce new soil or fresh water, to stem the inexorable chopping down of trees, or to lessen the increasing global appetite for more meat in the diet or additional private motor vehicles.

More cautious voices suggest that further advances in science and technology are not the whole answer. In addition, human society needs to embrace a conservation ethic with regard to nonrenewable resources, to improve the efficiency and sustainability of existing agricultural, industrial, and transportation systems, and, most of all, to rethink the relationship of human beings to the natural world. Through the power of human intellect and the technological achievement it allows, human beings have gained dominion over Earth and its nonhuman inhabitants. This dominion has encouraged a sense of invincibility that may be dangerously misplaced. Despite our achievements, we are still part of Earth, and our intrinsic biological nature cannot be denied. Our viability as a species still depends on the viability of the global ecosystem and its natural resource base. We must find ways to strike a balance between our desire for the continued advance of material culture and our biological need for responsible management of Earth's resources. Ultimately, our own survival depends on it.

Veterinarians can make important contributions in helping to strike this balance. As practitioners at home or as advisors abroad, veterinarians can work with farmers to improve production efficiency in existing animal management systems and introduce, where appropriate, new and improved sustainable livestock management practices, including even new forms of livestock. Veterinarians with interests in both animal production and wildlife conservation can help to develop land-use management schemes that accommodate wild animals and livestock in compatible, rather than competitive, ways. Veterinarians committed to the protection of endangered species and their habitats can help, through their professional activities, to promote a conservation ethic and cultivate new societal perspectives for sharing resources with nonhuman life forms on the planet.

Global Environmental Health Concerns

The human transformation of Earth not only consumes finite resources. Human activity also generates wastes and pollutants that foul the air, water, and soil; damage the health of people, animals, and plants; and even disrupt the normal function of the global ecosystem itself. Some of these pollution-associated problems have been recognized for a long time. Some have even been addressed in effective ways. Obvious examples include reduction of environmental contamination with lead by mandating the use of lead-free gasoline in motor vehicles, limitations on the use of chlorofluorocarbons to slow atmospheric ozone depletion, and prohibitions on the use of DDT to rectify its deleterious effects on wildlife and aquatic ecosystems.

Today, new environmental threats are emerging that are more complex, more pervasive, and less completely understood. They represent truly global problems. Most notable and dramatic among them are global warming and global climate change. The International Panel for Climate Change (IPCC), a group of 2500 atmospheric, biological, and physical scientists working through the auspices of the United Nations, believes that the Earth's atmosphere is warming and that the change is affecting global climatic patterns. These changes have profound implications for the human use of Earth, and indeed, for Earth itself. Numerous potential impacts of global warming have been identified, most notably

- Melting of the polar ice caps,
- Higher sea level, with widespread coastal flooding and submersion,
- Changes in planetary rainfall and temperature patterns,
- Shifts in growing seasons and geographic redistribution of prime agricultural lands,
- Changing patterns of arthropod vector distribution, helminth parasite survival, and microbial pathogen proliferation resulting in new patterns of animal and human disease and the possible emergence of previously unknown diseases,
- Deep ocean warming leading to more intense El Nino events and the redistribution of fishing stocks, and
- More unpredictable and violent weather patterns leading to economic losses, social disruption, and environmental degradation.

While the increase in carbon dioxide and other greenhouse gases that contribute to global warming is well documented, the source of these greenhouse gases remains a disputed and contentious issue. Most climate scientists believe that the major source of increased carbon dioxide in the atmosphere is the burning of fossil fuels. Representatives of the fossil fuel industries and allied interests resist this notion and downplay the contributory role of man-made gases to global warming. Livestock have also been implicated as contributors to the increase in greenhouse gases, a situation that should be of concern to veterinarians.

Whether man-made or not, global warming and climate change are real phenomena, and their implications are too serious to ignore. There is growing recognition that such problems transcend national boundaries and that cooperative, international efforts are required to better understand the source of these problems and to effect appropriate solutions. Veterinarians will have a key role to play in the coming years to monitor, document, explain, and alleviate the effects that global warming will have on agroecosystems, livestock productivity, and the changing patterns of diseases in domestic animals, wildlife, and humans around the globe. Atmospheric warming, climate change, and other global environmental problems that present professional challenges and opportunities for veterinarians are summarized in Table 1-2 and discussed further in Chapter 6.

Degradation of Natural Habitats

Perhaps the most serious challenge of the environmental era, beyond the consumption of nonrenewable resources and environmental contamination with man-made pollutants, is the widespread destruction of natural habitat. Best-publicized is the rapid destruction of tropical rainforests of Central and South America and Asia and the related loss of biodiversity. Worldwide, the net loss of forest converted to other uses is approximately 161,200 km² per year. This is an area roughly equal in size to all of New England. Only eight countries in the world-Canada, Russia, Brazil, Colombia, Venezuela, Suriname, Guyana, and French Guiana-currently possess large tracts of undisturbed, original forest that remain ecologically intact, and many of these are threatened.

Yet it is not only tropical rainforests that are being lost. The coral reefs of the world's oceans, the African savanna, the old-growth temperate forests and wetlands of North America, and countless small ecological niches around the world are threatened with obliteration or sufficient reduction in size that they cease to function as viable ecosystems. Most habitat destruction can be linked directly, or indirectly, to human activity, though the driving forces behind the destruction of habitat are complex and sometimes contradictory. For example, extreme poverty and extreme affluence both drive the destruction of tropical rainforests. The most distressing aspect of this accelerated dismantling of the world's natural landscape is that major ecosystems may be completely destroyed before we even begin to fully understand the ultimate consequences of such destruction.

One major consequence may be the destabilization of the planetary biosphere. Scientists are beginning to elaborate the

Table 1-2 Global Environmental Problems and Their Implications for Veterinary Medicine

Global warming and climate change	Changing patterns of arthropod vector distribution, helminth parasite survival, and microbial pathogen proliferation resulting in new patterns of animal and human disease; the contribution of livestock to greenhouse gas emissions needs to be addressed
Ozone depletion	Increases in ocular and mucocutaneous neoplasias of animals, associated with increased ultraviolet radiation; increased genetic mutations in organisms exposed to light
Land degradation/ desertification	Decreased productivity of agricultural and grazing lands; often associated with overgrazing by ruminant livestock; requires improved animal management
Deforestation	Contributes to global warming; increased loss of biodiversity; increased extinction rates of wild animals; forest clearing often associated in the public mind with cattle raising; requires new approaches to sustainable, multipurpose use of forest resources
Chemical pollution	Multiple sources and types from industrial, agricultural and consumer use; adverse affects on animal health and/or contamination of foods derived from animal sources; ecosystem perturbation, especially aquatic ecosystems, with adverse impacts on biodiversity and commercial fisheries
Endocrine disruptors	Special class of chemical pollutants; these are breakdown products of pesticides and other chemicals in the environment that mimic hormones; disruption of normal reproductive patterns in wildlife, domestic animals, and possibly humans
Livestock wastes	Intensive livestock production systems producing excessive amounts of manure; runoffs into water supplies causing eutrophication, disruption of aquatic ecosystems, fish kills, and possibly human disease
Nuclear radiation	Nuclear tests, terrorist acts, and accidents, such as Chernobyl, releasing radiation into the atmosphere; acute and chronic effects on animal and human health; contamination of animal-derived food, especially milk

important roles that various ecosystems such as wetlands and forests play in the regulation and maintenance of global environmental health and the impact that disruption of these processes may have not only on human society, but also on the ability of the planet itself to support life. The world's wetlands, for example, play an important role in fresh water purification and help to stem the loss of soil into the oceans. Forests too, play multiple roles. They retain water from rainfall and thus aid in recharging aquifers; they help to reduce flooding following heavy rainfall or snow melt, thus controlling soil erosion. Trees also consume carbon dioxide, and collectively, the world's forests act as a sink to regulate the excessive accumulation of carbon dioxide in the atmosphere, a key factor in the control of global warming.

Still, there is much that is not fully understood about the intricacies of global ecology. The limits of our knowledge about how ecosystems function was made clear by the Biosphere 2 project in Oracle, Arizona, carried out from 1991 to 1993. The project was designed to assess the feasibility of creating a self-sustaining habitat for human occupancy as a model for possible future space colonies. Eight people were sealed into a 3.15-acre structure near Tucson, Arizona, with over 3500 different plants and animals selected to reproduce five ecosystems-desert, grassland, marsh, ocean, and rainforest. The human inhabitants were to grow their own food, recycle their wastes, and maintain their own stable and viable living envi-

ronment. From the outset they were permitted electricity from external sources, and the experiment was to last 2 years. Nevertheless, before the intended completion date, carbon dioxide levels in the system's atmosphere began to rise, and it was necessary to pump external oxygen into the structure to keep the experiment and its participants alive.

The Biosphere 2 experience is a valuable one. It informs us about the limits of our knowledge of how ecosystems function.[5] In contrast to our increasingly powerful knowledge of how life functions at the genetic and molecular level, our understanding of complex, interactive ecological systems remains crude. Creating a "human terrarium" such as Biosphere 2 to sustain four men and four women for 2 years exceeded our technological ability and our ecological understanding. Yet, our collective behavior as a species suggests a stubborn conviction that no matter how much people disturb Earth's natural structure and operation, the planet will continue to support an ever-expanding, ever-demanding, human population that is projected to reach over 11 billion people by the middle of the next century.

As we begin the 21st century, the cautionary observation of the respected American naturalist John Burroughs, made near the beginning of the 20th century, seems especially insightful. Burroughs wrote that "One cannot but reflect what a sucked orange the Earth will be in the course of a few more centuries.

Our civilization is terribly expensive to all its natural resources: One hundred years of modern life doubtless exhausts its stores more than a millennium of the life of antiquity." Our last century, certainly is bearing out his prophesy.

Loss of Biodiversity

In addition to the disruption of global maintenance functions, habitat destruction leads to significant loss of biodiversity. We have reached a point where species of living organisms are being eliminated from the planet faster than scientists can identify and catalog them. For anyone who has ever derived personal or spiritual satisfaction from the simple pleasures of finding a bird's nest built of mud and twigs, watching a mimosa tree fold its leaves in repose as the daylight wanes, or seeing a meadow come alive on a summer evening with the blinking of fireflies, the prospect of so many of nature's unknown treasures disappearing before they have even been revealed is both troubling and saddening. Even more acutely painful is our seeming inability to prevent the destruction of living things that we already have come to know and to celebrate for their beauty, power, and uniqueness, such as the rhinoceros, the orangutan, the panda, the tiger, or the monarch butterfly.

While the loss of biodiversity may diminish us spiritually, appreciation of, or even reverence for, the beauty of nature has not been a sufficient social force to defend against the accelerating rate of biodiversity loss associated with human transformation of the global landscape. There is growing awareness, however, that biodiversity loss may also deprive humanity of myriad opportunities for greater physical and material well-being, and this realization may serve as a greater impetus to stem the tide of species disappearance. Scientists and "bioprospectors" are discovering a stunning array of beneficial compounds in the plants and animals of the world's forests and oceans that can offer profound benefits to humanity, if only the living things that produce these treasures can be protected from destruction. It may, after all, be in our own material self-interest to share the planet with other species.

Of particular appeal and importance to human society are potential new medicines derived from living organisms and new models for understanding and managing disease that are based on the evolutionary adaptations of living organisms to their environments. At a symposium on biodiversity and human health held in April 1998 at the American Museum of Natural History in New York, a diverse array of fascinating and important medical discoveries was presented that represent some of the benefits to be derived from the rainforests, oceans, and other ecological niches of our planet:

- Denning bears remain inactive for months without adverse physical effects. Studies of their physiological adaptations have improved our understanding of conditions such as osteoporosis, renal failure, obesity, and diabetes mellitus and are providing new approaches and products for the management and treatment of these conditions in human beings. Yet, around the world, many species of bears are threatened or endangered.

- Thermophilic bacteria found in association with natural hot springs provided the heat-stable DNA polymerase enzyme that made PCR possible-an essential research tool that has facilitated the rapid advance of biotechnology in the last decade.

- Marine cone snails have evolved protective venoms that contain anywhere from 50 to 200 pharmacologically active neuropeptides. Research into their mechanism of action has led to the development of analgesics more powerful than narcotics but whose precise specificity of action produces no side effects or chronic dependency.

- The potent anticancer drug Taxol, now approved for ovarian and breast cancers, was first isolated from the bark of the Pacific yew (*Taxus brevifolia*) tree. The existing population of Pacific yew trees was not sufficient to permit commercial production of Taxol, and alternative modes of production had to be developed.

- Fungi growing on the damp leaf litter of tropical rainforest floors in Costa Rica have yielded potent compounds with strong therapeutic potential against plasmodia, cryptosporidia, toxoplasma, and other protozoal pathogens.

- Amphibians possess a wide array of poisonous alkaloids that concentrate in their skin. Study of these alkaloids has enhanced knowledge of how neurotransmitters interact with their receptors. Alkaloids from the skin of poison dart frogs of the tropical rainforest have served as the basis for developing new and potent analgesics.

The power and promise of each protein or process now being revealed to scientists results from thousands to millions of years of evolutionary adaptation. Each living organism has slowly, through millennia of mutation and chance, worked out a survival strategy for its particular ecological niche and produced a remarkable array of adaptive molecules and mechanisms to support that survival. Now, human society has the power to either destroy this storehouse of natural wisdom in a matter of decades or exert the collective will to protect it and learn from it.

Veterinarians have important contributions to make in the area of protecting biodiversity. As scientists trained in comparative medicine, veterinarians can help to identify and elucidate new disease models in nonhuman species and work to bring new therapies to light. Veterinarians committed to wildlife conservation also can work to protect threatened and endangered species. They can participate, *ex situ*, in the development and improvement of captive breeding programs for species at risk, or become involved, *in situ*, with animal translocation and reintroduction programs. Veterinarians are needed to develop and carry out health management programs for endangered species in the wild and in captivity and to develop training and outreach programs that promote awareness and respect for the importance of biodiversity. Veterinarians should also be working with conservation biologists, ecologists, and other concerned scientists to help identify ecosystems at risk and develop management and surveillance plans to ensure ecosystem health. Various ecosystems may have their own indicator species of animals that reflect the overall health of the ecosystem. Veterinarians are needed to help identify these indicator or sentinel species and develop programs to monitor their health and, thereby, the health of their habitat. Conservation medicine, or veterinary conservation biology, is a new, emerging interdisciplinary field of veterinary medicine that encompasses these various professional activities in an effort to understand human and animal well-being in the context of ecosystem health. Conservation medicine and the role of veterinarians in the preservation of biodiversity are discussed further in Chapter 7.

Resurgence of Infectious Diseases

After the last case of human smallpox was documented in Somalia in 1977, the disease was officially declared to be eradicated. This event was widely heralded as a symbol of the power of modern medical science over the scourge of microbial infection. Starting with the establishment of the germ theory of disease, through the discovery and manufacture of antibiotics, to the global implementation of mass vaccination programs, it appeared that humankind, in a little over a century, had developed the knowledge and tools to eliminate infectious disease as a cause of human suffering. There was, indeed, justification for pride and optimism.

Yet, in recent years, something has gone very wrong. Since the conquest of smallpox, there has been a disturbing upsurge in infectious diseases. In the last 25 years, about 30 new microbial infections have been recorded that were not previously known to occur in human beings. Among the better-known of these conditions are human immunodeficiency virus (HIV) infection, Ebola virus infection, human rotavirus infection, hantavirus infection, Lyme disease, and Legionnaire's disease. In addition to new diseases, there has been a resurgence in the occurrence of previously known infections, such as cholera, malaria, tuberculosis, and sleeping sickness.

This pattern has been repeated in domesticated animals. Many previously unknown diseases have emerged in the same time period, including BSE, porcine reproductive and respiratory syndrome (PRRS), caprine arthritis encephalitis (CAE), canine parvovirus, and contagious equine metritis. New diseases and old diseases in new hosts are being reported in wild animals

as well. These include flaccid trunk disease in African elephants (cause unknown), canine distemper in lions of the Serengeti, calicivirus infection of sea lions off California, and fibropapillomas of sea turtles at various sites around the world.

Why is this happening? There is no single answer. To understand the factors at play, it is useful to think of the occurrence of infectious disease as a disruption of the balance that usually occurs between the susceptibility of host species and the pathogenicity of organisms that potentially cause disease. Usually, the normal equilibrium is maintained like a well-balanced seesaw whose fulcrum is the sum of the environmental conditions that prevail for a particular host and potential pathogen (Fig. 1-3). When the environment is disturbed in ways that shift the balance toward increased microbial pathogenicity or decreased host resistance, the host drops into the disease state. There is increasing evidence that environmental perturbation is functioning as the critical balance point between health and disease in our complex, modern society. Some examples are as follows:

- Extensive deforestation and incursion of humans into previously deforested and ecologically degraded areas increases the risk of new human disease. For example, HIV was historically restricted to nonhuman primate hosts in Africa. Decimation of indigenous African primate populations through extensive deforestation and hunting, accompanied by human incursion into former forested areas, is believed to have facilitated the initial adaptation of the virus to human hosts.

- Irrigation channels introduced onto previously nonarable lands increases the proliferation of disease vectors that require stagnant water to complete their life cycle. Expanded mosquito populations promote the spread of human malaria and of Rift Valley Fever in humans and animals. Expanded water snail populations promote the spread of liver fluke disease in livestock and schistosomiasis in animals and humans.

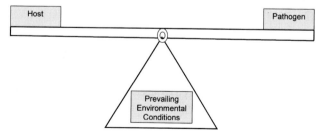

Figure 1-3. Schematic representation of the role of the environment in balancing host susceptibility and microbial infectivity in relation to the occurrence of infectious disease. When environmental perturbations shift the balance toward microbial infectivity or decreased host resistance, the host drops into the disease state.

- Increased atmospheric temperatures associated with global warming allow the expansion of arthropod vectors into new ranges where host populations are immunologically naive and therefore especially susceptible to diseases transmitted by the vectors. Warmer atmospheric temperatures also increase the rate of proliferation of some pathogenic microorganisms and favor the persistence of some species of helminth parasite larvae on the land.

- Runoff of chemical fertilizers and animal manure from agricultural enterprises into waterways encourages eutrophication and resulting algal blooms that may contain organisms, such as the dinoflagellate *Pfiesteria piscicida*, which are toxic for marine life and humans.[3]

In addition to environmental disturbances, other factors also are at work encouraging the resurgence of infectious disease. Pathogenic organisms and disease vectors are inadvertently being transported across the globe in a matter of hours via jet airplanes, putting new host populations at risk. Bacterial pathogens, such as *Salmonella typhimurium*, are developing increased resistance to antibiotic drugs. More and more animals are being raised under intensive confinement conditions that can facilitate the rapid spread of highly contagious diseases such as avian influenza or foot and mouth disease through large populations of poultry or livestock. Such passaging through large populations may also serve to enhance the virulence of infectious agents. Similarly, large-scale urbanization in developing countries concentrates people without adequate sanitation and public health services and favors the spread of tuberculosis and other infectious diseases. Malnourished and stressed refugee populations may flee from civil strife only to succumb to cholera in overcrowded and unhygienic refugee camps.

Despite the optimism fueled by our experience with smallpox eradication, infectious diseases have returned with a vengeance. Emerging infectious diseases represent a major challenge to the skill and determination of all health professionals, including veterinarians. Practicing veterinarians have always been attuned to the role of environment in the elaboration of disease. It is part of veterinary training to consider air quality in a barn as a predetermining factor of pneumonia in cows or to evaluate calf housing in outbreaks of diarrhea. Veterinarians are well positioned to broaden their concept of environment to include natural ecosystems and to consider human populations, domestic animal populations, and wild animal populations in the dynamic equation of health and disease. Veterinarians with professional interests in infectious disease research, disease ecology, and epidemiology and a commitment to the health of Earth and its diverse inhabitants will have much to engage them professionally for years to come and will make a significant contribution toward securing a healthy future.

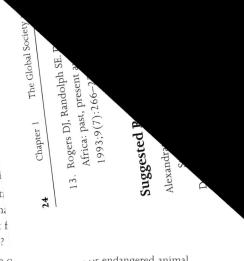

Discussion Po

1. Do you thi
   implication:
   identified in
   they affect v

2. What is your
   perils of biote
   to animal agri

3. Can you identi
   humans that ha
   5 years? What f
   these diseases?

4. Are you aware o .....ed or endangered animal species in your area? Are there any veterinarians involved in efforts to protect these species? In what ways can veterinarians become more involved professionally?

5. What is the current prevailing theory about global declines in amphibian populations? How might human activity be contributing to this catastrophic loss? How can veterinarians become involved in defining the problem and preventing further declines?

References

1. Berquist NR. Vector-borne parasitic diseases: new trends in data collection and risk assessment. Acta Trop 2001;79(1): 13–20.

2. Brown LR. Who Will Feed China? Wake-Up Call for a Small Planet. New York: WW Norton, 1995.

3. Burkholder JM, Mallin MA, Glasgow HB Jr. Impacts to a coastal river and estuary from rupture of a large swine waste holding lagoon. J Environ Qual 1997;26(6):1451–1466.

4. Carson R. Silent Spring. Boston: Houghton Mifflin, 1962.

5. Cohen JE, Tilman D. Biosphere 2 and biodiversity: the lessons so far. Science 1996;274:1150–1151.

6. Delgado C, Rosegrant M, Steinfeld H, et al. Livestock to 2020: The Next Food Revolution. Washington, DC: International Food Policy Research Institute, 1999.

7. Gladwell M. The mosquito killer. New Yorker, July 2, 2001:42–51.

8. Grace ES. Biotechnology Unzipped. Promises and Realities. Washington, DC: Joseph Henry Press, 1997.

9. MacLuhan M. Understanding Media: The Extensions of Man. New York: McGraw Hill, 1964.

10. Ormerod WE. Ecological effect of control of African trypanosomiasis. Science 1976;191(4229):815–821.

11. Reichardt T. Will souped up salmon sink or swim? Nature 2000;406(6791):10–12.

12. Robinson TP. Geographic information systems and the selection of priority areas for control of tsetse-transmitted trypanosomiasis in Africa. Parasitol Today 1998;12(11): 457–461.

13. Rogers DJ, Randolph SE. Africa: past, present a 1993;9(7):266–

Suggested

Alexandra

istribution of tsetse and ticks in
nd future. Parasitol Today
1.

eadings

tos N, ed. World Agriculture: Towards 2010. An FAO
tudy. Chichester, UK: John Wiley & Sons, 1995.

aily G, ed. Nature's Services: Societal Dependence on Natural
Ecosystems. Washington, DC: Island Press, 1994.

Garrett L. The Coming Plague: Newly Emerging Diseases in a World
Out of Balance. New York: Penguin Books, 1994.

Grifo F, Lovejoy TE, eds. Biodiversity and Human Health.
Washington, DC: Island Press, 1997.

McMichael AJ. Planetary Overload: Global Environmental Change
and the Health of the Human Species. Cambridge, England:
Cambridge University Press, 1993.

Symposium on biotechnology-the next revolution in veterinary
medicine. May 15, 1994. J Am Vet Med Assoc 1994;204(10):
1595–1625.

Suzuki D, McConnell A. The Sacred Balance: Rediscovering Our
Place in Nature. Amherst, NY: Prometheus Books, 1998.

Chapter 2
Animal Domestication and Human Society

OBJECTIVES FOR THIS CHAPTER

After completing this chapter, the reader should be able to

- Recognize the role that the use of animals for food, labor, and other purposes has had in the evolutionary and cultural development of human beings

- Appreciate the origins and history of the world's domesticated animals and the various factors that influenced the domestication process

- Perceive the major role that plant and animal agriculture has played in transforming human society and the human use of the earth

- Understand why certain domestic animals continue to predominate in certain regions and cultures of the world

- Recognize the opportunities and needs for new animal domestication efforts and the role that veterinarians can play in these efforts

Introduction

The relationship of human beings to animals is complex, dynamic, and essentially a work in progress. Human beings, as individuals and as societies, are constantly redefining their relationships with animals in cultural, economic, moral, legal, and spiritual terms. As there are many distinct human societies and a huge diversity of animal life, it should come as no surprise that a tremendous range of attitudes and practices is encompassed by the ever-evolving relationship of humans and animals.

A detailed examination of all aspects of the human-animal relationship is beyond the scope of this text. Nevertheless, for a better understanding of contemporary issues concerning the human use of animals, it is helpful to review some of the key developments in the history of that relationship, in order to illustrate the essential role that domestication of animals has had in the shaping of human civilization.[2] This chapter provides a brief overview of the prehistoric interactions of early humans with wild animals and the subsequent, gradual process of domestication of various animal species in relation to significant developments in human society, most notably the development of agriculture and commerce.

The Origins of Human and Animal Interactions

What differentiates humans from other animals? This is a timeless question that continues to generate enormous debate in philosophical and religious contexts. For the sake of the present discussion, however, an essentially anthropological and utilitarian answer will be offered: The differentiating characteristics of humans are the ability to modify the natural environment systematically to suit their own purposes, to develop symbolic written and spoken language that facilitates social cooperation, and to create as well as use tools. These processes and faculties evolved only gradually over the 4 million years of hominid evolution that is currently represented by the human species, *Homo sapiens*.

In critical ways, the evolution of humans (i.e., the expression and refinement of those characteristics that make us human) was greatly influenced, and perhaps even catalyzed, by the ever-changing relationship of humans to the animals around them. To understand the complexity of the human-animal relationship, it is helpful to review the key historical developments in that relationship from simple utilitarian purpose to complex social interaction.

The Prehistoric Phase

While there are many unanswered questions about the details of human development, a general scheme and timeline is known and is briefly summarized in Tables 2-1 and 2-2. The tables no doubt contain information subject to debate, as much remains unresolved in the fields of paleontology and archaeology, and they are intended to provide a general frame of reference for the following discussion.

In evolutionary terms, human beings derive from hominid ancestry, the hominids being primates with bipedal gait, vertical or erect posture, and the passageway for the spinal cord to

Table 2-1 Timetable of Early Phases of Animal and Human Development

Years in Past	Paleontological Period	Milestone, Activity, or Development
3.8 billion	Pre-Cambrian era	Oxygenation of the atmosphere, first simple life forms develop
700 million	Paleozoic era	Age of Invertebrates
230 million	Mesozoic era	Age of Reptiles
65 million	Cenozoic era	Age of Mammals begins
14 million	Miocene epoch	First indications that primates and hominids begin to evolve along different lines (*Ramapithicus* spp.)
4.0 million	Pliocene epoch	First evidence of bipedal hominids, *Australopithecus anamensis*, inhabiting Africa
2.6 million		First known use of stone tools
2.5 million		First evidence of ancestors of direct human lineage; *Homo habilis*, a small hominid, but with proportionately large brain to body size
1.8 million	Pleistocene epoch	First evidence of *Homo erectus*, a taller, longer-limbed hominid, with a heavy brow ridge
1 million	Lower Paleolithic culture	First known use of controlled fire; *H. erectus* beings to extend out of Africa into Europe and Asia
800 thousand		Archaic form of *Homo sapiens*, a large-brained human ancestor
350 thousand		First evidence of shelter use
300 thousand		Anatomical structures for speech in place
200 thousand		Cold-adapted Neanderthal form of *H. sapiens* populates Europe
100 thousand		Anatomically modern form of *H. sapiens*

extend from the brain (foramen magnum) occurring at the base of, rather than the back of, the skull. The first, reasonably well documented hominids, classified in the genus *Australopithecus*, were initially inhabiting the earth between 4.2 and 4.0 million years ago. Eastern and southern Africa have been, and still remain, the most fertile sources of fossil evidence of the earliest human ancestry known to paleontologists, archeologists, and paleoanthropologists. Africa appears to have been the chief venue for the development of human life.

Like other animals, the earliest humans must have spent a considerable amount of their time and effort in food gathering. Early food sources, collected through simple gathering, were predominantly of plant origin, supplemented with insects, shellfish, and other, easy-to-gather, nonplant foodstuffs.

The initial relationship of humans to vertebrate animals was probably a predator/prey relationship, with humans serving as the prey. One of the earlier and more noteworthy fossils chronicling the human prehistorical record is the 2.5 million year old skull of the so-called Taung child, an Australopithecine hominid found in South Africa in 1925. The skull contained puncture marks and was found amidst a pile of numerous bones from other small animals. It is presumed that the boy was carried off by an eagle or other large predatory bird and brought back to the nest for consumption.

The gradual role reversal of our human ancestors from prey to predator and the increasing inclusion of animal foodstuffs in the human diet occurred over millions of years. From simple gathering of insects, invertebrates, and the occasional small lizard, hominids probably first advanced to scavenging, picking shreds or scraps of flesh from the carcasses of predatory kills after wild canids, vultures, and other scavengers had abandoned the bones or been chased off. It is not difficult to imagine that hominids began to associate certain sights and sounds with the location of a kill and cautiously began to seek them out.

By following these natural cues, early hominids probably began to recognize the habits of the prey animals themselves and could begin to track or follow herds or groups in anticipation of a kill. Such behavior would set the stage for opportunistic hunting, wherein hominids might encounter young, aged, sick, or injured animals and be able to subdue them without much need for strategy or use of tools. As knowledge of terrain and prey behavior increased, early hominids may have been able to hunt animals strategically without tools,

Table 2-2 More Recent Advances in Human Development in Relation to Animals in Neolithic and Modern Times

Years Ago	Period	Milestone, Activity, or Development
100–40 thousand	Paleolithic period (Old Stone Age)	Nomadic hunter-gatherers living in caves, using fire and making stone tools; humans first reach Australia from Asia
40–15 thousand		Communal hunters, using man-made shelters having magic and supernatural belief systems; cave paintings depicting animal prey
15 thousand		Domestication of dogs and reindeer
12 thousand	Mesolithic period (Middle Stone Age)	Earliest confirmed human inhabitants, the Clovis hunters, populate the Americas, moving southward from Canada; their antecedents originated in Asia and crossed over what was a land bridge at the present Bering Straits
10 thousand		End of last Ice Age; domestication of sheep and goats begins in Near East; beginnings of agriculture in Near East
8 thousand	Neolithic period (New Stone Age)	Domestication of pigs in Asia
7 thousand		Domestication of cattle in Near East; beginnings of agriculture in Mesoamerica
6 thousand		Domestication of horses in Central Asia, donkeys in the Near East, and the cat in Egypt; beginnings of agriculture in South Asia
5 thousand	Bronze Age	Domestication of water buffalo in South Asia, camels in Near East (one hump) and Central Asia (two hump); and probably chickens in South Asia
4 thousand		Domestication of the elephant in Asia and probably the llama and alpaca in South America; first humans arrive in Polynesia, probably from New Guinea
3 thousand	Iron Age	Distinct cattle breeds developed in Europe
2 thousand		Domestication of yak
1 thousand		Goldfish cultivation developed in China; first humans reach New Zealand, from Polynesian islands
Present	Age of Globalization	Cloning and transgenic manipulation of domestic animals; rapidly accelerating rate of wild animal extinction; emergence of animal rights movement

driving them, through fear and the use of fire, to their deaths. The evidence to support this includes numerous sites where piles of ancient animal bones representing many individuals of a single species lie at the bottom of cliff edges, with only a few of the animals showing signs of butchering. The next likely phase was the development of strategic hunting, which required both social cooperation and tool use.

Some paleoanthropologists reason that there was a strong link between the development of tool use, the enlargement of brain size, and the inclusion of animal-derived food in the diet of evolving humans.[9] Enlarging brain size increased caloric requirement at the same time that it allowed increased reasoning power. Animal fat and protein were a dense source of the nutrients required to support brain development, and in turn, the expansion of brain size allowed hominids to think

of new ways to obtain such foods. Gradually, hominids began to use simple stones and then crude stone tools to cut through tough hides and to break open skulls and bones to access brain and marrow left behind by predators and other scavengers. By eating marrow and brain, they might access more nutrients in an hour than they could in a full day of extensive foraging.

Later, stone tools were also used to cut meat into mouth-sized chunks, and then sharpened stones were used as spear tips for thrusting into prey. Eventually, the notion of projectile weapons took hold, first as stone-tipped spears and later as stones shaped into arrowheads and launched from bows. Through their increased reasoning power, fueled in part by consumption of animal food, evolving humans learned to hunt more safely and more efficiently.

In the long period of human development before agriculture, the concentrated energy and protein of animal origin was the nutritional fuel that evolving man used to support his ever-expanding thinking capacity. Each gram of brain tissue requires 22.5 times the energy to keep it alive as an equivalent amount of muscle tissue at rest. There is evidence of butchering of deer and other animals in what is now Spain by early hominids (probably archaic *Homo sapiens*) close to 1 million years ago, indicating that meat consumption was important in the diet of hominids almost from the time they first migrated northward to Europe from Africa. One reason that meat in the diet of prehistoric humans inhabiting Europe may have been especially important was climate. In contrast to Africa, European winters were severe and many plant food sources were seasonal. This was strong motivation for developing technology and social organization that facilitated successful hunting year round.

The Paleolithic Period

Early human development is interpreted largely through the scant record of bones and stone tools left behind by prehistoric hominids. It is not until about 35,000 years ago that early humans, in Europe, begin to contribute to the telling of their own stories through symbolic and artistic representation of their daily lives. The most dramatic and earliest examples of such expression are found in the remarkable cave paintings of southern France and Spain. The almost exclusive subject of these hauntingly modern paintings is animals, indicating the central importance of wild beasts in the daily lives of early, preagricultural humans. Though not the earliest of such works, the cave paintings at Lascaux cave, near Montignac, France, are probably the best known. They were created by Cro-Magnon humans about 17,000 years ago, toward the end of the Upper Paleolithic period.

Paleolithic cave art is intriguing for a number of reasons: it provides a direct and palpable connection to our human ancestors and their daily lives; it offers an insight into the sophistication of a so-called primitive culture capable of creating the tools and techniques of artistic expression; it provides clues about the origins of spiritualism and the religious symbolism of animals; it underscores the central importance of animals in the Paleolithic human's cosmos; and, not least, it presents a museum gallery of evocative and well-executed artistic works. For a virtual tour of Lascaux cave, see http://www.culture.fr/culture/arcnat/lascaux/en/. The famed 20th-century artist Pablo Picasso, after viewing the cave paintings at Lascaux, was moved to pronounce, "We have invented nothing!"

Beyond their anthropological and artistic significance, the paintings also tell us some important stories about the dynamic nature of ecosystems and the forces that modify them. Virtually all the animals depicted on the cave walls of southern Europe roamed the area in large herds 17,000 to 20,000 years ago. Now, they are either extinct or occur in much restricted ranges. The definitive causes of these extinctions are not known, but global climate change, in the form of warming temperatures associated with the end of the last Ice Age 12,000

years ago, played a significant part. The open grasslands that supported large herds of Paleolithic herbivores such as the bison, red deer, and wild horses were gradually replaced by forest as temperatures increased. These grazing animals were pushed northward into ever-shrinking and inhospitable habitat or toward extinction. Human influences, in terms of hunting and environmental modification, are also presumed to have contributed to the demise of many of these large herbivores and the animals that preyed upon them.

The more recent of the European cave paintings show a more naturalistic and detailed rendition of the animals depicted than do the earlier, more schematic paintings. It is speculated that as the animals became more scarce over time, these graphic representations became specific evocations for their return, a spiritual hope that the drawing itself might become the animal, successfully brought forth from the "womb" of the deep cave through symbolic induction. If these paintings do indeed represent an attempt to bring back animals whose populations were diminishing, then the paintings may signal the first expression of a conservation ethic in human society, an ethic born out of a recognition of the need to actively maintain the wild species on which our material and spiritual fulfillment depends.

Despite these possible appeals to the spirits, the powerful forces of climatic change gained the upper hand. As the last Ice Age began to wane in southern Europe about 10,000 years ago, populations of prey species inexorably declined and the hunter-gatherer way of life declined along with it. In the world today, there are still so-called Stone Age societies based on the hunter-gatherer strategy of food procurement, for example, the Aborigines of Australia, and the "Bushmen" of the Kalahari in southern Africa. However, the trespasses of the modern world, including habitat encroachment, cultural intrusions, and overt hostility, have distorted the traditional lives of these people and threatened the existence of their cultural identity.

The Neolithic Period

As tools and techniques became more advanced during the Paleolithic era, hunting emerged as a successful survival strategy. It offered its practitioners a dependable and abundant supply of highly concentrated calories and protein nutrition from animal sources. For these successful hunters, fertility, offspring survival, and longevity are likely to have improved as a result, leading to increasing populations of human hunters. Therefore, the period of glacial recession in the northern hemisphere presented a serious challenge to Cro-Magnon peoples; a decreasing animal food supply in the face of an expanding human population. Not surprisingly, this dilemma coincides historically with the beginning of a significant period of change in human development with regard to food procurement, namely, the rise of agriculture and settled society in the Neolithic period.

The Neolithic period, or New Stone Age, is a critical period of accelerated human cultural growth that began roughly 10,000 years ago in the Old World and lasted for approximately 4,500 years. Knowledge about human cultural development during the Neolithic period comes from three main areas, all of which are associated with major river systems: the Tigris and Euphrates in the Near East (Mesopotamia), the Nile in North Africa (ancient Egypt), and the Indus in South Asia (Mohenjo-Daro and Harrapa).

Neolithic culture is generally defined by the development of pottery and weaving, the formation and use of writing, the establishment of towns and cities, the domestication of animals, and the development of agriculture. In short, it was a period of intense technological innovation that transformed the structure of human society, the relationship of humans to animals, and the human use of the earth itself, in profound and lasting ways. Arguably, the most fundamental of these achievements was the development of agriculture, or the cultivation of plants. Many of the intrinsic characteristics of modern human society are traceable back to the socially transforming power of crop cultivation, which shifted the basic strategy of human survival from food procurement to food production.

The revolutionary aspect of agriculture was that it allowed a comparative few to provide food for the many, primarily through the production of abundant and relatively nonperishable food grains that could be stored for extended periods. This freed up considerable segments of the population to develop ancillary skills and pursue other activities, giving free rein to human imagination and creativity. While this led to technological and artistic advancement, it also gradually led to the development of class structure, with agricultural workers, in the categories of peasant and slave, toiling for and increasingly controlled by ruling and priestly classes whose interests were also served by an expanding artisan and commercial "middle" class. The use of slaves as agricultural labor, of course, is not only a chapter of ancient history. The practice persisted in the United States until only a century and a half ago as an economic underpinning of plantation agriculture geared toward cotton production. The practice was only terminated as the result of a bitter, bloody civil war, which serves to underscore how fundamental agriculture and its practices are to shaping the social and political history of human civilization.

While Paleolithic hunting was characterized by small clans of hunters moving through the landscape in search of prey, cultivation necessitated tending plants for extended periods during growth. As a result, human settlements began to develop and expand in the Neolithic period, leading to advances in architecture, engineering, and social integration but also to crowding, poor sanitation, and overuse of land and water. The preparation of a specific piece of land for planting and harvesting produced the concepts of private property and land ownership. This in turn required systems of boundary measurement, calculation of land areas, and codes and laws of property rights and means of enforcement, all of which began to develop during the Neolithic period.

The production of surplus, stored foods for subsequent distribution required the development of storage technology, inventory methods, and accounting skills. Management of grain inventories is believed to have been a direct stimulus for the creation of writing. The earliest known writing samples, the cuneiform from ancient Sumer in the Mesopotamian region, were bookkeeping records of grain inventories.

The existence of stored grain surpluses no doubt also attracted the attention of groups outside the community who reasoned that it just might be easier to steal grain than grow it. This led to the development of walled cities, defense establishments, a military class, and the beginning of organized warfare fought fundamentally over food and the land on which to grow it. It is interesting that the stereotypical view of the Paleolithic hunter is one of aggression and fierce belligerence. More-recent anthropological studies would suggest, however, that conflict resolution among hunting groups is often achieved by a parting of the ways between adversaries and a search elsewhere for resources. The human capacity for organized aggression seems to have achieved a fuller expression as a byproduct of agriculture, which involves ownership of fixed parcels of land and the need to defend them.

As agriculture increased in importance during Neolithic times, new technical innovations emerged. These included identification and domestication of new grain crops, plowing and other methods of land preparation, selection for higher- yielding crops, the use of animals for agricultural labor, the fertilization of soil with manure, and irrigation of fields. Some of these innovations also led to the emergence of serious problems such as soil erosion, water-logging and salinization of soils from irrigation, and the extension of farming into marginal land areas at the expense of forests and grazing lands. Today, many of these same problems persist and, in some cases, have been aggravated by advances in mechanized agriculture and limitations on the availability of arable land.

The origins of cultivation remain unclear. Necessity being the mother of invention, it is presumed that experimentation with domestication of plants and animals began in an effort to bolster food sources in the facing of waning wildlife populations. At least in southern Europe and the Near East, which was to become the "cradle of civilization," this process was intensified by the ecological changes brought about by the receding glaciers at the end of the Ice Age. There is speculation that fishing peoples in the newly warming regions may have been first to initiate developments in agriculture. Fishing peoples were already sedentary. They may have accumulated refuse piles at their settlements that sprouted new vegetation from discarded seeds, roots or tubers brought from food-gathering forays into more distant locations. The more curious of these people may have experimented with replanting some of the more palatable or prolific of these plants so as not to have to travel to collect them. Some scholars speculate that cultivation may have been secondary to animal domestication rather than the other way around, as is commonly thought. The rationale is that early herders of sheep and goats, the first domesticated livestock in the Near East, recognized that their animals could eat considerable portions of plants that were unpalatable to humans and therefore experimented with the cultivation of forages or fodder as a noncompetitive source of foodstuffs for their animals.

Whatever its specific origins, formalized crop agriculture did not spring up overnight, nor was there any predestined blueprint for its linear development. It was undoubtedly a cumulative process of serendipity, casual and detailed observation, trial and error, adaptation, and accommodation.[4] A number of innovations can be identified for the gradual development of agriculture, and these are presented, for both animals and plants, in Table 2-3. In different areas of the world, with different resources available and different peoples present, the details and timetable of agricultural development no doubt varied.

For instance, the use of animals for agricultural labor was an early development in the Old World, with oxen used for plowing in ancient Egypt. The use of draft animals did not occur in New World Mesoamerican agriculture until thousands of years later because there were no large indigenous mammals suitable for domestication and use in animal traction in the Western hemisphere. Mayans and Aztecs devised novel ways to cultivate crops, such as the use of raised, aquatic gardens known as *chinampas*, and only integrated livestock into agriculture after draft animals were introduced during the period of European exploration. Today, many of the earliest agricultural innovations are still practiced in different parts of the world, alongside the most modern methods, as discussed in more detail in Chapter 4.

The Domestication of Animals

In modern times, human society has developed the capacity to set lofty goals for technical and scientific achievement and then methodically sets out to accomplish them. We say we want to land on the moon or map the human genome, and then we do it. Domestication of animals is arguably an achievement of equal stature in the annals of human social progress. It is unlikely, however, that our early ancestors set out intentionally to domesticate the particular species of animals that we have come to know today as our pets and livestock. Instead, domestication evolved as a social and biological process of mutual adaptation over thousands of years. The motivations and

Table 2-3 Key Developments in the Use of Plants and Animals by Humans as Food[a]	
Use of Plants as Food	**Use of Animals as Food**
Foraging for wild plants	Foraging for stationary invertebrates
Trial and error identification of edible plants	Simple scavenging from carcasses killed by other predators
Harvesting wild grasses	Scavenging with carcass manipulation using stone tools
Tending wild plants	Opportunistic hunting of vulnerable individuals
Domestication of genetically distinct plants	Following or driving wild herds for trapping
Swidden or slash and burn planting of roots and tubers that propagate vegetatively	Strategic hunting with hand-held tools
Planting of seeds for cropping	Strategic hunting with projectile tools
Use of plow for field preparation	Loose herding of wild animals
Animal traction for agricultural labor	Semidomestication of wild species
Irrigation of cropland	Full domestication of non-wild species
Selective breeding of seed for crop plants for desired production characteristics	Close herding and extensive grazing of livestock
Large-scale monoculture cropping	Seasonal confinement of animals
Mechanization and intensification of chemical inputs for increased production	Killing of wild animals as pests
Genetic engineering of food crops for desired characteristics	Continuous confinement of domesticated animals
	Intensive, industrial livestock production
	Genetic manipulation and cloning of animals
[a]While presented in a sequential fashion, each new development did not fully replace the preceding one. In fact, to varying degrees, numerous peoples and cultures around the world continue to use the earlier derived methods of food acquisition and production.	

circumstances for specific animal domestications changed over time and were often tied to other developments in the history of human cultural progress. The regional origins of important plant and animal domestications are represented on the map in Figure 2-1. In the following sections, the process of domestication and the historical phases of that process are discussed.

The Process of Domestication

Given the multitude of animal species inhabiting the earth, how is it that the cow, sheep, goat, pig, horse, donkey, dog, and cat have emerged as the eight most common domesticated mammals on the planet? Consider, for example, the fact that archeological evidence from the Near East in Upper Paleolithic and Mesolithic times indicates that gazelles and red deer were enormously abundant animals, actively hunted, and favored for meat by hunters. Furthermore, deer antler was highly valued as a raw material for tool productions because it was solid, pointed, strong, and resilient. Sheep and goats, in contrast to cervids, have hollow horns of relatively little value as tools. Yet, the first domesticated ruminants to emerge from the Near East in this era were the goat and the sheep, not the gazelle or the deer. The deer and gazelle could be tamed if individuals were captured when young, but in herds, people were not able to domesticate them.

A number of factors affect the suitability of a given species for domestication, i.e., the integration of that species into human society. A key element is the social structure of the species. With the exception of the cat, all of the successfully domesticated species mentioned above come from wild ancestors that were social animals, adapted to life in herds or packs. While different social organization patterns occur in different species, the wild ancestors of successfully domesticated animals maintained social structures that were strongly hierarchical, rather than territorial. In other words, these species clearly defined positions of dominance and submissiveness for individual animals within the group. This dominance hierarchy allowed humans to assume a dominant leader role within the animal group, with the animals recognizing and accepting the dominant human position. Successfully domesticated ancestral animals were not territorial, in that they did not defend a specific geographical area for breeding or food collection, though they would vigorously defend their group status relative to each other. This characteristic was attractive to Mesolithic humans, who, as essentially mobile hunters themselves, might have a home range but no well-defined territorial allegiances.

For these reasons, as well as other physiological and behavioral factors, wild sheep and goats were likely more amenable to human interaction than gazelles and deer. Similarly, these behavioral characteristics help to explain why domestic dogs derived from wolves rather than jackals or hyenas and why wild horses and asses were more conducive to domestication than their equid cousins the onagers.

Once the potential for mutual adaptation is recognized between humans and a specific wild species, a gradual process of domestication ensues that results in the transformation of the wild progenitor into the domestic animal we recognize today.

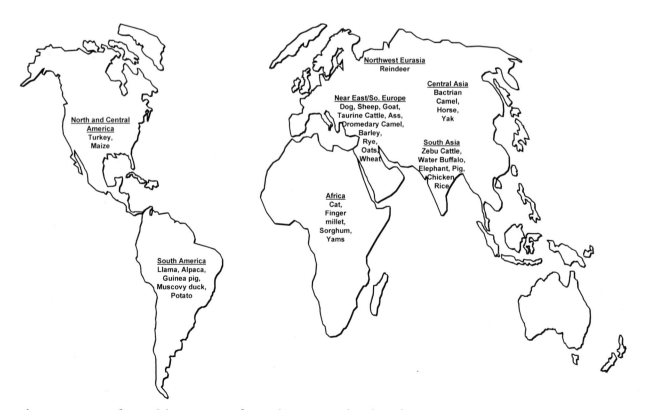

Figure 2-1.   Sites of original domestications of major domestic animals and cereal crops.

Though the details obviously differ among species, a general pattern with distinct phases is identifiable.[11] The key phases are as follows:

- In the initial phase there is a loose association between humans and the wild progenitor, with no control of the animal's breeding by humans.

- In the next phase, there is confinement or voluntary entry of the progenitor to the human environment, with breeding occurring in captivity.

- In the third phase, there is selective breeding controlled by humans to develop certain desired characteristics, but some cross breeding with wild progenitors is still permitted.

- In the next phase, specific breed traits are conceptualized to promote specific, economically advantageous modifications to the animal. This requires strict management of selective breeding and careful attention to artificial selection.

- Finally, there is banishment or killing of wild progenitors to avoid their coming into contact with domesticated breeds to avoid uncontrolled breeding.

The historical record offers an intriguing variety of associations between humans and animals that suggest that a successful domestication process occurred with many species of wild animals. Yet, today, we see no lasting evidence of these domestications. For example, the hieroglyphic record of ancient Egypt shows human attendants handling the beautifully horned antelope, the oryx, and elsewhere shows striped hyenas being shepherded by men. Why do we not see people walking their hyenas on the streets of Cairo today? It is most likely that these animals were never fully domesticated in the first place but, rather, were tamed. For taming, young individuals were taken from the wild, raised in captivity, and habituated to human contact. The critical distinction from complete domestication is that controlled breeding to produce subsequent tame generations was not successfully accomplished.

The Situation Before Domestication

Though a human society may depend directly on animals, those animals may not be domesticated. Paleolithic hunters, with a social organization that did not extend beyond family clans, were generally mobile, following wild animals through their habitat in pursuit of food. They left few traces of their cultural development beyond the bones and stone tools left behind at hunting camps. It must be assumed that these hunters were keen students of natural history, gradually learning a great deal about the behavioral habits, migratory movements, and life cycle events of their favored prey animals.

Gradually, sedentary hunting cultures did evolve that focused on prey species that allowed hunters to establish permanent bases for their food procurement activity. The archeological record of such cultures is richer than that of mobile hunters and includes remains of settlements, art, and evidence of religion, technological advances, and complex social structure. Interestingly, these cultural developments often occurred independent of any developments in agriculture, though cultivation is often credited as the catalyst of rapid human cultural advances in the Mesolithic and Neolithic periods.

Some such sedentary hunting cultures still exist today, though modified by contact with the modern world. In Arctic and northern latitudes, for example, there are indigenous social groups, such as the Inuit, or Eskimos, that settle in villages and fish or hunt marine mammals under harsh climatic conditions that essentially preclude agricultural activity. In these cases, the animals on which the society focuses are not domesticated, but the overall pattern and structure of the human society is intimately adapted to the natural history and life cycle of the chief prey animal, be it the whale, the seal, or the salmon.

For example, the Makah Indians of the Pacific Northwest region of the United States, lived for thousands of years in coastal villages of long houses, traditionally hunted the great gray whale in cedar log canoes with 18-foot harpoons, and used sealskin floats to track and move the whales after harpooning. The Makah, who now live primarily in the state of Washington, were banned by the federal government from hunting whales in 1926 because of declining whale populations due to overtaking by non-Native American whalers. In 1997, the Makah tribe once again won the right from the International Whaling Commission to begin hunting the great gray whale, with a permitted take of four whales per year. The whale was removed from the Endangered Species List in 1994 because vigorous conservation measures had led to increasing populations. Few, if any, contemporary Makah have first-hand experience with traditional whale hunting, and they will have to relearn their ancestral heritage.

Just 10,000 years ago, virtually the entire human population of the earth, though small, survived as hunter-gatherers. By the 16th century, when Europeans "discovered" the New World, the area of the world populated by hunter-gatherers was down to about 15%. Today, hunter-gatherers exist only in isolated pockets of the world, and less than 0.001% of the world's burgeoning population of close to 6 billion sustain themselves primarily by traditional methods of gathering and hunting, either sedentary or mobile. This marginalization of hunter-gatherers is linked to the Neolithic transition from a system of food procurement to one of food production. This shift to food production is one of the most profound developments in human cultural history. It was driven primarily by the development of crop cultivation and animal domestication.

Domestications Preceding Agriculture

Four key species were domesticated prior to the development of agriculture in the Neolithic period. These were the dog, the reindeer, the goat, and the sheep. All of these domestications evolved out of needs or opportunities related to hunting and are associated with pre-agriculturists in the Upper Paleolithic and Mesolithic periods. A brief discussion of these various domestications follows.

Dogs

The progenitor of the domestic dog, *Canis familiaris*, is now believed to be the wolf, *Canis lupus*. Formerly, it had been held that the wild jackal also contributed significantly to the development of the domestic dog. However, this theory essentially has been discarded. Recent studies on mitochondrial DNA sequences of wolves and dogs around the world suggest that domestication of the dog from the wolf began over 135,000 years ago.[10] Despite such scientific evidence, there will no doubt remain many people who will look at the tremendous phenotypic diversity of the modern dog breeds and wonder seriously how they could all come from a single source!

The relationship of early humans to the wolf was no doubt complex and contradictory. The wolf was at the same time a hunting competitor and a potential hunting partner. It was a predator to be feared, but also a potential prey to be pursued for food. Wolves were extensively distributed around the northern hemisphere in Paleolithic times. There is little question that wherever early humans hunted large game, they came into contact with wolves and undoubtedly got to know the behavior of wolves very well. Wolves likely frequented the margins of human hunting camps, scavenging for scraps from successful hunts. Humans may have tossed scraps to wolves, in what is a natural human gesture, and encouraged their association. When hunting, they may have killed nursing female wolves and brought pups back to their hunting camps for entertainment or for future food. Women may have even suckled wolf cubs, as there is much precedent for the nursing of animals by women in hunter-gatherer societies that persist today. Some of these tame, raised pups probably bonded to humans and began to accompany them on hunting forays and proved themselves useful in locating and capturing game. Out of this evolving utilitarian partnership coupled with the likely satisfaction humans derived from this animal companionship, the domestication of the dog was probably born.

Wolves show virtually all of the behavioral and social characteristics that make a species amenable to domestication. They are social, and their social structure is one of hierarchical dominance. Individuals show both dominant and submissive behaviors. These behaviors are based on posture and visual cues that are readable by, and transferable to, humans, who can then join into the dominance hierarchy as group leaders. They work cooperatively in hunting, and they are natural herders, as their instinctual hunting patterns involve controlling the movement of prey groups to cut out susceptible individuals for attack. Early humans apparently identified these characteristics and recognized the potential of tame wolves and, later, domesticated dogs as cooperative partners, first in hunting and then in herding.

The earliest archeological remains that can be definitely identified as domestic dogs rather than precursor wolves come from Mesopotamia, in what is now Iraq, and date back 12,000

years. While most early remains are found in western Asia, there is evidence of prehistoric human-dog association from Europe, North America, Southeast Asia, and Japan, indicating that domestication of dogs was an idea with almost universal appeal to early humans. In Australia, there was a human-dog association in prehistoric times between the aborigines and the dingo. Of interest is the fact that there is no fossil record of dogs in Australia, suggesting that dingoes reached the island continent from Asia in the company of humans from cultures unknown. The physical similarity of the dingo to the so-called common Asian Pariah dog is marked.

By 2000 BC, the pictorial record shows that ancient Egypt had different distinct dog types, both large hunting dogs and small lap dogs. In ancient Rome, systematic breeding of dogs was well established, though the variety of breeds does not approach what exists today. There are currently an estimated 450 to 850 breeds of dogs worldwide, with the American Kennel Club recognizing 150 breeds in the United States alone. Dogs continue to provide utilitarian services to people around the world as guardians, herders, and in some places, food. However, the overriding role of the dog in modern society has become that of companion and family member. The role of the dog as pet and how it shapes attitudes toward animals in general is discussed further in Chapter 3.

Reindeer

More than any other domesticated animal, the reindeer provides us with a window to our Paleolithic past. This is because the contemporary domesticated reindeer essentially appears unchanged from its wild ancestors, and the people who herd reindeer still draw on traditional practices that span the millennia.

The wild reindeer, *Rangifer tarandus*, is an unusual member of the Cervidae, or deer family. It has some distinctive traits that make it exquisitely adapted to arctic environments. It is unusual among deer in that both males and females have antlers. The antlers point forward and are used by the animals to dig in the snow for food. The nose is completely hair covered to protect against frigid temperatures, and the bony structure of the foot is unique in allowing the hoof to splay widely to help distribute the animal's weight and support it for snow walking. Reindeer, also known as caribou in North America, are at home in the Arctic tundra, where food is scarce and the openness of the landscape makes them easily noticed by their main predators, humans and wolves. Over time, the reindeer evolved social organization and behavior that helped protect them from their predators and meet their nutritional needs. They are gregarious and move in large herds to provide many eyes and ears for safety. They have naturally synchronized their breeding so that an entire herd calves within a 2-week period, thus reducing vulnerability of mothers and young. They migrate extensively in search of food, which consists primarily of lichens but also includes lemmings when they can catch them.

Currently, in the Old World, the wild reindeer is found only in northern Norway and northern Russia, but it formerly ranged extensively through the tundra and taiga regions of Asia, North America, and Europe. During the last glacial period, the reindeer was found as far south as France and Spain, and the Paleolithic cave paintings found in these countries depict reindeer. In North America, the range of the wild caribou is Alaska and Canada, dipping down into the north central United States.

The reindeer was an important prey species for Paleolithic hunters, and the early stages of domestication evolved out of hunting, though the details are lost in history. It is believed that initially, individual young reindeer were captured and tamed to use as hunting decoys. The captive reindeer would be tethered to attract wild reindeer with hunters hiding in ambush nearby. Later, hunters developed closer associations with herds, moving regularly with them and encouraging the reindeer to become habituated to them. Humans had a powerful lure to help them accomplish this, as the reindeer craves urine in its salt-deficient diet and is especially disposed to human urine. Gradually, humans took full advantage of the gregarious nature of reindeer social organization and assumed leadership roles in the herd, taking over control of the herd movements. Out of this process were born arctic herding cultures that depended exclusively on reindeer for food and raw materials.

These herding cultures still thrive today among the Lapps, or Saami, people of Scandinavia, Finland, and the Kola Peninsula of Russia as well as other groups in the Siberian and Asian Arctic. In contemporary times, the process of domestication has extended beyond simple herding. Today, reindeer are used to pull sleds, are ridden, and are even milked. These developments occurred much later than herding, probably inspired by contact with peoples who had domesticated cows and horses. The reindeer industry has also been commercialized. It is estimated that there are currently about 3 million domesticated reindeer. Russia produces over 30,000 tons of reindeer meat per year and over 600,000 hides. The domesticated reindeer has also been introduced to Alaska, Canada, Iceland, Greenland, and Scotland.

Goats

It cannot be known with certainty from the patchy archeological record whether the sheep or the goat was the first ruminant species to be domesticated. Both domestications, however, occurred in the Near East, beginning over 10,000 years ago, under presumably similar circumstances. As the climate began to warm with the receding glacier, wild game populations decreased. Hunters had to travel farther and for longer periods in search of prey, with diminishing chance of success. It is speculated that these hunters began to take goats and sheep with them, as a reliable source of meat on their extended journeys.

How this process of domestication was initiated is unknown. Wild goats and sheep were among the species commonly hunted, so the social behavior of these animals was known to humans. It is possible that inventive hunters drove wild goat or sheep herds to a desirable location, such as near a water source or salt lick, and then remained in the area with them for extended periods, encouraging habituation and acceptance of humans into the social hierarchy of the herds. Alternatively, lambs and kids could have been taken from the wild and raised as captive or tame animals that imprinted on humans as leaders.

The domesticated goat, *Capra hirca*, derives from the bezoar goat, *Capra aegregus*, a wild goat of western Asia, with a historical range from India west to Crete. Bezoar goats possess long, backward-curving, scimitar-shaped horns with a sharp anterior keel. The goat was most likely domesticated in what is now the Middle East. There is good evidence that the Nastufians, an early culture of the region, kept domestic goats 10,000 years ago, which means that the domestication process likely began before Neolithic or agricultural times.

Today the goat is one of the world's most ubiquitous domesticated animals, found on virtually every continent save Antarctica. There are many highly specialized breeds, selected for specific economic purposes including mohair and cashmere fiber production, milk production, and meat production. This selective breeding is an ongoing process that began thousands of years ago. The high-producing milking breeds of goats that are most familiar to us in the United States, such as the Alpine, Saanen, or Toggenburg, were developed in Europe only as recently as the 19th century. Wild goats were never indigenous to the western hemisphere. They had a more southerly range than sheep and appear not to have crossed the ancient land bridge at the Bering Straits from Siberia to North America. The mountain goat of North America is not in fact a true goat in the genus *Capra*. It is classified taxonomically as *Oreamnos americanus* and has never been domesticated.

Most of the world's goats, however, are of less specialized breed type and are multipurpose goats serving the needs of agriculturists, villagers, and herders in much of the developing world. The goat persists as a valued species of livestock for the rural and urban poor in all regions of the world, but particularly in Africa and South Asia. Goats are especially common among people trying to eke out a living under harsh conditions of difficult terrain, scant vegetation, and marginal rainfall, as the goat is well adapted to adversity and is recognized as a survivor, primarily because of its diverse eating habits. The goat is a browser as well as a grazer and can use a much wider variety of plant material as food in an environment of scarcity. Goats are even able to climb into trees to eat leaves when there is no food available at ground level (Fig. 2-2). Improperly managed, goats can cause serious damage to vegetation, leading to landscape degradation. The subject of goats and land degradation is examined in more detail in Chapter 6.

Sheep

The domesticated sheep, *Ovis aries*, is derived from the wild Asiatic mouflon, *Ovis orientalis*. This is a dark-colored, small-bodied, long-legged sheep. It has a short tail and backward-curving horns that are horizontally ringed along their length. The original range was western Asia from the Black Sea to the western Mediterranean. The bighorn sheep of North America, *Ovis canadensis*, has never been domesticated. Domesticated

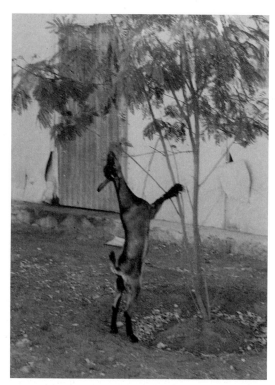

Figure 2–2. Young goat in Ethiopia standing on hind limbs to consume tree leaves. When necessary, a goat can climb into the tops of small trees to browse. (Photo by Dr. David M. Sherman)

sheep found in the New World are introductions derived from Old World stock.

While initial efforts at sheep domestication, as with goats, began more than 10,000 years ago, morphological changes that we associate with modern domesticated sheep are first documented at later Neolithic sites dating 7,000 to 8,000 years ago. These include shortening of the limb bones, hornlessness, and, based on a small statue from Iran, the wooly fleece, which does not occur in wild mouflon. By 3000 BC, sheep with wooly white fleeces were common, as indicated by artwork from Mesopotamia.

The wool fleece is an interesting example of early efforts at selective breeding. The main hair covering of wild sheep is not wool. It is guard hair produced in the predominant, primary hair follicles. The wool fiber in wild sheep is produced by secondary hair follicles, which are less represented in wild sheep. The secondary follicles produce a finer type of hair that grows out in colder weather to serve as insulation and then is shed during the warmer seasons. In producing wool fleeces, early breeders essentially eliminated primary hair follicle growth, replaced it with abundant secondary hair follicle growth, and eliminated the seasonal shedding. This is an impressive achievement for livestock keepers working several thousand years before Mendel explained the principles of genetic inheritance.

Today, domestic sheep, like goats, are widely distributed on the planet. There are many specific breeds, selected for wool pro-

duction, specific wool characteristics, and meat production. There are also milking breeds of sheep, used primarily for commercial cheese production, mainly in Europe and the Near East. Milking sheep were very much in the news in the United States in 2001, when some flocks in Vermont, imported from Europe, were seized and destroyed by the United States Department of Agriculture because of concerns that they might carry a transmissible spongiform encephalopathy related to bovine spongiform encephalopathy, or mad cow disease.

The sheep is a grazing ruminant, eating primarily grasses at ground level. Like the goat, it is commonly kept by herders, landless villagers, or small-scale farmers in developing countries, frequently in mixed flocks with goats. People living in Europe and North America may be surprised by some of the physical attributes of sheep breeds developed elsewhere in the world. Many local breeds have long straight hair rather than a wool fleece. There is also significant variation in the tail conformation. In Asia and Africa, many fat-tailed breeds of sheep are common and highly valued. The tail fat serves as a source of high energy food and tallow for lighting and other practical uses. The tail of a fat-tailed Mongolian sheep can weigh over 10 kg. Afghan herders still relish a soup made from sheep's tail fat, and you would no doubt be invited to partake of it should you visit an Afghan herding family in their traditional, felted, goat-hair tent.

Domestications in the Early Agricultural Phase

The animals that were domesticated in association with early agricultural development have been classified as crop destroyers, suggesting that these animals, notably the progenitors of swine and cattle, were recognized as a threat to cultivated fields-the wild boar because of its omnivorous scavenging behavior and the aurochs, or wild bull, because of its sheer size and aggressiveness. Both animals were valued by Neolithic people and their hunting ancestors as sources of meat but were simply too dangerous to have nearby once cultivation began in earnest. The response of early settled societies seems to have been to undertake the process of domestication of pigs and cattle while extirpating wild boar and aurochs from areas around cultivation. More details on the domestication process of pigs and cattle follow.

Pigs

The European wild boar, *Sus scrofa*, is the progenitor species of the domesticated pig. It is an even-toed ungulate in the family Suidae. It was widely distributed in prehistoric times, and early humans had considerable contact with the species throughout Europe, Asia, and northern Africa. The wild boar was a major prey species of Paleolithic hunters, sought primarily for meat but also for tusks and hide. At least 25 subspecies of *S. scrofa* existed, with variations based on localized climatic and environmental conditions. There is some evidence that a separate focus of domestication occurred in Asia from a different progenitor species, variously identified as *Sus vittalus* or *Sus cristatus*.

The modern, commercial domesticated pig is a thorough blend of breeding derived from both European and Asian stock, making its specific origins difficult to establish. So-called wild pigs in the New World are actually feral descendants of escaped domesticated swine introduced from Europe.

The earliest indications of efforts at domestication of the pig are from the Near East, where swine bones smaller than those of wild boars have been identified from excavations at Jericho dating to 7000 BC. Definitive evidence that farmers were breeding and keeping pigs in association with agricultural activity date from as early as 3500 BC at sites in Mesopotamia and by 2500 BC in ancient Egypt. It is generally accepted that domestication of the pig followed that of sheep and goats and required the settling of peoples in villages before full domestication could be achieved. This is because the domesticated pig is essentially a household animal and not a herd animal. Compared with small ruminants, it is relatively difficult to drive pigs or move them over great distances.

While the primary use of domesticated pigs is for meat, early efforts at domestication may have been driven by other uses. The pig is a single-stomached, omnivorous animal with a feeding behavior based on the scavenging of a wide variety of vegetable and animal foodstuffs. This scavenging behavior may have been used to good advantage by early agriculturists, to help in clearing fields of weeds and other debris in preparation for cultivation. There is evidence that the early Egyptians used pigs as living seed drills, walking them across irrigated or flooded fields prior to planting. The pointed depressions made by the pigs' feet in the soft soil were ideal for the subsequent sowing of seed.

As domestication took hold, two types of pigs and two types of pig-keeping emerged—forest pigs and sty pigs—both kept essentially as meat animals. Forest pigs were longer legged and rangier and were taken out for grazing under management of a swineherd. As pigs are difficult to herd, forest pigs were trained to return to the swineherd at the end of the day for penning in response to an audible signal such as a bell or horn, with grain as a reward. Sty pigs were short-legged and more compact. They were kept contained in farmyards or sties and fed a wide range of materials including kitchen wastes, crop residues, refuse, and whatever they could scavenge from the farmyard. The pig emerged as a favored source of meat for poor peasants wherever it was kept. The animal produced large litters of offspring, required little supervision, had impressive growth rates, and could be raised on a variety of feedstuffs not fit for direct human consumption.

It is of cultural interest that society has relegated the pig to the realm of food-producing animals, as it is an animal of relatively keen intelligence. Pigs are capable of being trained to work and also are reasonably suitable as companion animals. In the 11th century, in England, William the Conqueror banned the use of large dogs for hunting game to reduce the off-take by peasants from the New Forest. The more resourceful peasants trained pigs as retrievers and used them effectively for the next 400 or so years for hunting and retrieving. In contemporary France, muzzled pigs are still used to sniff out and dig truffles from the earth. In the past decade or so. there has been a growing practice in the United States of keeping Asian pot-bellied pigs as pets. This creates something of a conundrum for veterinarians who have been trained traditionally to see swine as food-producing animals and are now called upon to treat them as companion animals. The dichotomy raises deeper philosophical and anthropological questions about why some domesticated species are invited into the family room as friends and others only into the kitchen as food.

Cattle

How and why cattle came to be domesticated remains a curious puzzle. The progenitor of domesticated cattle, the aurochs, was actively hunted by prehistoric peoples in Europe and the Near East as an important source of meat, bone, horn, and hide. It was also well known as a fierce and dangerous adversary, standing over 7 feet tall at the shoulder, with a massive head and neck; sharp, curved horns; and an aggressive temperament as depicted in the cave paintings at Lascaux and elsewhere (Fig. 2-3). Nevertheless, Stone Age hunters pursued the aurochs with dogged determination and at great personal risk. Anthropologists have studied patterns and frequencies of bone fractures in skeletal remains of Neanderthal men and compared them with modern medical records of occupational injury. The occupation that exhibits a pattern of injury most similar to the Neanderthal pattern is the modern day rodeo competitor!

What motivated the early agriculturists to take on the formidable task of domesticating such an imposing beast? Cattle ultimately have turned out to be the most versatile of domestic animals, providing meat; milk; hides; manure for fertilizer, fuel, and building material; and draft power for transport and agricultural work. However, during the early stages of domestication, these potential uses, beyond those of meat and hides, were probably unrealized or unimagined, as soil enrichment through fertilization, the need for alternative fuels

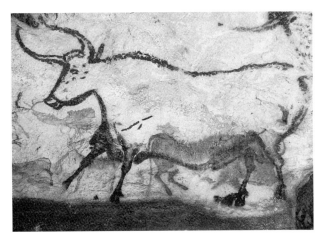

Figure 2-3. Aurochs depicted in a cave painting at Lascaux cave, France, dating from 15,000 to 10,000 BC.

because of deforestation, or the invention of the cart and plow were later developments. As the domestication of cattle is believed to have followed that of goats and sheep by about 1000 years, early agriculturists already had access to small ruminant animals that could provide meat, milk, fiber, and manure.

Some suggest that early domesticators tackled domestication of the aurochs for the sheer challenge and satisfaction of it, as an expression of collective courage, determination, ingenuity, and achievement. However, there were no doubt more practical reasons as well. As cultivation and settled societies increased in the Neolithic period, the aurochs grew increasingly problematic as a crop robber and destroyer, and some form of control was necessary. Killing wild aurochs that trespassed was one approach, but domestication also may have emerged as an alternative solution to allow exploitation of large ruminants while eliminating their threat to agriculture.

Religious or spiritual impulses rather than agricultural concerns may have been at the heart of cattle domestication. The magnificent power embodied in the aurochs had apparent spiritual connotations for humans from prehistoric times, and the bull and cow developed as potent mystical symbols in many early cultures.[8] The sacrifice of cattle evolved as an important religious rite, and it may be that some early cultures recognized that it would be much easier to provide tractable, domesticated cattle for sacrificial purposes than to have to capture wild and dangerous ones for each religious rite.

Whatever the reasons, people with experience in the domestication of sheep and goats were able to apply their experience to the domestication of cattle. Wild aurochs may have been lured to specific locations or natural enclosures such as ravines with water and/or salt to habituate them to humans. The smaller and more manageable of these individuals may have been subdued, captured, and penned. Newborns were likely snatched away and raised by people to encourage taming and human association. Early breeding was probably by the tethering of tamed cows for coupling with wild aurochs bulls. Whatever the specific details of the domestication process, it is likely that the full potential usefulness of cattle to evolving human society was not recognized until well after the domestication process had begun in earnest.

There are two main categories of domesticated cattle in the world, nonhumped and humped. The aurochs, *Bos primigenius*, is well established as the antecedent of *Bos taurus*, the domesticated species of nonhumped cattle that gives rise to the various breeds of dairy and beef cattle most familiar in temperate regions of the world, such as the Friesian and the Hereford. The humped, or Zebu-type, domesticated cattle breeds com-

mon in tropical regions, such as the Brahman, derive from *Bos indicus*. This species is believed to originate from a separate ancestral source, classified as *Bos namadicus*, an extinct form of aurochs of the Indian subcontinent. Some authorities consider this a distinct prehistoric species, while others consider it a clinal variant of the European aurochs. No ancestral wild cattle occurred in the New World, so all cattle in the Americas today are descendents of imported cattle.

The earliest evidence of full domestication of taurine cattle comes from the Catal Huyuk site in Turkey, dating to 4600 BC. Ceremonial benches adorned with cattle horns at Catal Huyuk lend force to the premise that early domestications had spiritual motivations. For Zebu-type cattle, the earliest evidence of full domestication comes from the Indus River valley cultures of Mohenjo Daro and Harrapa, where humped cattle are depicted on ceremonial seals dating back to 2500 BC. In Nile valley agriculture, the earliest indications of plows drawn by oxen occurred around 3000 BC (Fig. 2-4). Techniques for the castration of bulls must have preceded this date for oxen to be widely used by this time. Distinctive breeds of cattle were well established in ancient Egypt and Mesopotamia by 2500 BC. By about 500 BC, selective breeding of cattle was so well established that agriculturists in ancient Rome were recommending specific breeds for the effective plowing of different soil types found within the empire.

Cattle domestication has been, and continues to be, a powerful force in shaping human culture. Societies built around the practice of cattle keeping persist today. The Maasai in East Africa

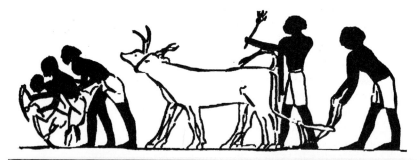

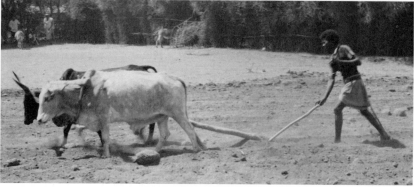

Figure 2-4. *Top,* An ox-drawn plow and hoeing in ancient Egypt from decorations on a tomb at Beni Hasan, Egypt, approximately 1900 BC. *Bottom,* A farmer in the Ethiopian Highlands in the 1990s using the same basic technology almost 4000 years later. (Top illustration courtesy of Egypt Exploration Society. Bottom photo by Dr. David M. Sherman.)

are perhaps the best known to outsiders, but there are many such tribes and societies, such as the Nuer and Dinka of Sudan and the Karamojong of Uganda, to name but a few. Virtually every aspect of daily life in these societies is structured around cattle. Cattle are revered in these tribes at the same time that they are exploited. Yet one does not need to travel to Africa to observe cattle culture. The development of the United States, particularly with regard to the opening and settlement of the western frontier, is largely a story of cattle keeping, and cattle culture is still an integral part of the American West.

Asian Water Buffalo

Cattle of *Bos* origin have become the predominant large domesticated ruminant in the world. They are, however, not the only such animal. Though not as widely distributed, there are several other large ruminants that have been successfully domesticated and integrated into human culture, primarily as sources of food and labor. All of these animals are derived from progenitors in the family Bovidae and the tribe Bovini, but most represent other genera in the family. The most important of these is the water buffalo.

The domesticated water buffalo, *Bubalus bubalus*, was most likely domesticated in India over 5000 years ago. It is believed to have been derived from the wild Asiatic water buffalo, or arni, *Bubalus arnee*, which still survives, though dwindling wild populations are now limited to the states of Assam and Madhya Pradesh in India and in Nepal. It is listed as an endangered species. The species was hunted in prehistoric times by early humans, so its behavior and nature were known, and the animal was valued for its meat and hides. While the original motivations for domestication are not known, the value of this animal for agricultural work evolved as a major asset.

The water buffalo is a wallower by nature and requires year-round access to wading water to thrive. As such, it is found most commonly in the humid tropics. This may explain why the use of the animal spread relatively quickly from the Indian subcontinent eastward and southward into Asia but rather slowly westward and northward into the Near East and Europe. Despite extensive trade between Rome and Indian civilizations, the water buffalo did not reach Italy until about AD 700, where its milk is currently used in the production of mozzarella cheese.

Currently, there are an estimated 165 million domesticated water buffalo worldwide. They are of major economic importance in most of tropical Asia, where they are used primarily as draft animals, particularly in the production of paddy rice. The animal is especially well adapted to work in muddy fields. They are also good milk producers and are the principal dairy animals in India and Pakistan, producing large volumes of milk of high butterfat content (Fig. 2-5). In modern times, the water buffalo has been successfully introduced to a number of other countries with climates and economies amenable to its well-being and usefulness, notably Egypt and Brazil. The water buffalo has never caught on as a valued domesticated animal in sub-Saharan Africa, nor has there ever been any successful ef-

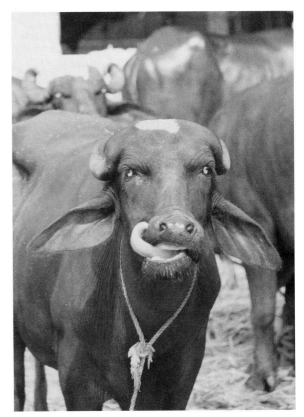

Figure 2-5.   This water buffalo is typical of the animals kept widely throughout India and Pakistan for milk production. Twelve of the 18 major breeds of water buffalo in the world are kept primarily for milk production. (Photo by Dr. David M. Sherman)

fort to domesticate the notably aggressive, indigenous African buffalo, *Syncerus caffer*.

Other Large Ruminants

Other large ruminant animals have been successfully domesticated for use in agriculture. They are generally less well known because they remain geographically and culturally localized. Their domestications probably occurred well after that of cattle, with foreknowledge of the experience of cattle domestication serving as a motivation and guide. These animals include the mithan, the domesticated banteng or Bali cattle, and the yak, all originating in Asia.

The mithan, *Bos frontalis*, is a domesticated bovid indigenous to northern India, Burma, and Bangladesh. Its origins are not completely clear. It is most likely derived from the wild gaur, *Bos gaurus*, but some authorities suspect it is a guar-cattle cross or a gaur-banteng cross. The wild gaur is still found in reduced populations from India south to Indonesia and Malaysia. The mithan, also known as the gayal, is very agile in mountain terrain. The animal is highly valued by local farmers for working fields on steep slopes. It is also a very good milk producer. A clue to the process of domestication persists to the present day. Many mithan remain only semidomesticated. They keep to the forests and only come to the villages when tempted by salt, and will eat salt out of people's hands. The mithan is important to the Nagas tribe of Assam as a sacrificial animal, again suggesting that the motivations for domestication, as with cattle, may have been grounded as much in religious ritual as in utilitarian need.

The domesticated banteng, or Bali cattle, resemble Jersey cows in stature and color. As the name implies, the animal is found in Indonesia on the island of Bali and other nearby islands. Bali cattle make up about 20% of Indonesia's total livestock population. Because of their appearance, the term "cattle" has been applied, but the animal is not derived from *Bos taurus* or *Bos indicus* progenitors, but rather the wild banteng, *Bos javanicus*, a large, strikingly attractive wild bovid of southeast Asia. The history of domestication is not well known. It is thought that indigenous people turned to domesticating the banteng after cattle introduced to Indonesia through trade failed to thrive under local conditions. The animals are used mainly for meat and also for light fieldwork (Fig. 2-6).

The domesticated yak, *Bos grunniens*, derives from the wild yak, *Bos mutus*. The range of the wild yak is limited to the high mountain areas of Asia, mainly within the boundaries of Tibet, Mongolia, and China. The wild yak is an animal of high elevations, found usually between 6,000 and 20,000 feet. It is well adapted to the rigors of steep terrain, severe cold, and snow. The animal is associated more with extensive grazing than with settled agriculture. There is little known about the process of domestication, which is thought to have occurred between 1000 and 2000 BC. The mountain people who live and work with yaks depend on them for a wide variety of services. Though infrequently used for meat, the yak is exploited widely for its milk and its hair, which is felted into tents. It is used both for riding and as a pack animal. Yaks are also frequently crossed with cattle. These yakow crosses are better adapted to lower elevations and have a somewhat wider distribution in Asia, found as far west as Afghanistan and Pakistan. They are used primarily as beasts of burden and for fieldwork.

Later Domestications Linked to Animal Traction

As agricultural societies became well established and grew more socially complex, different needs emerged that came to be met by additional species of domesticated animals. The expansion of agricultural activity brought new croplands into production that were increasingly distant from town centers and centralized grain storage facilities. This posed new challenges for transport of harvests. Development of trade between distant settlements also increased, requiring new methods for transporting goods. As communities became wealthier and more productive they grew increasingly subject to attack and plunder, calling for new strategies and weapons for defense and retribution. Hence, a number of wild species familiar to hunters and early agriculturists were enlisted into the domestication process, ultimately to serve as beasts of burden or participants in conflict. These included the horse, donkey, mule, camel, llama, and elephant, discussed in the following sections.

Horses

Millions of years before the advent of hominids, horselike species originated in North America, Their descendents migrated across the land bridge, at the present Bering Sea, into Asia and subsequently died out in North America. The wild horse, *Equus ferus*, was a creature highly adapted to temperate grassland habitat. As a denizen of open grassland with relatively little access to cover, the ancient horse evolved with speed and power as its main means of escape and survival from predators. Wild horses flourished on the steppes and grasslands of Asia and Europe up to the time of the last Ice Age about 10,000 years ago.

In the Paleolithic era, the wild horse was a major prey species of early humans, hunted essentially for meat, but with the hides and tail hair also used. The Cro-Magnon cave paintings of France and Spain show numerous horses, whose appearance is strikingly similar to that of the endangered wild Przewalski's horse of Asia, *Equus ferus przewalskii*, which persists into modern times, though in precariously low numbers (Fig. 2-7).

The interval between the Paleolithic and Neolithic eras was a difficult time for wild horses. The warming period associated with the regression of the glaciers also promoted the conversion of grassland to forest in much of Europe and Asia. As other prey species moved northward or died off because of climatic change, there likely was increased hunting pressure on herds of horses. As settled agriculture took hold in earnest, additional grasslands became unavailable to horses for grazing. Some scholars of

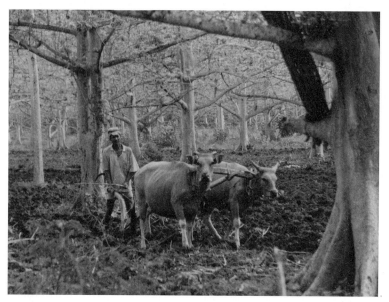

Figure 2-6.   A farmer in Bali, Indonesia, plowing a field with Bali cattle, derived from the wild banteng. The field is in a grove of kapok trees, the seed of which is used for filling in life preservers, so this piece of land, in a densely populated nation, yields multiple outputs. (Photo by Dr. David M. Sherman)

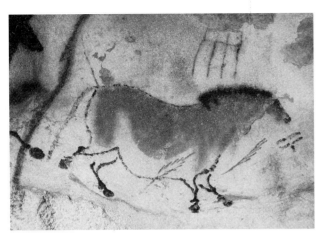

Figure 2-7. Cave painting of a so-called Chinese horse from the Lascaux cave, France. Note the short bristly mane, stocky physique, and relatively short legs similar to those of the surviving wild Przewalski's horse. Efforts to reestablish wild herds of Przewalski's horses in Mongolia are currently under way.

animal domestication believe that the horse was in fact in danger of extinction at this time, and it was only the intervention of humans, intent on domesticating the horse for their own purposes, that saved it from oblivion.

The history and origins of the domesticated horse, *Equus caballus*, are difficult to determine from the archeological record, in part because the bony differences between wild and domesticated horses are not easily distinguishable. The progenitor species is not clearly established. It is most likely an extinct European wild horse, possibly the Tarpan, classified as *Equus ferus gmelini*. Wild progenitor species were believed to have short, bristly manes, as seen in the surviving Przewalskii horse. Domesticated horses, through artificial selection, possess long, flowing manes. Otherwise, the horse, in general, is the domestic animal least physically modified by artificial selection relative to its wild ancestors.

Early efforts to control the horse were most probably related to its identification by hunters as a source of food. Trapping and luring horses into natural enclosures with subsequent killing for meat was the likely first step in the domestication process. Subsequent developments in the process may have been delayed until much later, after the domestication of cattle. The use of oxen as beasts of burden is thought to have served as a model for the use of horses as pack animals, with goods loaded on their backs. This was followed by the use of the bridle and harness for pulling loads, first by sledge and then by wheeled cart. The horse was also used, as were oxen, for plowing. The full domestication of horses is considered to have been achieved by about 4000 BC. It is believed to have centered primarily in the region surrounding the northern shore of the Black Sea, in present day Ukraine, radiating eastward into Asia and westward into Europe through trade.

The use of the two-wheeled, horse-drawn chariot for transportation and warfare was a pivotal event in the development of human civilization. The innovation spread steadily throughout various ancient cultures of Europe and Asia, mainly in the period between 2500 and 1000 BC. Horses drawing a war chariot are shown in Egyptian art by the 16th century BC. The use of the chariot for transportation was essentially restricted to the nobility in all of the cultures that adopted it. It is believed that this association of horses and chariots with the ruling class lent a cultural connotation of nobility to the horse itself, and this reverent attitude may have led to the gradual transition away from the use of the horse as a source of meat for human consumption.

The historical record suggests that the widespread use of the horse to carry a rider directly on its back is a later development in the domestication process, occurring after the use of horses to pull chariots. This innovation was nothing short of revolutionary for human societies of the time, with profound effects on the speed of transport and communication and for the conduct of warfare. The use of mounted cavalry added a savagery and strategic advantage to warfare that was previously unimaginable. The military might of mounted riders was even further enhanced by the invention of the stirrup, first described in China in writings dated AD 477. Stirrups provided excellent stability and allowed the rider to stand and hurl projectile weapons while moving, offering even greater superiority in battle. For centuries, the world essentially belonged to the warrior on horseback. From the time that the nomadic Huns swept down from the steppes of Asia to invade Europe in AD 360 to the time that the Mongols did the same in the 13th century, the peace and security of settled agriculturists in Europe and Asia were at the mercy of mounted cavalry.

The role of the horse in human society was greatly transformed in the 20th century. Its use as a draft animal was virtually eliminated in the developed world by the invention of the internal combustion engine. Police and military cavalry are maintained largely as ceremonial units. Horsemeat is eaten in relatively few countries, notably France and Belgium, though recent concerns about the wholesomeness of beef, related to mad cow disease in Europe in 2001, spurred a resurgence of horsemeat consumption. Nevertheless, the main functions of horses today, at least in western society, are as companions, performers, and athletes. If it is in fact true that the horse was headed for extinction at the time of the last Ice Age, then it would seem that the process of domestication has been, on balance, very good to the horse.

Asses and Mules

Ass and *donkey* are synonyms for the same domesticated animal, *Equus asinus*. A third synonym, *burro*, is simply the Spanish word for donkey. The donkey is the only major livestock species that has its origins in Africa. The progenitor species is identified as the African wild ass, *Equus africanus*, a hardy equid adapted to arid and semiarid environments. Three races of this wild ass—the Algerian, the Nubian, and the Somali—were known to exist, but only the Somali wild ass survives to the present, and its status is endangered. Taken together, the original range of the three races was from present-day Morocco in the east, across north Africa, and up into the Arabian peninsula.

There has been much debate about the role of the Asian wild ass, E. hemionus, as a progenitor in the development of the domesticated donkey. Also known as the onager, or hemione, the Asian ass ranged from modern day Syria eastward to Mongolia. While there are pictorial representations on archeological artifacts that suggest early domestication of the onager, strong evidence argues against the Asian ass as a progenitor of the modern donkey; an onager bred to a domesticated donkey produces sterile offspring, while the mating of an African wild ass to a domesticated donkey produces fertile offspring.

The first domestications of the donkey likely took place in the Nile valley or Libya, between 4000 and 3000 BC. Donkeys are frequently depicted in Egyptian art, starting about 2500 BC, mainly as beasts of burden. As the wild ass was a hunted species, the earliest motivations for domestication of the African wild ass was likely as a source of meat. However, the value of the donkey as a draft animal, particularly in arid regions, became increasingly evident. The donkey was hardy and resilient. It could survive well on poor-quality forage and could go longer without water than horses or oxen. It was sure footed on rough terrain and mingled easily with other forms of livestock. As the horse became increasingly associated with the nobility and grew more important in warfare, the demand for horses outstripped supply. The donkey increasingly filled the niche for agricultural power and commercial transport in early civilizations. It is as the "poor man's horse" that the donkey continues to function in much of Africa, Asia, and Latin America today—a puller of carts and carrier of loads.

The mule is a domesticated hybrid animal, a cross between a male donkey (jackass) and a female horse (mare), which was developed primarily as a beast of burden. The offspring of this mating, the mule itself, is infertile. The opposite cross, a female donkey (jenny) and a male horse (stallion) also produces an infertile offspring, known as a hinny. The hinny is less popular and less frequently used than the mule. One reason may be that it was historically easier to maintain the more tractable male donkey for breeding than the stallion. Mules are truly excellent draft animals. They are larger than donkeys and have more stamina and endurance. They can carry heavier loads than the donkey and most types of horse. If it were not for their legendary stubbornness and their infertility, they would have no doubt become even more popular in ancient and modern times.

As it was, the mule represents an important development in the domestication process. It served developing civilizations well as a plow animal, cart puller, and beast of burden, the latter especially well in difficult mountainous terrain. The origins of equid hybrid breeding are not well known. Hinnies are pictured pulling a two-wheeled cart in Egyptian tomb paintings dated 1400 BC, and mules are represented in art from Mesopotamian cultures, dating to the first millennium BC. The use of the mule was widespread in the daily civilian and military life of ancient Rome, and detailed accounts of husbandry and breeding techniques were recorded by the agriculturist Columella in the 1st century AD. The use of the mule persists up to modern times. Within our own century, the mule was a mainstay of agricultural work in the United States, depended on by poor farmers and sharecroppers before the widespread availability of tractors. Though less common today, there are still specialized niches for the mule. In the 1980s, in addition to the well-publicized gift of Stinger missiles that they provided, the United States also supplied mules to the Afghan mujahadeen to help maintain supply lines in the rugged mountainous terrain of northern Afghanistan in the struggle against Soviet occupation.

Camels

The early history of domesticated camels and their origins are not well known. There are two types of domesticated camel in the Old World, the one-humped camel, or dromedary, and the two-humped camel, or Bactrian. To underscore the mystery surrounding the camel's origins, it is not even fully clear if these camels are two distinct species or different races of the same progenitor species. The fetus of the one-humped camel has two humps, but one is reabsorbed prior to parturition. Both animals have the same chromosome number, $2N = 70$, and they readily interbreed, producing fertile females but sterile males. At any rate, they are at present taxonomically named as separate species, the one-humped dromedary, Camelus dromedarius, and the two-humped Bactrian, Camelus bactrianus.

Camels are even-toed ungulates (Artiodactyla) in the family Camelidae. Camels ruminate, in that they regurgitate and chew their cud, but their forestomach configuration differs from that of the true ruminants such as the bovine. Their dental structure differs from that of the true ruminants as well, with the retention of some upper incisors and canines and anterior placement of tusklike first premolar teeth. On the feet they have a broad cutaneous pad rather than a hoof. Taxonomists place the camels intermediate between ruminants and swine. Early prehistoric camelids the size of rabbits originated in North America millions of years ago but had long since become extinct on that continent prior to the arrival of humans. Evolutionary descendents of these early camelids crossed to Asia to become the wild precursors of the modern domesticated camels and also migrated southward to become the progenitors of the South American camelids known today—the wild guanaco and vicuna and the domesticated alpaca and llama.

Today there are no wild one-humped camels, though their extirpation is fairly recent, occurring only about 2000 years ago. The natural range of these wild camels was primarily the Arabian peninsula, reflecting their remarkable adaptation for the harsh, arid desert environment. It is from these wild camels in Arabia that domestication of the dromedary likely began 3000 to 4000 years ago. This represents a fairly late start relative to the other large domesticated mammals and suggests that camel domestication did not have its origins in agriculture. In fact, the reverse may be true.

It may have been the decline of agriculture in the Near East that spurred interest in the camel. As a domesticated farm animal, the camel did not compare favorably with the more readily available ox or donkey. While undeniably strong, the camel is an obstreperous animal that is difficult to train and to maintain in confinement. Males become aggressive and dangerous during the rutting season. Female camels only give birth every 2 years, and the young have to reach 4 to 5 years of age before they can effectively be put to work. Assuming that farmers have always been practical people, only the unusual farmer would have kept a camel if an ox or donkey could be had for agricultural work.

There is good evidence that agricultural development in the Near East experienced a reversal during the late Neolithic era. As human populations expanded, overpopulation became a problem in settled areas. Crop cultivation extended increasingly into marginal lands that required extensive irrigation. In some places, irrigation led to salinization and decreased productivity, resulting in the annexation of even more marginally productive lands for cultivation. At the same time, the herding of sheep and goats had become a major human activity in the region, leading to overgrazing and land degradation. The impact of all of these human activities on agricultural productivity may have been exacerbated further by a climatic change that brought increased temperatures and decreased rainfall to the Near East between 5000 and 3000 BC.

It is in this context that domestication of the camel likely began in earnest. The camel had long been known as an animal hunted for meat. Herders, pushed increasingly to marginal grazing areas, may have recognized the ability of the camel to flourish on grazing lands that would not support sheep and only barely keep goats alive. Thus, integration of the camel into grazing herds allowed humans to pursue food production activities in arid areas formerly considered uninhabitable. Once the camel had become tractable as a grazing animal, its potential as a beast of burden was easily recognized, and as the "ship of the desert," the camel became critically important in the development of human civilization, facilitating trade and communication between scattered ancient civilizations in the Near East and Asia separated by expanses of desert, semidesert, and difficult terrain. The camel was adopted by many cultures and steadily was disseminated from Arabia into the Nile valley and across North Africa and to South and Central Asia. It opened up vast areas of territory that would have been totally unusable to human beings without the aid of the camel.

The camel also found its uses in human conflict. The Bedouin nomads used the camel to great advantage to make surprise mounted raids into settled communities of Mesopotamia and ancient Palestine for general plunder and then return swiftly into the desert where their pursuers in horse-drawn chariots could not follow them. Some early military strategists also used the camel as an element of surprise against horse cavalry. Horses unfamiliar with camels are easily frightened by the smell and appearance of camels and will bolt at the sight of them. A detailed account survives of this tactic being used to great effect in 546 BC at the battle of Sardis.

Though their military role is diminished, camels are still in wide use today in arid regions of the developing world as draft animals and for agricultural work such as carrying the belongings of desert nomads, pulling heavy wagons laden with bricks or timber, plowing fields, threshing grain, and drawing water from wells. They are also used for meat, milk, hides, and hair. Camel hair is a highly valued fiber in the textile industry. Camel racing has become an important sport in the Arab world, and the breeding, care, management, and training of camels has become a high-profile, specialized area frequently requiring sophisticated veterinary expertise.

Very little is known about the domestication of the Bactrian camel. The wild two-humped camel ranged from the highlands of central Asia eastward to Mongolia. The status of the wild progenitor today is unclear. There are reports of a small wild herd existing in Mongolia, but it is not known if these are truly wild or are feral descendants of escaped, domesticated Bactrian camels. The Bactrian is hardier than the dromedary and more tolerant of cooler climates. Its use as a draft animal to open trade across the vast expanses of Asia along the Silk Route is legendary, and it is still used today in parts of China, Mongolia, and the Central Asian Republics primarily as a beast of burden.

Llama and Alpaca

The family Camelidae is well represented in the New World with both wild and domesticated species dwelling in the mountainous regions along the western edge of South America. The wild camelids of the area are the guanaco, *Lama guanicoe,* and the vicuna, *Vicugna vicugna.* Both are found in Bolivia, Chile, Peru, and Argentina and are classified as endangered species. The domesticated species are the llama, *Lama glama,* and the alpaca, *Lama pacos.* These camelids represent the only major mammalian domestications to have originated in South America, apart from the guinea pig.

It is well established that the domesticated llama is derived from the guanaco. The origins of the alpaca are less clear. Traditionally, the alpaca also was considered to have derived from the guanaco. However, more recent, detailed analysis of mitochondrial and microsatellite DNA of the various wild and domesticated South American camelids suggests that the alpaca is derived from the vicuna or from cross-breeds of vicuna and guanaco.

The domestication of llamas is believed to have been fully achieved in Peru 3000 to 4000 years ago. As with other species, the domestication process probably occurred in stages before full domestication was realized. The guanaco was a hunted animal, and it is speculated that guanacos were driven into natural enclosures, with groups kept in captivity as they were progressively culled for meat. This may have led to confinement of tamed individuals with breeding to wild mates and finally controlled mating and full domestication. Some contemporary insights into the early stages of domestication are available with regard to the vicuna as an example. Today, as has been done for ages, wild vicuna are periodically herded by mountain peoples into enclosures where they are shorn of their valuable fleece and then released. Though the vicuna is a territorial animal not conducive to domestication, the practice of capture and release was a likely phase in the domestication process of the more tractable guanaco.

The domesticated llama has proven to be extremely valuable as a beast of burden in mountainous terrain, and to this day, its primary use is as a pack animal, carrying loads of 80 to 100 pounds on steep slopes. The alpaca is used primarily for its fiber in textile making and also for meat. Both the llama and alpaca have become popular as pets, pack animals, and fiber producers for hand spinning in the United States over the past 20 years. However, the general impact of the New World camelids on human civilization has been limited relative to the Old World camelids. This is largely a function of geography. The llama and alpaca are indigenous to a region that is hemmed in between the Amazon rainforest to the east and the Pacific Ocean to the west, while movement north and south is constrained by the treacherous Andes mountains. The opportunities for geographical and cultural dissemination that existed for the dromedary and Bactrian camel in Asia simply did not exist for the llama and alpaca.

Elephants

Elephants have been used by human society for entertainment, war, and work. Their heyday in the military context was in the 3rd and 4th centuries BC. Ptolemy III in Egypt, Alexander the Great in Greece, and Hannibal of Carthage are all famous military and political leaders of the time who valued the elephant as a weapon of war. Metaphorically, elephants were the B1 bomber of their day. They were impressive, costly, and touted to provide great strategic advantage through the element of surprise, In practice, however, they were not quite as effective or useful as their advocates claimed. While there are a number of well-documented battles from the period in which the elephant played a decisive role in victory, there are a comparable number of accounts in which mounted elephants were ineffectual or actually deleterious to the outcome of the battle, turning around in response to archery attacks and trampling their own ranks of infantrymen bringing up the rear.

The elephants trained for use in warfare during this era were both the Indian elephant, *Elephas maximus*, and the African elephant, *Loxodonta africana*, the two species of elephants that survive in the wild today. In our own times, it is often presumed that the larger African elephant of the African savanna is not trainable, as virtually all circus elephants and the working elephants of Asia are the smaller Indian elephants. The historical record suggests that a smaller race of the African elephant, the African forest elephant formerly had a wide distribution in northern Africa, and it was this smaller African elephant that was trained for use in warfare as well as for use in the Roman circuses. The forest elephant, *Loxodonta africana cyclotis*, still persists today in a much reduced range, mostly in the Congo and western Uganda. The elimination of this elephant from its northern range is attributed to the demands of the Romans who took live elephants for their circuses but also exploited the elephant for its ivory. At any rate, the African elephant is indeed trainable. As recently as the early 1900s, African forest elephants in the Congo were trained for logging work, but the practice died out.

Elephants are not really domesticated animals by the strictest definition, but rather are trained, wild animals, because captive breeding is not carried out in populations of working elephants. There are simply too many obstacles to make it worthwhile for the exploiter of elephant labor to breed the animal in captivity. The breeding bull is an extremely dangerous and unpredictable animal. Even if the bull were manageable, there are management problems with the cow as well. The female elephant does not reach sexual maturity until her teens, produces a single calf only once every 3 or 4 years, and keeps the calf by her side for 5 years, interfering with work; the calves themselves cannot be put to work until age 14. It is less problematic for the user of elephants to capture young adults in the wild and train them for work. Though training is an arduous and difficult process for both the elephant and the trainer, the effort is justified by the longevity of the elephant. Once trained, their working life may span decades. Breeding, when it occurs, is carried out by allowing the captive cow to return to the wild for mating with wild bulls. She is then enticed back to captivity by a mahout who specializes in this task.

Contemporary use of the Indian elephant persists in Asia, mainly in India, Sri Lanka, and the forested nations of the southeast Asian peninsula. Uses include ceremonial and ritual activities and labor. In New Delhi, the bejeweled and silk-draped elephant is a standard feature at the poshest weddings, frequently seen in the parking lots of the five-star hotels on the day of the wedding celebration. Elephant rides are also a popular tourist activity. In the forests and timber plantations, elephants are used for land clearing and to carry, load, and unload logs for the timber industry, but these activities are becoming increasingly mechanized, and the role of the elephant is diminishing, as are the forests themselves (Fig. 2-8). In Thailand, opportunities for working elephants and their keepers have dramatically diminished, and many elephant keepers have, out of desperation, taken their elephants to Bangkok to earn a few baht as street corner performers. The number of working elephants in the country is down to about 2,000, compared with about 11,000 in the mid 1960s.

Both the wild Indian elephant and the wild African elephant are considered endangered species. The greatest threats to them, particularly the African elephant, have been the ivory trade and the loss of habitat. In recent years, the ivory trade has been in the public eye, and protective legislation has eased this pressure somewhat. However, the pressure on habitat from encroachment by expanding human activity goes on essentially unabated.

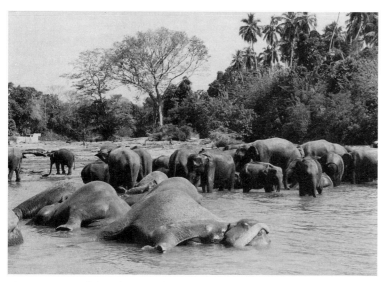

Figure 2–8.   Adult and young elephants during bathing time at the Pinnawala elephant orphanage in Sri Lanka. The expansion of agricultural development into traditional elephant habitat has brought elephants and farmers into conflict. The killing of elephants has led to increased numbers of elephant orphans, many of which are cared for at this orphanage. (Photo by Dr. David M. Sherman)

Domestication of Pest-Destroying Mammals

Once societies became settled, established households and began to store grains, these activities invited pests in the form of rodents, snakes, and insects. The domestication of several animals is closely intertwined with the need to control such pests. These animals include the ferret, the mongoose, and the cat.

Ferret and Mongoose

The origins of domestication of the ferret are not well known. Some authorities believe it occurred in Europe about 500 BC, while others cite evidence to suggest it began 1000 years earlier. Ferret nomenclature is a bit confusing. The progenitor species is considered to be the European ferret, or European polecat, *Mustela putorius*, a member of the weasel family, Mustelidae. The domesticated form may be referred to as the *stoat, ferret, polecat,* or *fitch ferret.* This is a true domesticated animal in that control of breeding is under human supervision. As late as the 5th century BC, it was the ferret, and not the cat, that was feared by the mouse, at least according to Greek fables of the time. While reasonably effective in controlling household pests, ferrets found particular use in ancient times for the control of rabbits, which periodically threatened crops. The ferret was sometimes muzzled and placed in rabbit warrens to drive the rabbits out for capture. There has been a surge of popularity in keeping domesticated ferrets as pets in the United States in recent years, accompanied by concerns in the public health community over the issues of infant bites and rabies control.

The mongoose, also referred to as the *ichneumon,* is not a true domesticate, in that breeding is left to the animals themselves.

Mongooses are basically tamed wild animals that enter into commensal relationships with human beings. They will move freely in and out of homes and interact with human beings and are demonstrably affectionate. Yet they remain wild animals, undifferentiable from their free-living kin. There are 32 different species of mongoose in the family Viverridae, which also includes civets and genets. Throughout much of Asia and Africa, people open their homes to the mongoose, sometimes as a diversion, but mainly to control rodents and snakes. The first people to do so in any consistent manner were probably the Egyptians, and the Egyptian mongoose was included in the pantheon of animals held sacred by this ancient civilization. The mongoose is an excellent snake hunter and is indelibly linked with the cobra in popular culture, thanks to Rudyard Kipling's famous tale of the mongoose Rikki Tikki Tavi. The traveler to India and Pakistan is constantly reminded of this story. Virtually every tourist shop has a shelf full of dusty, crudely wrought, taxidermic specimens of a cobra and mongoose perpetually entwined in a frozen tableau of fierce combat, their glass eyes pleading for release.

Cats

The domestic cat, *Felis catus,* is derived from the wild cat, *Felis sylvestris,* a small, felid carnivore of Europe and Asia with a striped tabby pelage. The animal shows some clinal variation in body size, being shorter and stockier in northern climates and longer legged and rangier in warmer southern regions. This accounts for some of the variation in body size and shape for domestic cats, which, apart from some highly selected breeds, are remarkably unchanged from their wild ancestors.

The domestication of the cat is a relatively late development in human society. The earliest records come from ancient Egypt about 2500 BC, but cats begin to figure prominently in depictions of everyday life much later, during the New Kingdom, after 1600 BC. Cats fared very well in Egyptian culture. They were kept in households but were also considered sacred to the goddess Bast, and killing them was forbidden. Cats that died were taken to the city of Bubastis for mummification and burial in sacred sites. The number of cats treated in this way is staggering. In the early 20th century, 19 tons of cat mummies were excavated in Egypt by entrepreneurial opportunists, shipped to Britain, ground up, and used for fertilizer! One cat skull from this shipment sits in the British Museum as mute testimony to this feline journey from the sacred to the profane.[3]

Historically, few cultures celebrated the cat with the enthusiasm and respect of the Egyptians. As Christian doctrine evolved and Christianity spread through Europe, the cat came to be a reviled creature. It was believed to be an agent of the devil, and cats were mercilessly persecuted and abused for centuries. As late as the 17th century, witches were identified and brought to trial on the basis of their association with the keeping of cats, which were labeled familiars. Familiars were regarded as demonic animal companions that carried out the evil intentions of the witch. Only in recent times in western society has the cat regained favorable status as a beloved pet. If no longer deified, cats at least are treated royally in many households.

The cat is unusual as a domesticated animal for two reasons. First, the wild cat is a strongly territorial animal, solitary in its behavior. This is in contrast to most other domesticated animals, which move in herds or packs, are nonterritorial, and maintain social dominance hierarchies. The domesticated cat was not a workable concept for mobile societies. Once people settled, however, the domestic cat could be accommodated, for it is willing to adopt the household as its territory and share control, albeit begrudgingly at times, with the human head of household. Secondly, at the time of domestication, the cat offered no clear utilitarian advantage to its domesticators. While the cat has pest control ability, it is, in fact, less efficient in this line of work than the mongoose or the ferret, which were also domesticated for this purpose. It is the cat's undeniable attraction as a companion animal, appreciated by the Egyptians almost 5000 years ago and rediscovered in our own culture, that has ensured its comfortable place in human society.

Notable Nonmammalian Domestications

Hunter-gatherers identified a wide range of potential foods of animal origin that extended beyond mammals. Birds' nests were robbed of eggs, fish were pulled by hand from shrinking ponds during hot periods, and beehives were looted for honey. However, domestication of nonmammalian species did not develop in earnest until the Neolithic period, as the nomadic lifestyle was not compatible with tending bird flocks, fish ponds, or beehives. These developments required the sedentary lifestyle that was born of land cultivation and the conversion from food procurement to food production. A brief history of the domestication of some significant nonmammalian species follows.

Birds

Domesticated chickens, turkeys, ducks, and geese are well known to us in our own age as poultry, i.e., domesticated land and water fowl raised primarily for meat and eggs. With over 8000 species of birds on the planet, why were these four the birds chosen for domestication? One part of the answer, no doubt, is their suitable size—recognized to this day as appropriate for a family meal, especially in places where there is no access to refrigeration. More important, perhaps, is their nesting behavior. All of these birds are ground nesters, which made their eggs and chicks relatively easy to locate and obtain for even the most casually observant hunter-gatherers. Given the fact that a newborn hatchling will imprint upon and follow the first parental figure it observes, it is not difficult to imagine how easily the progenitor species of these land and waterfowl came into association with human beings and subsequently became domesticated. A brief history of each domestication follows.

Chickens The domestic chicken, *Gallus domesticus*, has its origins in Asia. The progenitor species is the red jungle fowl, *Gallus gallus*, which is distributed widely across the continent. Recent evidence suggests that domestication was under way in Vietnam over 10,000 years ago. Until this discovery, conventional wisdom held that the chicken was domesticated in India by about 2000 BC, associated with the Indus valley civilizations. Given the ease with which wildfowl could be captured and confined, multiple sites and times for domestication are likely. The early motivation, at least in India, may have been for spiritual and entertainment purposes more than for food, since reading the entrails or bones of chickens was an accepted form of divination, and there is evidence that cockfighting was practiced in the Indus valley cultures.

From India, the chicken was introduced through trade and conflict into Persia, the Near East, and Greece, sometime between 800 and 700 BC. The first evidence of chickens in ancient Egypt came from the tomb of King Tutankhamen, dating their arrival from the East sometime before 1350 BC. The chicken reached Rome after 500 BC, and poultry breeding was a well-documented science there by the 1st century BC. The chicken probably did not enter the New World until the 16th century, when it was introduced by European explorers and conquerors.

Today, most of the eggs and chicken meat produced in the industrialized world comes from intensively reared birds maintained in highly mechanized and carefully managed confinement units. This intensive approach to production has been spreading rapidly in recent years to developing nations in Africa, Asia, and Latin America, to meet growing demands for animal protein as economies expand. Nevertheless, the free-ranging chicken remains a ubiquitous feature of the rural village landscape wherever people settle to work the land. Chickens are excellent scavengers and can provide meat, eggs, feathers, and cash income to small farmers and villagers who need to expend very little to sustain them. Roosters also continue to provide traditional entertainment in the form of cockfighting, a blood sport still practiced in many countries throughout the world, including the United States.[1]

Turkeys The turkey is the only animal originally domesticated in the New World that has achieved a worldwide distribution of economic importance. There are two indigenous turkey species in the New World, the wild turkey, *Meleagris gallopavo*, whose original range was North America, and the ocellated turkey, *Meleagris ocellata*, more restricted to southern Mexico and Central America. *M. gallopavo* served as the progenitor of the domesticated bird. The history of domestication is not well documented. It is believed that indigenous people in what is now Mexico and the southern United States kept turkeys, at least captive turkeys, before the development of the great Aztec civilization. The turkey was well domesticated by the time Cortez reached Mexico and had been brought back to Europe by 1524.

How the turkey got its English name is unclear. At the time it was introduced into England, there was considerable trade going on with Turkey, and the peafowl had been introduced around the same time. The birds, both new to the populace, may have been confused in people's minds. Turkeys now have a worldwide distribution and, like chickens, are raised both under free-ranging traditional systems as well as intensively managed systems. Artificial selection has produced a bird quite different phenotypically from its wild ancestor. The selection for increased breast meat has created a conformation in the modern commercial turkey that interferes with natural breeding, and these birds must be propagated by artificial insemination.

Other Gallinaceous Birds The turkey and the chicken are classified as gallinaceous birds—large land-dwelling birds that nest on the ground. Other members of this group have also been used by humans, including peafowl, guinea fowl, partridge, quail, and pheasant. These birds, though bred in captivity, have not been subjected to much artificial selection, so their status as true domesticates is nebulous. The reason they have not been manipulated is that their attraction to human society is embodied in their wild characteristics. For example, the extraordinary beauty of the tail feathers of the male Indian peafowl, *Pavo cristatus*, cannot be improved upon. The peafowl is indigenous to the Indian subcontinent, and traders early on realized that the peacock made an excellent gift of introduction when trying to establish new markets in the Near East and Europe, where the showy birds appealed to the nobility as status symbols and objects of splendor. They continue to serve today as living lawn ornaments whose aesthetic appeal is somewhat undermined by their loud, squawking call.

The guinea fowl, *Numidia meleagris,* is indigenous to Africa and was introduced to ancient Greece in the 5th century through trade with Carthage. Curiously it did not persist and was reintroduced to Europe 1000 years later by the Portuguese, who rediscovered the bird in their explorations of West Africa. The bird is still common in the wild state in Africa and is often seen scurrying into the brush along the roadside to hide from approaching cars. The bird has an attractive spotted plumage and, like the peacock, is sometimes raised in captivity and kept as an ornamental bird. Guinea fowl have been consumed as food throughout history, but the bird does not lend itself to mass production as it does not adapt well to confinement.

Partridge, quail, and pheasants, as well as turkeys, are raised in captivity primarily for release into the wild as game birds for hunting. Again, these birds are not modified by artificial selection, as it is their "wildness" that is the attraction to hunters. One particular partridge, the Chukar, *Alectoris chukar,* of south Asia is prized as a fighting bird. It is a common sight in western Pakistan to see turbaned men passing by on bicycles with a characteristically domed and cloth-covered structure fastened securely to the back fender. This is the wooden Chukar cage, and the man and the bird are on their way to the fighting competitions. The Chukar has been introduced into North America as a game bird and is found in rocky arid regions of the western states, a habitat similar to their natural habitat in Asia. The ring-necked pheasant that is now common in the woods and farmlands of the northern United States is also an introduced

species from Asia, successfully established in the United States in the late 19th century.

Ducks Most varieties of domesticated ducks have been derived from the well-known and widely distributed Mallard duck, *Anas platyrhynchos.* The main center of domestication is considered to have been China, and indeed, to this day, duck remains a more popular form of poultry in the far East than in the western world. The white Peking duck is the variety most often raised commercially in the United States for meat production. One specific duck domestication is known to have occurred separately in the New World, that of the Muscovy duck, *Cairina moschata,* whose natural range is from Mexico south to Uruguay. Interestingly, this duck is a tree nester, and the circumstances under which its domestication occurred are not well known. Nevertheless, it is a common farmyard bird in Latin America and is also seen in parks in the United States. The domestic form has variable colors from dark purple to black and white to all white, and the male has a red fleshy mask around the eyes.

Geese and Swans Geese have been kept by humans since Neolithic times, first as captives, then as domesticates. There are likely more than one progenitor species, but the principal one is considered to be the greylag goose, *Anser anser,* a wild northern Eurasian species and subject of intensive behavioral studies by the famed ethologist Konrad Lorenz.[5] Goose domestication most likely occurred independently at several locations, with evidence coming from China, ancient Egypt, and later, Greece. The Romans valued the goose primarily for its feathers for use in arrow making. In our own time, the goose feather, in the form of down, has gained popularity as a natural insulating material for outerwear in cold climates. The goose is not a major poultry type, its use as a meat bird is often restricted to holiday use, though the specialty market for goose liver pate persists. The goose is highly alert. Its keen hearing, loud honking, and aggressive territorial attitude made it an excellent home security system long before the invention of electricity, and it is still in use in rural areas today.

The domestic swan is the aquatic equivalent of the terrestrial peafowl, i.e., a bird prized for its beauty above all else. The mute swan of Europe, *Cygnus olor,* is the species that has been domesticated or at least bred in captivity. As with the peafowl, there has been little attempt to alter the original form of the bird through artificial selection. After all, who could improve on the swan?

Other Birds Birds, even more than mammals, have provided the most diverse services to human society. Some of the traditional uses of birds have been rendered obsolete by technological advancement, but their place in the history of the human-animal relationship deserves mention.

The domesticated pigeon (rock dove, rock pigeon), *Columba domestica,* served a critical role in communications. The homing instinct of the pigeon (or synonymously, dove) was recognized in biblical times. Noah first sent a raven from the ark to determine if dry land could be found, but the raven did not return to the ark. When he sent the dove, the dove returned with the olive branch, signifying dry land. The Romans used pigeons extensively for communication in warfare. Both the Arabs and the Europeans used them during the Crusades. Not until World War I was the pigeon effectively replaced by modern communication technology. Pigeons also have served as a source of meat and remain a feature of some cuisines, notably in Arab countries. The ancient Romans apparently pioneered some disturbing practices in relation to pigeon husbandry. It is recorded that the birds' legs or wings were broken to keep them easily in confinement while they were fattened with chewed bread and other rich feeds.

Falconry, or the training of captive raptors for hunting game, has a long and noble history, noble in the sense that the practice was associated mainly with kings, sultans, emirs, princes, and other various nobility. The art of falconry was developed and advanced mostly by the Arabs but was enthusiastically adopted by European royalty as well. The birds most commonly captured and trained were peregrine falcons and gyrfalcons, but a wide range of raptors has been used or at least tested over the years. Traditional falconry practices are still an important aspect of Arabian culture (see Chapter 7, sidebar, Houbara Brouhaha in Pakistan). Elsewhere, the practice persists mostly as a hobby.

The ostrich, *Struthio camelus*, is well known to us as the large, flightless, wild bird of the African savanna. They have always been hunted by indigenous people. The Romans exploited them cruelly in their circuses as entertainment, decapitating them and watching them run around headless. Ostrich feathers have been valued for adornment, both by local tribal groups and by the international millinery trade. Only in recent history have efforts have been made to use the ostrich in any organized way as a meat and leather-producing animal. The French first bred ostriches in captivity in Algeria in the 19th century to supply feathers for the European fashion market. In recent times, the South Africans have taken the lead in developing husbandry and management practices for the commercial production of ostrich meat and leather. In the last 10 years, ostrich farming has become established in the United States, Australia, and several European countries. Similarly, the native ratite of Australia, the emu, is also now raised in captivity to provide a variety of products, and emu farming has also been embraced in the United States. Veterinarians have had to add two new species to their list of animals about which they are assumed to be thoroughly knowledgeable.

A great variety of bird species have been kept by people throughout history as companions, prized either for their song (e.g., canaries), their intelligence (e.g., crows), or their ability to talk (e.g., mynahs and parrots). The penchant for keeping birds still runs strong in many cultures (Fig. 2-9). In towns and villages around China, for instance, it is common to see the elderly gathered at outdoor teahouses whose proprietors have hung numerous cages of songbirds amid the trees to attract customers. It is a peaceful and picturesque scene, appealing to the eyes and the ears.

Some species of caged birds, like canaries have been modified notably by artificial selection to produce different breeds and can be considered truly domesticated. Others have been bred in captivity but left unaltered. Many species are simply captured from the wild. The illegal trade in wild birds such as parrots and macaws has increased in recent years in response to consumer demand for exotic pets in affluent societies like the United States. This has become a major issue in wildlife conservation, as some species are threatened with extinction. This issue is discussed further in Chapter 7. Smuggled birds also pose a potential health threat to poultry and wild birds in the countries where they are introduced and have been responsible for major economic losses due to avian disease outbreaks.

Fish

Fishing is a very early development in the history of human innovation in the search for food. Fishhooks and fishnets date back about 25,000 years. It is not well established when humans first hit upon the notion of stocking fish in ponds, but there is evidence that early settled agricultural civilizations, including Mesopotamia, Egypt, and the Incas of Peru developed at least rudimentary methods of maintaining fish ponds. The most detailed record of such activities comes from China, where the Eurasian carp, *Cyprinus carpio*, was domesticated at least 3000 years ago, primarily as a food fish. The carp was well integrated into farming activities. It was kept in ponds and fed household garbage and agricultural wastes on which it thrived to produce fish for consumption and sale. The Chinese also domesticated a second carp, *Curassius vulgaris*, initially for food, but subsequently for aesthetic reasons. This became the domestic

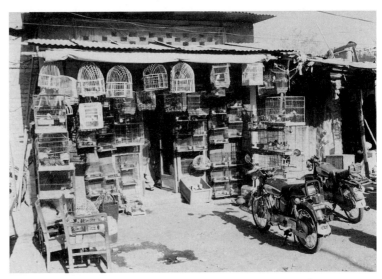

Figure 2-9. Songbirds and fighting birds are a major source of pleasure and entertainment for people in much of Asia. This is a typical bird shop in Quetta, Pakistan, one of many specializing in the sale of birds and bird-related supplies. (Photo by Dr. David M. Sherman)

goldfish. Through the breeders' art, the goldfish has been transformed into a tremendous array of ornamental breeds, frequently the subject of traditional Chinese art. The Romans successfully domesticated the moray eel, *Muraena muraena*, as a food fish and developed appropriate husbandry techniques to maintain them in saltwater pools.

Currently, there is an upsurge of interest in the captive rearing of fish, for both commercial and recreational purposes. The major thrust is in aquaculture, in which new techniques and new industries are being developed for large-scale production of a wide variety of fish and shellfish species for human consumption. This activity is spurred, in large part, by the fact that fish catches of wild commercial species are on the decline worldwide, largely because of overfishing. Technical developments in aquaculture are discussed further in Chapter 4. In addition, the demand for ornamental tropical fish by aquarium hobbyists is expanding, at the same time that the world's coral reefs, the main source for such fish, are being degraded by pollution and overexploitation. The profit motive as well as conservation concerns are encouraging efforts to develop new capabilities for the captive breeding of such tropical fish for the aquarium market.

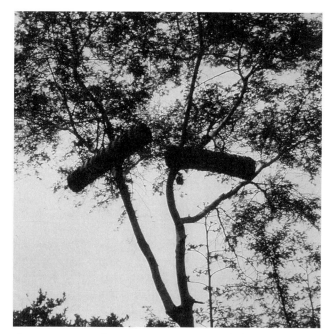

Figure 2-10. Hollowed-log beehives hung by villagers for a source of honey in Ethiopia. (Photo courtesy of Dr. Michael Goe)

Insects

Even insects have been the focus of domestication efforts. As much as prehistoric humans liked honey from the wild bees' hive, they no doubt did not enjoy being stung. By at least 2600 BC, the ancient Egyptians had figured out that they could suppress the bees' defense of their hive by smoking them out. The Egyptians understood the social organization of the honeybee and began the practice of providing hive space to prevent swarming and leaving some honey in the hive after harvesting so the bee colony would persist. These practices were disseminated widely throughout the early civilizations. Even with the advent of sugar production from cane and beets, beekeeping survives to this day in both the developed and developing world. When you drive along the roads in parts of Africa, you will see hollowed logs hanging from tree limbs by a rope or thong. These are beehives tended by local people (Fig. 2-10). The practice persists from ancient Egypt. Some technologies are so elegant in their simplicity that they last forever.

Though the number of insects that have been domesticated is limited, very few animals of any kind have had the broad social impact of the domesticated silkworm. Silkworms are the caterpillars of several genera of moths, most notably the genus *Bombyx*. These caterpillars feed solely on leaves of the mulberry tree and spin cocoons of fine silk thread that can be over a mile in length when teased out into a continuous strand. Silk is, and always has been, a highly desired raw material for textile production since the Chinese began to use it in this fashion probably close to 4000 years ago. It is the desire for silk from the East, more than any other commodity that encouraged early trade across central Asia between Europe and China. In the process, an enormous amount of intellectual, technical, and cultural exchange took place. The distribution of domestic animals themselves, such as the horse, donkey, and camel, grew more widespread as a result of this trade. These are considerable accomplishments for a caterpillar.

Other Domestications, Present and Future

In important ways, the history of animal domestication reflects the history of human social development. As illustrated in the previous discussion, there were right times and right places for specific domestications to take place, depending on the state of human society. For Paleolithic hunters, the dog was a useful partner in the hunt. For the emerging nomads, the sheep and goat were suitable replacements for diminishing wild prey. For the Neolithic agriculturists, the ox was an excellent work animal for preparing the soil for cultivation. For the merchant class that developed out of agricultural settlement, the donkey and the camel represented a better way of moving goods to facilitate trade. For the generals and politicians of city-states intent on empire building, the camel and the elephant represented tactical advantage in warfare.

Human cultural evolution is a dynamic process, and it will continue to include animals, both domesticated and wild. Technological advances will continue to diminish human dependency on animals for labor. However, the increased leisure time that labor-saving devices produce stimulates interest in animals from the recreational perspective. Colorful coral reef fish and talking birds of the rainforest are but two examples of creatures now in the early phases of domestication (i.e., captive breeding) to meet increased recreational demand.

Increasing affluence, or mass buying power, also creates new demands for consumer goods of animal origin. This also stimulates new efforts in captive breeding and domestication. Fancy leathers and luxury fibers such as cashmere and silk are no longer extravagances restricted to royalty and robber barons. The legendary Silk Road now leads to your neighborhood mall. Alligator and ostrich farming are becoming established industries to meet the growing demand for fine leathers, and there is renewed interest in domestication of the vicuna, whose soft, fine hair is highly valued as a textile fiber and status symbol. However, the animal product for which demand is most increased by affluence, is meat.

As discussed in Chapter 1, the emergence of growing middle classes in countries of the developing world has led to increased meat consumption. Not unexpectedly, this demand is being met largely through expansion of existing meat animal industries such as intensive swine and poultry production and expansion of cattle ranching. However, economic, environmental, and ethical issues are frequently associated with the introduction of intensive livestock production and ranching in developing countries, and alternative approaches need consideration, including new domestications. For example, in many parts of Africa, particularly in west Africa, cane rats (*Thryonomys* spp.), also known as grasscutters, and giant rats (*Cricetomys* spp.) are traditionally prized as a source of meat. Obtaining these rats means trapping and hunting in the forests, with the result that many other species, some endangered, are opportunistically captured by the hunters. There are currently efforts ongoing to domesticate these rats for caged production by villagers, a small-scale economic opportunity akin to rabbit raising, which would increase the availability of meat for urban markets and reduce hunting pressure in the shrinking forests. An analogous situation exists in central America, where cattle ranching has had a negative impact on the environment. Two Central American rodents, the diurnal agouti (*Dasyprocta mexicana* and *D. punctata*) and the nocturnal paca (*Agouti paca*) both offer potential for domestication as a source of meat. In Costa Rica, the paca is highly prized for its meat, preferred to beef by many people.[7]

Persistent poverty and population growth are also stimulating new frontiers in domestication. In many parts of the world, rural peasants still depend on animals for draft power and food. There are local wild animals that may still provide the basis for successful domestications to meet localized needs, consistent with local climate, terrain, and culture. Animal breeders, scientists, and development workers, for example, have identified a number of little-known Asian animals with promising economic futures.[6] These include wild bovine species such as the gaur, kouprey, tamaraw, and anoa as well as wild and feral pigs and piglike species, including the Sulawesi and Javan warty pigs, the pygmy hog, and the babirusa. In Russia, the large wild herbivore, *Alces alces*, known in Russia and Europe as the elk, but in North America as the moose, has been successfully domesticated to provide a domestic animal with economic potential for the indigenous people living in the inhospitable taiga regions of Russia. The animal fills a similar niche for taiga people that the reindeer fills for the tundra people further north. The animals are herded like reindeer, and the females are regularly milked by hand.

Veterinarians should be actively involved in all efforts to domesticate a new species. Though the situation of each new domestication will differ, veterinarians have the fundamental knowledge to advise and assist in the initial efforts to capture, restrain, and move wild animals; identify and manage stresses associated with captivity; and anticipate, identify, and manage disease problems that arise from the placement of animals in new systems of management and production. Incredibly, teams of scientists working together today may be able to accomplish in the span of a few generations, what our ancestors accomplished through extended observation and trial and error over the span of millennia.

Discussion Points

1. Why was the North American bison decimated instead of domesticated? What advantages were perceived for grazing cattle on North American rangelands in the 19th century instead of bison? At present, there is still conflict between cattle and bison around Yellowstone National Park, ostensibly over the issue of brucellosis transmission. Is brucellosis in bison a genuine threat to cattle? What other factors may be at play in this conflict?

2. Historically, Africa has not been a productive source of domesticated animals. However, there is interest today in the potential for domesticating some wild ruminant species of the African savanna as potential sources of meat production. Which animals might lend themselves to domestication? What advantages might they offer over cattle in Africa as a commercial source of meat? What disadvantages? What opportunities and challenges do such domestications offer to veterinarians?

3. How has the increased popularity of ornamental fish, psittacine birds, and other exotic creatures affected the practice of veterinary medicine in your area? Does veterinary school prepare you to deal with these species? What resources are available to increase professional knowledge in relation to exotic animal practice?

4. Despite their great strength and versatility as timber workers, elephants are subject to serious traumatic injuries from this heavy work. Do such injured animals receive adequate veterinary care in the countries where they work? If not, what are the obstacles to adequate care? How could you find this out? How can veterinarians in your country contribute to the health care of working elephants in other countries?

5. What is the current situation regarding efforts to domesticate the vicuna? What is the status of the wild vicuna in South America? Identify some instances in which domestication efforts could actually assist in protecting threatened and endangered species.

6. In your own society, how are attitudes and values changing concerning the human use of domesticated animals, particularly as a source of food? What challenges do these changing attitudes and values present for the veterinary profession?

References

1. Bilger B. Enter the chicken. Harper's Magazine 1999;298(1786):48–57.

2. Caras RA. A Perfect Harmony, The Intertwining Lives of Animals and Humans Throughout History. New York: Simon & Schuster, 1996.

3. Clutton-Brock J. Domesticated Animals from Early Times. Austin: University of Texas Press, 1981.

4. Heiser CB Jr. Seed to Civilization, The Story of Food. New Ed. Cambridge, MA: Harvard University Press, 1990.

5. Lorenz K. The Year of the Greylag Goose. New York: Harcourt Brace Jovanovich, 1978.

6. National Research Council. Little-Known Asian Animals with a Promising Economic Future. Washington, DC: National Academy Press, 1983.

7. National Research Council. Microlivestock: Little-Known Small Animals with a Promising Economic Future. Washington, DC: National Academy Press, 1991.

8. Schwabe CW. Cattle, Priests, and Progress in Medicine. Minneapolis: University of Minnesota Press, 1978.

9. Stanford CB. The Hunting Apes: Meat Eating and the Origins of Human Behavior. Princeton, NJ: Princeton University Press, 1999.

10. Vila C, Savolainen P, Maldonado JE, et al. Multiple and ancient origins of the domestic dog. Science 1997; 276(5319):1687–1689.

11. Zeuner FE. A History of Domesticated Animals. New York: Harper & Row, 1963.

Suggested Readings

Allman JM. Evolving Brains. New York: WH Freeman, 1999.

Clutton-Brock J. A Natural History of Domesticated Animals. 2nd Ed. Cambridge, England: Cambridge University Press, 1999.

Dunlop RH, Williams DJ. Veterinary Medicine, an Illustrated History. St. Louis: Mosby, 1996.

Parsonson I. The Australian Ark: a History of Domesticated Animals in Australia. Collingwood, Australia: CSIRO Publishing, 1998.

Stanford CB, Bunn HT, eds. Meat-Eating and Human Evolution. Oxford, England: Oxford University Press, 2001.

Chapter 3
Cultural Attitudes Concerning the Use of Animals

OBJECTIVES FOR THIS CHAPTER

After completing this chapter, the reader should be able to

- Identify key historical, cultural, and geographical factors that influence attitudes concerning the use of certain animals for food and other purposes in society

- Recognize contrasting patterns of human-animal interaction in developed and developing countries and some key reasons for these differences

- Appreciate the importance of understanding this diversity of attitudes and practices, to be able to work effectively in a global context

Introduction

As discussed in Chapter 2, early humans initially used domesticated animals such as the sheep and goat for the same reasons they used wild animals—to provide materials to meet their basic needs, including meat for food, skins for clothing and shelter, and bones for tools and weapons. With settlement and the beginning of plant cultivation, came new utilitarian roles for domesticated animals, with oxen, donkeys, and water buffalo providing draft power in support of agricultural activity. As societies became more complex, the use of animals in war and commerce also grew, with horses and camels assuming significant roles.

Agriculture, by facilitating food surpluses, spurred the diversification of human society. Bands of hunter-gatherers became villagers. Villages expanded to towns and to city-states. Civilizations with distinct identities developed, replete with codes of behavior, class structures, systems of governance, and distinct religious practices and beliefs.

Animals, which played such important utilitarian roles in people's daily lives, also took on significance in the cultural practices and religious doctrines of these emerging civilizations. It is beyond the scope of this book to detail the spiritual and cultural functions of animals in the ancient civilizations—the Sumerians, Babylonians, Assyrians, Egyptians, Greeks, Romans, and others all had their specific beliefs and practices involving animals. A useful resource on the symbolic role of animals in religion and society through history is *Animals with Human Faces: A Guide to Animal Symbolism* by Beryl Rowland.[4] The extent to which animals defined the spiritual and social life of ancient peoples is suggested by the example of Egypt, which is described here only briefly.

Animal-centered beliefs in ancient Egypt were rich and varied. This may not have been the first civilization to express such diversity in the human-animal relationship, but it is certainly the best documented among early civilizations. Divine associations with animals were a major aspect of ancient Egyptian religious practices. Many gods assumed animal forms, such as Ra, the falcon; Thoth, the ibis; Apis, the sacred black bull; Bast, the cat; Amun, the ram; and Anubis, the jackal. People gained merit by worshipping and caring for animals. Animals were ascribed human spiritual characteristics. Astronomical events were linked to animals as well, suggesting an awareness of the importance of the daily solar cycle to agriculture and human life. For instance, the crescent moon was believed to represent the curved horn of the aurochs or wild bull. The solar eclipse was explained as the serpent god, Apep, principal enemy of the king of gods, Ra, allegedly swallowing the barge that daily carried the sun across the skies over Egypt.

The Egyptians maintained wild animal preserves and stocked them with wild game for hunting. They trained cats as hunting partners to retrieve game birds. Many wild mammals, if not domesticated, were routinely tamed. Pet keeping was widespread, and lap dogs of small stature were favored, suggesting fairly extensive knowledge and application of selective breeding programs.

Vestiges of ancient Egyptian customs still persist today among peoples of the Nile river basin. Healing priests of the Nuer tribe, a pastoral people of the Sudan, still wear leopard skins as an indicator of their professional status, just as healing priests did in the Nile delta thousands of years ago.[6] In ancient Egypt, the hippopotamus was considered a goddess of fertility, revered by pregnant women. Today in Queen Elizabeth National Park in Uganda, the source of the Nile, park rangers report problems with poaching of hippopotamus by local tribesmen who sell the hippo meat in nearby villages as a treatment for female infertility.

As the Egyptian case points out, ancient polytheistic religions frequently represented their gods in animal form or associated certain animals with them. As some gods were good and some were bad, the animals too, were perceived as benign or evil. In Egypt for example, the cat, associated with the benevolent goddess Bast, was held to be so sacred that if a cat died naturally in a house, the household members mourned by shaving their eyebrows. If someone killed a cat, it was considered a capital offense. Alternately, the pig, associated with the malevolent god Seth, was shunned. If a person accidentally was brushed by a pig, that person would run to the river and plunge in fully clothed for cleansing. Pig herders made up an "untouchable" class, and no one outside that class would offer a daughter in marriage to a pig herder.

Among the monotheistic religions, with their proscriptions against idolatry, the representation of God in animal form was no longer acceptable, and animals were less likely to be considered representative of certain types of moral behavior. Nevertheless, Judaism, Islam, and Christianity have made value judgments concerning the social acceptability of specific animals, particularly with regard to an animal's suitability as food. Religious prohibitions against eating certain types of animals are generally considered articles of faith, i.e., doctrines handed down directly by God to the faithful. However, more-secular explanations for these beliefs are worthy of consideration. Anthropologists studying the evolution of human culture have asked if these proscriptions are obeyed because they are religious doctrine or, rather, have these proscriptions found their way into religious doctrine because they serve the culture in some important and rational way? This is not merely an academic question. It has practical significance for anyone intending to work cross-culturally. This would include veterinarians who believe that animals have a significant role to play in feeding the world's hungry. Sensitivity to the foodways of different cultures and a basic understanding of their origins are critical to making appropriate decisions in the selection, planning, and implementation of efforts concerning the development of animal agriculture.

The anthropologists' perspective has special value here. It suggests that there are distinct geographical, climatic, cultural, political, and even genetic forces that helped to shape beliefs concerning the use of animals as food. Ultimately, the acceptance or avoidance of a specific animal food source may represent an economic decision by a social group. Such decisions are economic in the sense that they weigh the costs of using an animal as food against the benefits of doing so. Considered in such decisions may be the cost of raising a certain animal for food against the resource base available to produce it; the opportunity cost of using that animal for food as opposed to another type of available animal; or, the value of alternative societal uses for the particular animal other than as food, for example, draft power.

Food Preferences and Prohibitions

In the following sections, the development of important animal food preferences and prohibitions are reviewed, and the factors that contribute to a society's collective view of that animal are identified, with emphasis on the decision to use it or not use it as food. The topics include Judaic and Islamic proscriptions against pigs, Hindu deification of the cow, cultural attitudes about eating horse meat, the geography of milk drinking, the eating of insects, and the keeping of dogs as pets.

Proscriptions Against Pigs

For the Jews, pigs are identified as unclean, and the consumption of pork is an abomination. The ban is part of a whole set of dietary rules and restrictions spelled out in Leviticus, the third book of the Torah, the written law of the Jews as revealed to Moses and Aaron by God. With regard to the animals that dwell on land, God commanded that the Jews could eat only an animal that "has true hoofs, with clefts through the hoofs, and that chews the cud." Specifically proscribed, as not belonging to that category are the camel, which chews its cud but does not have a true hoof, and the pig, which has a true hoof but does not chew its cud. Acceptable for consumption were the true-hoofed, cud-chewing ruminant animals, sheep, goats, and cattle. From a strictly religious perspective then, the ban on pork is accepted as the word of God. However, some anthropologists contend that the biblical prohibition against pigs can also be interpreted as a logical decision concerning the use of marginal resources among a people living in a difficult environment.[2]

The early Jews were essentially a herding society who kept sheep and goats in the semiarid grazing lands of the Near East, beyond the eastern shore of the Mediterranean Sea. Though pigs existed in the Near East, they were kept by people in forested areas of the region. Pig keeping was not consistent with the lifestyle of nomadic herders engaged in extensive grazing of their flocks on grasslands. Swine are difficult to herd and potentially dangerous, with long, sharp tusks and an aggressive disposition. Furthermore, the pig is not well adapted to hot, dry conditions, requiring water and mud for wallowing to dissipate heat, a difficult requirement for herders with animals on the move. Finally, pigs, though highly efficient converters of grain, do not perform as well on the high-fiber, cellulose-rich diets of grass, to which ruminants are so well suited. In summary, the pig was not a very useful animal for the early nomadic Jews. Having no use for it, they had little familiarity with it and were, therefore, likely suspicious of it.

As with other peoples in the region, the Jews gradually settled and took up crop cultivation, and the aversion to the pig took on even greater significance. Ruminant animals continued to prove their worth under conditions of settlement. In addition to meat, they produced milk for human consumption, fiber for textiles, and draft power for agricultural work. The pig, in contrast, was not a multipurpose animal—its main, if not sole, use was for meat production. The farmer-generated, grain-eating predilection of the pig also became more problematic since now the Israelites were cultivating grain for human consumption, and the pig was seen as a crop destroyer and food competitor. As forests were cut and more land came under cultivation, the natural foraging areas for pigs were reduced, bringing them more commonly into conflict with cultivators who increasingly had to protect their fields from raiding pigs.

Finally, religious differences between the Jews and other settled peoples in the region probably solidified negative attitudes toward the pig. The Jews were committed monotheists. They wanted to have a distinct identity from the pagan and polytheistic religions of other cultures who ate pork and sacrificed swine in ritual and celebration. Identifying swine as unclean and pork as unfit for human consumption was a way to distance the Jewish culture from that of the polytheists. From an ecological and agricultural systems perspective, given the fragile semiarid environment of the Near East, the Jews' attitude toward the pig-first indifferent and then overtly hostile-made good sense. The pig was inappropriate for the evolving conditions of geography, climate, and land use in their region, and the Israelites likely recognized this. When cultural and religious identity was added to the mix, it is not difficult to perceive how aversion to the pig came to be seen as the word of God.

For veterinarians, the story of Jewish aversion to pork is also of interest from the perspective of medical science. It has been frequently suggested that the ancient Hebrew leaders recognized the risk of trichinosis from eating pork and, therefore, discouraged consumption by religious proscription for public health reasons. This seems highly unlikely. The muscle cysts from *Trichinella spiralis* in swine muscle are microscopic, so pork meat would not be readily identifiable in ancient times as a source of illness. The early signs of infection, which occur within 1 or 2 days of ingestion of larva-infected pork, are nonspecific signs of enteritis, namely, diarrhea, nausea, and abdominal pain, which could just as easily be caused by bacterial food poisonings from the meat or dairy products of ruminant animals. The clinical signs of muscle involvement in trichinosis do not occur until 1 to 6 weeks postingestion, so it would be difficult to establish a causal relationship between pork consumption and the delayed onset of muscular disease. Finally, most cases of human trichinosis are subclinical, so clinical disease would be infrequent enough that it would not likely rank high in peoples' minds as a major disease concern. In fact, a number of diseases that produce more-consistent clinical illness, with shorter incubation periods and higher mortality rates, are readily associated with the religiously acceptable ruminant animals that were the lifeblood of early Jewish nomadic culture. These diseases include brucellosis, anthrax, and food poisoning due to *Salmonella* spp. or *Staphylococcus aureus*. Crediting ancient Hebrews with formulating public health policy on the basis of an understanding of the transmission of trichinosis is probably unwarranted. Nevertheless, the 12th century Jewish philosopher and physician Maimonides has been called the founder of veterinary public health for his observations on the role of saliva in the transmission of rabies and his recognition of tuberculosis in slaughtered animals.[1]

Islam also emerged as a monotheistic religion with its roots in the Near East, several millennia after Judaism. The earliest Muslims were Arabs, a Semitic people of the Arabian peninsula, whose culture involved herding and nomadic activity. Therefore, the same ecological constraints on pig raising that existed for the early Jews also existed for the early Muslims at the time that Islamic doctrine and practices were being formulated. In fact, the Near East had become significantly less favorable for pig raising. By the time the Prophet Mohammed was born, in the 6th century AD, the forest habitats suitable for pigs in the Near East were almost completely gone. Land degradation from agricultural use was also widespread, and Arab people, such as the Bedouins, had long since adopted the use of the camel to make the deserts accessible to them in support of their livelihood as herders and traders.

The sacred book of Islam, the Koran, is believed by Muslims to be the word of God revealed to the Prophet Mohammed over his lifetime. From the secular point of view, it is not surprising then that the Koran retains the prohibition on pigs established by the monotheistic Jews, as the ecological justifications for proscribing swine production had grown even stronger with the passage of time. More notable is that the Judaic prohibition against eating the camel is not retained in Islam. This decision not to proscribe camels may have a pragmatic explanation. Arabs did not routinely eat camels as a matter of course. The camel was too valuable as a draft animal. However, Arabs of the time depended on the camel for all manner of survival under harsh desert conditions. If lost in the desert, an Arab's life might depend on eating the accompanying camels. It would not have been conducive to winning converts to Islam, if camel consumption had been proscribed in the Koran.

As with Judaism, cultural and religious factors likely contributed to strengthening the Muslim bias against pigs. A major factor was the ongoing cultural, religious, and political competition with Christianity, the other monotheistic religion that followed Judaism. The Christians ate pork, and the Muslim ban on pork may have been one of many effective strategies for distinguishing the adherents of Islam from those of Christianity. It was only about 500 years after the establishment of Islam that the protracted conflict for control of the Holy Land took place. It can well be imagined that during this period of the Crusades, the depiction of Christians as "unclean" eaters of pork likely had considerable propaganda value.

Islam has been widely embraced over the centuries, with about 1.1 billion Muslims currently living in the world. There is a remarkable concordance between the geographical distribution of Muslim populations and the ecological suitability for traditional pig raising. For the most part, Islam radiated from the Arabian peninsula mainly eastward and westward through a zone of low rainfall sandwiched between temperate zones to the north and tropical zones to the south. The Muslim world stretches from dry Morocco in the west, across northern Africa and the Arabian Peninsula, into the arid zones of central Asia, and south to the dry zones of India. Some countries, such as Sudan and Nigeria, for example, have large Muslim populations in the drier, northern zones but Christian or animist peoples in the wetter, southern zones. It would appear that peoples living in environments not suitable for pig raising were more amenable to embracing Islam than people in environments conducive to raising pigs. The most obvious exception to this pattern is the tropical nation of Indonesia, which has the largest Muslim population of any country in the world. Pork consumption occurs in Indonesia, mainly among the non-Muslim citizens, including the Hindu Balinese and the urban Chinese.

The Hindu Sacred Cow

Hinduism is the principal religion of India. It has its origins in the religion of the Aryan people, warlike pastoralist/farmers from Persia and Turkmenistan who invaded India sometime between 2000 and 1200 BC and settled the northern plateau and Ganges river valley regions. The practices of the Aryans mixed slowly over time with the rituals and beliefs of indigenous peoples of the region to produce the beginnings of Hinduism. The Aryans and early Hindus were polytheistic and worshipped a variety of nature gods. They also believed in a caste system that included a priestly class, the Brahmans. A key duty of the Brahmans was to conduct animal sacrifices that served as propitious offerings to the gods. It was the exclusive right of the Brahman priests to kill animals. No one ate meat unless the Brahmans had conducted the ritual slaughter and had identified a suitable occasion to justify the sacrifice and to distribute the meat among people for feasting. It is this same priestly class of the Hindus today, the Brahmans, who most steadfastly uphold the Hindu abstention from eating meat, and who teach that the cow is sacred. How did this dramatic turnaround occur?

The Aryans were hard working and industrious, and their agricultural efforts in the Ganges River valley were successful to the point that expanding human populations, extensive deforestation, and progressive land degradation began to undermine the well-being that had been achieved. Farmers living close to the river and irrigating their lands were increasingly subjected to floods aggravated by the extensive deforestation of the Himalayan foothills. Farmers who had moved to peripheral lands beyond the reach of irrigation fell victim to crop failures from prolonged periods of drought. Earlier prosperity was replaced by a marginal, subsistence existence. Animals for slaughter became scarcer, and the Hindu Brahmans, who had been responsible for the slaughter of animals for redistributive feasting, became increasingly selfish. Animal slaughter persisted, but the benefits accrued only to the priestly class, who continued to eat meat in the face of scarcity for the common people.

By about AD 500, the situation was calamitous for farmers. Survival on the land became a tenuous prospect. As populations expanded, farms became smaller. Farmers found that they could not maintain the diverse forms of livestock that were familiar to them, because they could not justify feeding them. Only one animal figured favorably in the cost/benefit analysis of survival. That was the cow. The cow could give milk and could bear male offspring that as oxen were essential for plowing to break up the tough, sun-baked soils of the northern Indian plateau for crop cultivation. Cattle also provided manure in sufficient quantity to enrich the soil.

Around this time, new religious sects arose in the region that posed serious threats to the hegemony of Hinduism. Both Jainism and Buddhism had wide appeal for common people. These religions eschewed the caste system, rejected hereditary claims to priesthood, linked poverty to spirituality, and suggested that the path to achieving spiritual fulfillment lay with prayer and reflection rather than animal sacrifice. Jainism and Buddhism were both noteworthy in their respectful and benign attitudes toward animals. The Jains disapproved outright of killing any animal, even insects. The Buddhists permitted flesh eating, but only if non-Buddhists carried out the slaughter. In the face of this new thinking and the threat it posed to the status quo, it is not surprising that the Brahman priests also gradually adopted and promoted Hindu prohibitions on the eating of meat to retain religious dominance in the region.

Yet, a prohibition on eating meat falls short of outright sanctification of the cow. What purposes were served in elevating the cow to godlike status? One explanation is that the deification of cattle may have served as a hedge against disaster. During periods of severe drought, when peasants truly faced the prospect of starvation, the temptation to slaughter the family cattle for meat to ensure short-time survival was painfully real. However, in fending off starvation in the short term, farmers who ate their cattle were courting disaster in the long term. Without cattle, farmers could not plow, plant, and fertilize their fields when the rains returned and would, therefore, surely starve in the long run. Since rational decision making in the face of starvation is not easy, raising the cow to the level of a god in the minds of farmers may have helped those farmers to fend off temptation and spare their cows. After all, even under the direst circumstances, one could not risk eternal unrest by slaughtering a sacred cow. The Brahman priests may have recognized the importance of this reasoning in dire situations and codified the sanctity of the cow in Hindu teachings.

The sacredness of cattle is a core feature of Hinduism today, and no foreigner travels to India without being struck by the seemingly curious spectacle of full-grown cattle wandering unattended through villages and towns and even on busy city streets. Despite appearances to the contrary, relatively few of these animals are unclaimed. Cattle continue to be relied upon as an essential element of production by the vast majority of Indian farmers with small landholdings. That the cattle wander freely, reflects the low level of input that many farmers can invest in their cattle. Indian Zebu cattle are tough and resilient, bred and selected not for high production of milk or meat, but for endurance and survival. Many survive by scavenging and foraging on their own but are available to farmers when needed for plowing. The keen observer will also note that the animals' droppings are not wasted. People, often children, follow behind the cattle and pick up the manure for use as cooking fuel and fertilizer. It remains too valuable to leave in the streets.

Horses As Food

The eating of horse meat is traditional in central Asian societies where horse keeping is common, and the practice continues in developing nations of the region, such as Kazakhstan and Mongolia. In developed countries, there are varying attitudes toward consumption of horse meat. It is acceptable in France, Belgium, and Japan but virtually taboo in the United States, to the point that there are active campaigns currently under way by horse welfare advocates to ban the export of slaughter horses from the United States to other countries where they are used as food. Historically, the willingness of a culture to consider the horse as food has been based on economic and political considerations. Today, in the United States, ethical and emotional considerations have become the dominant factors, largely related to the emergence of the horse as a friend and companion in American culture.

Wild horses were hunted for food in Paleolithic times, but the domestication of the horse was a postagricultural event that was motivated primarily by the need for a powerful animal for traction and transport rather than for food. In fact, the horse would have been a poor selection for domestication by early agriculturists had the prime motivation been to develop a source of animal protein for human consumption. This is because horses are less efficient converters of grass to muscle mass than ruminant animals. Though the single-stomached horse is able to digest cellulose in the cecum, it does so less effectively than the true ruminants. With this higher nutritional energy cost, the horse was far more valuable as a work animal than a food animal.

The traditional horse-based cultures of the Asian steppes valued the horse as their principal means of production. First and foremost, the horse provided the mobility necessary to herd huge flocks of sheep over wide areas of marginal grasslands. It also became an effective weapon of war, facilitating the Mongol conquests of Europe and China. However, for both the herder and the soldier, the horse also served as an emergency food supply. Most often taken was mare's milk, but under conditions of great hardship, when supplies were short, soldiers would drink the blood of their horses, and when the horses weakened or died, they would eat their flesh as well.

Similarly, in Europe, horses were never principally raised for food. Again the reason was primarily economic. Abundant forests favored the raising of pigs, and the grasslands of Europe could be more efficiently used by ruminants, so meat for human consumption was relatively abundant. Horses were simply too valuable as work animals to compete with swine and ruminants as a regular source of animal protein. Nevertheless, the prevailing philosophy was "waste not, want not," and when horses reached the end of their productive lives as work animals, they found their way to the livestock markets and onto the dinner plates of the poorer classes.

When Islam was introduced by Mohammed to the Arabian peninsula in the early 7th century, the Arabs were already accomplished equestrians and horse breeders, and the horse became an important instrument for spreading the Islamic faith. Within 100 years of the death of Mohammed, Muslim Arab cavalry had, through conquest, spread their religion throughout north Africa and into Spain. By 715, they had crossed the Pyrenees Mountains into southern France. The Frankic kings to the north were well aware of the tactical advantage of the Arab mounted cavalry and began to train their own armored cavalry. At the Battle of Tours, in 732, the Christian Franks defeated the Arabs and put an end to the further spread of Islam into Europe. The role of the horse in this decisive battle was not lost on the leader of the Christian world, Pope Gregory III, who, in the same year, declared the practice of eating horse flesh unclean, detestable, and no longer permissible by Christians.

This prohibition of Pope Gregory's on eating horse flesh is noteworthy in that it represents the only specified food taboo in Christianity. Early Christian leaders recognized food proscriptions as obstacles to proselytism and avoided invoking them. Therefore, the Pope's decree underscored the extreme military value of the horse to the state and the church. This was not an animal to be sacrificed for the table. For the next 1000 years or so, this attitude prevailed, and the horse became increasingly associated with knights, generals, nobility, and the wealthy. For the most part, horses that found their way into the human food chain were the infirm and lame, and they usually arrived there surreptitiously.

The association of the horse with the elite classes of society took on particular significance in Europe during the social and political upheavals of the 18th century. In the aftermath of the French Revolution, it became acceptable again to eat horse meat, a convenient and nutritious way for the proletariat to express their victory over the ruling classes. By this time, horses, which had been scarce in the era of Pope Gregory III, were now abundant in Europe, and a proper trade in horse meat began, complete with butchers and restaurants that specialized in horses. The practice was most evident in France and Belgium, but much of northern continental Europe embraced the practice of eating horse meat.

The horse meat industry remained strong until the beginning of the 20th century, when motorized vehicles replaced the horse in the spheres of war, commerce, and agriculture. Horse numbers fell precipitously, and the price of horse meat rose accordingly, so people switched to other forms of meat, largely on the basis of price and availability. However, specialty horse butchers still exist in Belgium and France (Fig. 3-1). While many Europeans, like Americans, have come to view the horse as a companion animal, the latent acceptance of the horse as a source of food has become manifest in the resurgence of horse meat consumption around Europe in 2001, following concerns about the wholesomeness of beef associated with mad cow disease. This increased demand has led to an increase in the price of slaughter horses in the United States destined for European markets, which in turn has resulted in a spate of horse thefts by criminal profiteers and redoubled efforts by horse welfare advocates to ban the sale of horses for slaughter.

The Geography and Genetics of Milk Drinking

The production of milk to nourish their offspring is a defining characteristic of mammals. Milk is an excellent food for the neonate, offering a wide array of nutrients in an easily accessible and usable form. Milk provides abundant, concentrated energy both as fat and carbohydrate, protein for tissue building, and a variety of vitamins and minerals to promote proper metabolism and growth. Most notable among these is calcium, essential for bone formation and development. Milk is the most concentrated dietary source of readily available calcium. For the hoofed mammals, milk also provides early and immediate immunity against disease for neonates in the form of immunoglobulin present in the first milk, or colostrum.

While the mammary secretion of milk is an excellent adaptation for rearing mammalian young, continuous lactation by the dam and ongoing consumption of milk by the mature offspring does not offer survival advantage for any mammalian species in

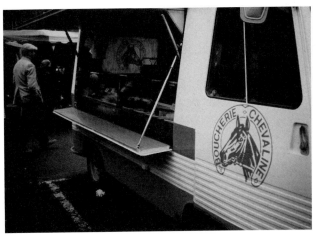

Figure 3-1. Mobile horse meat purveyor in rural France. The vehicle travels from town to town to be present on the designated weekly outdoor market day of each town on the route. (Photo by Dr. David M. Sherman)

an evolutionary sense. It places an ongoing nutritional burden on the female for continued production of milk and encourages the mature offspring to stay with the mother rather than move off to its own territory and seek alternative food sources. As such, lactation after parturition is relatively short-lived, and offspring are weaned well before reaching maturity.

The proper digestion of milk requires the digestive enzyme lactase. Lactase, produced in the small intestine, is responsible for the breakdown of the milk sugar, lactose, a disaccharide composed of glucose and galactose. Without the action of lactase, lactose remains in the gut. It induces an osmotic influx of fluid into the bowel lumen, and instead of being absorbed, the lactose is fermented by colonic bacteria. These events lead to diarrhea, cramping, bloating, and abdominal pain. The cessation of production of lactase in humans after childhood can be viewed as another adaptive mechanism to discourage continued milk consumption beyond normal weaning age.

However, starting about 10,000 years ago, the domestication of lactating ruminants such as the cow and goat began to influence the course of natural selection. Societies that kept lactating domesticated animals suddenly had the capacity to continue to consume large quantities of milk into adulthood, long after their own mothers had stopped producing milk. The consumption of milk into adulthood may have offered a selective advantage, particularly for women. Calcium deficiency adversely affects bone growth through the development of deficiency diseases such as rickets and osteoporosis. The resulting bone deformities and associated fractures can, if involving the pelvic bones, result in a narrowed or partially obstructed birth canal, with increased risk of dystocia and death in childbirth. Therefore, consumption of milk, as a concentrated form of calcium, may have had survival advantage. The genes for production of lactase in adulthood exist, but historically, they had not been expressed. There was now a new factor in the selection process, namely the milk supply from domestic animals, which favored the expression of these genes.[5]

As a result, a very interesting demographic pattern of lactose tolerance and intolerance among human populations has emerged over the last 10,000 years that roughly mirrors the history of cattle domestication. Those cultures that did not have access to cattle, such as the indigenous peoples of the New World, and those cultures that did not embrace cattle widely because they had access to other domesticated animals that better suited their needs, such as the Chinese, remain mostly lactose intolerant. In contrast, the people of the Near East, who domesticated the cow, and the people of Europe, who readily accepted and disseminated cattle, are more lactose tolerant.

Even within Europe there is gradation in the prevalence of lactose tolerance. Lactose tolerance increases in a northward direction, with the lowest level of tolerance in the Mediterranean region and the highest in Scandinavia. This may be explained by geography and the mechanisms of calcium metabolism. The absorption of dietary calcium from the intestine is facilitated by the action of vitamin D. Cholecalciferol, the active mammalian form of vitamin D is produced by sunlight striking

the skin. It is subsequently carried to the liver and then the kidney for modification and, ultimately, to the intestine where it induces synthesis of calcium-binding hormone to improve the efficiency of calcium absorption.

As one moves north in Europe, away from the equator, the overall amount of sunlight decreases, especially in winter. In addition, temperatures get colder so that people, to survive, have to keep themselves covered with insulating clothing for considerable portions of the year. As a result, northern Europeans have less opportunity to produce vitamin D in the skin than do southern Europeans. However, lactose itself is a very efficient facilitator of calcium absorption from the gut, involving both passive and active mechanisms of absorption. As such, milk is an especially good source of dietary calcium because the calcium is present in high concentration and the lactose ensures its proper absorption and use in the face of potential shortages of vitamin D. Therefore, northern Europeans have been more consistently selecting for expression of lactase production in adulthood than southern Europeans have, and accordingly, the proportion of the population with lactose tolerance is larger in the former group than in the latter.

In summary then, individuals of northern European extraction are least likely to show lactose intolerance, while southern European populations show variable levels of intolerance. Groups with high levels of lactose intolerance include Native Americans of North America, Mesoamerican Indians of South and Central America, natives of China and other southeast Asian nations, and many of the peoples of Africa, particularly West Africa. In East Africa, there are numerous cattle-based pastoralist cultures for whom milk represents the principal staple food, and these groups have a lower level of lactose intolerance. Not surprisingly, in places like Brazil, which has a very diverse and mixed ethnic population of native Indian, African, and European heritage, the occurrence of lactose intolerance is quite variable.

This is not to say that many of the world's people cannot or do not use milk in the diet, because they do. For example, in India, with a population of relatively high lactose intolerance, the inclusion of dairy products in the typical Indian diet is widespread (Fig. 3-2). However, much of the milk is used in fermented form, as yogurt or yogurt-like products. Through the fermentation process of yogurt making, lactose is broken down to lactic acid, and the digestive upsets associated with the consumption of fresh milk are avoided. It is important to realize that much of the world's adult population is not inclined to gulp down a big tall glass of cold milk enthusiastically or to associate the act with any particular sense of well-being. In fact, the opposite is often true. The aversion to milk drinking in China is particularly strong. Many Chinese, particularly the older generation, find the notion of drinking a glass of milk absolutely revolting. Nevertheless, the Chinese government in the 1970s made a decision to promote dairy development and milk consumption in China, targeting their campaign to increasing health and nutrition of children. The strategy is sensible. Children are

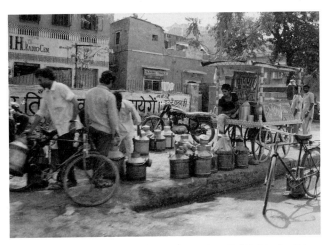

Figure 3–2. Milk dealers on the street in New Delhi. Much of the milk consumed in India is used in cooking as ghee, a liquid butter valued as cooking oil, or as fermented milk products such as yogurt and lassi, a sweetened, fermented milk drink. (Photo by Dr. David M. Sherman)

much more likely to be influenced than adults in this traditionally milk-averse society.

Insects in the Diet

Many readers may have had the experience as children of being coaxed and cajoled into eating a worm or a bug. Some older sibling or friend told you that the object in question tasted good and was good for you and that plenty of people ate them. In fact, the sibling or friend probably claimed to have just eaten a handful of the things when you, conveniently, were not looking. Then, when you, trusting soul, actually put the thing in your mouth, your tormentor would shriek with laughter and deride you for being foolish enough to listen to such extravagant lies. The truth is, however, that these were not lies. Insects can taste good and are highly nutritious, and in fact, millions of people do eat them. Those people just happen not to live in highly industrialized countries. Why do people in developed countries find insect eating to be so repugnant when so many people in developing countries routinely eat them? As with the abomination of pigs or the sanctification of cows, strong emotions follow from pragmatic judgments about the food in question.

Historically, insects always have been a part of the diet of people living in zoogeographical regions with few large mammals suitable for hunting or domestication. In general, these are tropical zones rather than temperate zones. For example, in the Amazon basin of South America, where few animal domestications took place, anthropologists have identified Indian tribes that gather and eat up to 20 different specific insects, which constitute as much as 14% of their daily protein intake. Another major group of insect eaters are the landless, rural poor, who often cannot afford to keep animals. As such, insect eating is common today in much of Africa and parts of Asia.

Insects are quite nutritious, as the comparative data in Table 3-1 illustrate. They are particularly valuable as a source of protein, since they contain many calories from fat, which spares protein for tissue building rather than for use as energy. For hunter-gatherers, decisions about the quantity and variety of insects to include in their diverse diet were probably based on consideration of the time spent pursuing and capturing a specific food relative to the caloric reward it provided. This would favor the pursuit of rarer items of high nutritive value, such as small mammals, over the pursuit of commoner items of less nutritive value, such as earthworms. However, in times of scarcity, new food items would likely be included in the diet if a favored food item with high nutritive value becomes so rare that the time spent in pursuit of it was perceived as excessive. Under such conditions of scarcity, insects get added to the menu. Not all insects are equally favored though. If one considers the criterion of time invested relative to calories provided, it is not surprising that even today, the insects usually favored in diets of scarcity are the social insects, such as termites and ants, who build large nests with concentrated quantities of larvae and adults, and locusts, who swarm in huge numbers, permitting large accumulations of calories in short periods (see sidebar "Eating Locusts").

In the temperate zones, which include Europe and America, larger mammals have always been relatively abundant, and conditions for raising domesticated livestock are favorable. In addition, swarming insects and large colony-building insects are less common in temperate zones than in the tropics. Therefore, compared with the tropical situation, there was little motivation and comparatively little opportunity for temperate zone people to include insects in their diet.

When a culture decides not to eat something it is not unusual for some favorable or unfavorable value judgment to follow. In the case of the Jews and Muslims, the pig, not used for food, was vilified as an abomination. However, in the case of the Hindus, the cow, not used for food, was revered as a god. The difference lies in the residual value of the animal beyond its

Table 3-1	Comparative Food Values of Various Insects With Hamburger		
Food (100-g portions)	**Calories (approx.)**	**Protein (g)**	**Fat (g)**
Cooked, medium-fat hamburger	245	21	17
African termites	610	38	46
Moth larvae	375	46	10
Housefly pupae	475	63	15
Bee pupae	440	90	8

Adapted from Harris M. Good to Eat. New York: Simon & Schuster, 1985.

Eating Locusts in Uganda

The desert locust, *Schistocera gregaria*, is the swarming locust of the Bible, one of the 10 plagues visited upon the Egyptians to persuade Pharaoh to release the Israelites from slavery. A member of the grasshopper family, the desert locust occurs normally in the arid regions of northern Africa, the Middle East, and southwest Asia. When swarming, the range often extends

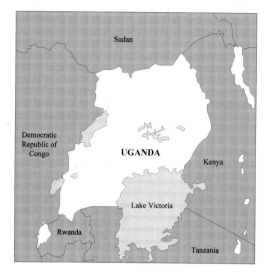

further southward. Normally the desert locust behaves very much as other grasshoppers do. However, under certain environmental conditions, there will be simultaneous hatching of eggs and a short-winged migratory form of the locust will gather into huge swarms, numbering up to 100 billion insects, with up to 80 million insects per square kilometer. Each insect can eat up to 2 g of plant material a day. An invasion of locusts, therefore, wreaks enormous agricultural destruction and subsequent human misery due to lost crops.

While clouds of locusts are a nightmarish threat to farmers with crops in the fields, they can be, at least momentarily, like manna from heaven for the urban poor in Africa. I have seen the locusts come to Kampala, Uganda. They arrived in early evening, blackening the skies in their multitude and obscuring even the light from the street lamps. They rained from the sky and were soon ankle deep in the roads. Almost immediately, throngs of eager people poured into the streets, running to and fro with all manner of containers, furiously stuffing locusts into burlap bags, coffee tins, plastic pails, and pillow cases. Soon the smell of burning charcoal filled the air, and the glow of a thousand curbside fires illuminated the night. Large, circular, blackened metal pans were filled with palm oil and balanced precariously on top of the charcoal fires. All night long, the locusts were brought to the fire tenders for frying. Almost miraculously, by morning there was not an unclaimed locust to be seen lying on the streets. All were fried and carefully spread out on canvas tarps and colorful cloths for sale to passersby. For many days to follow, locusts were being eaten on the streets, enjoyed by children and adults alike. The locust is highly nutritious. On a dry weight basis, it is about 62% protein, 17% fat, and rich in minerals, including copper, iron, and manganese. And yes, they do taste like chicken, but crunchier.

The occasional, impromptu locust feast aside, what is the general quality of life for children in Uganda today? Ugandan babies born in 1996 had an average life expectancy of 44 years. One reason this is so low is that 8 of every 100 children born die before 1 year of age, and almost 15 of every 100 die before the age of 5. Though up to 80% of Uganda's children receive an appropriate complement of childhood vaccinations during their first 2 years, only 65% of them receive adequate nourishment during the same period. In rural areas, only about 30% of the population has access to safe drinking water supplies and sanitary waste disposal. The number of orphaned children in Uganda is unusually high, resulting largely from the HIV/AIDS epidemic of the last 15 years. At the end of 1999, the orphan population in Uganda was reported by the Joint United Nations Program on HIV/AIDS to be 997,426. An estimated 110,000 Ugandans died of AIDS that same year.

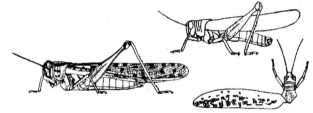

Desert locust phases of development. (From Knauserberger W, ed., Shear B, illus. Crop Protection Clip Art Book, vol 1. The Sahel. Washington, DC: USAID, 1990. Electronic version available copyright free from ICIPE Web site www.icipe.org/clipart.)

value as food. Cows had tremendous value to Hindus as draft animals, so the ban on eating was reinforced by sanctification. The pig had no residual value to the arid zone dweller, rather, it was a food competitor. Therefore, the ban on pigs was reinforced by revulsion. So it is with insects in the western world. Insects are associated with a variety of negative attributes including crop destruction, biting and stinging, transmission of disease, and unwanted invasion of personal space. Not needed for food and threatening in these other ways, insects have come to be culturally despised.

The Keeping of Pets

Seeking personal enjoyment from animals is a human urge that probably found expression about 135,000 years ago, when humans first began to domesticate the dog. Imagine a group of our primitive ancestors seated around the cook fire at night, gorging themselves on a deer or wild pig captured earlier that day. They have been eating for some time and finally begin to feel sated. They relax a bit, when some nearby movement catches their attention. At the periphery of the encampment, faintly illuminated by the fire are some wild jackals, hyenas, wolves or other such canid carnivore, attracted by the aroma of the cooked meat wafting through the night air. The dogs slowly and warily circle the camp when one hunter, seeking to amuse himself, begins pulling scraps of gristle and tendon from the scattered bones of their meal and tosses a scrap toward the animals. First he throws it far away and laughs as he sees the dogs scramble for it. Then he begins tossing the scraps gradually closer, making a game of it to see how close in he can entice these suspicious, but hungry, creatures. Eventually, many campfires later, he actually succeeds in having one of the bolder animals come close enough to take food from his hand. As entertainment, this is capital stuff, but this pioneering hunter, to his surprise, also feels something other than amusement. There is a certain curious satisfaction that comes from this demonstration of mutual trust with the animal, a new emotion, different from the adrenaline-charged feelings the hunter feels in pursuing animals for the kill. A more calming and enriching sensation is induced by this benign contact. This beginning of companionship with non-human creatures has a magical appeal. The sense of bonding it promises feels deeply gratifying. The notion of companion animals is born.

Harris identifies three stages of pet keeping in human societies.[2] The first is simply as entertainment or amusement with no lasting attachment developing between animal and human. There are numerous reports from New World explorers and anthropologists of hunter-gatherer societies in which the men bring home young animals of all types from their hunting forays. The smallest ones were handed to children as living toys, and the larger ones were tethered in the encampment as entertainment for as long as they lasted. In neither case were the animals tended to, fed, or nurtured.

The second stage of pet keeping is physical communion, in which a definite, even intimate, attachment is developed between people and animals, but the relationship does not preclude the subsequent use of the animal as food. It was a regular practice of indigenous Hawaiians to raise dogs and eat them. Yet, the dogs were treated in a manner that expressed strong personal attachment. Women nursed puppies at their own breast. Men commonly carried their dogs with them in their arms or on their backs to social and religious gatherings. The willingness of Hawaiians to eat their dogs, in spite of their obvious attachment to them, reflects the zoogeography and resulting foodways of the Polynesian Islands. There are very few indigenous mammals on the island archipelagoes suitable for hunting, and domesticated herbivores did not reach the islands until modern times. With limited access to animal protein, many Polynesian peoples, including Tahitians and Maoris as well as Hawaiians, were able to culturally accommodate the apparent paradox of enjoying the company of dogs but using them for food as well.

The third stage of pet keeping is spiritual communion, which precludes the use of the animal for food. This is the operative case in most of the western world and especially the United States. Clearly, in contemporary western society, dogs and cats are not needed for food because an unprecedented and abundant array of foodstuffs is available for human consumption. Dogs and cats have always provided useful services to western cultures as hunting companions, sentinels, and pest controllers, so a tradition of eating these animals never developed. This again was reinforced by the availability of alternative game and domesticated animals in temperate regions and the fact that as carnivores, dogs and cats themselves eat high on the food chain and would therefore be costly to raise as food. Today, we collectively expend considerable amounts of money to feed dogs and cats. However, the goal is not to fatten them for the table, but to care for them as friends and family members, with all the respect, rights, and privileges that the status of family member implies.

The reasons that pets, especially dogs and cats, have achieved this special status in western societies are complex, and a thorough discussion is beyond the scope of this book. An excellent analysis of the subject is offered by James Serpell in his book *In the Company of Animals*, which explores historical, psychosocial, and philosophical bases of pet keeping.[7] Justifiably, Serpell sees pet keeping as a healthy expression of human spiritual growth, a shift away from the anthropocentric view that put humans at the center of the universe with dominion over all living things, toward a more egalitarian view of animals and the natural world.

Pet keeping is so strongly established in affluent western cultures that it has come to be perceived as the natural order of things by those who embrace it. However, pet lovers living or working overseas need to be sensitive to the fact that pet keeping is not universal and that many people do not feel any special affection for either dogs or cats. On the contrary, dogs and cats may be reviled or feared for a variety of reasons. In some countries, dogs may have been used by repressive governments in an abusive manner to intimidate people. In the countryside, rabies may be common and rabies control programs nonexistent, so people rightfully fear any approaching dog. In Islam, it is taught that dogs are unclean animals, and though dogs may be used for work, herding or guarding, they are rarely kept as pets in Muslim countries. In Pakistan, for instance, it is not unusual to see children throwing stones at stray dogs on the street, and the furtive demeanor of these thin, often mange-infested dogs suggests that they have come to expect this hostile reception. In a number of Asian countries, including China and South Korea, dogs and cats are still used as food by some segments of society, a practice rooted in a long, past history of food scarcity.

Finally, many people in developing countries just cannot come to terms with the economic investment that westerners make in pet keeping, nor can they, in their own cultural context, understand how we can accord animals a level of care and comfort that they themselves cannot afford to offer to their own human family members or fellow citizens (see sidebar "Babies and Puppies"). In 1995, Americans purchased over $9.3 billion worth of dog and cat food within the United States. This dollar amount exceeds the total annual gross national product (GNP) for 1995 of over 80 countries in the world (Table 3-2). The GNP is a measure of the value of the total output of goods and services for the nation and includes all consumer purchases, private investment, and government spending.

Pet keeping can become symbolic of the disparities in wealth that exist between societies and can be a source of frustration and even anger for people without economic opportunity. In some developing countries, where the extended family remains a strong social institution and pet keeping is viewed as a curiosity, visiting Americans may be asked, "How it is that Americans bring dogs into their houses but put their own parents into nursing homes?" It is a question that does not lend itself to an easy answer, but which genuinely merits consideration. Yet even in the developing world, the habit of pet keeping is on the rise. As the global economy has improved, affluence, education, and increased exposure to other cultures have encouraged increasing numbers of people to consider the

prospect of animals as companions. The practice of pet keeping often finds expression first among the urban elite, who are most likely to have contact with westerners who own pets and to have the financial wherewithal to care for themselves and their pets. In 2000, for instance, a government-sponsored program was established in Taipei, the capital of increasingly affluent Taiwan, which supports the rescue of dogs from the city pound by high school classes. The program teaches schoolchildren respect and responsibility for keeping pets and helps the city to reduce the burden of stray dogs. It also allows children of families living in apartments too small for a pet to experience the pleasure of having a pet at school.

Human-Animal Relationships in Transition

Throughout history, human-animal interactions have been shaped by physical factors of geography and climate, ecological factors such as the variety of species present in a given area, and cultural factors such as religion. Such influences are still operative today. For instance, swine represent an important form of livestock in largely Christian nations in temperate re-

Babies and Puppies in Afghanistan

In 1994, I worked in the Quetta, Pakistan, office of the United Nations Development Program (UNDP) to provide animal health support services to herders and farmers inside Afghanistan. The country had been at war since the Soviets invaded Afghanistan in 1979 to prop up the communist government that had seized power in the capital, Kabul. Virtually the whole nation mobilized against the Soviet-backed government, and the armed resistance, the Mujahadeen, gradually took control of the countryside. Veterinarians who had worked for the government in earlier times were now unable to carry out their duties, because, as government representatives, it was unsafe for them to travel outside the cities and large towns. Many left their positions and fled the country, seeking refuge in Pakistan.

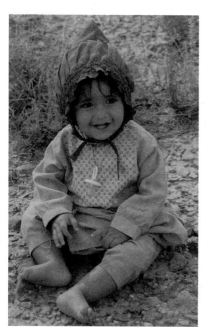

Young Afghan child. (Photo by Dr. David M. Sherman)

Dr. S, who worked in the UNDP Program office with me, was one such Afghan veterinarian. When obliged to abandon his government post, he went straight to the Mujahadeen and worked as a field medic for several years, tending to wounded on the battlefield. In the meantime, his extended family had fled to Pakistan, so he too finally left Afghanistan and crossed into Pakistan seeking work, as he had become the sole supporter of the family. His medical skills helped him to land a job with a relief agency that provided maternal/child health care services to women and children in the Afghan refugee camps in Pakistan. Eventually, he was able to secure a position with the UNDP program, so he could once again work in his chosen profession as a veterinarian. In the UNDP program, Dr. S trained and equipped Afghan paraveterinarians to provide basic animal health care services to farmers and herders, and he traveled inside Afghanistan at regular intervals and at significant risk, to monitor their performance in the field and provide additional on-site training. Dr. S was a conscientious and capable veterinarian. He was a patriot, deeply committed to the liberation of Afghanistan and the health and well-being of its people. He was also a devout Muslim.

The war had been very disruptive for Dr. S. He had obtained his veterinary degree in Kabul and then a masters degree in India. He had hoped to get a Ph.D. in the West and

gions where climate and technology support abundant grain production. Swine remain absent in largely Muslim countries in arid regions with conditions that do not support grain production. Even when the same animal is present in two different societies (e.g., the dog), each society will have its own distinct attitudes and practices toward that same animal. In some societies, the keeping of animals itself is the defining characteristic of the culture, for example, the Maasai cattle herders of East Africa or the Sami reindeer herders of Finland and the Kola Peninsula of Russia.

Today, one factor has emerged that tends to override the traditional influences that have shaped the human-animal relationship within individual cultures throughout history. That factor is industrialization. Industrialization has a strong, generalizing effect on patterns of animal use in the world. The degree to which a society is industrialized and the attendant social transformations that industrialization produces have increasingly come to determine the role of animals in society. Such transformations include the mechanization of agriculture, motorized vehicular transportation systems, increased personal wealth, the shift to urban population centers, the emergence of a dominant middle class, and increased consumer choice in the marketplace. These societal changes pro-

foundly affect the use of animals in society and attitudes toward them. As a result, two broad patterns for the human-animal relationship are identifiable today, one for the industrialized or developed nations and one for the nonindustrialized or less-developed nations.

There is no strict, universally approved, definition of a less-developed country. It is a relative term that suggests a yet unrealized potential for a nation's economic growth, social development, and citizen well-being compared with those of more affluent nations. A variety of terms have been used through the years to draw this comparison: have and have-not nations; rich and poor nations; high-income and low-income nations; developed and developing nations; industrialized and nonindustrialized nations; the North (developed nations) and the South (less-developed nations); and, the First World (developed nations) and the Third World (less-developed nations).

Some examples of criteria used to contrast the status of a nation's economy and its citizens' well-being are given in Table 3-3. Obviously, "developed" and "less-developed" are not absolute categories. Individual nations may be at different stages of economic and social growth that place them in an intermediate or transitional position with regard to overall

teach at the veterinary faculty in Kabul. We had spoken over lunch one day about the difficulties that Afghan refugee veterinarians had staying up to date professionally. There were virtually no continuing education opportunities. It was rare even to find a professional book or journal that was reasonably current. A few weeks later, I received a package from home that contained several recent American veterinary journals. I remembered Dr. S's comments and brought them into his office, offering them for his perusal. He was very grateful and said he would be most happy to look at them.

About 20 minutes later, he came into my office carrying the journals. He looked obviously out of sorts, either distraught or angry. The reason quickly became apparent. He handed me an open journal that contained a full-page advertisement that prominently featured pictures of a human infant side by side with a puppy, with the large-print statement "Like all growing babies, puppies may need special protection, too." Dr. S slumped into the chair across from me, and holding his head in his hands, he said, on the verge of tears, "How can you Americans value the life of a dog equally with that of a child? For Muslims, dogs are unclean. Dogs are nothing here. Children are everything in my culture. When I worked in the refugee camps, I saw dozens of infants die of tetanus because the birth attendant did not have even a small piece of soap to wash her hands or a few drops of iodine to put on the umbilical cord. I saw babies shrivel and die from diarrhea and dysentery, with no clean water or hydration salts to treat them. We have no vaccinations for our children, barely enough to feed them, and you say that a dog deserves the same care as a child? Is the world turned upside down?"

He did not wait for an answer. He stood up, and walked from the room, leaving the journals in a pile on my desk. Though we worked together well for the rest of the year and remained friends, he never referred to his outburst, and he never touched those journals again.

Table 3-2 Countries of the World Whose Annual Gross National Product (GNP) in 1995 Was Less Than the Total Retail Sales of Dog and Cat Food in the United States in 1995 ($9.3 Billion)

Area/Country	$US (billions)	Area/Country	$US (billions)
Asia		**Former Soviet Union**	
Bahrain	4.5	Albania	2.2
Bhutan	0.3	Armenia	2.8
Cambodia	2.7	Azerbaijan	3.6
Laos	1.7	Estonia	4.3
Maldives	0.2	Georgia	2.4
Mongolia	0.8	Kyrgyzstan	3.2
Nepal	4.4	Latvia	5.7
		Lithuania	7.1
Africa		Moldova	4.0
Angola	4.4	Tajikistan	2.0
Benin	2.0	Turkmenistan	4.3
Botswana	4.4		
Burkina Faso	2.4	**Oceania**	
Burundi	1.0	Fiji	1.9
Cameroon	8.6	Micronesia	0.2
Cape Verde	0.4	Papua New Guinea	5.0
Central African Republic	1.1	Solomon Islands	0.3
Chad	1.4	Vanuatu	0.2
Comoros	0.2	Western Samoa	0.2
Congo	1.8		
Democratic Republic of Congo	5.3	**Central America and the Caribbean**	
Equatorial Guinea	0.2	Bahamas	3.6
Ethiopia	5.7	Barbados	1.8
Gabon	3.8	Belize	0.6
Gambia	0.4	Costa Rica	8.9
Ghana	6.7	El Salvador	9.1
Guinea	3.6	Grenada	0.3
Guinea Bissau	0.3	Haiti	1.8
Ivory Coast	9.2	Honduras	3.6
Kenya	7.6	Jamaica	3.8
Lesotho	1.5	Nicaragua	1.7
Madagascar	3.2	Panama	7.2
Malawi	1.6	St. Kitts/Nevis	0.2
Mali	2.4	St. Lucia	0.5
Mauritania	1.0	St. Vincent	0.3
Mauritius	3.8	Trinidad/Tobago	4.8
Mozambique	1.4		
Namibia	3.1	**South America**	
Niger	2.0	Bolivia	5.9
Rwanda	1.1	Guyana	0.5
Sao Tome/Principe	0.1	Paraguay	8.2
Senegal	5.1	Suriname	0.4
Seychelles	0.5		
Sierra Leone	0.8	**Europe and the Middle East**	
Swaziland	1.1	Albania	2.2
Tanzania	3.8	Iceland	6.7
Togo	1.3	Jordan	6.4
Uganda	4.7	Macedonia	1.8
Zambia	3.6	Qatar	7.5
Zimbabwe	6.0	Yemen	4.0

Information from the Pet Food Institute, Washington, D.C., and Wright JW, ed. New York Times 1998 Almanac. New York: Penguin Reference Books, 1998.

Table 3-3 Comparative Characteristics of Developed and Developing Nations	
Developed Nations	**Developing Nations**
Industrial and/or service-based economy	Agricultural and/or natural resource-based economy
Majority of population living in urban/suburban areas	Majority of population living in rural areas
Low percentage of population directly involved in food production	High percentage of population directly involved in food production
Static or slow population growth	Steady or rapid population growth
High gross national product	Low gross national product
High annual per capita income	Low annual per capita income
Well developed communication and transportation infrastructure	Limited communication and transportation infrastructure
High literacy rate	Variable literacy rate
Average life expectancy more than 70 years	Average life expectancy less than 70 years
Widespread access to primary health care	Variable access to primary health care

development, and this will be reflected in the changing status of its human-animal interactions.

Currently, according to the United Nations, there are about 45 countries categorized as developed nations. These are located mainly in Europe and North America and also include Japan, Australia, and New Zealand. As most are in the northern hemisphere, they are sometimes collectively referred to as the North. These are highly industrialized nations with a high standard of living, well-developed infrastructure, and advanced science and technology. They are highly urbanized societies, with only a small proportion of the population directly involved in food production for the society at large, often less than 5% of the workforce.

The United Nations places approximately 125 nations in the less-developed nation category. These are countries with a lower level of industrialization, a lower standard of living, poorly developed infrastructure, and limited access to advanced science and technology. Most people in these nations live in rural areas, and a considerable proportion of the population is directly involved in food production, either at the subsistence or commercial level. This is frequently more than 50% of the total workforce. Most of the less-developed nations are in the southern hemisphere and are sometimes collectively referred to as the South.

The Situation in Less-Developed Countries

When traveling in the less-developed countries of Africa, Asia, Latin America, or the Caribbean, you quickly realize that animals are everywhere in the landscape-part and parcel of everyday life, both urban and rural. Interaction between animals and people are constant and commonplace. Drive along a dusty rural highway in Ethiopia, and you will see drovers on foot leading groups of fattened bullocks down the road to the city

market for sale (Fig. 3-3) or groups of donkeys carrying enormous mounds of sorghum straw on their backs from the harvested fields to the village for use in home construction or to feed livestock. In western Pakistan, you may get stuck on the road behind camels with bells on their ankles, pulling enormously heavy carts full of clay bricks to town from the brickworks. In New Delhi, you may be late for an appointment because your taxi is stuck in traffic made more knotty by cows lying in the main thoroughfare. In downtown Cairo, traffic may be slowed by flocks of urban sheep and goats being herded across the city streets in search of garbage piles in which to forage (Fig. 3-4).

In rural China, sit by the side of the road and you will be passed by young girls on foot with large woven baskets out to collect grass from the roadside to feed their livestock back on the family compound. From the same roadside perch, you may see poultry vendors on bicycles with saddle baskets chock full of live geese and ducks (Fig. 3-5), or a farmer off to market with an adult hog ingeniously, though not very humanely, tied to the frame of his bicycle. If you can sit until evening, you are likely to see tired peasants walking their water buffaloes back home after a day's work of plowing in the rice fields outside the village.

On the mountain roads of Guatemala, you would see chicle gatherers returning from the rainforest, their donkeys loaded with the natural gum. In Myanmar, it might be working Asian elephants dragging bundled logs out of the teak plantations to the roadside for pickup. In Zimbabwe, you will see throngs of rubber-tired carts on the red dirt roads, hauling people or goods, all pulled by thin, tired-looking horses. In southern Afghanistan, with no other vehicles around for miles, you still might have to come to a full stop as a group of Koochi nomads crosses the highway with enormous flocks of sheep and goats,

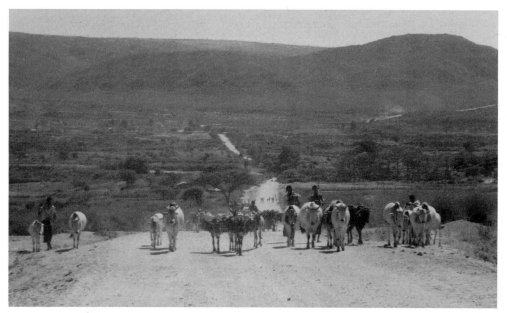

Figure 3-3. Cattle being driven long distances to market on foot in eastern Ethiopia. (Photo by Dr. David M. Sherman)

along with dozens of camels and donkeys piled high with their possessions, including children and baby lambs, still too young or frail to make it on foot. In northern Afghanistan, you might see farmers using oxen to thresh grain (Fig. 3-6).

Follow farmers in almost any less-developed nation to the town market and you will see all manner of live animals offered for sale as food. Where refrigeration is uncommon, smaller animals such as poultry, rabbits, guinea pigs, or cane rats are frequently offered live for sale or slaughtered at the time of purchase. In some places, you may be shocked or outraged by what you find offered for sale as food. In Cameroon, you might see a primate head set in front of a market stall, advertising smoked gorilla or chimpanzee meat for sale inside.[3] In South Korea you might find the traditional dog meat soup, *poshintang*, on a restaurant menu, though this is increasingly unlikely because of government sensitivity to growing international outcry against the use of dogs as food and an increase in animal welfare activism within South Korea itself (see http://www.kore-ananimals.org/dogs.htm).

Travel to rural villages in much of Africa and south Asia and you will be struck by the ubiquity of goats. They are lying under parked buses to avoid the afternoon sun or may be tied to the top of the bus, as so much additional luggage. They wander freely around the main streets, sometimes slyly, but often boldly, snatching vegetables and greens from the produce displays of vendors seated on the ground. Incredible as it may seem to the outsider, ownership of these free-roaming goats is well established. Groups of male goats may be seen butting heads on the verandahs of shops, establishing their pecking order, while the occasional, unfortunate, tethered goat waits forlornly in front of the butcher shop, destined for slaughter. In Muslim

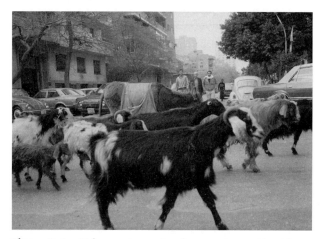

Figure 3-4. Urban goats crossing the street in a residential neighborhood of central Cairo, Egypt. (Photo courtesy of Dr. Laurie C. Miller)

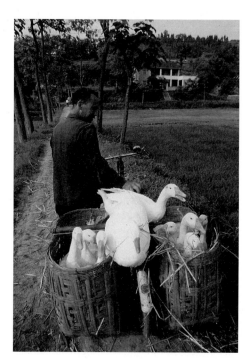

Figure 3-5. Geese going to market by bicycle in China. (Photo courtesy of Heifer Project International, Little Rock, Arkansas. Photographer, Matt Bradley)

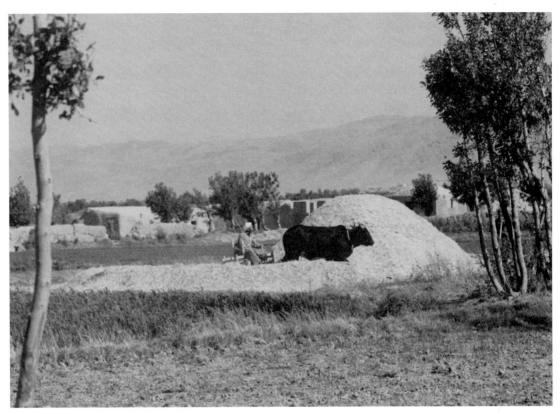

Figure 3-6. Farmer threshing wheat by use of a weighted pallet pulled by an ox outside of Herat, Afghanistan. (Photo by Dr. David M. Sherman)

countries, during the month of Zil-Hajj, the streets of villages may literally run red with the blood of goats and sheep ritually slaughtered for the holiday feasting of Eid-ul-Adha, which commemorates the willingness of Abraham to sacrifice his son to God.

Go to a farm in a less-developed nation and you will be surprised by the variety of animals present. Diversification rather than specialization is the strategy of most of the world's subsistence farmers. A fortunate farm family may own a draft animal for farm work or to transport goods to market. This might be an ox, a donkey, a horse, a buffalo, or a camel, depending on location. Even if they do not have a draft animal, they are likely to have small flocks of mixed poultry including chickens, ducks, turkeys, and/or geese. Depending on their religion, they may have a sow with piglets kept in a wallow near the house and fed household garbage or agricultural refuse. Alternatively, they may have some small ruminant stock, sheep and/or goats, which often sleep with the farm family at night to reduce the risk of theft or predation. There may be some rabbits in cages or, in Peru, perhaps guinea pigs. In the Middle East, it might be pigeons.

Entertainment in the less-developed countries may also frequently involve animals. In the Philippines, you might come upon a crowd of village men gathered together in a tight circle to watch and wager on a cock fight to the death between two aggressive and brightly colored roosters, each armed with a sharpened steel spur. In the Afghan refugee camps in Pakistan, the bird fighting competition is between Chukar partridges rather than roosters. The birds are not armed, and both birds, doted on by their owners, live to compete again. Inside Afghanistan itself, you might see teams of men on horseback playing the rugged, rugbylike game of *buzkashi*, in which two loosely organized teams of competing riders try to take possession of a headless dead calf and break free of the pack to score a goal. The game is often seen as a metaphor for Afghan culture itself—fierce, individualistic competition played out in the context of cautious but necessary cooperation. Many cultures have traditional annual festivals that revolve around animals. If you arrive at the right time, you can witness remarkable displays of equestrian skill at yearly celebrations in Tibet or Mongolia. On the Indonesian island of Madura, you can watch the annual bull races; on the island of Tobago in the Caribbean, the annual goat races.

The purpose of this brief travelogue is to convey how animals continue to fulfill important, practical daily functions for vast numbers of people throughout the developing world-people whose lives have not been transformed by industrialization and the economic development it spawns. Thus, where tractors and other mechanized farm equipment are scarce, animals are still widely used for plowing, threshing, or drawing water for irrigation. Where roads are poor and trucks uncommon, animals are still used to transport goods to market. Where private cars are unavailable or beyond the means of average citizens, people continue to move around on the backs of animals or in carts pulled by them.

Where farms remain small, conditions remain difficult, and life is precarious, farmers plant a variety of crops and raise several types of livestock to minimize risks of failure due to drought or disease and to provide diverse food supplies and possible cash income for their families. Where chemical fertilizers are expensive and supplies limited, animal manure still serves to enrich the soil. Where electricity does not reach homes, animal manure is used for cooking fires (Fig. 3-7). Where banks are nonexistent or untrustworthy, livestock serve as living savings accounts. Where veterinary services are unavailable or costly and animal protein in the diet is limited, sick livestock often are quickly slaughtered for food, and even dead animals are willingly eaten, despite public health risks such as anthrax. Where commercially prepared pet food is hardly conceivable, let alone available, dogs and cats may be chronically malnourished and often survive by their wits. Where television sets or radios are rare, animals persist as a source of recreation and entertainment.

For many people in the developing world then, animals mean livelihood or survival—as food, as labor, as transport, as a source of fuel, as liquid capital, as insurance against destitution, and, occasionally, as diversion. For such people, who are figuratively, if not literally, in harness with animals every day of their lives, the attitude toward their animal companions is largely utilitarian, practical, and unsentimental. This is not to say uncaring. It is clearly in the interest of those who critically depend on animals to care for them, and most people do. They can do so, however, only within the limits that their resources and circumstances allow. Unfortunately, these circumstances are often constrained and sometimes dire. Therefore,

the level of care received by some animals in the less-developed world may be shocking to animal lovers from developed countries who are unfamiliar with the hardships that daily confront most of the world's people.

Consider, for example, a poor citizen of Quetta, Pakistan, a married man with five children of his own and also responsible for the wife and four children of his deceased brother. A poor and illiterate, but decent and God-fearing man, his sole means of livelihood is a donkey and a wooden cart available for hire. After weeks of bad luck, he has been able to find temporary work hauling loads of lumber along the airport road on the outskirts of the city to a building construction site in the center of town. He travels back and forth on the airport road with the donkey and is paid per load. If he works steadily, for 10 hours each day, he can earn about 100 rupees per diem, a little over US$3.00. The donkey, who is thin to begin with, is having a tough go of it. The harness straps have been rubbing over his back and have broken the skin over the withers. A festering wound has developed and is quite painful, but every time the donkey balks and attempts to rest, the man snaps his whip on the donkey's neck and exhorts the donkey to keep moving.

Finally, on the morning of the 9th day of this routine, the donkey collapses on the road and refuses to get up. The man is in a panic. He has a dozen mouths to feed, his landlord is threatening eviction, and his brother's youngest son is ill. He has earned only 30 rupees so far today, and that simply will not do. He knows the donkey needs rest and its wounds need attention, but these are acts of kindness the man cannot see clear to offer. The consequences of idleness right now are just too onerous for him to imagine. He hollers at the donkey to get up and begins to strike at him repeatedly on the rump with a piece of lumber pulled hastily from the cart. Just then, a group of western tourists passing in an air-conditioned, hotel courtesy bus, observe this desperate man and his suffering donkey in their painful drama of shared misery. As the foreigners pass this scene, they burst forth in a heated chorus of indignation and protest against the callousness of this dreadful man beating his donkey.

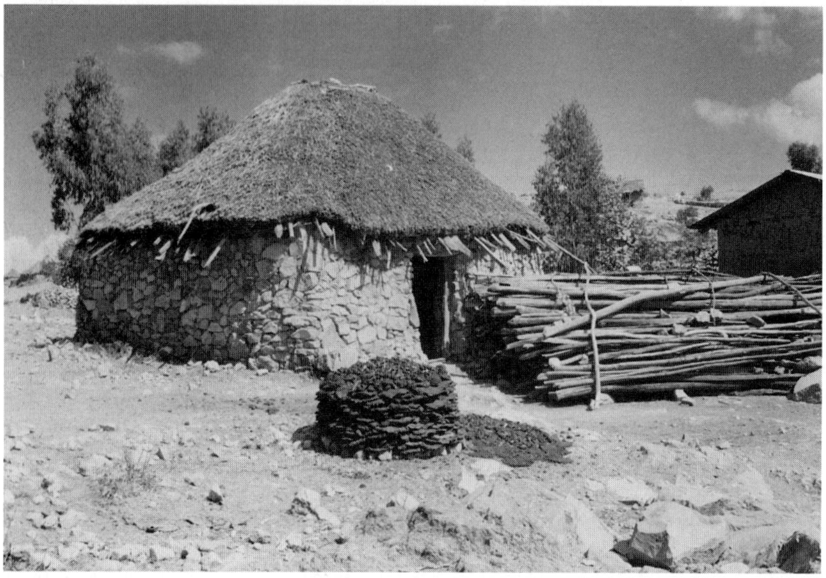

Certainly, this donkey was suffering and abused. The objective evidence is clear. Nevertheless, it remains difficult to pass judgment fairly on the character or behavior of the man. Sympathy for the animal, without empathy for the man, is itself another form of callousness. In the developing world, improvements in the welfare of animals can only be meaningful and lasting if they are linked to the social and economic development of the people who care for, and critically depend on, those animals (see sidebar "Pity the Poor Donkeys").

Figure 3-7. A neat stack of dried manure cakes to be used for cooking sits in front of a hut in rural Ethiopia. The rough lumber shown in the picture is too scarce and therefore too valuable to use as fuel. It will be used in building construction. (Photo by Dr. David M. Sherman)

Pity the Poor Donkeys

Probably no other domesticated animal in the world experiences the hardships known by the donkey. Today, as it has for millennia, the donkey serves as the principal beast of burden for the world's poorest people. The suffering of the donkey is especially poignant, in that the animal is intelligent, gentle, and patient and endures its hardships with a noble grace and humility that call forth our compassion and respect.

There are at least 44 million donkeys, or asses, in the world at present. The vast majority are in the developing world, particularly in those nations of Africa, Asia and Latin America with mountainous terrain and a semiarid climate. Donkeys are used primarily to carry loads, either directly on their backs or by pulling carts and wagons. The weight and bulk of these loads often appear preposterous. Donkeys are also used for plowing and other farm work, often filling in for oxen that have died during conditions of drought, which the donkeys are better able to survive.

The donkey's lot is often difficult, at best. Donkey owners usually have few resources to allocate to the well-being of their animals, let alone themselves. Feed for donkeys is often limited to poor-quality grass or straw with no supplementation. Donkeys usually carry heavy burdens of internal parasites and rarely receive effective anthelmintic therapy. As a result of poor diet and parasitism they are usually very thin, with no fat cover and little muscle mass. Consequently, they commonly develop skin abrasions from harnesses, saddles, and pack

Donkey clinic at the University of Addis Ababa Faculty of Veterinary Medicine, Debre Zeit, Ethiopia, supported by the International Donkey Protection Trust (IDPT). (Photo by Dr. David M. Sherman)

frames, which often lead to deep, festering wounds. Poorly designed equipment exacerbates this problem, for example, poorly designed carts and harnesses that make the donkey pull from the neck rather than the chest.

The International Donkey Preservation Trust (IDPT) is a charitable organization established in the U.K. in 1976 by Dr. Elizabeth Svendsen, M.B.E. to reduce suffering in the world's donkeys, increase awareness of their condition, and provide help to their owners to improve the well-being of the animal and the people who depend on them. The IDPT currently has four in-country programs in addition to their activities in the U.K. in association with its parent organization, The Donkey Sanctuary. The countries include Ethiopia, Kenya, Mexico, and Jamaica. A main activity of country programs is to provide veterinary services for donkeys through clinics managed by the IDPT, especially for internal parasite control and wound management. In Ethiopia, the IDPT clinic is at the University of Addis Ababa, Faculty of Veterinary Medicine, in Debre Zeit. This affiliation with the veterinary faculty allows veterinary students to develop awareness and expertise concerning the problems of the donkey during their professional training. Public awareness and educational campaigns are also undertaken by

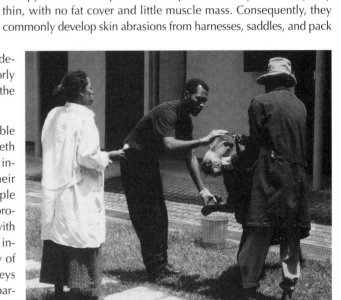

Staff treating a farmer's donkey for an infected traumatic injury of the head at the IDPT clinic in Ethiopia. (Photo by Dr. David M. Sherman)

IDPT, including efforts to encourage the passage and enforcement of legislation to encourage humane treatment of donkeys. In addition, the IDPT supports research into improved harness, saddle, and pack frame design to reduce trauma and stress on working donkeys. The Donkey Sanctuary website is www.thedonkeysanctuary.org.uk.

The Situation in Developed Countries

By comparison, in the developed world today, animals are scarce in the landscape. In the cities and on the highways, beasts of burden have essentially disappeared, fully replaced by motorized vehicles in just the last 60 years. Animals are usually banned from modern highways and city streets as dangerous traffic hazards. The urban horse-drawn carriage has become a nostalgic tourist attraction, carefully regulated and restricted to city parks and specific routes. The occasional mounted police officer may be observed in the city. While still useful in crowd control, they are often present as a concession to tradition. Even pet animals, though present in urban areas in large numbers, are not widely seen. For reasons of health, sanitation, and decorum, laws prohibit the unrestricted movement of dogs and cats on the streets, and salaried animal control officers are present and equipped to impound stray animals. If you see a pack of dogs on a city street, they are all likely to be leashed and under the control of a professional dog-walker. To see cats, you might have to look upward at the high-rise buildings and notice them perched on the window ledges. On the occasional rooftop, you might notice a pigeon fancier exercising a flock of birds. Food-producing animals are essentially nonexistent in the cities, again because of zoning and health restrictions, though many of the urban poor might welcome chickens or goats into their neighborhoods. In supermarkets, well-equipped with refrigerators and freezers, it is rare to see live animals, except lobsters, for sale as food.

Travel to the suburbs and the situation is essentially the same. Draft animals and livestock are virtually nonexistent, and pet animals are largely restricted to homes and fenced yards or contained by electric shock collars. Many suburbanites are now more likely to have contact with wild herbivores and omnivores than domesticated ones, as suburban growth and development extends into previously rural areas. Deer wander into vegetable gardens from nearby woodlands, bears break into kitchens, raccoons crawl out of sewers to turn over garbage cans, and skunks dig holes in suburban lawns in search of grubs. Beavers arrive at a nearby pond and threaten to flood portions of the new country club golf course, while duffers navigate gingerly through a veritable minefield of Canadian goose droppings.

Drive out of the suburbs to the countryside, and still the relative lack of animals is evident. Many small commercial farms have ceased to operate. Pastures that once contained herds of commercial livestock now sit empty, awaiting development for nonagricultural purposes, or are simply reverting to brush. A few farms, near to cities, may be converted to horse facilities for recreational purposes. The horses also fulfill an aesthetic function. It is surprising how hungry the eye becomes for the image of four-legged creatures grazing in a green, fenced field.

Even in rural areas where livestock production is thriving, the animals are becoming invisible to passersby. The raising of animals for food in much of the developed world is becoming increasingly consolidated and moving indoors. The number of animals raised for food is tremendous, but they are kept in fewer herds and flocks of larger size, with fewer people directly involved in livestock production. For example, between 1985 and 1995, the number of hog producers in North Carolina fell from 23,000 to 8,000, but in the same period, hog production in the state tripled. These changes result from the implementation of intensified management practices that include total confinement housing of production animals in climate-controlled buildings and the feeding of scientifically formulated rations tailored to specific production needs.

Swine and poultry production have been especially transformed by intensive management, and these practices are becoming more common in dairy production as well. Beef cows and their calves are still seen on pastures and grazing lands, but steers also are finished for market under intensive management conditions in large feedlots. When any of these animals or their products go to market, it is not on foot, but in enclosed trucks. When they appear in retail stores, it is increasingly in processed and packaged forms that are difficult to link with the animal of origin. A shrink-wrapped, Styrofoam package containing chicken breast meat with both the skin and the bone removed evokes little connection with the living and breathing birds which produced that flesh.

So it has come to be that the vast majority of people living in the developed world no longer have any direct contact with animals that produce food or perform work. This disassociation has occurred within the last century, largely as a result of the intensification of agriculture, the mechanization of labor and transportation, and the shift of populations from rural to urban centers. Now, when people in the developed world have direct, daily contact with animals, that contact is most often with dogs and cats, animals that essentially have been integrated into the human household and are loved and cared for as family members.

This relationship with companion animals is, however, essentially sentimental. The notion of sentimentality is used here in a positive sense, meaning that the relationship with the companion animal is influenced more by emotion than by reason and that the relationship inspires people to act on their feelings about animals rather than from purely practical motives. This is in sharp contrast to the practical and largely unsentimental attitudes toward animals that still prevail in much of the less-developed world, where peoples' lives are often lived close to the bone, and the exploitation of animals remains a critical element in the physical survival of many human beings.

The Challenge of Changing Attitudes

In the developed countries then, the sentimentality that people feel in their relationships with companion animals is emerging as the paradigm that defines their relationship toward all types of animals. This paradigm affirms the dignity of an animal by affording it essentially equal status in a mutual partnership with humans, while meeting a human need for interaction, caring, and play with other sentient beings. It acknowledges an animal's capacity for feeling and expression, and it conveys respect for the animal as an individual. As the vast majority of citizens in developed countries no longer have any direct contact with domestic animals used primarily for food or work or with wild animals that may threaten their crops or families, there is little in their own experience to suggest that this new paradigm may not be universally appropriate or applicable in all other societies or even to other segments within their own society.

Given the long history of human exploitation of animals, this new, sentimental perspective is nothing short of revolutionary. As with any revolution, its supporters can range from the zealous and doctrinaire to the level headed and pragmatic. Such is the case with regard to the human-animal relationship, where expression of support for the new paradigm ranges from the criminal destruction of animal research facilities by radical groups, with loss of life, to the quieter and more personal choice by caring individuals to adopt a vegetarian diet. Regardless of the mode of expression, issues surrounding animal welfare and animal rights have become rallying points for public discussion, social activism, and legislative lobbying within the mainstream of western societies. The general trend is toward decreased tolerance for the exploitation of animals by humans. This is already having profound effects on how many developed countries view the use of all types of animals, not just companion animals.

Among the more prominent issues drawing attention and action are the use of animals for food and the conditions under which food animals are kept. Some people have begun to question altogether the exploitation of animals for food of any sort, even if the animal does not have to be killed to produce the food, for example, milk. More-moderate voices call for a re-examination of the conditions under which food-producing animals are managed in "factory farms." Particular attention has been drawn to veal calf, poultry, and swine production systems, and their effect on the animals' well-being. The conditions of transport of livestock to market and their treatment at slaughter are also increasingly scrutinized for evidence of animal neglect and suffering.

Social concern about the conditions under which animals are raised, managed, and used extends beyond animals used for food. The conditions of exploitation of fur-bearing animals has evoked criticism. This includes industry practices for the handling of domesticated animals such as mink as well as harvesting and trapping practices for wild animals such as seals and beaver. The wearing of fur garments has been essentially stigmatized in the United States. The use and treatment of animals in medical research and product testing has also received extensive public attention, resulting in legislation leading to greater oversight of laboratory animal care and spurring a search for effective, alternative research methods and models that do not use animals.

The welfare of companion animals themselves is also an issue. More people are choosing not to declaw housecats or to dock tails or trim ears on their dogs just to conform to a particular breed standard. There has been public outcry over the poor treatment of dogs in so-called puppy mills, the large-scale, commercial facilities that provide puppies for the pet shop industry. In the recreational world of horses, traditional practices have come under scrutiny, such as soring Tennessee Walking Horses to induce their characteristic high-stepping gait. Rodeos have been picketed as inhumane to horses and other livestock, and animal welfare advocates have campaigned aggressively to outlaw all forms of blood sport involving animals, notably bull fighting, dog fighting, and cock fighting. Even racing has come under scrutiny. Recently, in Massachusetts, animal welfare advocates, concerned about the treatment of racing greyhounds, sponsored a referendum on the state ballot to outlaw greyhound racing altogether.

The compassionate stance concerning animals extends beyond domestic animals to wildlife as well. Through contemporary print and electronic media, citizens of the developed world are barraged with images and information concerning the lives of wild animals and the threats wild animal species face throughout the world. These stories evoke strong emotional responses. As a result, there is unprecedented financial support for wildlife conservation organizations, broad support for legislation to protect endangered species, and increased public awareness of the links between wild animal survival, habitat destruction, and human activity. Animals in zoos have also benefited from this increased awareness and activism, with greater public interest and financial support allowing zoo managers to remove animals from cages and offer them more-natural habitats to live in. Many zoos also have responded by expanding their education and wildlife conservation programs.

Of course, no society speaks with one unified voice, nor should it be expected to. Within developed nations, contradictory tendencies persist concerning human attitudes toward animals. Often, there is a notable discrepancy between rhetoric and reality. Collectively, we voice concern over the welfare of food-producing animals but continue to eat meat in substantial amounts. Paradoxically, we have reduced our level of beef consumption because of health concerns but have largely replaced the deficit with increased consumption of pork and poultry, thus increasing the demand for meat supplied by the very industries usually singled out for "factory farm" abuses. We decry the plight of wild species facing extinction in developing nations but increasingly view the wildlife in our own suburbs as nuisances and pests. Furthermore, we indirectly encourage the poaching and smuggling of threatened species through our growing appetite for increasingly exotic companion animals, including rare parrots, tropical fish, snakes, and lizards. While we proclaim the dignity of animals and have ceased to exploit them for work, we now exploit and demean them in new ways for profit, notably in the entertainment industry.

Redefining the human relationship with animals is obviously a work in progress. A lot of sorting out remains to be done, as different societies and different groups within societies evaluate competing needs, interests, attitudes, and goals. This is true within a given society but even more challenging between different societies. The needs and priorities of developing countries with regard to the use of animals are strikingly different from those of developed countries. It would not be an exaggeration to say that many of the ideas expressed by citizens in developed nations concerning the welfare of domesticated animals or the conservation of wild animals would be perceived as hostile by citizens of the developing world because these ideas appear to put the well-being of animals before their own well-being.

Veterinarians themselves are not of one mind on issues concerning the use of animals in society. When the ban on greyhound racing came to the ballot in Massachusetts, there were veterinarians speaking out publicly and with sincere conviction on both sides of the argument. Importantly, these veterinarians, regardless of their position on the issue, recognized the professional responsibility that veterinarians have to address issues concerning the use of animals and animal well-being in society and to assume a leadership role in public debate surrounding such issues. Surveys in the United States have indicated that the public holds veterinarians in high regard with respect to their knowledge, professionalism, and integrity. People look to veterinarians for guidance on complex issues involving animals. As societies work through their shift in attitudes concerning the use and status of animals, veterinarians need to be in the forefront, leading the debate, not only as respected community members, but as scientists, able to inform the debate with the results of scientific inquiry on issues of animal well-being. In the global context, particularly with regard to the role of animals in developing countries, veterinarians must be dispassionate, careful to balance the needs of people who depend on animals for their livelihood against the needs of the animals themselves. The welfare of both people and animals must be considered together.

Discussion Points

1. Goats are an important form of livestock in much of the developing world. Even in the developed world, particularly in Europe, a sizable dairy goat industry exists. In the United States, however, goat numbers are insignificant compared with other major livestock species. Except for an Angora fiber goat industry in the Edwards Plateau region of Texas, goats contribute relatively little to the national economy. What are the historical, cultural, physical, and economic factors that resulted in the marginalization of the goat in American life? How and why did the specialized Angora goat industry take hold in Texas? What new markets and opportunities exist to expand goat production in the United States today?

2. You graduate from veterinary school and join the Peace Corps. You are assigned to an upcountry region in Ghana to work on a women's poultry cooperative project. Shortly after arriving, you befriend a stray dog in the village where you are living. After a few days the dog is living in your house and you have developed a companionable relationship with it, typical of what you would do back in the United States. It becomes evident however that the villagers find your behavior to be quite extraordinary, and your relationship with the dog has become a major topic of conversation. What might be some of the villagers' issues concerning your relationship with the dog? How would you explain your relationship with the dog to them? Would you keep the dog?

3. People in the developed world continue to consume vast quantities of meat but also express concern about the management conditions under which meat-producing animals are kept. Most people also expect meat to be available at low prices. Issues of ethics are often weighed against economics. Is it possible to improve the welfare of meat-producing animals significantly and still deliver the same volume of product without increasing the consumer price significantly? Is society at large prepared to pay a higher price in exchange for knowing that food animals are being treated more humanely?

4. Do you eat insects? If not, why not? Is their anything that you are comfortable eating based on your background or experience that others around you might find objectionable? Discuss the reasons why. Identify a country in which insects or rodents contribute to the food supply, and formulate a development project for managed production of insects or rodents to improve food security.

5. Why is it more likely that South Koreans will abandon the tradition of eating dogs than that Cameroonians will abandon the practice of eating primates? In the current, integrated global economy, why is international pressure more likely to influence the former rather than the latter nation's behavior?

6. Identify some examples of recent legislation, proposed or enacted, that reflect growing societal concerns for the welfare of domestic or wild animals. As a veterinarian, do you support or oppose the legislation you have identified? Identify a classmate or colleague with an opposing view and, working together, draft the wording for a legislative proposal on the subject that is acceptable to both of you.

References

1. Dunlop RH, Williams DJ. Veterinary Medicine, an Illustrated History. St. Louis: Mosby, 1996.

2. Harris M. Good to Eat: Riddles of Food and Culture. New York: Simon & Schuster, 1985.

3. McRae M. Road kill in Cameroon. Nat Hist 1997;106(1):36–47,74,75.

4. Rowland B. Animals with Human Faces: A Guide to Animal Symbolism. Knoxville: The University of Tennessee Press, 1973.

5. Sahi T. Genetics and epidemiology of adult-type hypolactasia. Scand J Gastroenterol 1994;29(Suppl 202):7–20.

6. Schwabe CW. Cattle, Priests, and Progress in Medicine. Minneapolis: University of Minnesota Press, 1978.

7. Serpell J. In the Company of Animals: A Study of Human-Animal Relationships. Oxford: Basil Blackwell, 1986.

Suggested Readings

Harris M. Cows, Pigs, Wars and Witches: The Riddles of Culture. New York: Random House, 1974.

Harris M. Cannibals and Kings: The Origins of Cultures. New York: Random House, 1977.

Manning A, Serpell J, eds. Animals and Human Society. London: Routledge, 1994.

Menzel P, D'Aluisio F. Man Eating Bugs: The Art and Science of Eating Insects. Berkeley, CA: Ten Speed Press, 1998.

Simoons FJ. Eat Not of This Flesh: Food Avoidances from Prehistory to the Present. 2nd Ed. Madison: University of Wisconsin Press, 1994.

Singer P. Animal Liberation. A New Ethics for our Treatment of Animals. New York: Avon Books, 1977.

Chapter 4
Animal Agriculture and Food Production Worldwide

OBJECTIVES FOR THIS CHAPTER

After completing this chapter, the reader should be able to

- Recognize the diverse roles of animals in agriculture and daily life, particularly in developing countries

- Appreciate how climate, landscape, and culture affect animal health and husbandry practices

- Identify the various animal management systems used by farmers and herders worldwide

- Discern the relative merits of local (indigenous) and imported (exotic) breeds of livestock

- Understand the different approaches available for improving animal health and productivity

Introduction

As discussed in Chapter 2, the domestication of animals began in earnest during the Neolithic era, often in relation to the development of crop agriculture. For the next 10,000 or so years, domesticated animals played an integral part in the daily lives of most of the world's people. The Industrial Revolution, which began in the mid-18th century, changed that relationship dramatically, as mechanization in all facets of human activity began to reduce the direct dependence of people on domesticated animals. Nevertheless, in developing countries,

where the effects of industrialization have not been as pervasive, a large proportion of the human population continues to reside in rural areas and is still directly responsible for their own food production. For these people, livestock continue to provide many of the goods and services with which they have been traditionally associated since the time of domestication.

While many of the functions of animals in human society have been diminished by technological advances, one traditional use strongly persists—the use of animals as food. Global demand for foods of animal origin increased steadily over the last half of the 20th century and continues unabated. Meeting this growing demand for foods of animal origin has strongly influenced how animals are raised and, importantly, how they will be raised in the future. In 1999, the world's population reached 6 billion people, and it is expected to reach 7.2 billion by 2010. Most of this population increase will occur in developing countries, particularly in urban centers within these developing countries. It is estimated that demand for meat will grow by 0.6% per annum in developed countries and 2.8% per annum in developing countries, while demand for dairy products is projected to grow at 3.3% per annum over the next decade. Significant challenges exist to meeting this relentless demand. Veterinarians will play a pivotal role in meeting these challenges by developing new approaches for improved animal health and productivity around the world.

For veterinarians to work effectively in animal agriculture in a global context, they must appreciate the diversity of approaches to livestock production that still exist in the world today. Veterinarians must be cognizant of the underlying influences and constraints that dictate the persistence of traditional approaches to livestock keeping and must understand the factors that determine acceptance of, or resistance to, change among animal keepers around the world. They must recognize when technology transfer between the developed and developing word is appropriate and beneficial and when it is not. To assist in creating such awareness, this chapter provides a review of the following topics: factors that influence the use of different types of livestock in different locations, the pattern of distribution of the world's livestock species, the varied uses of animals and animal products, the types of management systems under which animals are kept, constraints that exist on animal production, and different approaches to improving animal production, including improvement of animal health.

Factors Influencing the Agricultural Use of Animals

The various species of domesticated livestock are not uniformly distributed around the world. A variety of factors determine their presence in different locations. Among these factors are history, culture, geography, climate, economic conditions, and the physiological adaptability of the animal themselves.

History

The presumed geographic origins of the various species of domesticated animals were shown in Figure 2.1. Over time, domesticated species spread from their centers of origin to new regions. This process occurred either gradually or abruptly, depending on historical circumstances. The introduction of cattle from the Near East into Europe, for example, occurred gradually over millennia, as climate change, expanding human populations, degraded agricultural lands, armed conflicts, and later, commerce and trade, pushed people northward and

westward with their livestock. Similarly, the domestic pig and chicken spread gradually from their centers of origin in Asia.

In contrast, the period of exploration, global navigation, and colonization that began in Europe in about the 15th century led to the abrupt introduction of domesticated animals into new lands. In the case of South America, for example, cattle and other domestic species were introduced during the period of Spanish exploration and conquest in the 16th century. In Australia, cattle and sheep were introduced in the late 18th century, in association with the establishment of the British penal colony there. In both South America and Australia, cattle keeping, and sheep raising took hold because the local conditions, notably, extensive grasslands, were amenable to the establishment of cattle and sheep industries.

Likewise, the introduction of new types or breeds of livestock occurred throughout the period of colonization of Asia and Africa by Europeans, particularly in the 19th and early 20th centuries. European settlers often recognized landscapes and climates that suggested conditions suitable for commercial farming activities similar to those they knew at home. Even near the equator, highland plateaus or hill country could offer milder temperatures, adequate rainfall, and suitable grazing conditions for high-producing dairy cattle imported from Europe, and commercial dairy farming became established in places such as South Africa, Kenya, and India.

Some modern introductions have become anachronistic. Camels were introduced into Australia in the mid-19th century, with the idea that they would be useful in the development of the arid regions of the country and help to link the more developed east with the developing west. The camels were used in the construction of the overland telegraph and the transcontinental railway, and they provided reliable transport to railheads for wool from remote sheep stations. Many camels became feral, and wild herds reached numbers as high as 100,000. Police in the outback patrolled on camelback as late as the 1950s. Today, however, the use of camels has been superseded by mechanized transport and the development of highways, and their role has been relegated to recreational uses such as camel racing and tourist safaris.

Culture and Religion

As discussed at length in Chapter 3, culture and religion greatly influence which species of animals are used in a given society and for what purposes. India, for instance, with close to 1 billion people, has the highest cattle populations of any nation in the world, yet also has one of the lowest per capita rates of beef consumption, because the slaughter and eating of cattle is prohibited in Hinduism. Yet cattle remain critically important to the agricultural economy of that nation by providing much-needed draft power for the cultivation of small farmers' croplands.

Such cultural influences on the use of animals are widespread. In some parts of Africa, farmers would not dream of plowing with a single ox, convinced that a pair of oxen is essential for the task. In other parts of Africa, certain tribes will not work with cattle at all, believing that it suggests an inferior social status. Likewise, some groups perceive goat's milk as having medicinal properties, while others consider it unpalatable for any reason. Clearly, the success of efforts to improve animal production will depend in good measure on a basic understanding of the cultural and religious preferences of the society involved. Cross-cultural education is a necessary prerequisite to any such effort.

Geography and Climate

Geography and climate are important factors in defining the distribution of livestock species and their use. Among the important features that determine the presence of domestic animals in a given region are rainfall, temperature, terrain, and vegetation cover. In turn, these factors may be influenced by other important variables such as soil type, altitude, humidity, and day length. Overall, these factors are used to define different agroclimatic zones on the earth.

Rainfall is a key determinant of the species of domesticated animals present in an area. The pattern and amount of rainfall strongly determines the existence and types of vegetation cover that are possible in a region. This, in turn, influences land use patterns for that region, such as the grazing of animals versus the planting of crops. In many natural grassland areas, rainfall is neither sufficient nor distributed appropriately to support the growing of crops, but it will support growth of indigenous vegetation such as grasses, forbs, and shrubs. In such areas, the grazing of ruminant animals, capable of converting natural vegetation to animal protein, represents the only human use of that land for the purpose of food production. Approximately 60% of the world's land mass is composed of grasslands and rangelands. By comparison, only 11% of the world's land mass is suitable for crop agriculture, which underscores the vital importance that grazing animals have in expanding the capacity of the Earth to feed people.

Sere and Steinfeld of the Food and Agriculture Organization of the United Nations (FAO) have classified the world's agroclimatic zones with special reference to livestock production systems. In their classification, growing season is used as the frame of reference, with growing season being a function primarily of rainfall volume and pattern, balanced against the rate of evapotranspiration, the latter being an important factor in determining the availability of soil moisture.[20] The following categories are defined:

- Arid: Growing period of less than 75 days
- Semiarid: Growing period in the range of 75 to 180 days
- Subhumid: Growing period in the range of 181 to 270 days
- Humid: Growing period of more than 270 days

As temperature and day length also influence the length of the growing season, geographical location is also factored into classification schemes for patterns of livestock distribution and use. Hence, the following categories are included:

- Tropics: The region of the world lying between the Tropic of Cancer (23°26' North latitude) and the Tropic of Capricorn (23°26' South latitude), an area generally characterized by persistently warm temperatures and minimal seasonal fluctuation in day length.
- Subtropics: Regions of the world directly bordering on the tropical zone, with greater seasonal variation in day length and temperature.
- Temperate: Generally, the region of the globe between the subtropics and the polar regions. More specifically, in the context of growing seasons, it indicates areas in which mean monthly temperatures fall below 5°C for one or more months.
- Tropical highland: Areas in the tropical zone in which, because of altitude, daily mean temperatures are cooler than in low-lying areas and range between 5 and 20°C during the growing season.

Various agroclimatic and ecological categories may be combined to characterize a production system in a certain area. A quick look at any atlas indicates, for example, that in the tropics there are arid, semiarid, subhumid, humid, and highland areas roughly equivalent to areas of desert, seasonal grasslands, permanent grasslands, forests, and croplands. Within these different areas, different systems of livestock production may be practiced in accordance with the potential for grazing and/or growing crops in each area. In the semiarid tropics, where cropping is severely constrained by rainfall, extensive grazing of cattle, sheep, goat, and camel herds by pastoralists may be the major human activity in the region and the principal source of food. In the humid tropics, on the other hand, mixed cropping by sedentary farmers is likely to be the principal form of food production. Small livestock, such as pigs and chickens, are included on such farms for diversification of risk, food, and income, while large livestock, such as oxen or buffalo, serve primarily as draft animals and sources of manure for fertilization.

Economic Development

The degree of economic development has a profound influence on the use of animals in any given society, both for agricultural and nonagricultural purposes. The level of technical modernization, the degree of prosperity and extent of urbanization, and the availability of credit and capital flow are among the economic factors that influence the use of animals and the demand for animal products.

Technical Modernization

In general, the greater the technological advance in a society, the less likely it is that animals are used for labor. Modern farm machinery reduces the need for animal draft power for plowing, seeding, harvesting, threshing, and other cropping activities, while chemical fertilizers diminish the use of manure as a soil enricher. Railroads, highways, and automotive transport reduce the use of animals to bring farm produce to market.

At the same time, technological advances significantly influence how food-producing animals are raised and animal food products are marketed. The intensification of livestock production, with large numbers of animals raised under carefully controlled, uniform conditions of housing and nutrition is made possible by the application of industrial technology and the exploitation of modern transportation infrastructure. Animal production is no longer tied directly to the land. Feeds can be imported from great distances, and animal production can be moved closer to major markets. In addition, refrigeration technology, modern container ships, and air transport open up distant markets for otherwise perishable animal and vegetable foods.

In less-developed countries, animals still play a considerable role in providing agricultural power and overland transport. Animals also remain an important food source in developing countries, but many animal production systems remain closely tied to the land, either through extensive grazing or by the integration of animals into cropping systems so that crop byproducts can be used as animal feed and the manure from animals can, in turn, be applied to croplands for fertilization.

Prosperity and Urbanization

Economic growth in recent years has led to greater per capita income in many developing nations. This has resulted in increased demand for foods of animal origin consistent with the cultural preferences and religious practices of a given nation, be it demand for dairy products in India, pork in China, or goat meat in Africa and the Middle East. In most countries, economic development is closely linked to urbanization, so consumer demand is increasingly concentrated in urban centers distant from food-producing areas. This has focused critical attention on the capacity of traditional domestic livestock production systems to meet growing demand and the effectiveness of traditional marketing systems and rural infrastructure to deliver goods reliably to urban markets.

Credit and Capital Flow

Improving production capacity and efficiency often requires the investment of capital and the availability of credit. Poor farmers in developing countries commonly have little or no access to credit and very limited cash resources, which severely constrains their ability to innovate and improve productivity. In such cases, animals themselves become an important form of capital, serving many of the roles of a modern finance system, including risk diversification, investment, savings, and liquidity. Cattle and goats may be grazed together in semiarid

regions, because cattle, though more highly valued, are more likely to be lost during periods of drought when the grasses disappear. Goats, which can survive the loss of grazing resources through their capacity to browse trees and shrubs, are more likely to survive. Since goats are also more prolific than cattle, with a shorter reproduction cycle, goats serve in effect as an "insurance policy," allowing the herder to survive the drought and recover more rapidly when the rains return. For settled farmers, poultry, pigs, small ruminants, or rabbits often serve as a living savings account and a ready source of cash in emergencies, through the sale of eggs, birds, meat, milk, or young stock.

Animal management systems are shaped to a great extent by economic conditions. In developed countries in which capital is available and labor is expensive or in short supply, investment in buildings, equipment, and automated systems for intensive livestock production is favored by economic circumstances. Likewise, in many developing countries in which labor is abundant and cheap but capital flow is limited, low-input, low-cost, labor-intensive animal-production systems such as grazing or mixed small-scale farming reflect a rational use of available economic resources. However, as demand for animal products grows in developing countries, there is increased pressure to improve the productivity and output of traditional systems as well as to introduce more-modern, capital-intensive systems.

Physiological Adaptation

The suitability of different species of domestic animals and different breeds within a given species for a specific geographical and climatic situation will vary depending on intrinsic characteristics of the animal itself. The attributes that determine an animal's usefulness in a given setting include feeding habits, ability to conserve water, disease resistance, and its production characteristics.

Feeding Habits

The feeding habits of animals are a critical determinant in their distribution. Ruminant animals, through the action of the rumen and its microflora, can break down cellulose in plant materials and use it as a nutrient source. Not only does this allow vast areas of grassland and scrubland not suitable for crop production to be exploited for food production through the grazing of ruminant animals, it also allows crop stalks and other fibrous agricultural byproducts to be used as animal feed, ensuring a role for ruminant animals in mixed farming systems.

In addition to true ruminants, including cattle, sheep, and goats, the camelids, which have compound stomachs, and equids, with an enlarged cecum adapted for cellulose digestion, also can use grass and fibrous plants efficiently as a food source. Monogastric animals such as the pig and poultry, however, are less well adapted for cellulose digestion and will not perform well with diets based on grasses or stover. Traditionally, pigs did well in woodland settings, where they foraged on the forest floor for a wide variety of feedstuffs. Similarly, chickens are well adapted to village life where they can forage freely for grain, insects, household wastes, and other food sources.

One of the many reasons why pigs and poultry are so widely used in intensively managed, confinement production systems is that they will thrive on a concentrate or grain-based ration in contrast to ruminant animals, who require significant roughage in their diet for proper digestive function and health. In such confinement systems, where animals may be housed distant from the croplands where feeds are grown, it is easier and cheaper to ship concentrate feeds than bulk roughage feeds.

Within the group of true and functional ruminants, there is considerable variation in diet selection, and this contributes significantly to animal distribution. For example, cattle and sheep are essentially grazers, requiring grass as the principal foodstuff. Goats and camels, however, are grazer/browsers, capable of consuming a wider array of fibrous vegetation including brush, shrubs, cacti, and various parts of trees. This gives them a greatly increased foraging range compared with that of cattle and sheep. It also favors their survival in semiarid regions and during periods of drought. In areas where grasslands contain abundant trees and shrubs, goats are frequently kept in mixed herds with cattle and/or sheep for more efficient use of the nutrients available. Furthermore, goats are being used increasingly as an alternative or adjunct to chemical spraying for weed control in pastures, while at the same time improving the offtake of livestock products in the form of goat meat and fiber. The Australians and New Zealanders have been most active in using goats in this way.

Water and Energy Conservation

The ability to conserve water also influences the distribution of livestock. Camels are well known for their usefulness in arid and semiarid regions, in large part because of their ability to go for long periods without drinking. During periods of lush grass growth and cool temperatures or when succulent plants are available, camels may not need to consume any free water at all, being able to meet their water needs through the moisture present in green feed. Because of their ability to clear large quantities of salt in the urine, camels are also able to consume and tolerate brackish water that would be toxic or fatal to humans or other livestock. How long a camel can go without water varies, depending on a number of factors, including the succulence and availability of feed, air temperature, and the amount of work being performed. There are reports of camels going 30 days under drought conditions without water and surviving, but this is extreme. Working or lactating camels should be watered every 6 days or more often as long as water intake does not result in reduced feed intake.

Some goat breeds have adapted very well to desert conditions, such as the black Bedouin goat of the Middle East.[21] These goats also show notable water-conserving ability, though the mechanisms may differ from those in the camel. Black Bedouin goats can consume large amounts of water in a short time, up to 40% of their dehydrated body weight, after an extended period of water deprivation. They do not, however, absorb the water rapidly. Instead the rumen serves as a water reservoir, with as much as 80% of the water consumed remaining in the rumen for up to 5 hours. During this time, glomerular filtration rate, renal blood flow, and urine output all decrease, with the kidneys working in concert with the rumen to conserve water. Desert goats frequently go up to 4 days without drinking, with no ill effects. Cattle are more likely to show ill effects from dehydration within 2 days of water deprivation. These differences in water conservation affect herd composition in arid and semiarid areas. In Afghanistan, for instance, pastoralists graze mixed herds of sheep and goats and carry their belongings on camels and sometimes donkeys. Cattle are not included in the dry pastoral grazing systems of this country, though cattle are found throughout the country in settled farming areas where water supplies are more reliable.

Conservation of energy in the form of fat storage is another adaptation that allows livestock to survive in semiarid or drought-prone areas where grazing can be scant or absent for extended periods. Camels conserve fat in their humps, which can visibly shrink as fat is metabolized during periods of metabolic need (Fig. 4-1). Less well known to westerners are the fat-tailed breeds of sheep that store large fat reserves in their tails. These sheep are common in much of Asia, particularly the colder and drier regions from Mongolia southwestward into the Indian subcontinent and the Near East. Herders may demonstrate a preference in winter to consume the fat tail of the sheep rather than the flesh, recognizing that the fat provides a higher concentration of calories (Fig. 4-2).

Disease Resistance

The ability of certain species or breeds within a species to resist disease has been recognized and exploited by livestock keepers around the world, and therefore, disease resistance or,

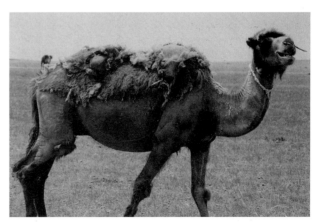

Figure 4-1. A two-humped, or Bactrian, camel in the Gobi region of Mongolia during an extended period of drought and poor grass growth. Note the shrunken, flopped-over appearance of the humps, indicating that the camel has been drawing on its fat storage for energy during a period of nutritional shortages. (Photo by Dr. David M. Sherman)

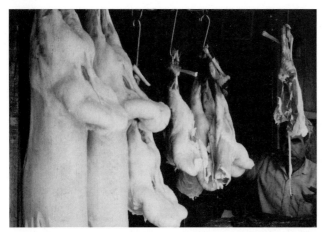

Figure 4–2. Fat tail sheep carcasses. The fat tail sheep breeds are usually found in harsh, marginal environments of Asia, the Middle East, and northern Africa, where low and unpredictable rainfall makes grazing unreliable. The fat deposited in the tail serves as a reserve store of energy for the animal. It is also a highly prized and important source of fat calories for people living in the same harsh environments. The fat tail is prized by hard-working people as a concentrated source of energy in the diet. (Photo by Dr. David M. Sherman)

notably, the lack of it, affects the distribution of domestic animals. Some examples are given below.

Trypanosomiasis The presence of tsetse flies and the risk of trypanosomiasis associated with this insect vector has effectively closed off vast areas of grassland otherwise suited for cattle grazing, thus limiting the potential for livestock to contribute to the food supply in Africa (see sidebar "Trypanosomiasis Control in Africa" in Chapter 1). There are, however, some local breeds of ruminant livestock that show trypanotolerance. N'dama cattle for example, are *Bos taurus*-type cattle of the humid coastal regions of West Africa. This is a long-horned, compact breed with good beef conformation but relatively poor milk production. While trypanotolerance is considered to have a genetic basis, the expression and mechanisms of trypanotolerance are not completely understood. It is clear however, that these animals can withstand a much greater challenge with trypanosomes and express milder clinical disease than other breeds when infected. Many development agencies, governments, and commercial enterprises have introduced N'dama cattle into tsetse-infested regions to take advantage of their disease resistance, and they are now widely present on savanna grazing lands in the Central African Republic, Gabon, Nigeria, and the two Congos. In addition to N'dama cattle, West African Shorthorn cattle breeds (*Bos taurus brachyceros*) such as Muturu are also considered trypanotolerant, as are Djallonke sheep and West African Dwarf goats.

Tick Resistance Ticks are a major constraint on livestock production, particularly in tropical regions. In addition to producing direct damage to skin, ticks serve as vectors for many important infectious diseases, transmitted to hosts during feeding by ticks. Among these economically important diseases are East Coast fever, heartwater (cowdriosis), anaplasmosis, and babesiosis. Managing tick burdens on extensively grazed cattle in the tropics requires significant effort and expense. It has become clear over time that *Bos indicus* breeds of cattle demonstrate a significantly greater capacity to acquire resistance to tick attachments than *Bos taurus* breeds. This is one reason why *Bos indicus* breeds of cattle such as Zebu, Brahman, and Sahiwal have found favor in grazing systems in the more humid, tropical regions of Australia, South America, and the southern United States.

Resistance to Toxins Different species vary in their susceptibility to plant toxins, which may limit their distribution for grazing. Goats, for example, show far greater tolerance for consumption of oak (*Quercus* spp.) leaves, stems, and acorns than cattle and sheep. Serious clinical disease including hemorrhagic enteritis and nephrosis can occur in the latter species when oak is consumed. Goats have higher levels of tannase enzymes in the rumenal mucosa able to break down the gallotannins responsible for the toxic effects in cattle and sheep. This is likely to have resulted as a selective advantage linked to the goat's browsing behavior. At any rate, this makes goats valuable to farmers and herders with access to land containing scrub oak. Goats can clear oak from such pastures effectively and safely, making them safe for grazing cattle and sheep. In semiarid regions, goats often eat a wide variety of plants that are potentially toxic and only get into trouble with them during periods of drought when alternative feed sources become scarce and the goats are obliged to consume considerable quantities of the potentially toxic species.

Production Characteristics

Certain traits possessed by different species and breeds of animals make them suitable for use in certain agroclimatic zones, production systems, or specific activities. The foot structure of the water buffalo, for instance, makes the animal more suitable as a draft animal than cattle for working in the mud of wetland rice-production systems in southeast Asia. The camel, so well adapted to arid conditions and so vital as a source of transportation, also provides excellent quality fiber, ample quantities of milk, and, at slaughter, hides and meat under conditions in which other animals might not survive. Cattle breeds in India are characterized by strong necks and forequarters, consistent with their primary use in plowing, compared with beef breeds elsewhere, which have strong, well-muscled hindquarters. Sheep breeds with hair instead of wool are better adapted to tropical conditions, both humid and semiarid, than the wool sheep breeds so well known in temperate regions. Hair sheep are indigenous to tropical west Africa, including the Sahel, where they are most abundant, but are also found in the Caribbean, Brazil, southern India, and parts of southeast Asia and are used primarily for meat production. Animals adapted to cold mountainous regions, such as the cashmere goat and the yak, allow herders in Central Asia to exploit grazing areas that might otherwise be unproductive.

The selective breeding of domestic animals to suit the needs of society is not a new phenomenon. There is pictorial evidence that the ancient Babylonians and Egyptians had developed definitive breeds of dogs, cattle, and sheep by the beginning of the second millennium BC.[3] However, breeding livestock to increase production of foods of animal origin was intensified dramatically under the stimulation of the Industrial Revolution as a response to the expanding market demand for meat and milk among the growing population of city dwellers. Great Britain was especially active and successful in producing new breeds of production animals. One advantage Great Britain had was its status as an island nation. While breed improvement also was occurring in continental Europe, serious animal plagues during the 1800s, such as foot and mouth disease, contagious bovine pleuropneumonia, and rinderpest, periodically wiped out large numbers of animals, including improved purebred breeding stock. As an island, Great Britain was relatively protected from these plagues, and its steady progress in animal breeding was preserved. Major breeding advances were made with dairy cattle such as the Guernsey and Jersey, mutton-producing sheep such as the Suffolk and Southdown, and also swine. In the 19th century, when consumer tastes in pork began to change from fat pork and bacon to lean ham and chops, breeders in Britain were able to transform the hog in record time, replacing large, roly-poly breeds like the Berkshire and Yorkshire with leaner, longer pigs such as the Large White. Thus many of the high-producing breeds of livestock common today are only 200 or so years old.

Animal Distribution and Use

The world census of major domesticated animal species in the years 1975 and 2000 is shown in Table 4-1. In the following sections, a brief status report on the various domestic animal species is presented, highlighting the importance of each species in different regions or nations and their principal uses. Statistical information and production rankings presented in these sections are for the year 2000 and are derived from the agricultural databases of the FAO, available on the internet at http://apps.fao.org/.

Cattle

Cattle continue to serve as multipurpose animals, used for draft power; food in the form of milk, other dairy products, meat, and blood; and hides for leather production. Historically, the distribution of cattle was closely linked to the availability of grazing lands, and a considerable portion of the world's cattle are still grazed extensively on rangelands. In certain regions, usually in developed countries, modern transportation infrastructure and high-yield crop agriculture have allowed intensification of cattle production. In these situations, grains are transported to feedlots for beef production and to large commercial dairies for milk production.

Cattle populations and cattle productivity are not always directly proportional. India, for example, with the largest num-

Table 4-1 World Populations of Different Species of Livestock in 1975 and 2000		
Livestock Type[a]	**1975**	**2000**
Geese	62,777,000	234,680,000
Ducks	295,953,000	884,532,000
Rabbits	180,143,000	474,828,000
Chickens	5,913,474,000	14,446,913,000
Goats	403,923,631	720,007,792
Turkeys	144,031,000	240,391,000
Buffalo	113,140,310	164,968,015
Pigs	685,705,556	908,104,421
Cattle	1,187,104,340	1,350,130,000
Donkeys	39,084,317	43,398,200
Camels	16,448,358	18,228,926
Sheep	1,046,298,160	1,057,908,000
Mules	13,459,667	13,571,414
Other camelids	6,229,200	6,200,000
Horses	61,870,259	58,807,504

[a]Species are listed in descending order relative to the proportional increase in their population between 1975 and 2000. Geese had almost a fourfold increase in their global population, while the world horse population actually decreased over the last quarter of the 20th century. Data from the FAOSTAT Agriculture Database of the FAO, accessible on the web at http://apps.fao.org.

ber of cattle of any single country, ranks eighth worldwide in beef and veal production. The largest national cattle populations, in descending order, currently exist in India, Brazil, China, the United States, Argentina, Sudan, Ethiopia, Mexico, Russia, and Australia. The countries with the highest outputs of beef and veal production, in descending order, are the United States, Brazil, China, Argentina, Russia, Australia, France, India, Mexico, and Germany. The countries with the highest outputs of cow milk production are the United States, Russia, India, Germany, France, Brazil, the United Kingdom, Ukraine, New Zealand, Italy, and Poland. The fact that countries such as Ethiopia and Sudan have high cattle numbers but do not rank highly in beef or milk production reflects the fact that most cattle in these countries are maintained for subsistence purposes and may not enter into commercial market channels.

There is a tremendous variety among the world's estimated 920 cattle breeds, and they can be categorized in a number of ways. A main distinction is the differentiation of *Bos taurus* and *Bos indicus* breeds. The *Bos indicus* breeds are cattle with a prominent hump over the withers and a loose, pendulous dewlap. They most likely originated in the Indian subcontinent and are well adapted to tropical and subtropical climates. *Bos taurus* breeds are the humpless breeds more familiar to Europeans and Americans. They can be longhorned or shorthorned. Cattle breeds used for food are also categorized according to their principal use, either as beef breeds, dairy breeds, or dual-purpose breeds.

Selective breeding, particularly over the last 200 years, has produced distinctly high-producing dairy breeds such as the Holstein, but even this breed is not always exclusively exploited for milk. In parts of Europe, the Holstein is considered a dual-purpose breed, and male offspring are routinely raised for beef production. Cross-breeding is widely used to develop breeds that meet specific local needs. Jamaican Hope cattle, for example, are derived from Zebu and Jersey crosses, with the intention of creating a high-producing dairy cow that is well adapted to climatic, nutritional, and disease conditions in the humid tropics. A useful resource for learning about the world's cattle breeds as well as breeds of other domestic animals is at the website of Oklahoma State University (http://www.ansi.okstate.edu/breeds/).

Sheep

Sheep are distributed throughout temperate, subtropical, and, to a lesser extent, tropical regions and are reasonably well adapted to regions of low rainfall, i.e., semiarid environments. Sheep are common in both developed and developing countries. Worldwide, sheep are exploited mainly for meat production. Wool production is also an important economic activity, though the development of synthetic fibers in the 20th century depressed global wool markets. There are specialized commercial sheep milk production and cheese-making industries, mainly in southern Europe, for instance, the production of Pecorino Romano cheese in Italy and Roquefort cheese in France. Sheep also serve as a source of milk in some pastoralist cultures and among subsistence farmers. The vast majority of the world's sheep are managed under extensive grazing conditions, either for subsistence or for commercial exploitation, though there is some intensive lamb production in feedlots in the western United States.

Countries with the largest numbers of sheep include, in descending order, China, Australia, India, Iran, New Zealand, Sudan, the United Kingdom, Turkey, South Africa, and Pakistan. The largest wool-producing countries in the world, in descending order, are Australia, China, New Zealand, Iran, Argentina, the United Kingdom, Uruguay, South Africa, Sudan, India, and Turkey. The 10 largest mutton or sheep-meat producing nations are China, Australia, New Zealand, the United Kingdom, Turkey, Iran, India, Spain, Pakistan, and Syria.

There are well over 650 breeds of sheep worldwide, only a small proportion of which are regularly exploited for commercial purposes. Most are local, indigenous breeds characterized by morphological features reflecting adaptation to local conditions, not necessarily linked to production characteristics. Wool breeds of sheep originated in cooler temperate regions where the wool coat served as protection against cold weather. Tropical breeds of sheep, used primarily for meat, lack the wool coat and possess a hair coat similar to that seen in cattle, as is common in the sheep breeds of Africa such as the Dorper. Breeds indigenous to semiarid regions where dry-season grazing may be sparse have developed fat tails as a source of stored energy. Selective breeding has allowed the manipulation of desirable traits to meet commercial demands. The Merino sheep, for example, is a fine wool breed originally developed in Spain. The extremely fine wool of small fiber diameter, makes it desirable for the production of high-quality woolen textiles. The medium-wool Merino is now the predominant sheep breed in Australia. Breeders there have been able to improve carcass quality so the animal has become dual purpose. Other dual-purpose breeds exploited commercially include Columbia, Corriedale, Finnsheep, Polypay, and Targhee. Other important wool breeds include Rambouillet for fine wool and Border Leicester, Cotswold, and Romney for longer, coarser wool.

Major commercial meat breeds include Cheviot, Dorset, Hampshire, Southdown, Suffolk, and Texel. In addition, there are many regional breeds adapted to local conditions, such as the Dorper sheep of South Africa and the Awassi sheep of the Middle East. The Awassi breed is a hearty, fat-tailed, long-wooled breed, well adapted to semiarid conditions and capable of producing considerable quantities of milk, as much as 725 kg over a 210-day lactation. Average nondairy sheep breeds in the United States produce about 45 to 90 kg of milk per lactation by comparison.

Goats

Goats are well adapted to a wide range of climatic and agroecological conditions and are widely distributed in temperate, tropical, subtropical, semiarid, and even arid environments. The diverse feeding habits of the goat, as a browser and grazer allow it to survive in niches unsuitable for cattle and sheep. While some goats are found in developed countries, often associated with commercial goat dairy and cheese-making enterprises, the vast majority of the world's goats are found in developing countries, where they are commonly held by subsistence farmers, nomadic herders, and landless rural people. Goats can be critical to the survival of these people. All 10 countries with the highest numbers of goats are categorized by the FAO as developing countries. In descending order of goat populations, they are China, India, Pakistan, Sudan, Bangladesh, Iran, Nigeria, Ethiopia, Somalia, and Mongolia. Four of these nations, Bangladesh, Ethiopia, Somalia, and Sudan, are further categorized by FAO as least-developed countries (LDCs). This designation is based on criteria of low income, weak human services, and a low level of economic diversification.

There are at least 265 breeds of domesticated goats in the world. As with sheep, a relatively small number of these breeds have been selectively bred for one or more specific production characteristics such as milk, meat, cashmere, mohair, or skin quality for leather production. The vast majority of goat breeds are local, indigenous breeds well adapted to survival in difficult conditions but with comparatively little selection for production characteristics. Ethiopia alone has 14 recognized indigenous goat breeds. Indigenous breeds serve a variety of needs. The Koochi nomads of Afghanistan, for example, rely heavily on their hearty, long-haired goats for numerous products and services. The coarse hair is shorn and felted for use in tent making. Finer fibers are separated for use in rug making and textile weaving. Skins are tightly sewn to produce leakproof water-storage containers. Goat milk and meat are consumed as food, and surplus goats are sold when necessary to provide cash for purchase of other basic necessities not produced directly by the Koochi themselves. Such reliance on goats is commonplace throughout much of Africa and Asia.

It is a curious fact of life that goats, frequently kept by the world's poorest people, produce a range of luxury products highly prized by the world's most affluent citizens. Such products include cashmere coats, mohair sweaters, kidskin leather goods, and chevre, or French-style goat cheese. Commercial industries have developed around these various products in different parts of the world, using selected breeds of goats. Goat dairying for the production of cheese is primarily a European enterprise, with intensively managed goat herds found primarily in France, Spain, and Italy. Dairy breeds of goats include Saanen, Toggenburg, Alpine, and Nubian. In South Asia, especially India, goat milk is also an important food product, and there are specialized dairy breeds of goats with high milk production, notably the Jamnapari breed.

Mohair is the fiber produced by Angora goats. These small, fine-boned, long-haired animals are found predominantly in dryland grazing areas of Turkey, South Africa, and Texas. Cashmere is an even finer-diameter fiber than mohair and is highly prized for textile manufacture. Goats have primary and secondary hair follicles. The primary follicles produce coarse guard hair, and the secondary follicles produce a downy, insulating undercoat, which is harvested as cashmere. Indigenous goats in the cooler Himalayan region of Asia produce varying degrees of cashmere fiber, which is sheared or brushed out in the springtime. Four countries, China, Mongolia, Iran, and Afghanistan, produce roughly 97% of the entire world supply of cashmere.

Goat meat is consumed widely in Asia and Africa and also in Latin America and the Caribbean. Most indigenous goat breeds serve as a source of meat, though more often than not, they are not selectively bred for improved commercial carcass quality. One notable exception is the Boer goat of South Africa, which has been bred as a meat-type goat and exhibits the blocky, heavily muscled phenotype usually associated with well-known beef cattle breeds.

Skins are a byproduct of goat slaughter, so comparatively little selective breeding has gone into production of quality skins. Nevertheless, some breeds are widely recognized for their superior skin quality, such as the Red Sokoto goat of Nigeria. Historically, raw skins, primarily from Africa and Asia, were shipped to Europe for production of finished leather goods, but increasingly, developing countries with large numbers of goats and other livestock, such as India, Pakistan, and Ethiopia, are developing their own tanning industries and expanding the manufacture and export of finished leather goods.

Buffalo

Asia, where the water buffalo was originally domesticated, remains the primary home of this versatile animal, where it is closely associated with wetland rice farming and milk production. The 10 countries with the largest numbers of water buffalo are, in descending order, India, Pakistan, China, Nepal, Egypt, the Philippines, Vietnam, Indonesia, Myanmar, and Thailand. Countries outside Asia with relatively large buffalo populations include Brazil and Italy.

The buffalo provides multiple products, and services including draft power for agriculture and transport, milk and meat. There are a variety of types and breeds. The Swamp buffalo, characterized by large, backsweeping horns is primarily a work animal, particularly for use in rice cultivation, and a source of meat. Swamp buffaloes originate in, and remain most common in, eastern Asia. River buffaloes, which originated in, and remain more common in, western Asia, are the dairy type of water buffalo, used both as a source of milk and for draft power. They are characterized by tightly coiled or drooping, straight horns, and as many as 18 different breeds are recognized in the Indian subcontinent, including Murrah, Nili, Jafarabadi, Surti, and Nagpuri. While cow dairying has increased in recent decades, in years past, as much as 60% of the milk consumed in India was buffalo milk, which still accounts for more than half of overall milk production in the country. In India and Egypt, demand for buffalo milk can be so high that buffalo calf survival is compromised by the aggressive collection of milk for sale. There is also a Mediterranean type of buffalo, derived over 1000 years ago from the River buffalo, with good meat and milk characteristics. This buffalo type is used in the mozzarella and ricotta cheese industries of Italy.

Buffalo do not tolerate extremes of temperature very well and do not adapt to cold climates. In hot climates, buffalo, with one tenth the density of sweat glands of cattle, require regular access to water, and preferably, opportunities to wallow. Though often perceived in the west as aggressive or dangerous animals, domesticated buffaloes are, in fact, usually quite docile and are frequently tended by children (Fig. 4-3). The buffalo is particularly well adapted for agricultural work in wetland or paddy rice farming. Consistent with its normal wallowing behavior, the buffalo suffers no ill effects from having its limbs and hooves submerged in water for extended periods, in contrast to cattle, who may develop foot rot or skin lesions. Its body weight is well distributed over the feet and legs for efficient traction, and its large, squarish hooves help it to move more easily in the soft mud found in rice fields. The buffalo is a slow-moving animal. Typically it is worked for about 5 hours

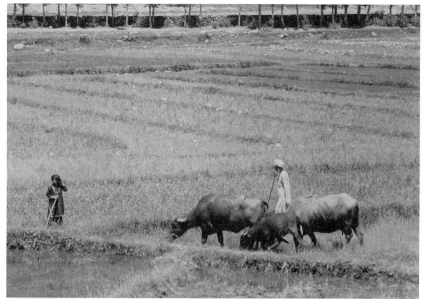

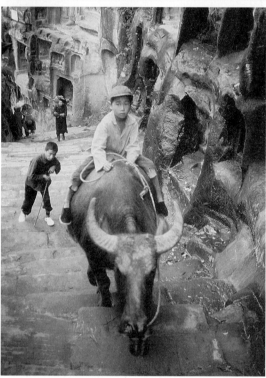

The two-humped Bactrian camel is more prevalent in east Asia, notably Mongolia and China, while the one-humped dromedary camel predominates in western Asia and North Africa. The camel is exploited as a multipurpose animal providing transportation, agricultural labor, milk, fleece, meat, and manure for both nomadic and sedentary peoples. There are numerous breeds of dromedary camel and a variety of ways of categorizing them. Many breeds are local and are given the name of the ethnic group of herders that keep them. Broadly, the breeds can be grouped according to their primary use—beef, dairy, dual purpose, or racing. Working camels perform many different labors from plowing, drawing water, and carrying riders to hauling heavy cargoes, either on their backs or harnessed to wagons. It is not uncommon to see camels in urban settings hauling heavy loads of basic materials such as timber, bricks, or crushed stone for road making. They are enormously strong and quite tractable.

Serious prolonged droughts in the Sahel region of Africa in recent decades have often been associated with considerable human suffering and loss of ruminant livestock. These events have prompted efforts by governments and development agencies to encourage Sahelian cattle herders to integrate camels into their herding practices as an effective buffer to catastrophic loss during severe drought. For example, during a severe drought in northern Kenya in 1984, Samburu people were obliged to sell or trade their starved, emaciated cattle for maize to survive, even though the loss of their cattle jeopardized their long-term future. However, nearby Rendille people, who herd camels, were still collecting an average of 5 L of milk per

Figure 4–3. Buffaloes are an important livestock species in Asia. Top, A landless herder grazes his milking buffalo on stubble in crop fields in Pakistan. Bottom, A young Chinese boy in Sichuan province rides his family buffalo home from work in the rice fields. (Both photos by Dr. David M. Sherman)

per day in southeast Asia and takes between 6 and 10 days to plow, harrow, and grade a 1-hectare (ha) rice field. For dry field work, cattle, mules, or horses are usually preferred because they are faster than buffalo.

Camels

Camels are closely associated with arid and semiarid regions of the world, as is reflected in the list of the 10 countries with the largest camel populations: Somalia, Sudan, Pakistan, Ethiopia, India, Kenya, Chad, Saudi Arabia, Niger, and Mongolia. The Sahelian region of Africa, the Middle East, the desert regions of the Indian subcontinent, and the Gobi region of central Asia are well represented in this list.

day from each of their lactating camels and were able to avoid short-term starvation and long-term economic disaster.[5] Camels can be successfully moved longer distances between water sources in search of available grazing sites than cattle and small stock, which may need to drink three or four times more frequently than camels. Furthermore, because of their diverse foraging habits, camels can find suitable browse to eat where cattle, sheep, and possibly even goats may not find sustenance.

Camel racing is a traditional sport in the Arabian countries of the Middle East, associated with weddings and special festivals. In recent times, however, camel racing has been organized into a formal industry with an extended racing season. Government leaders in the region have sought to bring modern veterinary science to this growing industry to improve the performance and breeding of racing camels. In the United Arab Emirates alone, three research centers have been established for this purpose, the Veterinary Research Center in Abu Dhabi, the Camel Reproduction Centre in Dubai, and the Embryo Transfer Research Centre for Racing Camels at Al-Ayn.

Horses, Donkeys, and Mules

There are at least 240 breeds of horses in the world, including ponies, warm-blooded horses, and working breeds. Countries with the largest horse populations, in descending order, are China, Mexico, Brazil, the United States, Argentina, Mongolia, Ethiopia, Colombia, Russia, India, and Kazakhstan. Many of these countries, notably in South America and Central Asia, have large, open plains where grazing animals are still managed extensively, and the horse continues to be an important work animal for herders and ranchers required to cover long distances. In other countries, such as Ethiopia, the horse serves as a beast of burden in field, village, and urban settings, while in the United States, the horse has become largely a recreational animal used for pleasure riding, showing, equestrian competition, racing, and rodeo.

Horse meat is eaten in Japan, central Asian nations, and some European countries, notably Belgium and France. France consumed 37,000 tons of horse meat in 1998, and 34,300 tons of the total were imported, principally from Poland, Canada, and the United States. Horse meat imported from Serbia in 1998 was responsible for a human outbreak of trichinellosis in southwestern France. The 10 biggest producers of horse meat are China, Mexico, Kazakhstan, Argentina, Italy, Mongolia, Australia, Kyrgyzstan, the United States, and Canada. Horse meat is also used as an ingredient in pet foods.

Donkeys remain critically important in the daily lives of many poorer rural and urban citizens in the developing world. A list of the 10 countries with the highest donkey populations underscores this dependency. The countries are China, Ethiopia, Pakistan, Mexico, Egypt, Iran, Brazil, India, Nigeria, and Afghanistan. As this list suggests, donkeys may be found in a wide range of climatic and ecological zones. However, they are particularly common in semiarid areas and in mountain areas, especially in Africa and Asia. The central highlands of Ethiopia, where donkeys abound, is a good example (Fig. 4-4). Donkeys are involved in agricultural work and transport, either carrying basic commodities, such as fuel wood, or agricultural goods on their backs, or by pulling carts and wagons. Donkeys in the developing world, like the people who commonly own them, are often overworked and undernourished and commonly lack access to health care (see sidebar "Pity the Poor Donkeys" in Chapter 3).

Mules are also used primarily as work animals. Bigger and stronger than donkeys, they are more likely to be used for plowing. Mule populations, like donkey populations, have been essentially static in recent years. While mules are often found in the same regions and under similar circumstances as donkeys and horses, they are more commonly found in Latin

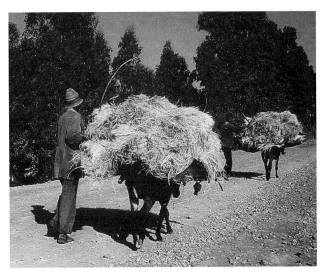

Figure 4-4. Donkeys in Ethiopia carrying straw that is used both as animal feed and as building material. Ethiopia has one of the highest donkey populations in the world. The animals are used extensively for transport. (Photo courtesy of FARM Africa-UK, London, England)

America and are not well represented in much of Africa outside highland regions. The 10 countries with the largest mule populations are China, Mexico, Brazil, Ethiopia, Colombia, Morocco, Peru, India, Argentina, and Iran.

Swine

Pigs are found throughout temperate, tropical, and subtropical areas. They are uncommon in semiarid and arid zones and, for religious reasons, are not kept widely in Islamic countries, though even in such countries, pigs are sometimes raised to meet market demands of non-Muslim minority populations or foreign visitors. In temperate zones, notably in Europe, North America, and China, swine raising has been historically linked to cereal crop production, with grain-fed swine being raised for commercial markets. Tropical pig raising has traditionally been more subsistence oriented, with pigs fed household wastes and crop byproducts to supplement rooting and scavenging. These pigs are destined for home use or for sale at local markets. Subsistence swine raising is especially common in southeast Asia, the Pacific Islands of Oceania, and Latin America.

While small-scale swine production remains a widespread activity, there has been an explosion of growth in intensive, commercial swine production around the world in places where economic growth in recent decades has increased consumer demand for pork, most notably in Asia. In China, for instance, meat consumption per capita per year increased fourfold from 1977 (8 kg) to 1994 (32 kg). Pork accounted for 75% of this increase. Currently, the 10 top swine-producing nations in the world are China, the United States, Brazil, Germany, Spain, Vietnam, Russia, Poland, India, and France.

There are many breeds of swine in the world. Many are indigenous breeds found only locally. Others have been widely adapted for commercial purposes. Modern-day swine breeding is a dynamic activity, as breeders work to develop new types of pigs with conformational characteristics and uniformity that adapt well to current production conditions and market demands. Custom breeders can work with producers to develop new hybrid types of pigs to fit specific niches of climate and consumer preferences for certain product characteristics.

Chickens

Domestic chickens are found throughout tropical, subtropical, and temperate regions. The production of chicken meat and eggs is one of the fastest growing sectors of the global livestock industry. Chickens are kept under a wide range of management situations from simple subsistence, where a few chickens may run free in the farmyard, to midsized commercial, family-run operations (Fig. 4-5), to large-scale intensive commercial production units where tens of thousands of layers or broilers may be maintained under carefully regulated conditions of climate and nutrition. The 10 nations with the highest populations of chickens are, in descending order, China, the United States, Brazil, Indonesia, Mexico, India, Russia, Japan, Iran, and Turkey.

At the subsistence level, village and farmyard chickens are usually multipurpose. They fit well into mixed farming systems, scavenging for grubs in farmyards and feeding on household wastes and crop gleanings. They provide eggs and meat for the family, as well as a ready source of cash when needed. When chickens are penned, their manure can be collected for application to gardens or into fish ponds.

Considerable research effort is put into improving production efficiency in the modern poultry industry. Today, a commercial broiler chicken can be brought to market at a weight of 1.85 kg in less than 6 weeks on a total input of 3.4 kg of grain. Not long ago, it took 14 weeks and 7.2 kg of grain. The 10 nations with the highest production of chicken meat are the United States, China, Brazil, Mexico, the United Kingdom, Japan, Thailand, France, Canada, and Argentina. The 10 nations with the highest hen's egg production are China, the United States, Japan, Russia, India, Mexico, Brazil, France, Germany, and Italy.

There are many different breeds of chickens in the world, including many locally distributed indigenous breeds. As with swine, commercial breeders have made tremendous gains in the creation of highly productive breeds that are well adapted to intensive commercial production under different environmental conditions.

Other Poultry

While the chicken is the major poultry species in the world, domesticated ducks, geese, and turkeys are also exploited by human society. Regional preferences for these other poultry species are marked. Duck raising, for instance, is important and common mainly in Asia. Seven of the 10 nations with the highest numbers of ducks are in Asia, mainly in the east and southeast regions of the continent. The top 10 countries are China, Vietnam, Indonesia, France, Ukraine, Thailand, Bangladesh, Malaysia, the Philippines, and Egypt.

The preponderance of ducks in Asia reflects the integration of duck production into wetland rice farming. Flocks of ducks are part of the rice production cycle, turned on to fields during the early rice growth period and again after harvesting. Being excellent foragers, ducks in the early period are useful in controlling weeds and insects while returning manure to the soil. Postharvest, they can effectively glean rice grains left behind in the fields, converting them to meat and eggs. It is common in rural Asia to see a duck herder guiding a large flock down a country road where the ducks can feed on roadside vegetation, from irrigation ditches, or in open fields. In addition to traditional methods, ducks are increasingly being raised in confinement and fed grain under commercial conditions. Australia, for example, has a growing commercial duck industry.

Goose production is also largely regional, with Europe and the Middle East predominating, though China has the single highest number of geese, where they may be herded like ducks (Fig. 4-6). The 10 countries with the high-

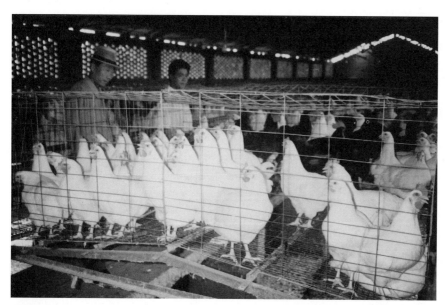

Figure 4-5. A private, family-run, cross-bred broiler chicken operation on the outskirts of the provincial capital, Chengdu, in Sichuan Province, China. The expansion of urban markets for foods of animal origin in Asia have stimulated the creation of many such poultry enterprises in periurban areas. (Photo courtesy of Dr. Pu Jiabi, Heifer Project International-China)

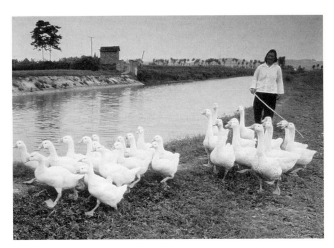

Figure 4–6. Herding geese along an irrigation channel in China. The goose is growing in popularity among landless villagers as a source of animal protein and cash income and also integrates well into subsistence farming systems to improve productivity and promote sustainability. (Photo courtesy of Heifer Project International, Little Rock, Arkansas; photographer, Matt Bradley)

est goose populations are China, Egypt, Romania, Russia, Madagascar, Turkey, Israel, Hungary, Iran, and Yugoslavia. Birds are raised for meat, eggs, and feathers. France, well known for its goose liver pate, or foie gras, industry comes in at number eleven.

The domestication of turkeys occurred in the New World, and current production reflects those origins, with the United States being the world's largest producer of turkeys. In addition to the United States, the countries with the largest turkey populations are France, Italy, the United Kingdom, Brazil, Germany, Portugal, Canada, Israel, and Mexico. Turkeys are raised primarily for meat. Commercial breeding reflects this use, with intense selection exerted over the years for enhanced breast meat production.

Aquatic Species

Animal protein derived from aquatic sources in the form of shellfish, finfish, amphibians, reptiles, or mammals has long been an important part of the human diet. Some of the earliest examples of complex social development and human cooperation are associated with ancient cultures that fished or hunted aquatic mammals. Today, many people situated near oceans, seas, lakes, and rivers continue to fish as a means of livelihood using traditional methods. There are an estimated 13 million artisanal fishermen registered worldwide.[11] Artisanal fishermen are subsistence or small-scale fishermen who work in family or community units. They are usually net or line fishers who use open boats such as canoes or other small craft that may be powered by small outboard motors. Usually men do the fishing, with women in the community involved in processing, transport, and marketing. This small-scale fishing is very common in developing countries and may play a critical role in sustaining poor communities both economically and nutritionally. In some island nations, the Maldives, for

example, the percentage of animal protein in the human diet derived from fish is, on average, 96%, and in the coastal nation of Bangladesh, it is 46%. In Uganda, which is landlocked, but which contains and borders many large lakes, people derive on average 40% of their animal protein from fish.

While traditional, subsistence fishing has persisted, commercial fishing has become such a highly efficient, technically sophisticated enterprise, that many global fish stocks are in peril of depletion due to overfishing. Many well-known commercial fish species have been overfished in recent years, including the Atlantic cod, Atlantic halibut, summer flounder, swordfish, red snapper, Atlantic salmon, bluefin tuna, orange roughy, and some species of groupers, rockfish, and sharks. The depletion of the Atlantic cod and other north Atlantic groundfish has had important cultural and economic ramifications for coastal communities throughout New England and the Canadian Maritimes.

As established commercial fish populations become depleted, commercial fishers shift to other species of fish, previously considered to be of lesser economic value, such as barn door skates, chub mackerel, and Alaskan pollock. These species in turn come under pressure of overfishing with potentially far reaching consequences. The taking of Alaskan pollock, for example, has already had an adverse affect on Stellar sea lion populations, which feed on the pollock. This has led to a reassignment of the mammal from threatened to endangered under the Endangered Species Act.

Even with the aggressive pursuit of less valuable fish species, overall catches are beginning to decline. The rate of increase has slowed considerably. In the 1950s and 1960s, global catches increased at rates reaching as high as 6% per year. In the 1980s, the rate of annual increase had fallen to about 1.5%, and in 1995–1996, the rate of increase was only 0.5%. In 1997, world fish catch actually declined slightly from the previous year, from 95 to 94 million tons.

A counterpoint to this gloomy picture has been the steady and dramatic increase in aquaculture in recent decades. Aquaculture is the controlled cultivation of aquatic species. It is more than "fish farming," in that a wide variety of plant and animal species are cultivated in various aquaculture systems around the world, including kelp and other seaweeds, mollusks, crustaceans, fin fish, and turtles. Over 300 cultured species or species groups have been reported to the FAO as being under aquaculture production since 1984. There are however, a smaller group of species that can be considered major aquaculture varieties in terms of overall production and the market value of the output produced. Among the finfish, these are carp, salmonids (salmon and trout), and tilapia. Among the shellfish, these are mussels, oysters, scallops, clams, and cockles, and among the crustaceans, these are shrimp, mainly of the *Penaeus* spp., such as giant tiger prawns.

In contrast to captured fish production, growth in aquaculture production has been strong. In 1989, cultured finfish and shellfish contributed 11.7% to total world finfish and shellfish production. In 1995, that contribution had increased to 18.5%. The annual percentage growth rate of cultured finfish and shellfish production increased from about 5.5% in 1991 to 14% in 1995.

The 10 cultivated species with the highest world production output in 1996 were kelp, Pacific cupped oyster, silver carp, grass carp, common carp, bighead carp, Yesso scallop, Japanese carpet shell, crucian carp, and Nile tilapia. When product value is taken into account, the list assumes a somewhat different character. Some of the high-value products, such as tiger prawns and Atlantic salmon are targeted for high-end markets in developed countries and demand a high unit price. The top 10 value products for 1996 were giant tiger prawn, Pacific cupped oyster, silver carp, kelp, common carp, grass carp, Atlantic salmon, Yesso scallop, Japanese carpet shell, and bighead carp.

Aquaculture has a long history. It is believed that the Chinese have been raising carp in ponds for at least 3000 years. Today, Asia still remains the major center of aquaculture, particularly with regard to carp and prawns. China is the world's largest cultivator of carp, though India, Indonesia, Myanmar, Thailand, Laos, Russia, and Ukraine also produce notable amounts of common carp. Thailand is the world's largest producer of giant tiger prawns. Other Asian countries actively involved in prawn production include China, the Philippines, Indonesia, India, and Bangladesh. Shrimp culture is expanding outside of Asia, however, particularly in Latin America, where Mexico, Ecuador, and Colombia produce prawns.

Tilapia production is strongest in China, the Philippines, Thailand, Indonesia, and Egypt. China alone is responsible for 48% of global tilapia culture. Production of Nile tilapia there increased from 18,000 metric tonnes in 1984 to 315,000 metric tonnes in 1995. Mexico, Costa Rica, and the United States also have active, albeit smaller, tilapia industries. The key area of aquaculture where Asia is not dominant is salmonid production, largely because the salmonid species are cold water fishes. The top three producers of cultured Atlantic salmon in 1995 were Norway, Chile, and the United Kingdom, which together accounted for 83% of world production. Forty-eight countries are involved in culture of rainbow trout, but four countries accounted for roughly half of all world production in 1995, namely France, Chile, Denmark, and Italy.

Other Species

A number of additional species of animals, both domestic and wild, are exploited by human society for food, labor, or other goods and services. Many are locally or regionally important. Llama and alpaca, camelids found in the Andean highlands of South America, remain economically important to local residents. The llama provides meat and draft power, while the lighter, finer-boned alpaca is used primarily for its fiber. In recent years, llamas and alpacas have become popular with breeders and hobbyists in North America, and populations are increasing in the United States and Canada.

Guinea pigs, or cavy, are raised in some South American countries for meat. Peru, for example, has over 20 million guinea pigs and produces about 17,000 tons of meat annually, almost as much as the country's sheep industry. Guinea pigs, though native to South America, have been adapted elsewhere in the world as well. It is estimated that 10% of households in southern Nigeria raise guinea pigs for food. These small, prolific, and tractable rodents are easily raised indoors on household wastes, and therefore can provide a source of animal protein to landless families, even in urban settings.

Like guinea pigs, rabbits offer tremendous potential for the landless or urban poor to supplement their diets with animal protein. Rabbits are also tractable and prolific and can do reasonably well on household wastes and forages cut from fields and roadsides and brought to the hutch. Rabbit production is reasonably well established in many places in the world. China produces the most rabbits, mainly through household or small farm production. Other countries with sizable rabbit populations include Korea, Uzbekistan, Italy, Kazakhstan, France, Germany, Egypt, and Ukraine.

There are numerous additional species of animals found in various places around the world that could be more widely exploited for food and adapted to more-productive management systems. Some may have the potential for a wider distribution and acceptance beyond the locale where they are currently known. These animals fall into a number of categories including birds, rodents, reptiles, and ungulates. Avian species with potential for wider use include Muscovy ducks, quail, guinea fowl, and pigeons. Underexploited rodents include the agouti, capybara, hutia, mara, coypu, paca, and vizcacha of South America and two African species, the cane rat, and the giant rat. Among the reptiles, the green and black iguanas of Central America have the potential to be raised for food production. A number of ungulates are prized for their meat and show potential for either domestication or at least controlled ranching. These include the duiker of sub-Saharan Africa, the mouse deer and muntjac of south Asia, the water chevrotain of west Africa, the musk deer of central Asia, the water deer of China and Korea, and several small deer of South America, including the pudu, the huemul, and the brocket.

Conservation-minded readers may bristle at the notion that these wild species should be exploited for food. However, the reality is that local citizens already put significant pressures on wild populations of these undomesticated species through an active "bushmeat" trade facilitated by hunting and trapping activities that are often illegal and widespread. If veterinarians and animal scientists can work with local people to develop ways to raise these animals productively under controlled management conditions, this would help to meet demand for animal products from these species while removing some of the hunting pressure on wild populations. The current status of these various animals and what is known and unknown about their management and production is presented in an informative publication entitled *Microlivestock*.[16] The use of game farming and game ranching as conservation tools is discussed further in Chapter 7.

Role of Animals in Agriculture and Daily Life

Domestic animals provide a wide range of goods and services to people in their daily lives. In the developed world, animals are an important source of food, but only a relatively small percentage of the population has direct contact with food-producing animals. For most citizens in developed countries, daily animal contact is with companion animals whose main function is to provide friendship and recreation. In the developing world, the situation is quite different. Direct contact with livestock is a regular feature of daily life, and many people in developing countries, especially in rural, agricultural areas, depend on livestock for a variety of goods and services including food, manure, draft power, herding, protection, financial services, and cultural and religious uses. Each of these functions is discussed below.

Food

The anthropologist Marvin Harris observed that many different cultures, from hunter-gatherers to complex industrial societies, express preferences for foods of animal origin, even when adequate foods of plant origin are available.[7] In his book *Good to Eat*, he notes that "virtually every band or village society studied by anthropologists expresses a special esteem for animal flesh by using meat to reinforce the social ties that bind campmates and kinfolk together."

Harris contends that the main reason primates, including chimpanzees and baboons, as well as humans, actively seek out foods of animal origin is that such foods have attributes that make them especially nutritious. Key among these attributes are abundant high-quality protein and a variety of essential micronutrients in relatively high concentrations and in readily absorbable forms.

Protein is an essential nutrient for growth and development of muscle and other body tissues. Human proteins are composed of 22 amino acids, 8 of which, the essential amino acids, cannot be synthesized by human beings and must therefore be consumed in the diet. Ideally, to optimize dietary efficiency, the essential amino acids should be available in the diet in quantities proportional to the amounts required for protein synthesis. Otherwise, any single essential amino acid in short supply becomes a limiting factor in the production of new protein, and other amino acids in excess supply are burned as calories rather than contributing to protein construction. The nutritional attraction of foods of animal origin, including meat, eggs, and dairy products, is that they are excellent sources of highly concentrated, digestible protein containing suitably balanced supplies of essential amino acids.

While all essential amino acids are available in foods of vegetable origin, they are not available from any single vegetable source in proportions suitable for maximally efficient use. For example, beans have a low protein efficiency because they lack the essential amino acid methionine. Similarly, whole wheat has a low protein efficiency because of a relative shortage of lysine. To achieve a suitable daily intake of lysine for adequate daily protein needs using bread alone, an 80-kg man would have to consume 1.5 kg of whole wheat bread each day. By contrast, 340 g of meat would provide sufficient quantities of all the required essential amino acids in proportional balance to meet daily protein production needs. By combining different foods of vegetable origin (e.g., rice with beans, or wheat breads with lentils or other legumes) the essential amino acids can be better balanced in the total diet. Nevertheless, foods of animal origin remain the best solitary source of protein, both qualitatively and quantitatively, and are valuable additions to the diets of individuals with higher protein needs, notably growing infants and children, pregnant women, and the infirm and convalescing.

Moderate protein and energy malnourishment affects one third of the world's children and results in low birth weight of infants, stunting of young children, deficits in cognitive functions, and decreased immune functions. Numerous international development organizations, including the FAO, the World Bank, and a variety of nongovernmental aid agencies, have recognized the major contribution that foods of animal origin can make in addressing protein and energy malnutrition in the young.

In addition to high-quality protein, foods of animal origin are excellent sources of iron, zinc, iodine, vitamin A, folic acid, and B vitamins. Vitamin B_{12}, or cyanocobalamin, an essential nutrient, is not available from foods of plant origin. In the case of the other micronutrients, they may be present in a variety of foods of plant origin, but concentrations and availability from such plant foods may make them less useful sources. For example, in the case of iron, cooked maize contains 0.5 mg of iron per 100 g, but only 5% is absorbed. Cooked beans contain 2.9 mg of iron per 100 g, but absorption is also only 5%. Beef contains 1.7 mg per 100 g, but absorption is 20%, so the iron available from meat is more than twice that from beans, even though the absolute concentration in meat is lower.

Iron deficiency is a serious nutritional problem in much of the developing world. For the average citizen in Bangladesh, for instance, only 2 to 3% of caloric intake comes from meat, and the overall diet is deficient in bioavailable iron. In that country, as many as 45% of preschool-age children are anemic, as are over half the adult women. Even small increases in meat or fish could improve overall nutrition and help to correct the problem of iron deficiency anemia with improved mental development of children and increased vitality and work capacity in adults.

The content and composition of fats in foods of animal origin has become a major issue in human diet and health in the last half of the 20th century. Foods of animal origin are relatively high in cholesterol and saturated fats, compared with foods of plant origin, and consumption of high levels of these compounds have been associated with increased risk for a number of chronic diseases. An enormous amount of scientific investigation has been carried out over the last few decades, much of it epidemiological. Hu and Willett of the Harvard School of Public Health have carried out a critical review of the literature on the relationship between consumption of animal products and the risk of chronic disease.[8] They examined dozens of studies, including correlational studies, case control studies, prospective cohort studies, and controlled clinical trials, in an effort to determine the health effects of specific types of animal food products on a variety of diseases including coronary heart disease, hemorrhagic stroke, breast cancer, colon cancer, and prostate cancer. A tabular summary of their findings is presented in Table 4-2. There were several notable conclusions:

- Foods of animal origin cannot be lumped together when discussing health effects. Different products can have different effects on the same disease, and the same product can have different effects on different diseases.

- Health effects of white meat from fish and poultry differ from those of red meat from beef and pork in epidemiological studies, and health policy

recommendations must take that distinction into account.

- Similarly, eggs and dairy products must be distinguished from meats. There is little consistent evidence that egg consumption contributes to chronic disease, despite the high cholesterol content of eggs. Dairy products can have both positive or negative effects relative to chronic disease, but some of the negative effects may be ameliorated through consumption of low-fat dairy products.

- Diets containing substantial amounts of red meat and red meat products probably increase risk of coronary disease and some forms of cancer, and substitution of white meat for red meat can have clear health benefits.

With ready access to the latest medical information, abundant food supplies, and a plethora of choice, many citizens in developed countries are altering their eating habits by increasing their intake of foods of plant origin, reducing their overall intake of foods of animal origin, or substituting some animal-

Table 4-2   A Qualitative Assessment of Associations of Animal Product Consumption with Risk of Chronic Diseases

	Red Meat (beef, pork, lamb)	Poultry	Fish	Eggs[a]	Dairy Products
Coronary heart diseases (CHD)	Probably ↑	Possibly ↓	Probably ↓	Probably no increase in risk	Probably small ↑[b]
Hemorrhagic stroke[c]	Possibly ↓	Possibly ↓	Uncertain[e]	Probably no increase in risk	Possibly ↓
Breast cancer	Possibly ↑	Probably no relation	Probably no relation	Probably no relation	Probably no relation
Colon cancer	Probably ↑	Possibly ↓	Possibly ↓	Probably no increase in risk	Probably no increase in risk
Prostate cancer	Probably ↑	Probably no relation	Probably no relation	Probably no relation	Probably ↑[d]

[a]Up to 1 egg per day.

[b]It is possible that substitution of low-fat dairy (e.g., skim milk) for high-fat dairy products (e.g., whole milk) decreases risk of cardiovascular disease for individuals, but this is largely irrelevant for population disease rates because the dairy fat produced is almost inevitably consumed.

[c]The associations between animal products and risk of ischemic stroke, which is more common in the U.S. than hemorrhagic stroke, are probably similar to those for CHD.

[d]It is unclear whether it is due to fat or calcium.

[e]Data are limited. It is possible that higher intake increases risk.

↑, increase in risk; ↓, decrease in risk.

Information provided by F. B. Hu, Harvard School of Public Health, Cambridge, MA, 1999, personal communication.

derived products for others. In the United States between 1970 and 1996, for example, there was a 15% decrease in red meat consumption and a 23% decrease in egg consumption, along with a 90% increase in poultry consumption, and a 143% increase in cheese consumption.[23] By 1996, total meat, poultry, and fish contributed nearly a third less saturated fat to the per capita American food supply, and fluid milk contributed 50% less saturated fat. Paradoxically, however, total per capita fat and oil consumption was up 21% over the same period, and overall caloric intake was up 15%. One third of adults in the United States were considered overweight by the early 1990s, compared with one quarter of adults in 1970. Overnutrition has emerged as an important public health and policy issue in the United States and other developed countries. Overweight and physical inactivity account for more than 300,000 premature deaths each year in the United States, second only to tobacco-related deaths.[14]

Meanwhile, in the developing world, undernutrition continues to be a major constraint on human, social, and economic development, with an estimated 800 million people worldwide not having enough to eat on a daily basis. A high value is still placed on foods of animal origin in much of the developing world, and whenever expanding incomes permit it, consumption of animal products of all types increases, within the framework of social, cultural, and religious preference and subject to availability. In areas of food scarcity, animal fat is still recognized and valued as a highly concentrated source of calories.

The increased demand for food of animal origin is closely correlated with economic development, industrialization, and urbanization. As such, Asia has seen the strongest growth in consumption of animal products. Latin America has also shown marked increases in consumption but not to the extent of Asia. Africa, which has lagged behind in economic development, has shown the smallest growth. Between 1967 and 1997, the per capita growth in meat consumption of all types in Asia increased by 293%, in Latin America by 50%, and in Africa, by 5%. It is instructive to note that meat consumption in Asia, despite its rapid expansion, still falls considerably short of meat consumption in the developed world, even though citizens in developed countries have ostensibly been scaling back on meat intake. In 1997, for example, per capita meat consumption in the United States was 118 kg, compared with 42.5 kg in China.

Sustaining the phenomenal growth in production for all types of animal products, illustrated in Figure 4.7, offers considerable challenges for the future. Policy analysts at the International Food Policy Research Institute (IFPRI) suggest that meeting the explosive demand for livestock products will require social and agricultural transformations equal in scope and magnitude to those that characterized the Green Revolution of the 1950s and 1960, which led to tremendous increases in crop productivity.[4] As early as 1975, scientists were warning that constraints on land and energy resources would make it impossible to feed the world population (4 billion at the time, now 6 billion) an American-type diet, in which 69% of dietary protein came from foods of animal origin.[19]

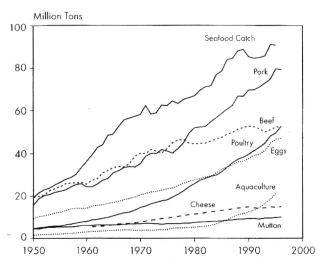

Figure 4-7. World production of animal protein by source, 1950-1996. (Reproduced by permission from WorldWatch Institute. Source: Brown LR. The Agricultural Link: How Environmental Deterioration Could Disrupt Economic Progress. World Watch Paper no. 136. WorldWatch Institute, 1997.)

Certainly, expanded livestock production, particularly intensive commercial production, will have significant ramifications on agriculture and the environment. Some of these effects are already becoming evident. Industrial livestock production requires considerable use of grain as animal feed for growing and finishing meat animals as well as for promoting egg and milk production. There is growing concern that the dedication of increased agricultural land for cereal grain production to feed livestock may actually reduce grain supplies for direct consumption by people. Even if grain supplies remain adequate, there is also concern that demand for cereal grains as livestock feed will drive up world grain prices, causing hardships for the poorest people in developing countries, particularly in countries that must import grains to feed their people. The impact of expanding livestock production in China alone has caused serious concern about the future of world grain supplies (see sidebar "The Challenge of Feeding China"). In addition, expanded animal production can potentially result in a number of environmental problems if such problems are not anticipated and properly managed. Environmental problems associated with both extensive and intensive livestock production, such as land degradation in the former and groundwater contamination in the latter, are discussed in more detail in Chapter 6.

Manure

Traditionally, manure has been an important and valuable byproduct of livestock raising, with varied uses, and in many situations today, manure continues to be a valuable commodity for use as fertilizer, fuel, and animal feed.

Use As Fertilizer

The chief limiting nutrient in crop agriculture is nitrogen. Much of the improvement in crop yields associated with the

The Growing Challenge of Feeding China

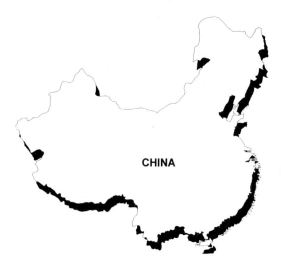

CHINA

China is a country with a history marked by periods of famine and food scarcity. Historically, food scarcity in China was associated with crop failures due to floods, drought, and other natural disasters leading to shortages of basic food for people in the countryside. Today, China faces a different sort of food supply problem, namely, the production of adequate supplies of grains to feed its growing livestock population. In the last 50 years, the challenge of feeding China has shifted from a context of overcoming rural hardships and poverty to meeting the demands of urban prosperity. In the last 30 years, China has become industrialized, its urban populations have expanded, the purchasing power of the populace has increased, and demand for foods of animal origin has skyrocketed. This has created an ever-increasing need for cereal grains to feed livestock. There is currently a serious debate about whether or not China has the capacity to produce enough grain domestically to meet this growing demand and, if not, what effect large-scale importation of grains into China will have on world grain markets, grain supplies and world hunger. Consider some of the following items:

- The Chinese economy is expanding rapidly and producing considerable prosperity for an expanding segment of the national population. Since 1978, the gross domestic product of China has quadrupled.

- Over the last 15 years of the 20th century, per capita income in China rose 170% for urban dwellers and 150% for rural dwellers.

- Per capita consumption of animal products in China has increased dramatically in recent decades. Between 1967 and 1997, per capita consumption of poultry increased by 781%, pork by 355%, whole milk by 394%, and eggs by 785%.

- China is urbanizing rapidly. The share of the urban population increased from about 23.7% in 1985 and is projected to reach almost 50% by 2030. The consumption of meat and other livestock products is 2 to 3 times higher in urban populations than in rural populations and has been steadily increasing.

- If the goals of population control policies in China are met, the population of the country in 2030 will be 1.6 billion. However, at the actual growth rate (1.4%) measured during the 1990s, the population of China in 2030 could be as high as 2 billion. If the latter number is reached, it represents a 25% greater need for food.

- Income elasticity, a proportional measure of the increased demand for goods as incomes rise, is very strong for livestock products in general and for certain livestock products in particular. Demand for milk and milk products, poultry meat, and fish have increased more than proportionally with income, with reported income elasticities of 1.5, 1.46, and 1.34, respectively. Income elasticity for pork, beef, and mutton were all 0.57, while income elasticity for crop products was low, 0.3 during the 1990s.

- Livestock production has risen dramatically in China, particularly after the agricultural reforms of the 1970s that allowed private livestock ownership. For example, between 1980 and 1995, poultry meat production increased from 1 million tons to 9.35 million tons, and egg production increased from 2.57 million tons to 16.77 million tons.

- During the same period, industrial feed production increased from 2 million tons in 1980 to 50 million tons in 1995. Pigs received 42% of this expanded production, layers and broiler chickens 50%, fish 5% and the remaining 3% was allocated as feed for cattle and other animals.

Green Revolution of the 1950s and 1960s is attributable to the increased use of chemical fertilizers containing nitrogen, phosphorus, and potassium to enrich soil and promote plant growth. Yet for many small farmers around the world, chemical fertilizer remains a costly, difficult-to-obtain, external input that they can neither afford nor acquire. When livestock are present in the farming system, the manure from these animals serves as fertilizer. Considerable manure is produced by animals. The weekly output for a 2-kg hen is 0.8 kg of manure; for an 80-kg pig, 40 kg of manure; and for a 650-kg cow, 150 kg of manure. In addition to providing nitrogen, phosphorus, and other micronutrients to soil, application of manure also helps to improve soil by increasing moisture retention and cation exchange capacity and by adding organic matter to the

- If grain is fed to livestock under commercial production systems, it takes approximately 2 kg of grain for each kg of poultry produced, 4 kg for each kg of pork, and 7 kg for each kg of feedlot beef.

- Grain production increased in China from 200 million tons in 1965 to 467 million tons in 1995 as a result of agricultural policy reforms and a number of technological improvements including increased fertilizer application, mechanization, irrigation, improved hybrid crop varieties, and multiple cropping. Nevertheless, China became a net importer of grain for both human and animal consumption beginning in 1995, including soybeans, maize, wheat, and barley.

- Arable land available in China for crop production decreased by approximately 8% between 1965 and 1995, from 103.3 million ha to 95.0 million ha, largely as a result of urban expansion and industrialization.

- Efforts to derive greater outputs from remaining lands are beginning to produce negative environmental consequences such as soil erosion from overcultivation, groundwater contamination from excessive fertilizer application, and depletion of water supplies through excessive or inefficient irrigation. This suggests that it is not likely that cereal grain production will continue to increase at the impressive rates reported between 1965 though 1995.

Some observers have expressed serious concern that the Chinese population, expanding in size and affluence and in its hunger for foods of animal origin, is indirectly creating a demand for cereal grain to be used as animal feed that will not be able to be met by domestic production within China. This will mean steady increases in grain importation into China. Lester R. Brown at the WorldWatch Institute cautions that this situation will have profound effects on world grain supplies and prices and ultimately influence the availability of grains available for direct human consumption.[2] Brown looked at various possible scenarios for grain consumption and production in China by the year 2030 and suggested that required Chinese grain imports may be in the range of 207 to 390 million tons. To put these numbers in perspective, the world's entire amount of grain exported in 1994 was 200 million tons. In 2030, Brown projects that 10 of the world's developing countries, themselves with expanding human populations, will need to import 190 million tons of grain for direct consumption by people to meet basic food needs. Grain is traded as a market commodity, so increased competition and demand will undoubtedly lead to higher prices. As a result, some of the least-developed countries of the world may be unable to afford to purchase the quantities of grain necessary to meet basic food needs.

Clearly there are challenges ahead and perhaps more questions than answers. Is it possible to meet the growing demand for livestock products in China without creating major distortions in world grain markets? Is it more rational for China to import finished pork and poultry products from the United States and developed countries to meet growing demand or to import the grains to raise their own livestock? Are there alternative strategies for feeding livestock that can reduce the pressure on grain supplies? In a country like China with a large rural population, inexpensive labor, and many small mixed farms, can small-scale sustainable pig and poultry production meet growing demand using a model similar to the Indian dairy industry or is intensive commercial production the only answer for improving efficiency? These are questions worthy of consideration by veterinarians interested in the challenges of international veterinary medicine.

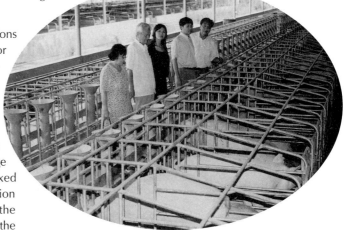

Commercial Swine Breeding Farm in Sichuan Province, China. (Photo courtesy of Dr. Terry S. Wollen, Heifer Project International, Little Rock, Arkansas)

soil structure. Even when chemical fertilizer is available, some of the costs of use can be offset by using manure as the foundation for fertilization and then purchasing only the additional fertilizer necessary to meet the supplemental requirements of the soil. In southeast Asia, for example, application of manure to fields for intensive rice production is important as a source of phosphorus. While meeting only 6 to 10% of the nitrogen requirement of the rice crop, it can provide up to 59% of the required phosphorus.

In traditional farming systems, animal management practices are often organized with an eye toward maximizing the capture of available manure. Housed animals may be kept in elevated structures with slatted floors so that manure and urine that drop below the animal house can be easily collected for distribution on fields. Animals that are routinely taken out to graze daily are still likely to be penned at night, in part for protection, but also to concentrate manure in a location in which it is easily collectible and not lost. In areas where pastoralists are present, farmers with croplands will strike deals with the herders, allowing them to turn their herds into harvested fields to glean stover and leftover grains, so that the farmer can have the benefit of the manure deposited in his fields while the animals are grazing.

Use As Fuel

In the developed world, there is reliable access to energy sources for commercial and household uses such as lighting, heating, and cooking. In much of the developing world, where energy infrastructure is lacking or the cost of energy is prohibitive for poor households, families often have to identify and procure their own energy sources for household use. Fuel wood from trees and shrubs is the most common source of household fuel where forest resources abound. However, in semiarid regions with large human populations and limited economic development, such as the Sahel region in Africa and many parts of south Asia, deforestation has been severe, and adequate fuel wood supplies are lacking. In these areas, manure has become an important source of fuel, primarily for cooking. It has been estimated that 50 to 60% of the animal manure produced in India and Pakistan is used as fuel rather than as fertilizer.

Manure can be used as cooking fuel in two ways, either burned directly or anaerobically digested to produce methane gas, which is then burned. Direct burning requires collection of animal manure, a task usually performed by children or women, who may follow grazing animals and pick up manure. The manure is then mixed with straw and water and formed into flat cakes that are laid out in the sun to dry, with intermittent turning. When dry enough for storage, they are stacked and set aside in a place safe from rain. Often, an actual mud or dung house is built to store the stacked cakes (Fig. 4-8). The dried cakes are burned as cooking fuel in simple stoves or pits. While the use of manure as a fuel has the advantage of reducing dependence on nonrenewable fossil fuels or limited forest resources, it has an adverse consequence as well, since manure burned as fuel basically becomes lost as fertilizer, thus reducing the fertility of local soils and their crop productivity.

Biogas production represents a more sophisticated and versatile approach to using manure as a fuel. Through the use of anaerobic digestion and related appropriate technology, methane gas can be produced, collected, pressurized, and piped for use as a fuel for heating, cooking, or lighting, while the digested, spent slurry can still be used as a valuable fertilizer. Such slurry is superior to fresh manure as a fertilizer because the digestion process converts a considerable proportion of the nitrogen present into forms more readily accessible for uptake by plants. Agricultural productivity can increase as much as 30% when digested slurry is used instead of fresh manure.

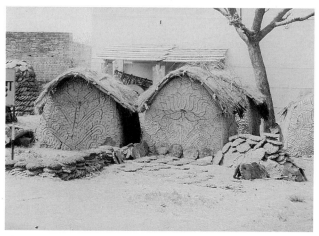

Figure 4-8.   Dung storage houses in India used for storage of manure. The manure is shaped into flat cakes and dried for storage as seen in the foreground. The dung is ultimately used as cooking fuel, especially in areas where fuel wood is scarce. Note the decorative patterns on the walls of the storage houses. (Photo by Dr. David M. Sherman)

The application of biogas technology has advanced considerably in a number of developing countries, notably China. Marchaim reports that China has over 9 million working digesters in place, providing as many as 25 million people with gas for cooking and lighting for 8 to 10 months a year, who then use straw and wood as fuel during the winter months.[13] India has at least 650,000 biodigesters, and South Korea has approximately 30,000. Many other developing countries have programs in place to increase use of biogas but have not reached this level of participation.

Biogas technology is not limited in its application only to single households. More-complex technology allows biogas to be applied in community settings, for large-scale commercial animal rearing operations, and even at the municipal and industrial level. Communal systems offer some economy of scale that make them more efficient than single-household digesters. China has 800 biogas electric stations producing electricity for over 17,000 households. The potential for expansion of biogas use as an alternative energy source in China and other countries with expanding livestock production systems is immense. Biogas technology may also offer solutions to the problem of manure waste management in developed countries where intensively housed livestock production systems generate large quantities of manure. In 2001, for instance, a dairy farmer in Oregon teamed up with the local utility company to install a biodigester on his 320-cow farm. Methane produced by the digester will be piped to a company generator to be burned as fuel to provide electricity for as many as 65 homes.[15]

Use As Feed

Under normal conditions of alimentation in animals, a significant portion of the nutrients available in feeds remains undigested or unabsorbed in the digestive tract and is passed in the feces, notably crude protein, B-complex vitamins, and some minerals. Therefore, manure possesses considerable potential nutrient value itself as a feed for livestock and fish. The use of animal manure as a source of nutrition for fish in fish ponds is a well-established, traditional practice in Asia. In the dike pond system of carp production practiced in South China, for example, pig feces and urine are routinely added to the pond as a principle nutrient source for the fish. Pig manure may contain over 20% crude protein.

The use of animal manure as a constituent of livestock feed in commercial production systems has expanded considerably in recent decades as animal production specialists and nutritionists have sought to develop balanced, least-cost rations that will keep production costs low. Additional impetus for the use of recycled manure as animal feed stems from efforts to alleviate the growing waste disposal problem associated with intensive livestock production. The potential of poultry manure and litter as animal feed has received considerable attention.

Poultry manure contains about 30% crude protein on a dry basis. Half of this is from uric acid. Rumen microbes, after a period of adaptation, can use uric acid to produce protein, and for adapted ruminants, the digestibility of crude protein in poultry manure approaches 80%, making it a valuable feed constituent for cattle, sheep, and goats. In commercial poultry production, deep litters are used under cages to absorb manure to reduce odors, moisture, and contamination. The litters themselves are frequently agricultural byproducts such as citrus meal, peanut shells, or sugar cane residue (bagasse), with some potential nutrient value. Manure-laden poultry litter removed from poultry houses can be dried and used as feed for both dairy and beef cattle, though it must be supplemented with more energy-rich feed constituents. It has no noticeable affect on the taste and smell of beef or milk. Poultry litter can also be ensiled, adding to its versatility as a cattle feed.

The practice of feeding manure to livestock offends some sensibilities and raises health concerns about both the livestock being fed and the people who ultimately consume livestock products. These concerns need to be addressed. However, in the face of growing demand for livestock products and the associated pressures on cropland to produce animal feed at the expense of human food, innovative approaches to livestock nutrition need to be developed and applied. The use of manure as a feed offers one such approach and also helps to address the problem of waste disposal from intensive livestock management systems.

Draft Power

Draft animals remain a critical source of agricultural and motive power in the developing world. The FAO estimates that 52% of the cultivated land in developing countries, excluding China, is farmed with draft animals. Only 22% of land is farmed with tractors, while 26% is still worked with hand labor. By contrast, in developed countries, 82% of cultivable land is now farmed with tractors. The use of draft animals is not uniform throughout the developing world. It is estimated that in Africa, 90% of agricultural power is provided by human

labor, 8% by draft animals, and only 2% by tractors. The potential for wider application of draft power in Africa is recognized by researchers, policymakers, and development agencies. The International Livestock Research Institute has been very active in promoting the acceptance and improved use of draft animals in different regions and farming systems of Africa.[10]

The persistence of draft power in the developing world is primarily due to economic constraints. Many poor farmers lack the capital for investment in mechanized farm equipment or have inadequate land holdings to justify the purchase of tractors or other farm machinery. Even with sufficient capital, additional constraints may exist, such as limited availability of equipment, replacement parts, qualified repair service, and reliable, affordable fuel supplies. When overall economic development in a country occurs and the buying power of farmers increases, rapid shifts away from draft animals to mechanized farming do occur. For instance, in Taiwan, one of the economic success stories of the late 20th century, rural prosperity resulted in increased mechanization of agriculture and an associated decline in buffalo numbers from 325,000 in 1960 to 123,000 in 1974, largely replaced by hand tractors (Fig. 4-9).

Nevertheless, draft animal use is still widespread and offers some practical and environmental advantages. Draft animals are, for the most part, self-repairing and self-propagating. They do not require nonrenewable fossil fuels to operate, but rather are fueled by renewable, locally produced energy sources, namely, forages and other crop products and byproducts. Draft animals can be integrated into small farming systems and provide additional services to the farmer in the form of manure, offspring, and milk when cows are used. In some situations, animal tillage actually may be preferable to tractor tillage in that it is less damaging to soils, resulting in less compaction than tractor use. For millions of cash-poor, hand-laboring, small-scale farmers in Africa and elsewhere, the introduction of sustainable draft power can reduce labor burdens and improve the overall productivity of small farms.

Animals used for draft purposes around the world include cattle, buffalo, horses, donkeys, camels, and elephants. Selection depends on local conditions of geography, climate, soil characteristics, farming system, animal adaptation and availability; the type of work required; and cultural preference. The advantages of water buffalo over cattle for use in wetland rice farming in southeast Asia, for example, was mentioned earlier in this chapter. When cattle are used for agricultural work, it is usually castrated males, known either as oxen or bullocks, that are used. Oxen are more tractable than bulls and are preferred over cows because of relative size and strength. However, the opportunity costs of maintaining draft oxen for agricultural work are high. They may be used intensively for short periods of the year but must be fed and cared for year round. During this time they will produce manure but may produce little else of value. There is much interest in promoting the use of cows as draft animals, as the animals can provide milk and offspring in addition to labor, thus offering the farmer and family greater returns year round for the investment in feeding and maintenance.

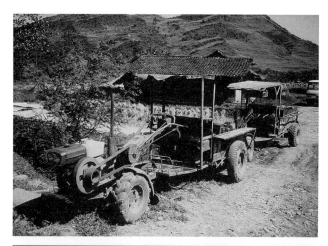

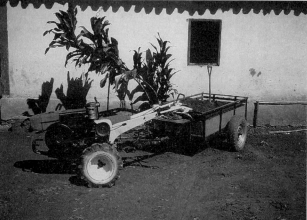

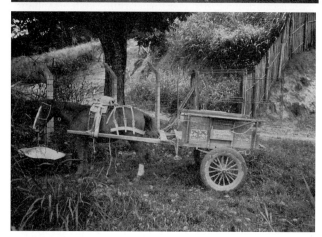

Figure 4–9.   Small tractors like the ones pictured here from China (top) and Brazil (middle) are replacing draft animals in many developing countries. The machines can be used for field work but can also be hooked to a wagon or trailer and used as road vehicles to transport loads to town. When draft animals are replaced by machines, feed resources can be used instead to feed food-producing animals. However, these small tractors are polluting, use nonrenewable fossil fuels, and are costly to purchase and maintain relative to draft animals such as the Brazilian horse shown at bottom. (All photos by Dr. David M. Sherman)

However, the successful use of cows for draft purposes requires much greater attention to health and nutrition if the animal is going to be able to provide all the various services that are expected. Fertility and milk production often decline in draft cows unless adequate supplemental feed of high quality is provided. Similarly, the use of draft animals in pairs rather than single animals for plowing may increase overall livestock numbers and put heavy demands on available feed supplies and the farmer's overall resources. There have been numerous efforts, notably in Ethiopia, to design single-ox yokes and plows and encourage the use of single-ox plowing.

The use of draft power around the world is not restricted to the farm. As recently, as 1980, it was estimated that as much as 60% of all goods taken to market in India and Pakistan were transported by draft animals. Today, that percentage is reduced, but it is still commonplace to see donkey carts, horse-drawn taxis, and large, heavily laden wagons pulled by camels jostling for position with cars, trucks, and buses in the congested urban streets of south Asia. In rural areas, draft animals continue to be used to carry burdens such as straw, fuel wood, and drinking water from the fields and countryside back to the village and to carry produce and other agricultural products to district or regional markets. In Latin America, donkeys and llamas are used to bring coffee and other mountain-grown products down from the slopes, and in India, the Army still uses mules to carry ordinance up to remote military outposts on the mountainous borders with China and Pakistan.

The successful use and ensured productivity of draft animals requires good health and access to veterinary services. There are numerous health constraints on working stock. Skin wounds associated with ill-fitting yokes and harnesses are commonplace, as is lameness associated with overwork and poor foot care. Undernutrition and parasitism are widespread. Regrettably, poor farmers and teamsters who use draft animals often lack the financial resources to obtain adequate veterinary service, or such service may not be available. Improving access to veterinary care for draft animals is an important and worthwhile goal for improving agricultural productivity and economic development in developing countries.

Herding and Protection

Livestock herders face a number of risks and hardships, including predation and theft of their stock. Dogs have long been used by herders in different parts of the world, as a means of reducing these risks, and a number of livestock-guarding dog breeds, such as the Aidi of Morocco, the Akbash and the Kangal of Turkey, the Komondor of Hungary, and the Ovtcharka breeds of Russia and Central Asia, have been developed over the years to specifically address this need. The use of dogs as protection naturally extended to sedentary farmers to defend their penned livestock and to villagers to protect their families and household goods.

Today, in an era of intense, accelerating, global urbanization, the dog as a protector of property has become widespread in the world's cities. It is difficult to obtain statistical information on urban dog populations or their rate of growth, but one need only listen to the incessant din of barking, howling, and other forms of canine expression that marks nightfall in any contemporary African city to be convinced that dogs are ubiquitous. In much of Asia, Latin America, and Africa, members of the expanding urban middle class increasingly live in single-family houses surrounded by a high wall with a metal gate. Worries about crime are widespread, and security is a common concern. While the number of home security options continues to expand, the use of dogs, turned out to patrol the walled compound at night, remains a preferred choice. From 1950 to the close of the 20th century, the number of people living in urban environments increased from 0.75 billion to approximately 2.75 billion people, or about 46% of the world's population. This increase has led to a concurrent increase in the number of urban dogs, many of which are used for protection purposes. This increase in turn has encouraged demand for small animal clinical veterinary services in urban centers around the world, a demand that so far, has not always been successfully met. The potential for increased small animal practice in urban areas of the developing world remains high. Urbanization also leads to increases in stray dog and cat populations, with attendant problems of animal suffering and public health problems such as rabies.

Financial Services

An Afghan friend visiting the United States in 1996 was asked what most impressed him about America. What most impressed him, he said, "was that you could stick a plastic card into a brick wall and in response, money came out." While citizens in developed countries can take the ATM machine and other financial services for granted, many citizens in the developing world have little or no access to even the most basic banking services, such as savings accounts or credit. This remains particularly true in rural areas, where animals serve the function of "cash on the hoof."

For farmers, herders, and landless villagers, livestock often serve a variety of financial functions. Steady income can be derived from regular sales of milk, eggs, or manure. Periodic income can be generated from sale of meat or hides from slaughtered animals, wool or hair from seasonally shorn animals, or from fees for services involving the use of their animals, such as breeding, plowing, or transport.

Farmers with excess cash income from the sale of crops and no bank to deposit it in may buy additional animals as means of savings. These animals serve as an investment of "principal," and the offspring they produce are the "interest" on the account, which can be held or spent. When cash markets are not available for crop surpluses, these crop surpluses will be fed to animals as a means of storing the surplus and drawing upon it later for food or cash to meet recurring demands such as purchase of seed, fertilizer, and equipment; payment of school fees; or unforeseen expenses such as medical bills. Small stock, such as sheep, goats, poultry, and rabbits are often used as savings accounts rather than larger, more-expensive animals such as cattle for practical reasons. Just as there is more opportunity and less risk in having a mixed investment portfolio, so it is with having a mix of small ruminants and poultry rather than owning a single cow.

Cultural and Religious Uses

Before humans domesticated animals, they observed and studied them. By learning the behavior and habits of wild animals, humans were able to draw them gradually into the sphere of human society as domesticated versions of their wild progenitors. During their study, humans reflected on the similarities and differences between themselves and various kinds of animals, and in the process, animals came to be imbued with spiritual and symbolic significance for human beings. Human ideas about animals and what they represented became an integral part of religious ritual and cultural expression. Specific animals became associated with certain human traits or came to represent significant deities in polytheistic religions. Animals were used in ritual to seek help, give thanks, purge sin, acquire virtue, or appease the gods.

Animals continue to serve a variety of cultural and religious purposes in human society. For instance, the use of animals in sport and recreation is almost universal, though it takes many forms, be it rodeo in the United States, bullfighting in Spain, hare coursing in England, Buzkhazi in Afghanistan, goat racing in Tobago, cock fighting in the Philippines, camel racing in Dubai, horse racing in Mongolia, or chukar partridge fighting in Pakistan. A considerable number of the sporting activities that involve animals are so-called blood sports that lead to injury or death of animal participants. Social and political pressures are increasing to curb bloodsports, but it should be recognized, in a cross-cultural context, that sentiments against such activities are by no means universal.

The breeding and showing of animals, though frequently serving a commercial purpose, also provides an important social function for the people involved. Fairs and festivals that focus on the display of animals and the awarding of prizes are commonplace around the world (Fig. 4-10). Pet keeping may also be considered principally a recreational activity, though the psychosocial benefits of animals serving in the role of companions are being increasingly recognized. This recognition has led to the increased use of animals for therapeutic purposes in a number of settings, including prisons, nursing homes, and hospitals.

In traditional societies, animals continue to serve a number of cultural and religious functions beyond recreation or diversion. In animal-centered cultures, such as the pastoralist societies of Africa, animals play a number of important social roles beyond providing a livelihood. The Karimojong of Uganda, for instance, use their livestock to cement social contracts between families or clans, such as occurs when cattle are offered as part of the bride price prior to marriage. The Karimojong also carry out ceremonial sacrifice of cattle in recognition of the spiritual significance of cattle in the culture. By drinking the blood and eating the meat of the sacrificed ox, Karimojong men ac-

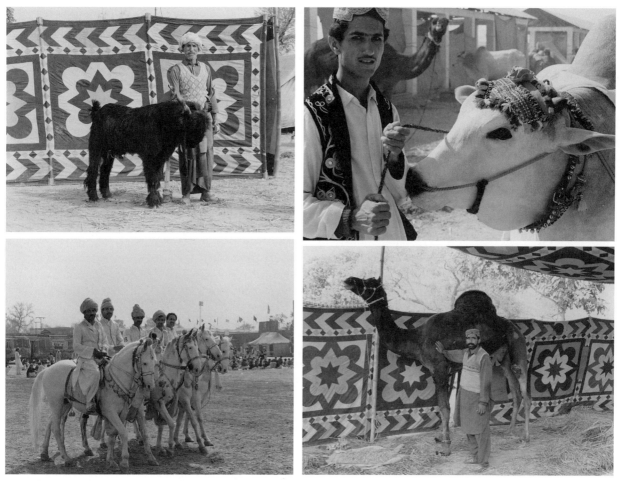

Figure 4–10.   Showing prized livestock at fairs has a worldwide appeal for animal keepers. At Pakistan's annual national agricultural show in Lahore, it was not difficult to get camel, goat, horse, and cattle owners to pose proudly with their animals. (All photos by Dr. David M. Sherman)

knowledge their dependence upon the God who provided them with the gift of cattle and allowed them to prosper. The sacrifice also serves to maintain the link with their forefathers, who also tended cattle received from God. The individuality and personality of young Karimojong men are closely linked to their cattle. Each Karimojong herder has a special relationship with a particular ox that was received from his father as a calf and whose name he adopts as his "name of respect" when addressed by his inferiors (Fig. 4-11). He will risk his life to save his special ox in the event of an enemy raid and might even commit suicide in the event of its death.[14]

Animal Management Systems

Livestock are managed under a variety of production systems around the world. The production system that prevails in any given place reflects the local available resource base. The key determining resources are land, labor, and capital, though climate, geography, and culture also play important roles in shaping the management system. Traditional systems, prevalent in developing countries, tend to reflect conditions of abundant land, cheap labor, and limited capital. However, in many areas of the world, population increases and economic development are placing new limits on land availability and forcing some changes in traditional patterns of animal keeping. The more modern, mechanized, and intensive systems of livestock management, seen primarily in developed countries, generally reflect the prevailing conditions of expensive or limited land, scarce or expensive labor, and abundant capital.

Brief summaries of the main animal management systems present in the world today are presented in the following sections. These systems include pastoralism, agropastoralism, transhumance, ranching, mixed subsistence farming, mixed specialty farming, intensive industrial livestock production, and aquaculture. In addition, the role of livestock in the lives of landless villagers and urban dwellers and the role of livestock in sustainable agriculture are discussed.

Pastoralism

Pastoralism is a mobile system of keeping livestock in which herders move repeatedly with their grazing animals in search of suitable pasture and water, usually on a seasonal basis. Pas-

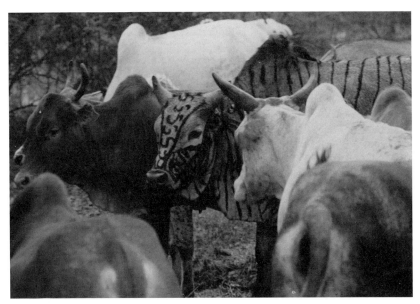

Figure 4–11. A favorite ox, decorated by a Karimjong herder in northeastern Uganda. The Karimojong are one of numerous cattle-based, pastoralist cultures in Africa that derive spiritual, social, and utilitarian value from their cattle. (Photo by Dr. David M. Sherman)

beest herds are still prevalent, herders will keep their cattle away from grasslands where wildebeest are calving to reduce the risk of exposure to malignant catarrhal fever.

The mix of species kept by pastoralists will depend largely on local conditions of feed and water availability. When there is sufficient water, cattle are usually present and are often the focus of the herding group. The Maasai, Dinka, and Karimojong of east Africa are, for example, cattle-based cultures (Fig. 4-12). However, in some pastoralist regions, conditions are too consistently dry or vegetation too sparse to support cattle. In these areas, for example, Afghanistan or Arabia, grazing herds are composed primarily of sheep, goats, camels, and possibly donkeys. Even in cattle-based cultures though, herds are often mixed, with sheep and goats maintained along with cattle. This represents a strategy for reducing and diversifying risk of catastrophic loss in drought-prone environments.

toralists are found primarily in semiarid regions of the world, where inadequate, erratic, or seasonal rainfall will not support reliable crop production. The grazing of livestock on these dry rangelands represents the most appropriate and practical way to use the land productively for food production. The traditional pastoral system depends on virtually no external inputs. Solar energy is converted to animal protein via the grazing of animals on natural, rain-fed grasslands . The main input is the labor of herders tending and defending their grazing stock. Connections to crop agriculture are minimal. Crop farmers, when present in pastoral regions, may invite herders to graze their animals in harvested fields to forage on crop residues so that the farmer may benefit from the animal manure deposited in the fields.

An estimated 180 million people worldwide are engaged in pastoralism, tending approximately 960 million ruminant livestock on some 10 million km² of arid or semiarid rangeland. Some of the world's pastoralist groups include the Taureg and Bororo of the western Sahel in Africa; the Maasai, Turkana, Samburu, Karimojong, and Dinka of eastern sub-Saharan Africa; the Bedouins of Arabia; the Raikas and Gujars of Rajasthan in western India; and the Koochi Pashtun of Afghanistan. Most pastoralists communities represent specific ethnic groups divided along tribal lines, with their own characteristic culture and preferences for animal species used.

The movements of pastoralists are not random. Rather, they represent accumulated experience about a variety of factors, including rainfall patterns, geography, forage quality, land rights, tribal conflicts, and disease risks. In consideration of disease, for example, African herders seasonally move cattle away from areas when tsetse flies are active, to reduce the risk of trypanosomiasis. Similarly, in eastern Africa, where wilde-

Maintaining large herds is another common strategy for minimizing risk in the face of harsh and unpredictable conditions. The rationale is that the greater the number of cattle present when a drought begins, the greater the proportion of cattle that are likely to survive the drought and serve as seed stock for repopulation. Furthermore, traditional pastoralism is a subsistence undertaking. Livestock are raised primarily for the use of herders and their families, for food as well as for a variety of cultural purposes. Traditionally there is not a great inclination to sell off animals to external markets for commercial purposes, though in more-recent times, considerable efforts have been undertaken by governments and development agencies

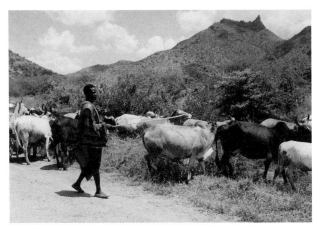

Figure 4–12. A Karimojong herder tends cattle in northeastern Uganda. Pastoralism represents the most rational use of semiarid rangelands for production of food through the grazing of ruminant animals. The Karimojong also tend sheep and goats, which may be herded with the cattle or tended separately by young boys. (Photo by Dr. David M. Sherman)

to encourage greater offtake from pastoralist herds. A key reason, beyond promoting economic activity, is that large herds are often cited by environmentalists as an important cause of land degradation and desertification in the fragile environments where pastoralists are generally found. The role of pastoralism in land degradation is, in fact, a complex issue about which there is still significant debate, as discussed further in Chapter 6.

The pastoral way of life is under siege. Many governments view pastoralists as backward and unproductive, and some have explicit policies to encourage pastoralists to give up their traditional way of life and pursue sedentary livelihoods. Even without the pressure of hostile governments, economic development and population growth are undermining traditional pastoral livelihoods. Traditional grazing lands have been annexed into protected wildlife areas, converted to crop production, switched over to commercial ranching, or simply disappeared under the advance of urban expansion. Complaints of land degradation intensify as livestock populations are increasingly crowded onto shrinking areas of traditional grazing.

The irony in the assault on pastoralism is that livestock grazing, as traditionally practiced by pastoralist herders, may be the most cost-effective way to exploit semiarid grasslands for food production. It is true that some grasslands can be converted to crop production, but this often requires intensive capital inputs in the form of irrigation, fertilizers, pest control, and other technical resources. Even ranching systems may not be as cost-effective or productive as traditional pastoralist systems. Recognition of the importance of traditional pastoralism has increased in recent years, and considerable efforts have been made to better understand pastoralist culture and practices, to recognize the productivity of pastoralism, and to develop support services to ensure its future. The current status of pastoralism and prospects for the future have recently been reviewed.[1] A good source for more information about pastoralism is the Pastoralists Development Network (PDN), which now functions through the internet under the auspices of the Overseas Development Institute. An extensive range of PDN papers is available on-line at http://www.odi.org.uk/pdn/index.html.

Agropastoralism

Agropastoralism is a form of pastoralist livelihood in which some crop agriculture is carried out in addition to extensive grazing of livestock. Livestock keeping remains the principal economic or cultural activity of the community, while cropping serves as a means to diversify risk by providing alternative sources of food or cash income as well as a source of supplemental feed for livestock during periods of poor grazing.

Some pastoralist groups, such as the Maasai, have been historically disdainful of crop agriculture and the neighboring peoples who practice it. Others, however, have electively incorporated cropping activity into their overall survival strategy, such as the Barabaig of north central Tanzania. While their culture is centered around cattle, and milk and blood are their preferred foods, the Barabaig have a long-standing practice of supplementing their diet with maize. Maize may be obtained by barter or purchase from sedentary farmers, but the Barabaig themselves engage in maize cultivation on small plots of one-quarter acre. Similarly, archeological and anthropological information on southern African tribes, notably the Tswana, Zulu, and Shona, suggest that these cultures have carried out extensive grazing in conjunction with crop production for at least 700 or more years. Agropastoralism is also traditionally practiced among people living around the oases of the Sahara desert, who use irrigation to grow date palms and extensively graze camels, sheep, and goats beyond the periphery of the oasis settlement.

While some pastoralist groups have chosen agropastoralism, other groups have been pushed into crop production by changing circumstance. Government policies promoting settlement, the loss of prime grazing lands to commercial agriculture ventures, urban sprawl, war or civil insecurity, and expanded populations within the herding communities themselves are just some of the pressures that have made herding more tenuous and increased the need for herders to seek modified means of livelihood. When possible, most pastoralist groups resist outright sedentarization. Instead, the family or clan may be split, with some members remaining behind in settlements to cultivate crops along with some milking animals and perhaps poultry, while others continue to graze mixed herds of livestock extensively. During dry seasons, livestock may be returned to the family settlement to consume crop residues as supplemental feed. In the Sahel region, many among the Taureg and Wodaabe pastoralists have made the transition to agropastoralism in response to many of the pressures cited above.

While subsurface water supplies may be available in some places, allowing continuous or rotational cropping, in most cases, crop cultivation in agropastoralist systems is rain fed, depending primarily on seasonal rainfall, which is often variable in semiarid regions. In Africa, millet and sorghum, which are relatively drought resistant, are preferred cereal crops, though in areas of higher rainfall, maize is also grown. Groundnuts may be cultivated as a cash crop, and vegetable gardens are also cultivated and assume greater importance when rainfall will support them.

Transhumance

Transhumance is a form of extensive livestock management in which herders and their animals move seasonally between two specific regions. In many transhumant cultures, one seasonal site may be a permanent settlement, as in Scandinavia, Austria, Germany, and Switzerland. Traditionally, cattle, sheep and goat herders in these countries would move their animals up into the mountains as the snow melted, to take advantage of summer mountain pastures between May and September. Access to the high mountain pastures was difficult, and herders would remain with their flocks in the mountains for the grazing season. They would frequently engage in cheese making to convert the summer milk into a storable form. In the winter, animals would be returned to the valleys below for winter grazing or to be housed and fed stored feeds, depending on the severity of winter conditions. The prevailing cold temperatures and short days of winter in these temperate countries generally required the construction of permanent animal housing in an established, settled site.

In other places, where winters are less severe, permanent settlements may not be part of the transhumant system. For instance, in Iran, tribal Bakhtiari, Basseri, Quashqai, and Lur herders may graze their sheep and goats on the grasslands of the central plateau during winter and then migrate as much as 1000 km to use the rich upland pastures of the Zagros Mountains in the summertime. As this example suggests, precise categorization of certain types of extensive grazing is sometimes difficult. Pastoralism and transhumance represent a continuum of adaptations rather than discrete categories of extensive livestock management.

Ranching

Ranching can be viewed as a commercial form of pastoralism. It involves the extensive grazing of livestock on large farms, estates, or leased rangelands. There is little or no relation between ranching and crop production. Ranching represents another means of using rangelands for food production by exploiting the capacity of ruminant animals to convert plant material not directly edible by humans to animal protein. While traditional pastoralists engage in livestock keeping as a subsistence activity, ranching is managed for profit, with the offtake and sale of livestock as the principle objective. The issue of offtake is important. In the 1960s, many foreign assistance programs in Africa were aimed at encouraging traditional pastoralists to take up ranching. Some of these programs failed, at least in part, because their advocates did not recognize that pastoralists are culturally disinclined to sell "excess" cattle. Ranching projects would identify specific carrying capacities for cattle on a given acreage on the assumption that the periodic sale of young and culled cattle would maintain a suitable, stable herd size. When pastoralists-cum-ranchers kept their cattle instead, as was their traditional practice, the overpopulated ranch lands soon became degraded and nonproductive.

Historically, ranching has been a low-input enterprise. It required low labor inputs and low capital investments but large areas of land. Since rangelands were generally perceived as not suitable for other uses, the cost of rangeland was generally low. This situation is changing in modern times, and ranching is becoming more costly. With the advent of modern irrigation technology, some rangelands have become suitable for cropping, increasing land value. Other rangeland may increase in value as it is eyed for commercial development, suburban expansion, or recreational use. In the face of encroaching development, most ranches now require fencing, which is relatively costly. Ranchers may also need to invest in pasture improvement through fertilization and seeding with more nutritious grasses and legumes to compensate for range degradation and to improve nutrition for grazing cattle. Grazing fees for ranchers using government-owned land are also increasing. In the face of higher costs, ranchers must become expert managers to protect profit margins.

Cattle ranching is a major form of livestock keeping in North America, Central America, South America, and Australia and has also been introduced into Africa with some success. The major sheep ranching area of the world is Australia and New Zealand, with considerable sheep ranching still occurring in South America, notably, in Uruguay and Argentina. Sheep ranching, though important in the 19th century, has declined in the United States. In general, goats are not kept in ranching schemes. They are more often kept under situations of traditional pastoralism. Fiber-producing goats, however, may be managed commercially under extensive grazing systems. For example, Angora goat ranching is practiced in the Edwards Plateau region of Texas, with mohair harvested for sale.

The best cattle ranching in South America occurs in the temperate Pampas region of Argentina and Uruguay, where fertile soils, warm temperatures, and adequate rainfall support good grass growth. Ranchers have been able to enhance productivity in the Pampas by introducing Hereford cattle and other imported European breeds and by sowing rye grasses, clover, and alfalfa in the more humid regions. In Brazil's Matto Grosso region, conditions are drier and harsher, and pasture improvement is more difficult to achieve. Cattle can take up to 6 years to reach slaughter weight under these conditions. Improved Zebu types of cattle are kept in this region, as they are more drought and disease resistant than the European breeds.

In Australia, the central desert is more or less surrounded by rough grazing land. In dry areas, it may take up to 400 ha (1,000 acres) to support a single steer, and ranches of 40,000 ha (100,000 acres) are not uncommon. Zebu-type cattle, such as Brahmin, are more common in the tropical northern regions of the country, while European breeds are raised in the more temperate, southern regions. Sheep ranches can also be up to 40,000 ha (100,000 acres). Merino sheep producing a fine-quality wool predominate, and Australia is the world's major producer and exporter of wool.

In Africa, ranching is most common in the southern nations of South Africa, Zimbabwe, and Namibia, where historically, white settlers developed commercial agricultural enterprises. Cattle, sheep, and Angora goats are raised under ranching conditions. Some cattle-ranching schemes have taken hold in eastern Africa as well. The savannas of Africa often represent a mixture of grasses along with shrubs and trees. Research has shown that cattle, sheep, and goats grazed together under ranching conditions can use such a diversity of forages more productively and increase the overall offtake. An even more efficient exploitation of the various plants available on savanna can be achieved by the inclusion of indigenous wild ruminants in ranching schemes, since over the evolutionary time frame, these various species have frequently identified noncompetitive feeding niches in the savanna ecology. Indeed, game ranching offers an alternative approach to commercial use of grasslands, and interest in game ranching, particularly in South Africa, has been increasing in recent years as discussed further in Chapter 7.

While ranching represents an important and useful means of producing food and fiber for human consumption, it has been associated in recent times with environmental problems, particularly land degradation and deforestation. Land degradation is associated primarily with overstocking of animals, excessive concentration of animals around specific sites such as watering points, and the failure to move animals regularly throughout the grazing area. Deforestation has become an issue in ranching, particularly in Latin America, where rainforest has been systematically cleared and then used, at least initially, for cattle ranching. The relationship of ranching to these environmental problems is discussed further in Chapter 6.

Mixed Subsistence Farming

In the spectrum of animal management systems under discussion, mixed subsistence farming is the first that represents a fully sedentary system. The primary focus is usually crop cultivation on a small parcel of land, sometimes as little as 0.2 ha (0.5 acre) as in some Middle Eastern countries, 1 ha (2.5 acres) in Bangladesh, or 4 ha (10 acres) in the Punjab region of northern India. In the 1980s it was estimated that there were over 100 million farms in the developing world with a size under 5 ha (12.5 acres) and an additional 50 million farms of less than 1 ha (2.5 acres).

Though crops may represent the main source of food for the farm family, animals play a vital role in supporting the overall farming operation. They provide animal traction for working the fields, manure to fertilize the soil, transport of goods to market, food, fiber, a savings account, cash income, and risk diversification. The integration of crop and animal agriculture is a key feature of the mixed subsistence farming system. Mixed subsistence farming relies on few external inputs, and there is a high value placed on the use and cycling of all available nutrient resources within the farming system. Animals are an essential part of this nutrient recycling, through consumption of household wastes and crop residues such as stubble and straw and the return of manure to croplands.

Mixed subsistence farming represents the most widespread form of agricultural activity in the world today. An estimated 440 million farmers in developing countries practice mainly subsistence agriculture, and subsistence crops cover more than 50% of land resources in most low-income countries. Subsistence farmers are found primarily in humid and subhumid tropical regions of the developing world, where rainfall volumes and patterns adequately support crop production. Mixed subsistence farming is constrained in semiarid regions by lack of rainfall, but the use of irrigation has allowed the system to take hold in some dry regions as well, notably in south Asian countries such as Pakistan and Afghanistan and north African countries such as Egypt. Historically, mixed subsistence farming was common in temperate and tropical highland regions

of the world, but economic development and new market opportunities have stimulated a shift away from subsistence farming to income-driven, specialty mixed farming, such as commercial dairying, as discussed in the next section.

Regional, climatic and cultural differences influence the mix of crops and livestock that are used in mixed subsistence farming. In much of Asia, rice is the principal crop, with water buffalo primarily used for draft power. Pigs, ducks, geese, chickens, and fish are well integrated into the farming system through various nutrient-cycling practices. In Latin America, maize, beans, potatoes, and rice are important crops, while oxen, donkeys, mules, or horses may be used for animal traction. In highland regions, llamas may be used for transport. Animals for food or cash include pigs, small ruminants, llamas, cattle, poultry, rabbits, and guinea pigs. In the Pacific Islands of Oceania, subsistence farmers are likely to grow root crops such as taro, yams, and sweet potatoes; keep pigs in the farmyard; and supplement their animal protein needs by fishing.

In dry north Africa, such as in Egypt, subsistence farmers commonly grow barley and wheat as staple crops plus a variety of fruit and nut trees as well as pulses such as beans, peas, and lentils. Fields are worked primarily by oxen, and small ruminants and poultry are kept. In the drier, low-rainfall regions of sub-Saharan Africa, sorghum and millet are the principal crops, with oxen, camels, or donkeys providing draft power, and small ruminants, chickens, and possibly a cow rounding out the farm animal population. In subhumid areas of Africa, maize is the predominant crop, and the animal populations are similar, though, for non-Muslims, pigs are more likely to be present, and the potential to sustain one or more dairy animals is higher than in drier areas. In humid Africa, bananas and root crops such as cassava and yams assume greater importance, and pigs, poultry, and small ruminants are common in the farmyard. The mixed farming systems of the developing world, both subsistence and commercial, contain approximately 67% of the cattle and 64% of the small ruminants in the world, and these numbers are increasing most rapidly in the humid and subhumid regions. Sheep and goat numbers are increasing at a much faster rate than cattle numbers, suggesting that human population pressure continues to reduce farm size and access to feed resources for larger stock.

In recent years, farming systems analysts and policymakers have begun to pay more attention to the farming practices of mixed subsistence farmers and the lessons that can be learned from them. The integration of livestock and crop production, the practice of nutrient recycling between crops and livestock, the maintenance of soil fertility through fallowing, the rotation of crops to reduce pest buildups, conservation of soil and trapping of rainwater through terracing, and the relative independence from nonrenewable external energy inputs are highly desirable aspects of subsistence farming from the standpoint of protecting environmental quality and promoting agricultural sustainability. At the same time, there is recognition that in the face of growing human populations, expanding pressures on arable land resources, and demand for increased quantity and diversity of food supplies, mixed subsistence farming systems need to become more productive and contribute more to meeting food demands beyond those of the immediate family. There is also recognition that population pressure is causing subsistence farmers to abandon some desirable practices, such as fallowing. Some critics contend that subsistence agriculture has become nonviable in the modern world and requires a radical overhaul, with strong emphasis on commercialization.

Nevertheless, the potential for improved production for many subsistence farmers is considerable and could be achieved if these farmers had, among other things, land tenure reforms to improve opportunities for land ownership; more available credit for improved seeds, fertilizer, and equipment; better access to improved animal genetics; better interaction with extension and veterinary services tailored to the needs of small farmers; better market information, organization, and access; and improved rural infrastructure such as bridges, paved roads, and phone service to support increased productivity and entry into a market economy. The challenge, of course, is to preserve the sustainable aspects of small mixed farms while increasing productivity to meet growing food demands in the marketplace. These aspects of rural development are discussed further in Chapter 5.

Mixed Specialty Farming

Mixed specialty farming is a sedentary system of agriculture that integrates crops and livestock for the primary objective of producing livestock and/or livestock products for sale and profit. Crop production is not geared toward feeding the farm family as in mixed subsistence farming, but rather toward feeding the livestock. Forage crops and cereal grains suitable as animal feeds predominate crop cultivation in this system. Typical livestock products may include dairy products, eggs, poultry, specialty fibers, and market animals for slaughter, such as hogs, sheep, or goats, the choice depending on production potential, market demand, and culture. With regard to dairy products, for example, a family with a specialized dairy farm in the United States is likely to produce cows' milk, a French family might produce goat milk, and a Pakistani family, buffalo milk.

Mixed specialty farming represents the transition of mixed subsistence farming into the commercial sector. The process occurs usually in response to external factors that create a market demand for livestock products along with the development of suitable infrastructure and public policies that enable farmers to move livestock products to market successfully and achieve a reasonable profit. Some of these factors include general economic development; increased population; enlarged urban markets; increases in per capita income; farm-to-market infrastructure improvements such as paved roads, mechanized transport, and refrigeration; and deregulation of prices paid to farmers for their products (Fig. 4-13).

The transition from small-scale subsistence farming to specialized livestock production has been going on in different

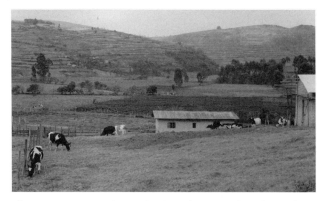

Figure 4-13. Mixed specialty dairy farm on the outskirts of Kampala, the capital city of Uganda. This farm demonstrates substantial capital investment in improved Holstein cattle, permanent buildings and fencing, as well as land for forage production and pasturing. Increased urban demand for milk products can stimulate the transition from subsistence farming to mixed specialty farming such as this. (Photo by Dr. David M. Sherman)

settings under different sets of circumstances for quite some time. An excellent example of this transformation occurred in what was to become the Corn Belt in the American Midwest during the second half of the 19th century. In 1862, to promote settlement of the hinterlands and land ownership among citizens, the U.S. Congress passed the Homestead Act, which offered ownership of a 160-acre parcel of land in the American prairie to any family willing to pay 10 dollars and work the land for 5 years. The response was enormous, and many easterners moved their families to the Midwest, including Iowa and Nebraska. These initial settlers, who came to be known as sodbusters, converted the dense grass prairies, formerly grazed by bison, into crop fields, in the process using the top layer of sod as building material to construct their simple cabinlike sod dwellings. Initially, these settlers engaged in mixed subsistence farming, not unlike what one would observe today in many parts of Africa, Latin America, or Asia. Crops of wheat and barley were planted, and vegetable gardens were cultivated, emphasizing root crops with good storage characteristics such as beets, squash, melons, and potatoes. A flock of chickens ran free around the sod house to produce eggs, along with several pigs to produce meat and lard. The more fortunate families had a milk cow and calf tethered nearby. A pair of horses or mules was present for field work and trips to town. (Fig. 4-14).

Then conditions began to change. The Civil War created a considerable demand for preserved meat products to feed the Union Army, which in turn stimulated growth and development of the meat-packing industry. By 1861, the city of Chicago had replaced Cincinnati as the main center of meat packing in response to this Civil War demand. By 1865, nine separate rail lines were converging in Chicago, and the Chicago Union Stock Yards were opened, with large pens capable of holding up to 100,000 hogs at any given time. Following the Civil War, demand for pork products remained high as a result

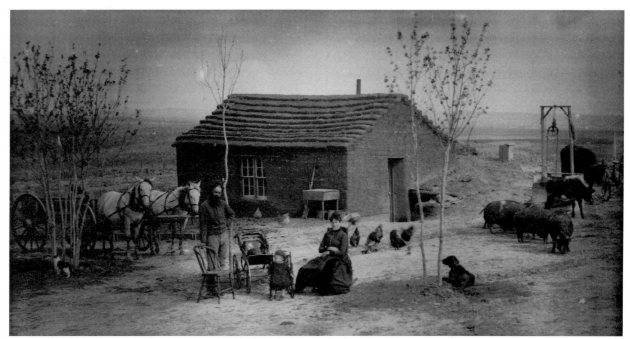

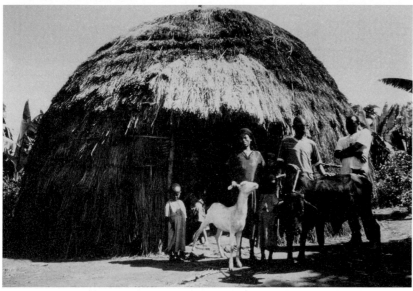

Figure 4–14. Top, Sodbusters in Nebraska in the 19th century. The mix of livestock and the rudimentary housing are not unlike what is often found in some rural areas of Africa, Asia, and Latin America in the present day. Bottom, A subsistence farm family in the Ethiopian highlands at the end of the 20th century living under similar circumstances. (Top photo with permission of the Nebraska Historical Society; bottom photo courtesy of FARM Africa-UK, London, England)

of urbanization and industrialization in the Eastern cities, a growing export market to Europe, and completion of the transcontinental railroad in 1869, which served growing markets in the West. In 1872, Armour & Company developed the first chill room at its Chicago slaughtering plant, to allow year-round slaughter and sale of fresh meat. By 1881, refrigerated rail cars were sufficiently advanced that shipment of dressed carcasses to coastal urban markets from Chicago was routine.

These developments were not lost on the homesteaders and their offspring in Iowa and Nebraska. The soils and climate of the region had proved excellent for production of feed corn, and hogs thrived on a corn-based diet. Many farmers in the region began to grow corn as the principal field crop and to feed hogs for sale to Chicago. By 1885, the U.S. corn crop exceeded 2 billion bushels, double what was produced in 1870. The vast majority of that corn went into hog feeding, and the subsis-

tence homesteaders of the prairie had become the specialty hog producers of the Corn Belt. In, 1867, following the end of the Civil War, there were approximately 1.75 million hogs in Iowa; a half-century later, following the end of World War I in 1919, there were 10.92 million.

The shift to commercial hog production in the Corn Belt underscores how external factors create opportunities for small farmers to enter commercial markets. The same situation is now being repeated elsewhere in the world, as economic development, increased market demands, and technological advances are stimulating change. The traditional rice/water buffalo subsistence systems of China and other south Asian countries offer an example. Many southeast Asian nations have undergone substantial urbanization and industrialization in recent years, with growing demand for food animal products in urban markets. Technological advance has also reached a growing number of subsistence farmers, who have purchased small, diesel-powered, mechanical tillers to prepare their rice fields, thus reducing or eliminating the need to maintain water buffalo. Many have given up their water buffalo and used the available feedstuffs instead to raise dairy cattle or hogs to produce income-earning commodities for domestic urban markets.

Another dramatic example of the shift to specialty farming is the growth and development of the small-scale dairy industry in India over the last 40 years (see sidebar "People Power: The Success of Cooperative Dairying in India"). Everywhere that urban demand for milk is rising, some farmers have taken the initiative to develop small specialty dairy enterprises.

The same forces that create new opportunities for mixed specialty farming can also create threats and challenges. Even the successful hog-producing descendents of the sodbusters in Iowa must continue to respond to changing market forces. In recent years, as the global market for pork continues to expand, competition has increased, production costs have risen, and the nature of hog farming has changed. Large corporations have entered the hog business to capitalize on economies of scale in large, industrialized, hog-production operations and have used their international marketing experience to establish a competitive edge. Many American family farmers have recognized that they must respond to these changes or lose their livelihood. Some have become hog-raising subcontractors to large corporations, while others have become involved in efforts to pass state laws that limit corporate farming.

Intensive Industrial Livestock Production

Intensive industrial livestock production is a commercial system of livestock raising in which animals are confined and fed in buildings or yards. The production process is carefully managed to achieve well-defined production and market goals. Intensive systems are found most commonly in highly industrialized countries, in which adequate capital, technological expertise, transportation infrastructure, and energy supplies are reliably available to support such enterprises. By 1996, industrial livestock systems were responsible for 43% of total global meat production. This included over half of world pork and broiler poultry production and 10% of beef and mutton production. The most highly developed countries, as reflected by membership in the Organization for Economic Cooperation and Development (OECD) were responsible for 52% of world industrial pork production and 58% of industrial broiler production. The OECD countries include most western European countries, the United States, Canada, Japan, Australia, and New Zealand.

In intensive industrial livestock production systems there is frequently a disconnection of the traditional link between crop and animal agriculture. A central characteristic of industrial production is the concentration of large numbers of animals into production units to achieve production efficiency through economies of scale. In many instances, the feed requirements of the animals in a large unit exceed what can be produced locally, so that feed, mostly in the form of cereal grains, may be produced in areas geographically separate from the animal-production units. As such, industrial systems are sometimes referred to as landless production systems, since decisions about crop production are dissociated from decisions about animal production, and the closed loop of nutrient recycling that characterizes mixed farming systems is often lost. Animal are not available to do work or consume crop residues, and manure from the animals is not readily available to return to the cropland as fertilizer. Feeds become a traded commodity, and manure potentially becomes a waste management liability.

Other economic, environmental, and marketing factors influence the location of animal production units at sites distant from crop production. In developing countries, for instance, where transportation infrastructure is poor, production units are frequently located close to urban markets where the livestock products will ultimately be sold. This is because relatively nonperishable, densely packed grains are more economical to transport than bulky live animals or perishable animal products requiring refrigeration. On the other hand, animal-production units cannot be too close to cities because odor and animal wastes may create social and environmental problems not acceptable to urban dwellers or government. Efforts to develop intensive swine production in Singapore in the 1970s were largely derailed because of such odor and waste considerations.

Farming systems analysts find it useful to distinguish between two main types of intensive industrial livestock production—monogastric systems and ruminant systems. Monogastric systems include swine and poultry, either for egg or meat production. Ruminant systems include sheep for meat production and cattle for meat or milk production. Physiological and nutritional differences between monogastric and ruminant animals strongly influence the management of industrial production systems. Monogastric species are more easily and advantageously used under industrial production. They have short growth and production cycles, have high prolificacy, and perform well on grain diets. In contrast, ruminants tend to have longer growth and production cycles, have lower prolificacy, and require roughage in their diet for optimal performance. As cereal grains are highly concentrated sources of energy and can be densely packed for shipment, the cost and logistics for transporting grain long distance to production sites are more favorable than those for transporting roughage in the form of hay, haylage, and silage.

Ruminants, on the other hand, can use grasslands more effectively than monogastrics. The beef feedlot system of the United States exploits this characteristic of cattle. Because rangelands are abundant, cow-calf operations are managed as extensive ranching systems to produce weaned calves that are then contracted or auctioned to feedlots for finishing on grain diets. Specialized beef breeds used in this system are selected for good survivability and growth under grazing conditions. In parts of Europe, on the other hand, grazing land is in relatively short supply. As a result, a high percentage of the cattle being

People Power: The Success of Cooperative Dairying in India

During the period of World War II and leading into the emergence of India as an independent democratic state in 1947, there was a sizable increase in urban populations within the country, and this was accompanied by a noticeable urban demand for dairy products. Several private entrepreneurs responded by opening dairy-processing plants and by contracting with city governments to provide milk to the cities. However, these businesses remained uninvolved in the milk-production side of the dairy business. Plant owners relied on middlemen to identify milk sources and deliver milk to the plants. As demand for milk, yo-

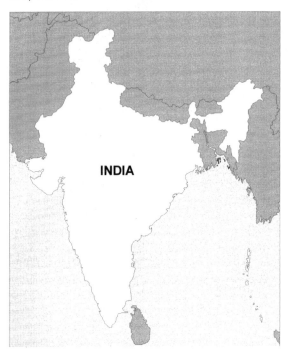

gurt, butter, and ghee increased, middlemen ranged deeper into the countryside to identify milk sources. In the mid-1940s, most cattle and milking buffalo were owned by small subsistence farmers or landless peasants who possessed only one or two milking animals. The animals were used primarily for draft purposes, but when milk was available, some was sold to neighbors or at local village markets for sporadic cash income. Many of these small farmers were approached by middlemen to sell to the private milk plants. The milk plants were enormously profitable, including the one serving Bombay, and in 1946, milk producers in the Kaira District of Gujarat, about 425 km north of Bombay, asked for an increase in their milk price to share in the prosperity. Their request was refused and, in response, they went on strike, organized themselves, and created the Kaira District Cooperative Milk Producers Union, composed of two village-level milk societies. In the first year of 1946, the two societies collected an average of 250 L of milk per day. In 1948, they were collecting 5000 L/day. By 1952 they were large enough to get the Bombay government to agree to sign a supply contract with the Union, and by 1955, they had built their own processing plant in Anand with help from UNICEF. By 1965, an expanded plant was processing pasteurized milk, milk powder, sweetened condensed milk, dried baby food, and cheese. The number of village societies in the cooperative had increased from 2 to 421, the number of farmer members swelled to 85,000, and 60 million kg of milk was collected in the year, about 160,000 L/day.

Society members received steady income from milk sales but also agreed to have the Union retain a portion to promote activities that would benefit all Union members. In turn, the Union developed and provided a variety of support services. On the business side, the Union provided services related to milk processing and quality, new product development, marketing and distribution, and price negotiations. On the production side, it offered farmer members access to organized veterinary service, genetic improvement through record keeping, bull selection, progeny testing, and artificial insemination and provided extension services related to health, nutrition, management, and other subjects geared toward improving productivity. Cropping strategies and feeding emphasis shifted toward improving milk production. Farmers who previously fed their animals roadside grasses, millet straw, and cotton seed began to sow alfalfa to feed to lactating animals. A shortage of alfalfa seed offered opportunities for some farmers to develop businesses cultivating alfalfa seed for other farmers. In 1964 the Union established its own feed mill to produce a low-cost,

finished in feedlots there are Holsteins purchased from dairy operations.

Monogastric species are also more efficient converters of concentrate feeds into animal protein than ruminants. It takes approximately 2.5 to 3.0 kg of grain to produce 1 kg of live weight gain in pigs, and 2.0 to 2.5 kg of feed to produce 1 kg of live weight gain in broiler chickens. By contrast, it takes 8.0 to 10.0 kg of concentrate feed to produce 1 kg of live weight gain in a feeder steer during the period of feedlot production, though one should remember that the steer achieved a considerable amount of growth and development on a grass or roughage diet prior to the finishing period.

Intensive industrial production of poultry and pigs has increased dramatically in recent years in response to growing market demand for livestock products, especially in Asia. Currently, about one third of world industrial pork production now occurs in Asia. Ruminant industrial production has not been as widely embraced, though in certain specialized cases, local economic conditions have facilitated the introduction of intensive production, for example, large-scale dairying in oil-rich Saudi Arabia, and beef production in Japan, where prolonged economic growth and a demand for beef has allowed consumer prices that are high enough to cover production costs in a country with very limited land available for cattle grazing.

balanced ration that farmer members could purchase to feed their buffaloes and cows. By 1970, the Union had a staff of 2000 people, including 39 veterinarians, 78 dairy specialists and 29 engineers serving the needs of farmer members.

Over the decades, with the support of their Union and with increasing demand in urban markets, thousands of subsistence farmers have been able to make milk production their primary activity, earn a steady income, and realize a level of prosperity and security that was previously unattainable for the rural poor. By 1996, 50 years after its conception and successful evolution, the Kaira District Cooperative Milk Producers' Union Ltd. has 943 village societies, has 513,280 farmer members, and produces well over 740,000 L/day.

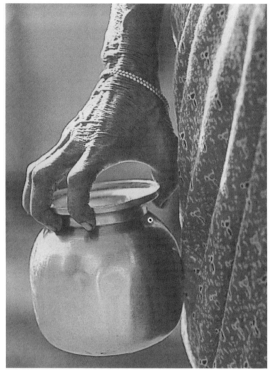

The value of the Kaira Cooperative should be recognized in both economic and social terms. Not only was it a great commercial success, it was also a phenomenal achievement in rural development. The Cooperative improved the quality of life for tens of thousands of the rural poor without serious dislocation of their traditional way of life. At the same time, it strengthened communities through democratic participation in the village milk societies. The Cooperative movement represented an indigenous approach to development that took into account the conditions that prevailed in India, namely a large rural population with limited capital for investment. Rather than consolidating and intensifying farming through capital investment, the dairy industry was developed through participation of legions of small farmers and livestock owners. These successes were not lost on government. In 1965, Prime Minister Lal Bahadur Shastri called for the creation of the National Dairy Development Board (NDDB) to disseminate the philosophy and accomplishments of the Kaira Union throughout rural India.

A village Indian woman carrying a milk pail. (Photo courtesy of Heifer Project International, Little Rock, Arkansas. Photographer, Matt Bradley)

The NDDB has been very successful in achieving its goals, creating a national network of dairy cooperatives through Operation Flood, a development assistance scheme supported by the World Bank and the European Union, largely through the donation of European milk powder and liquid butter. The sale of these commodities was used to create greater urban demand for milk products and to finance the establishment of cooperatives and dairy infrastructure throughout the country. By 1994, there were at least 70,000 village milk societies with 8.4 million farmer members in 170 milksheds throughout the country, collectively producing over 12.3 million L/day. Milk outputs have improved spectacularly in India over the last 50 years, in large part because of the promotion and establishment of producer cooperatives and the technical innovations and services that the cooperatives provided to farmer members. India proudly closed the 20th century as the world's largest milk producer, displacing the United States as number one with a 1999 production of 77.13 million metric tonnes, compared with a U.S. production of 73.48 million metric tonnes. More information about dairying in India and Operation Flood can be found at http://www.indiadairy.com/default_nondhtml.html, the website of the India Dairy Industry.

The development of livestock production as a high-technology business has increased the availability of low-cost livestock products for millions of people around the world. At present, industrial animal production is the fastest growing sector of the global livestock industry, far outpacing extensive grazing systems and mixed farming systems. Data reported in 1996 indicated that industrial pork production was increasing at a rate of 4% per year, broiler production at 5% per year, industrial egg production at 3.8% per year, and beef and mutton at 2.5% per year. Global averages mask some of the more dramatic regional growth in certain sectors, for example, 9% annual growth rates in poultry meat and egg production and 7% for pork production in Asia. In contrast, industrial production in the countries of the former Soviet Union has been shrinking, as centralized, state-supported enterprises have been broken up, and animal production has moved back into the hands of individual farmers.

Despite its obvious commercial success, industrial livestock production has its critics, and they represent a variety of perspectives and concerns. Those concerned with animal welfare express dismay about management conditions and practices in factory farms, which they believe result in unacceptable animal suffering. Such concerns include densely populated cages, inability of animals to turn around in their pens, and the debeaking of poultry. Environmentalists express serious concerns related to the contribution of animal wastes to water and air pollution and the high use of nonrenewable energy sources in industrial production. Consumer advocates and some public health officials decry the use of antibiotics and hormones as growth promotants during the production cycle.

Social policy analysts raise a variety of issues. Some express concern that the continued growth of industrial production, which depends so heavily on cereal grains, may result in increased amounts of arable land being converted to feed grain production, resulting in grain shortages or excessively high prices for cereal crops used for direct human consumption. Other social critics contend that industrial livestock production based near urban centers is inconsistent with overall development strategies in developing countries that are labor rich and cash poor because industrial production uses less direct labor than traditional livestock keeping methods and requires the use of limited foreign exchange to import grain as animal feed. Furthermore, there is concern that the growth of industrial production will reduce efforts to improve the production capacity of traditional subsistence farmers and may also remove incentives for government to improve transportation, communication, and marketing infrastructure in rural areas, if demand for livestock products is met by industrial production units close to cities.

Many informed analysts believe that there is considerable potential to improve animal production in traditional grazing and mixed farming systems, but that inevitably, the steadily increasing global demand for foods of animal origin will be met primarily by expansion of industrialized animal production. If this is indeed the case, then intensive, industrial livestock production systems will have to continue to innovate and address the environmental and social concerns that challenge their long-term sustainability. This will require new production efficiencies that reduce the requirements for grain and fossil fuels, greater consideration of animal welfare issues, new approaches to animal waste management, and careful planning in developing countries to ensure that industrial livestock production does not seriously undermine rural development and the livelihoods of traditional farmers.

Aquaculture

Aquaculture is the cultivation of aquatic plants or animals for human use. Various aquatic environments are used for aquaculture, with different farmed species being matched to their natural aquatic ecology. The main aquatic ecosystems affecting species selection are primarily fresh water, brackish water, and salt or marine water. Fresh water environments include lakes, rivers, irrigation canals, ponds (either natural or constructed), and flooded crop fields. Freshwater species of importance in aquaculture include carp, tilapia, catfish, and trout. Marine water environments include the open sea, protected coves and bays, and, more recently, constructed ponds and tanks with recirculated saltwater. Important species in marine water aquaculture include filter-feeding shellfish and salmon. Brackish water environments are linked to coastal areas and include

riverine estuaries, tidal marshlands, and mangrove swamps. These environments are used for the cultivation of crustaceans, notably prawns, as well as some finfish including tilapia, and some mollusks. Many of the natural environments listed include naturally occurring aquatic species as well, and a number of environmental concerns have been raised about aquaculture and its impact on natural flora and fauna, as discussed further in Chapter 6.

Like agriculture, its land-based equivalent, there are several approaches to the cultivation and harvesting of aquatic species, which can more or less be categorized in a manner similar to land-based farming systems. These categories include extensive aquaculture, mixed system or rural aquaculture, and intensive or industrial aquaculture. Taken together the output from these various forms of aquaculture is substantial. By 1995, over one quarter of the world's total food fish supply was derived from aquaculture activity. The value of aquaculture products in 1995, including seaweed and other plants as well as finfish and shellfish, was US$42.3 billion.

Extensive aquaculture, like extensive livestock production, requires few inputs and takes advantage of existing resources in the environment to support the growth of the target species. Stocking lakes and rivers with young salmon, trout, bass, or other fish is an example. These juvenile fish live freely in unmodified environments, grow to maturity by consuming naturally available feed, and are then harvested by fishermen. This pattern is not unlike the use of grasslands by pastoralists. The extensive aquaculture system however, does require the development and support of hatcheries, in which controlled reproduction provides the spawn and juvenile fish required for the stocking effort.

Mixed rural aquaculture is more akin to mixed subsistence and mixed specialty farming. In fact, aquaculture is often an integral part of these systems, especially in Asia. These are usually low-input systems, but they vary in their sophistication. Some may derive seed stock from the wild, while others use hatcheries. Some more-specialized enterprises may require supplemental feeds or a particular form of netting or penning to manage the production cycle of the target species. Mixed aquaculture systems generally try to fully exploit opportunities for nutrient cycling in which waste products from other crop and animal production activities are used to feed fish, and the manure from fish in turn is used to improve soil fertility of croplands.

A wide variety of mixed farming situations have been able to incorporate fish production, especially carp production, into the overall farming scheme. In China, for instance, small fish may be introduced into flooded rice paddies shortly after rice planting to help control potentially damaging insect pests. The fish also stir up the mud, increasing soil nutrient availability for the plants, and add their own excreta to enrich the soil. In these cases, paddies yield both a fish and a rice harvest. In other cases, separate fish ponds may be established into which manure of pigs or sheep and even silkworm droppings may be deposited to promote plankton growth, which serves as the basis of the fish diet. Ponds may be drained for harvesting fish, and the rich sediment at the pond bottom is transferred to garden plots and crop fields as fertilizer. In a development project in the Philippines, goats fed grass and legumes were kept in pens with slatted floors directly over fish ponds so their manure dropped directly into the water and increased overall fish yields in the pond.

Intensive aquaculture, like intensive industrial agriculture, is a strictly commercial enterprise. Intensive aquaculture requires more capital, equipment, feed, and technical expertise. Much industrial aquaculture is aimed at developing products for lucrative market niches, and the value of the final product in the marketplace can justify the high front-end investment involved. Such products include prawns and salmon. Salmon farming, for example, requires a significant investment in housing, in the form of sea cages that are predator proof and escape proof, as well as a considerable, ongoing cost for feed. Salmonids are carnivorous fish, and farmed salmon are fed a commercial diet of animal origin that is high in fat and protein. The ration may be composed primarily of fish meal and fish oil as well as blood meal, meat meal, and wheat, with a variety of vitamin and minerals added. A pigment may also be incorporated into the feed to impart a pinkish color to the salmon flesh. The feed may be offered in the form of an extruded pellet (Fig. 4-15). Stocking density in pens is very high, and not unlike intensive livestock units, disease problems are a major concern. When diseases occur, they can spread rapidly and widely through a population. Diagnostic services, preventive vaccinations, and tactical treatments are additional costs involved in such enterprises, and the growth of aquaculture has created enormous new opportunities for the veterinary profession.

Livestock Among the Landless/Urban Agriculture

It is common in rural villages and small towns in the developing world to find livestock wandering freely in the streets and alleys. Much of this livestock belongs to local citizens who have no land to cultivate. While some have regular employment or businesses in town, many are casual laborers or otherwise underemployed in the rural economy. Livestock offer the possibility of some supplemental cash income and improved nutrition. Small ruminants, swine, and poultry are the most common forms of livestock seen running free around villages, and as impossible as it may seem to the outsider, ownership of animals is usually well known to local people.

Many landless livestock keepers invest great effort in managing their animal charges. Children may tend a small group of sheep or goats and drive them along roadsides or fence lines to graze grasses, or the animals may be tethered along the roadside and moved periodically when they have grazed down a circle of grass. In other situations, particularly with milking animals, the animals may be kept penned in the family yard, while household members go out to cut forage and bring it back to the animals for feeding. Many smaller animals may also be kept in the yard or household and fed household wastes

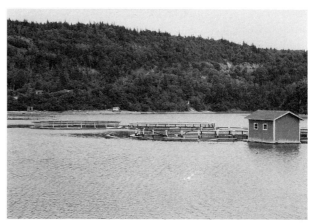

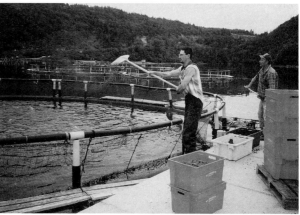

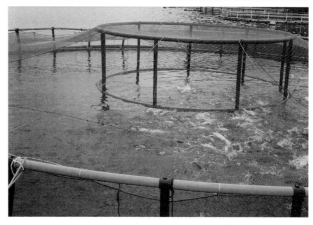

Figure 4-15. Feeding captive-bred salmon off of Grand Manan Island, New Brunswick, Canada. The fish are maintained in circular, netted pens suspended from large floating rings (top). Attendants visit each cage twice daily for feeding. Pelleted feed is tossed onto the surface of the pens by the shovelful (middle), and the fish roil the surface of the water as they come up to feed (bottom). A single pen may contain thousands of salmon. (All photos by Dr. David M. Sherman)

or gathered forage. These include, among others, pigs, rabbits, rodents, or poultry. These efforts are generally low-input and low-output systems. There is little or no investment in feed purchase or health care, and productivity of animals is relatively low. Indigenous breeds are usually involved, which are well adapted to local conditions and which can perform tolerably on less than optimal diets.

In recent decades, the practice of small-scale, landless livestock keeping has extended well beyond the villages and small towns of the countryside and has moved right into the heart of urban centers and periurban areas. This trend is part of a more general trend in urban agriculture that has grown in synchrony with the general trend of urbanization in the second half of the 20th century, especially in developing countries. In 1950, based on FAO data, an estimated 29.7% of the world's population (which was then only 2.5 billion) lived in urban areas. By 1995, 45.3% of the world's population of 5.6 billion lived in urban areas, and by 2025, it is projected that the proportion of urban dwellers will be about 60%.

The urban shift has been most dramatic in developing countries. Between 1975 and 1999, Lagos, Nigeria, added 10.2 million to its population; Bombay, India, 11.2 million; Sao Paolo, Brazil, 7.7 million; and Shanghai, China, 2.7 million. In Kenya, rural populations did not quite double between 1975 and 1999, moving from 11.9 million to 20.1 million. In contrast, urban population increased more than fivefold, from 1.7 million to 9.9 million. In 1964, the area of Nairobi, Kenya's capital, was 65 km². By 1998, that area had increased over tenfold to 690 km².

Providing adequate and nutritious food for expanding urban populations is a challenge in many developing countries. Despite the fact that a large proportion of the rural population is directly engaged in agriculture, there are numerous constraints on producing and delivering the variety and quantity of foods required by city dwellers in the same country. For one thing, commercial agriculture is simply not well developed in many countries. When it exists, it may be oriented toward production of cash crops such as tea or coffee for export to earn foreign exchange, while food crops are produced mainly by subsistence farmers who do not have the resources to produce much beyond what they need for their own families or to enter commercial domestic markets. Similarly, traditional herders may be more inclined to keep animals as insurance against hard times than to market them to the cities.

However, even when producers want to serve urban markets there are difficulties. A key problem is lack of adequate infrastructure. Inadequate feeder roads, poorly maintained highways, high fuel prices, high transport costs, and lack of refrigerated vehicles are examples of typical constraints. Even when such infrastructure is available, another obstacle has been government control of farm prices. There has been a strong tendency for politicians in developing countries to favor urban constituencies over rural ones, as historically, urban dwellers were better educated, more likely to vote, and generally were better able to make their opinions known to government, since it is relatively convenient for city folk to mass in front of the parliament building downtown and hurl stones through the windows when food prices become too high. As a result, prices paid to farmers for commodities such as milk have been held low to provide food to urban dwellers at lower prices. This has long proved a disincentive to farmers to invest in improvements to increase production.

One additional challenge to feeding urban populations is that many among them are poor. Many move to the city from rural areas, where employment and income opportunities are low, with the hope and expectation that the city will offer better prospects. For many it does not, and income remains low. Even for regular wage earners, inflationary pressures, devaluations of local currency, and increasing demand for food in urban centers mean that purchasing power has diminished, and an increasingly high proportion of salary goes toward the purchase of food. Surveys indicate that households in the largest cities in developing countries spend anywhere from 50 to 80% of their average income on food and that food prices were 10 to 30% higher in urban areas than in rural areas.

For all these reasons, the practice of urban agriculture has continued to grow along with cities themselves, especially in developing countries. In different countries of Africa, the percentage of households engaged in some form of urban agriculture ranges from 32 to 70%. Whether on rooftops and median strips or in window boxes, backyards, and empty lots, the cultivation of fruits, vegetables, and cereal crops has become a regular feature of the urban landscape. An estimated 200 million people are directly involved in urban agriculture worldwide. It has been projected that by 2005, urban agriculture will be responsible for 33% of world food production, and over 400 million people will be engaged in some urban farming. As much as 50% of the food consumed in cities is projected to come from the urban areas themselves.

While many municipalities have laws that specifically prohibit raising crops or keeping livestock, the practice has become so widespread and so critically important to the urban food supply that such laws are rarely enforced any longer. In fact, some city governments have begun to incorporate urban agriculture into long-range growth and development plans and have found international support for their efforts. For instance, the International Development Research Centre in Ottawa, Canada, supports a program called Cities Feeding People, which acts as a resource base for research on urban agriculture. Many interesting and informative reports, studies, and links can be found at the website (http://www.idrc.ca/cfp/). Much of the statistical information presented in this section comes from papers available through Cities Feeding People.

Not surprisingly, livestock raising is an important part of urban agriculture. A broad range of species and animal management systems are represented in urban and periurban settings. At its most basic, urban livestock keeping is a low-input, low-output subsistence system. As in the village situation, poor people with scant resources may keep some poultry and small ruminants, allowing them to range freely in open lots, on roadsides, or in alleyways. However, in urban settings, risks of loss due to theft and traffic accidents usually prompt more-careful control such as tethering, confinement to yards, or supervised grazing. Even in very large and cosmopolitan cities, such as Cairo, it is not unusual to see flocks of sheep and goats on the city streets being herded by boys on a regular tour of known rubbish piles and dumpsters. A survey done in the

1980s indicated that at least 80,000 households raised animals within the Cairo city limits.

Urban animal keeping is frequently constrained by a lack of space. Many animals are kept in cages, pens, sheds, or hutches within the walls of family compounds and raised on kitchen wastes, roadside cuttings, and possibly some purchased feed. These animals are for family consumption or informal sale. Choice of animals depends to some degree on geography and culture. Raising of chickens, rabbits, sheep, goats, and even cattle is fairly universal. Pigeon keeping is common in North Africa and the Middle East. Guinea pigs are commonly raised for food by households in the highlands of South America, while household pigs are common throughout east and southeast Asia. Urban and periurban beekeeping is practiced in much of Africa.

In addition to urban subsistence livestock raising, there are also smallholder and large-scale commercial enterprises.[22] Smallholder commercial systems are essentially family businesses, with family members providing the labor for animal keeping. The degree of investment in feed, housing, and health care depends on the income from sale of products. Animals commonly kept for sale include goats, swine, and chickens for eggs or meat. Of particular significance in the smallholder commercial sector are small dairies. In many cities, demand for milk is high and may outstrip supply through formal market channels. There is an important and growing sector of informal dairying in which families may maintain anywhere from 1 to an average of 10 cows or milking buffalo within the city limits, in a walled compound with zero grazing. Concentrate feeds are purchased, and forages are purchased or gathered from roadsides and brought to the animals. Sales are usually direct to customers at the "farm" gate or through middlemen in informal market channels.

Large-scale commercial systems tend to be periurban rather than in the heart of the city. They are either existing farms that have been surrounded by urban expansion over the years or new operations that have been purposefully sited to serve urban markets. Dairies, swine-production units, and poultry-production units are most common. While dairy units are sometimes linked to fodder production when land is available, swine and poultry units are likely to be zero-grazing confinement systems where purchased feeds are brought to housed animals.

In general, the urban livestock sector is underserved. Very little research or extension activity has been aimed at this sector, and existing laws and marketing policies often work against it. As a result, urban livestock production continues to grow in informal and haphazard ways and does not reach its full potential to contribute to the urban food supply. Veterinary issues include improved animal health and productivity as well as public health concerns. Access to veterinary services for urban producers needs to be improved. Preventive vaccination, mastitis control, and artificial insemination to cross indigenous breeds with more-productive, commercial breeds are some typical services that are frequently lacking. Similarly, sound ad-

vice on improved sanitation, housing, ventilation, and approaches to improving nutrition are frequently unavailable to urban livestock keepers, especially subsistence livestock keepers. Veterinarians also can play an important role in helping to develop standards for the health and management of new or unfamiliar species that may be introduced into urban household production, for example, the introduction of guinea pigs, a native South American rodent, into urban African households, where people are unfamiliar with their management. Increasingly, development agencies and governments have been looking at ways to improve access of urban livestock keepers to such service and advice. Heifer Project International, for example, has a number of projects aimed at providing technical support to small-scale urban livestock keepers in Peru, India, and even the United States.

Public health issues loom large in urban livestock production. First, in urban settings, livestock and people are often in very close contact due to lack of land. Secondly, many livestock enterprises are small scale and operate in the informal sector where they are not fully or properly regulated. Animal wastes may contaminate public areas and water supplies, and the risk of zoonotic disease by contact with or consumption of animals, animal wastes, and animal products is high. Of particular concern is the spread of tuberculosis and brucellosis to people consuming the unpasteurized milk of infected cattle. Unregulated slaughter of animals increases the risk of foodborne illnesses such as salmonellosis or campylobacteriosis. Similarly, zoonotic parasitic infections such as trichinosis and taeniasis can result from consumption of inadequately cooked meat from uninspected animals.

Livestock in Sustainable Agriculture

The tension that exists today between the growing demand for food and the finite amount of land available to produce it means that yields of crops and livestock from existing land must be increased to ensure an adequate food supply for future generations. Tremendous advances have been made in increasing agricultural productivity through technological innovation, particularly in the last half of the 20th century. The mechanization of agricultural production; the use of chemical fertilizers, herbicides, and pesticides; and improved techniques in plant breeding to create new, high-yielding varieties adapted to local conditions of climate and disease have all increased crop outputs dramatically in the last 50 years. Through these innovations of the Green Revolution, countries like India, which were grain importers at the beginning of the 20th century, are now able to export grain at the beginning of the 21st century. Similarly, the intensification of livestock management, scientific advances in animal nutrition, the application of selective breeding, and the increased use of sophisticated veterinary services have resulted in dramatic increases in animal production in recent years.

These gains in productivity, however, come at a cost. A number of environmental and social problems have come to be associated with modern agricultural practices. Mechanization, when inappropriately applied, can contribute to soil erosion and/or soil compaction. Crop monoculture, which is favored by the heavy investment in specialized equipment required to produce a particular crop, tends to exhaust soil nutrients and increase risk of disease and pests. The use of agricultural chemicals to counteract these effects is associated with a number of environmental and public health problems including contamination of water, land, and air; death of wildlife; and, most recently, the potential disruption of endocrine and reproductive functions in humans and other animals, as discussed in Chapter 6.

The mechanization and intensification of agricultural enterprises also have social consequences by reducing labor requirements and transforming market structures. As a result, traditional family farm units have become less competitive relative to corporate enterprises. This has had, in some cases, a disruptive effect on the viability of rural farming communities and the families that compose them. Also, modern animal and crop production depend heavily on a continuous supply of high energy inputs from nonrenewable fossil fuels, and some analysts have projected that the known supply of such fuels will be depleted by as early as the end of the 21st century.

Clearly, to make abundant food of high quality and variety reliably available to the coming generations, future agricultural practices must find ways to balance continued gains in productivity and output with concerns about environmental quality, the conservation of nonrenewable resources, public health, and social stability. The development of methods, strategies, and policy frameworks to achieve this balance is the essence of sustainable agriculture.

There is no single definition of sustainable agriculture. However, several key elements are frequently identified in discussions of the subject. In general, sustainable agriculture practices should

- Reflect a sense of stewardship for natural and human resources,

- Optimize the use of on-farm resources,

- Reduce the use of nonrenewable resources and other external purchased inputs,

- Take full advantage of natural biological cycles and biological controls in the farming system,

- Protect and renew soil fertility and the natural resource base,

- Minimize adverse impacts on human health, wildlife, and the environment,

- Be economically profitable and provide adequate and dependable farm income,

- Promote growth, development, and stability for family farmers and farming communities.

There has been considerable media attention in recent years about industrial livestock production or so-called factory farming. Much of this attention has been unfavorable, and some of the criticism has been justified. Nevertheless, this media exposure has contributed to a growing societal perception, especially in developed countries, that all livestock production activities are inherently inconsistent with environmental health, social welfare, and the wise use of natural resources. This is an unrealistic and erroneous assessment, especially when animal agriculture is viewed from a global perspective. Most of the world's livestock populations and the products derived from them are still found in subsistence and small mixed farming systems, in which the contribution of animals to agricultural sustainability is profound, and their potential for promoting greater sustainability is significant.

The inherent sustainability of subsistence and mixed farming systems derives from the fact that animal production and crop production remain directly linked and under the decision-making control of the same farmer-manager. This increases the chances that on-farm resources will be used and recycled within the production system, and it reduces the demand for external inputs in agricultural production. The presence of animals in the mixed farming system allows crop residues to be used for livestock feeding. Draft animals provide power for agriculture and transport without consumption of fossil fuels or the need to purchase and maintain costly equipment. Animals such as sheep, ducks, or fish provide weed control in row crops, while goats provide weed control in pastures, thus reducing the need for herbicides or brush-clearing equipment. All animals produce manure, which can be used to fertilize crops, provide fuel for cooking or heating, enrich ponds for fish cultivation or, in the case of poultry manure, be fed to other livestock. All of these uses of manure reduce dependency on external inputs such as chemical fertilizer, fossil fuels, fuel wood, or purchased feeds. In addition, livestock can improve the productivity of farmers and their families by improving overall family nutrition. They can provide a more dependable source of income through the sale of livestock or livestock products and offer greater opportunities for risk diversification in the event of crop failure. If cereal crops are cultivated and drought occurs after the plants have achieved some growth but before the seed heads have matured, the value of the crop to the farmer would be lost unless livestock were present to consume the drought-affected plants.

Such sustainable practices are part and parcel of traditional mixed farming systems. Yet the productivity of many mixed farming operations remains low, with many farmers continuing to function only at subsistence levels. Increasing productivity in these systems while preserving and enhancing their characteristic sustainability is the principal challenge for the future. This dual objective has become a driving force for much of the rural social and economic development activity being carried out in developing countries of the world. Many policymakers and implementing agencies are coming to recognize and understand the value of animals in improving both the sustainability and output of smallholder farmers. International development agencies, such as FARM Africa and Heifer Project International, frequently use the introduction of animals with improved production characteristics as the basis for rural community development projects that aim to improve rural livelihood by strengthening sustainable agricultural practices. Such programs are discussed in greater detail in Chapter 5.

Opportunities for promoting sustainability in mixed farming systems exist in the developed world as well. Consumer concerns about personal health, food safety, and environmental contaminants associated with the use of chemicals in agriculture have stimulated a dramatic growth in organic farming in recent years. Many family farmers have found organic farming practices to be both sustainable and profitable, especially with consumers prepared to pay prices as much as 20% higher than they pay for equivalent conventionally produced foods. According to the FAO, organic agriculture has come to represent up to 10% of the food system in Switzerland and Austria and is growing at a rate of over 20% annually in the United States, France, and Japan.

The potential for improving the sustainability of livestock production extends beyond mixed farming systems to extensive grazing systems. Efforts are needed to restore the inherent balance between pastoralism and the grazing lands that support it. One hurdle is to overcome the traditional practice of herders who keep large numbers of animals as insurance against livestock losses during extended periods of drought. Government policies aimed at providing a safety net for herders in difficult times and offering them reliable assistance for restocking lost animals could allow herd sizes to be stabilized at reduced levels. If such policies are linked to improvements in marketing infrastructure and attractive pricing, it could encourage greater offtake and allow more pastoralist livestock to enter commercial channels for meat production. In addition, the growing presence of crop agriculture in former grazing areas provides opportunities to integrate crop and livestock production through greater interactions between settled farmers and pastoralist herders. Crop residues can be grazed by pastoralist livestock in exchange for the manure left behind to fertilize fields, and herders could potentially earn income by renting out animals for agricultural work to farmers who cannot afford their own draft animals.

There are also opportunities to enhance the sustainability of industrial livestock production. In these landless systems, waste disposal poses a significant environmental problem. However, biodigestion of wastes to produce biogas can once again turn manure back from a problem to a resource by reducing the need for external energy inputs. When industrial livestock production units are concentrated in a geographic area, pooling wastes for biogas production can result in sufficient biogas output to substitute for fossil fuels in the commercial production of electricity.

Perhaps the most significant criticism of industrial livestock production systems, with regard to their lack of sustainability, is the reliance of producers on cereal grains as animal feed In the developed countries, the abundance of locally available domestic grain serves in part to justify the practice. However, there is considerable concern about the proliferation of grain-based intensive production systems in developing countries in which much of the feed required for animal production needs to be imported at great economic and social cost. In these situations, intensive production can be made more sustainable by research into the use of alternative feeds that are locally available and may be manipulated to improve their nutritional value, thus reducing dependency on grain.

Animal production also can be integrated into plantation agriculture, notably tree-based production systems, in which a forage crop can be planted between tree rows and animals grazed to produce a livestock output within the overall production system. In turn, the animals improve soil fertility by dropping manure. The principle of using locally available alternative feed for intensive animal production also merits further investigation and application. It represents an important tool for promoting sustainability in animal production.

Sustainable agriculture is based on a fundamental premise that the agricultural production unit represents an ecosystem and that it should be recognized and managed as such. Just as animals are an integral part of natural ecosystems, they are also a vital part of agroecosystems. In the developed world, livestock increasingly have become the target output of a specialized production system, a marketable commodity that results from the livestock-production enterprise. The epitome of this approach is the intensive monogastric production unit, which, while remarkably productive, depends heavily on inputs not contained within the production system itself. In the developing world, livestock remain an integral part of traditional agroecosystems. They are not simply products of the system; they are also active contributors to the system and add significantly to its overall sustainability. Veterinarians who can integrate their knowledge of production medicine with an appreciation and knowledge of agroecology can contribute enormously to increasing animal productivity around the world in sustainable ways.

Approaches to Improving Animal Productivity

The growing worldwide demand for foods of animal origin, the continued dependence of millions of people in developing countries on animals in their daily lives, and the important role that animals play in promoting sustainable agriculture all underscore the need for more vigorous efforts to improve the health and productivity of animals around the globe. There are five general areas in which such improvements can be achieved. They include improved access to veterinary service and disease control, improved animal management, improved nutrition, rational use of genetic resources, and improved marketing of livestock and livestock products.

Improved Veterinary Service and Disease Control

Ensuring the health of animals is an essential prerequisite for improving animal productivity by other means. Improvements in management, nutrition, breeding or access to markets are of little benefit if animals cannot be protected from debilitating or deadly disease. Disease can be a profound constraint on animal production. Vast areas can be rendered unsuitable for animal production as a result of disease risk, as is the case with trypanosomiasis in Africa. Not only does the risk of trypanosomiasis inhibit animal production in tsetse fly-infested areas by restricting access to potential grazing lands, it also encourages overstocking animals in tsetse fly-free areas. This contributes to degradation of grazing lands, reduced levels of nutrition, increased susceptibility to disease, and lowered productivity of livestock populations.

In addition to endemic diseases such as trypanosomiasis, epidemic disease outbreaks can cripple or destroy livestock industries. Perhaps the most notorious example is the rinderpest outbreak that occurred in Africa between 1889 and 1897. Previously unrecorded on the continent, rinderpest was introduced into northern Africa with cattle imported from Europe. The infection swept southward and killed millions of cattle and wild ungulates. This caused massive suffering among herders and farmers who lost their livestock, a direct source of food and needed labor to cultivate their crops, leading to instances of starvation. Efforts to control rinderpest on the African continent continue today through cooperative multinational efforts coordinated through the Interafrican Bureau of Animal Resources of the Organization for African Unity.

Such epidemics are not merely the stuff of history. In recent years, a number of important epidemics have undermined livestock industries at national or regional levels. An epidemic of Newcastle disease in domestic fowl in Northern Ireland in 1997 required the slaughter of over 1 million birds, resulted in direct economic losses exceeding US$15 million, and required suspension of export of poultry products for 8 months, until disease-free status could be reestablished. An outbreak of African swine fever in hogs in the Ivory Coast in 1996 cost the country an estimated $9.2 million. A foot and mouth disease epidemic in hogs in Taiwan in 1997 affected over 1 million pigs, led to the slaughter of over 4 million pigs, and cost the industry more than US$1.3 billion. The emergence of bovine spongiform encephalopathy (BSE) in the United Kingdom in 1986 has resulted in the slaughter of over 4.5 million cattle and has cost the cattle industry more than US$3.3 billion. The disease continues to generate serious public health, economic, and trade repercussions 15 years after it was first recognized. The subsequent outbreak of foot and mouth disease (FMD) in the U.K. in 2001 dealt a second devastating blow to cattle farmers in the nation. Between them, BSE and FMD have challenged the very survival of the cattle industry in the U.K.

Countries that are able to successfully control or eradicate infectious diseases such as rinderpest, FMD, or African swine fever achieve greater productivity for animals within the country. In addition, however, they also enjoy enormous economic advantages through access to international trade in livestock and livestock products. Such trade is severely restricted for countries with endemic, highly contagious livestock diseases, as a result of international agreements administered on behalf of member nations by the World Trade Organization and the Office International des Epizooties (OIE) in Paris, France.

Effective control of endemic and epidemic diseases remains an elusive goal in many developing countries in which many obstacles to effective veterinary service delivery exist, and the risk of disease still represents a serious constraint on improved animal production. Deficiencies exist in the delivery of services for both the public good and the private good. Public good services are defined as those that benefit society and the economy at large. Such public good services include national animal disease surveillance and control programs against endemic and epidemic diseases; the control of zoonotic diseases such as tuberculosis, brucellosis, and hydatid disease; and other public health services such as meat inspection, monitoring of drug residues, and assurance of pharmaceutical safety and quality. Private good services are those that primarily benefit the individuals who own or keep animals. Such private good services include the delivery of clinical diagnostic, therapeutic, and prophylactic interventions and other herd health services such as reproductive management.

Veterinary service delivery is such an important aspect of international veterinary medicine that a whole chapter of this book has been set aside to address it. The structure of veterinary service delivery around the world, the constraints facing veterinary service delivery in developing countries, and some possible solutions for overcoming these constraints are discussed in more detail in Chapter 8.

Improved Management

While the world is full of differences, there are some surprising similarities, even in the matter of livestock keeping. As a large animal medicine resident at the University of Minnesota in the late 1970s, the author had many occasions to treat outbreaks of pneumonia in young dairy cattle during the cold winter months. Farm visits revealed that the affected heifers and weaned calves were often kept in tightly closed barns. The smell of ammonia in the uncirculated air was powerful, and the lack of ventilation undoubtedly contributed to the buildup of pathogens and the outbreaks of pneumonia. When farmers were asked why they sealed the animals into these barns with closed windows and doors, the answer was inevitably that they were trying to keep them warm, as surely the cold, harsh winter temperatures would be harmful to them. Twenty years later, doing development work in Afghanistan, the author once again came upon young cattle with pneumonia in winter, sealed tightly in mud sheds with ammonia-laden air. Once again, when queried on the practice, Afghan farmers insisted that they were protecting their cattle from cold winter temperatures. In neither case had the extension message been effectively transmitted that while cattle can usually tolerate cold winter temperatures, they cannot tolerate bad air quality associated with inadequate ventilation.

The point of this anecdote is that there are certain basic animal health problems related to management deficiencies that are encountered regularly throughout the world and are readily correctable. Such predictable problems include a variety of situations that most experienced veterinarians are already familiar with at home, such as pneumonia of weanlings in poorly ventilated housing, neonatal mortality from diarrhea associated with dirty birthing areas and inadequate colostrum, coccidiosis in animals and birds kept in housing with excessively moist floors, nematode parasites in grazing animals on overstocked pastures, bloat or acidosis associated with abrupt feed changes in ruminants, mastitis associated with inadequate hygiene during milking, outbreaks of clostridial diseases such as blackleg and malignant edema from grazing unvaccinated animals on previously flooded pastures, and tetanus from poorly executed castrations or carelessly tended wounds. Each agroecological zone offers its own unique health challenges to the animals that reside there, as a result of the presence of certain disease vectors and specific endemic diseases not found elsewhere. Nevertheless, considerable opportunity exists to improve livestock health and production in traditional livestock management systems by implementing simple changes in basic animal husbandry and herd health management.

Another way to improve productivity is by ensuring that appropriate management expertise, technical support, and extension information are available when new animal-production systems are introduced into areas where they were previously unknown, for example, the introduction of intensive swine and poultry production into developing countries that are experiencing strong economic growth. Large-scale, intensive, confinement operations require high degrees of management experience to function properly and efficiently. Problems can arise when the appropriate technical expertise is not available locally or when foreign technical advisers providing support to the new industry are not fully aware of local conditions relating to temperature and humidity patterns, water quality, or indigenous disease problems. The rapid spread of disease is always a threat when large groups of animals are concentrated in confinement housing. This risk can be further increased when intensive systems are introduced into hot and/or humid environments, when nonindigenous breeds are introduced into the production system, when contagious diseases are endemic in local populations of the same animal species, and when local managers are relatively inexperienced in the daily operation of intensive systems. Proper management requires an adequate understanding of both the intensive production system itself and the local conditions that can affect that system when it is introduced into a new environment.

Improved Nutrition and Use of Local Feeds

The lack of reliable and nutritious feed supplies for livestock is a common production constraint in many livestock production systems around the world. Pastoralism, for instance, fundamentally represents a management strategy that evolved to deal with the reality of seasonal feed scarcity. Subsistence farmers, as a rule, generally do not grow nutritious fodder for their animals, as their small plots are allocated to the production of crops directly consumed by people. As a result, animals usually are left to make do on crop byproducts of relatively low nutritional value, such as straw. Commercial farmers in developing countries may import improved livestock such as Holstein dairy cattle hoping to capitalize on their dramatic production potential, but that potential is not realized because adequate energy and protein are not available to feed them at the level necessary to exploit their genetic potential for milk production fully.

Undernutrition not only results in the failure to reach production potential in animals, it has other consequences as well. Disease conditions such as pregnancy toxemia, rumen impaction, hypovitaminosis A, and other deficiency-related disease may result directly from poor nutrition. In addition, immune function is compromised, and animals become more susceptible to infectious diseases. Reproductive performance can be adversely affected, with increased infertility, low conception rates, and higher rates of fetal and neonatal mortality. The ability of animals to perform work is also affected, which can be a major problem for subsistence farmers who depend on animals for preparing fields for planting. In many tropical regions, the planting season, which is the rainy season, follows a long dry season by the end of which, draft animals may have little forage to eat. As a result, these draft animals are often in their worst condition at the very time that they must work the hardest to ensure a successful crop for the farmer.

Alternative feeding strategies need to be considered to address the nutritional needs of livestock in developing countries. Many innovative options have been explored and successfully implemented using locally available, alternative feeds. One option is the use of crop residues that have been manipulated to improve their nutritional value, for example, straw treated with urea. Urea is a simple nitrogenous compound of relatively low cost and reasonable availability. Urea provides ruminant animals with a ready source of nitrogen so rumen bacteria can take the carbohydrate substrate available from straw and use it to build much-needed amino acids. This simple technology has been widely adopted in developing countries to improve the diet of ruminant animals. The procedures for handling, mixing, and feeding the urea-treated straw are relatively straightforward, and adoption of the technique has been reasonably good where it has been introduced, though some farmers find the stinging odor of urea difficult to work with, and this sometimes interferes with acceptance of the practice.

Another option is the use of byproducts from food-processing industries such as sugar production, brewing, and fish canning and, in urban areas, discards from restaurants and food markets. Sugar cane has been used to feed cattle successfully in Cuba, Colombia, Mauritius, and Trinidad, where whole chopped cane is fed. In more than a dozen countries of tropical Asia and Latin America, pigs are being fed on diets that successfully replace grains with sugar cane juice, palm oil, sugar palm juice, and cassava tubers. Citrus pulp residues from juice making are also used for livestock feeding. In China, beef production systems have been developed that depend solely on straw treated with urea and cottonseed cake, with no cereal grains being fed.

In many developing countries, farmers are being encourage to integrate leguminous shrubs, trees, and forages into their plantings, both in the fields and in their gardens. Nitrogen-fixing legumes are an excellent source of protein as animal feeds. Leaves, twigs, and seeds of various leguminous plants can be used as feeds. The plants also offer other advantages. They improve soil quality through nitrogen fixing. Trees and shrubs can serve as living fences around fields and gardens and help to prevent soil erosion, and in addition to providing animal feed, these perennials can also provide fuel wood for heating and cooking. Table 4-3 identifies some leguminous plants that have been used to improve the productivity of subsistence farmers in the tropics.[18]

Duckweeds are another potential animal feed gaining increased attention for integration into smallholder farming systems. Duckweeds are small aquatic plants that form dense mats which float on the surface of still or slow-moving bodies of water. They have been recognized as very useful in removing certain mineral contaminants from wastewater and are being used increasingly at wastewater treatment plants to help clean wastewater stored in lagoons. Duckweeds are also very high in protein, which makes them desirable as animal feeds. Duckweeds can be substituted for cereal grains in pig and mature poultry rations and maintain a high level of feed efficiency. The use of duckweed as a fish feed has yielded dramatic increases in fish growth. Duckweed, like urea, can be mixed with crop byproducts in ruminant diets to improve the overall quality of the diet and enhance its protein content. Duckweed is also a good source of phosphorus, a critical nutrient that is deficient in certain livestock-raising areas, for example, in many parts of Africa. Duckweed production can be integrated into sustainable smallholder farming systems when farm ponds are present or can be constructed.[12]

Veterinarians need to be involved in the process of identifying and introducing novel feedstuffs to livestock, as such introductions, while offering the prospect of improved nutrition, can sometimes have unexpected metabolic or toxicological consequences that need to be recognized, explained, and overcome. For instance, the leguminous tree *Leucana leucocephala* was recognized as a potentially valuable source of protein in the diets of ruminant animals. However, when leucana was introduced into the diets of ruminant animals in some places, there were no unexpected effects; in other places, cattle, sheep, and goats exhibited a number of clinical abnormalities including alopecia or wool loss, salivation, poor appetite, cataracts, weight loss, and hypothyroidism. Researchers eventually figured out that the adverse effects were due to a breakdown product of a plant constituent known as mimosine. This breakdown product, DHP, was produced during mastication. In some places, cattle, sheep, and goats possessed rumen microflora that degraded DHP and rendered it harmless, while in other places, ruminants lacked the appropriate microflora, and the DHP persisted to act as a potent toxin and goitrogen. It was learned that leucana could be effectively exploited as a high protein feed by livestock in areas where there had been problems if animals received a rumen inoculation with the appropriate DHP-degrading microflora.[9]

Technological innovation also can improve the quality of feedstuffs or the animal's ability to use them. Take for instance the development of high-lysine corn. Normal dent corn has a protein content of about 9.4%. However, the levels of two essential amino acids, lysine and tryptophan, are low, which limits the nutritional value of corn for nonruminant animals and humans. Ruminant animals can produce these amino acids via the rumen microflora. In 1963, researchers at Purdue University, examining soft, opaque varieties of corn, identified a recessive gene, Opaque-2, which produced higher levels of lysine and tryptophan in opaque varieties, resulting in a more nutritionally balanced corn. Through cross-breeding, commercially adaptable strains of corn with higher lysine and tryptophan content became available. These high-lysine hybrids have demonstrated nutritional advantages over normal corn for swine feeding, allowing more-efficient use of the total amino acids available in corn for building tissue proteins.

With advances in genetic engineering, it is now possible to manipulate the animal as well as the feedstuffs being offered. In 1999, for instance, researchers at the University of Guelph produced a transgenic pig that can produce additional amounts of phytase, a salivary enzyme that enhances the digestion and absorption of phosphorus from ingested plant materials. The impetus for this research was to reduce the amount of phosphorus excreted in pig manure to reduce the adverse environmental impact of excess phosphorus entering groundwaters from pig manure associated with large-scale intensive hog-farming operations. However, the genetic innovation would presumably also be useful to increase the efficiency of phosphorus use by animals raised in areas of the world where phosphorus deficiency in soils and feeds is a major constraint on animal production.

Rational Use of Genetic Resources

The use of domestic animals often depends on two major attributes, both of which are controlled, to a large extent, by genetics. These two attributes are productivity and adaptability. In commercial agriculture, especially in developed nations, animals have been bred largely to improve their production outputs. In high-production livestock systems, problems of adaptability are largely dealt with by manipulating the animal's environment to provide suitable conditions of nutrition, housing, comfort, and health. In subsistence farming systems in developing countries, the reverse situation often prevails. Farmers lack the resources to transform environments to suit animals

Table 4-3 Leguminous Plants Useful for Integration into Small Animal Farm Sustainable Agriculture Enterprises[a]

Tree Legumes

Common Name	Scientific Name	Minimum Rainfall (mm/yr)	Drought Tolerance	Waterlogging Tolerance	Frost Tolerance	Nutritive Value
Pigeon pea	Cajanus cajan	300	Very good	Poor	Poor	Very good
Calliandra	Calliandra calothyrus	1000	Fair	Good	Poor	Good
Glyricidia	Glyricidia maculata	900	Fair	Fair	Poor	Good
	Glyricidia sepium	900	Fair	Fair	Poor	Good
Leucaena	Leucaena diversfolia	500	Good	Fair	Fair	Good
	Leucana leucocephala	400	Very good	Poor	Fair	Good
Sesbania	Sesbania grandifolia	600	Good	Good	Poor	Good
	Sesbania sesban	500	Good	Good	Poor	Good
Tree lucerne	Chamaecytisus prolifer	500	Good	Poor	Very good	Good

Herbaceous Legumes

Common Name	Scientific Name	Minimum Rainfall (mm/yr)	Drought Tolerance	Waterlogging Tolerance	Frost Tolerance	Nutritive Value
Calopo	Calopogonium mucunoides	700	Fair	Fair	Poor	Good
Cassia	Cassia rotundifolia	400	Very good	Fair	Fair	Good
Centro	Centrosema pubescens	900	Fair	Fair	Poor	Very good
Desmanthus	Desmanthus virgatus	500	Good	Fair	Poor	Good
Greenleaf desmodium	Desmodium intortum	700	Fair	Good	Fair	Very good
Silverleaf desmodium	Desmodium uncinatum	700	Good	Fair	Fair	Very good
Glycine	Glycine wightii	600	Good	Poor	Fair	Very good
Lablab	Lablab purpureus	400	Good	Poor	Fair	Very good
Lotononis	Lotononis bainesii	800	Fair	Very good	Good	Good
Siratro	Macroptilium atropurpureum	500	Good	Fair	Fair	Very good
Axillaris	Macrotyloma axillare	500	Good	Fair	Poor	Very good
Alfalfa	Medicago sativa	600	Very good	Poor	Very good	Very good
Tepary bean	Phaseolus acutofolius	300	Very good	Poor	Poor	Good
Puero	Pueraria phaseoloides	1000	Fair	Good	Poor	Good
Graham stylo	Stylosanthes guianensis	600	Fair	Fair	Poor	Good
Verano stylo	Stylosanthes hamata	500	Very good	Poor	Poor	Good
Seca stylo	Stylosanthes scabra	500	Very good	Poor	Poor	Fair
Red clover	Trifolium pratense	600	Fair	Poor	Good	Very good
White clover	Trifolium repens	600	Fair	Fair	Very good	Very good
Vetch	Vicia dasycarpa	400	Fair	Fair	Good	Very good
Cowpea	Vigna sinensis	300	Good	Poor	Fair	Good

[a]The qualities of the different plants vary, but in general these legumes provide fodder for animals, fuel wood, living fences, soil enrichment with nitrogen, and inhibition of soil erosion.

Adapted from Peacock C. Improving Dairy Goat Production in the Tropics: A Manual for Development Workers. Oxford, England: Oxfam/FARM—Africa Publication, 1996.

and traditionally have depended upon domestic animals that have largely been selected for their adaptability to survive under local conditions, frequently without concomitant increases in productivity.

To increase the contribution of domestic livestock to food production and economic development throughout the world, animal productivity must be enhanced. However, this should not be achieved by sacrificing adaptability. The finite availability of arable land on the planet continues to push farmers and herders into more challenging and difficult environments. The need for animals highly adapted to extremes of climate, limited access to water, or uncertain forage supplies remains strong. As such, the rational use of genetic resources for improved animal production requires both the use of selective breeding to improve productivity and the conservation of genetic resources among the world's domesticated livestock breeds to ensure continued adaptability to a wide range of agroecological conditions. Both approaches are briefly discussed in the following sections.

Selective Breeding

Over the centuries, livestock breeders have learned to identify desired, heritable traits, select and mate animals that express and transmit those traits, and thereby develop breeds of domestic animals that suit their needs. Through this process, wild fowl that produced a single clutch of eggs per year have given way to domesticated commercial laying hens that produce eggs on a daily basis. Through the same process, the wild and fierce aurochs cow, which likely produced just enough milk to suckle a single calf in a year, has provided the genetic basis for the modern Holstein cow, a docile beast capable of producing as much as 45 kg of milk per day over a 305-day lactation.

Today, the commercial swine industry is so responsive to consumer tastes and the need to improve production efficiency, that maintaining breed purity has taken a back seat to meeting production and marketing goals. Commercial herds are increasingly made up of mixed-breed pigs from a variety of purebred breeding stocks, such as Duroc, Landrace, Hampshire, or Yorkshire. The selection of purebred boars and gilts for use in a commercial herd is determined by managers and breeding consultants aiming to address such specific goals as reduced backfat thickness, faster rate of gain, and even aesthetic characteristics of concern to consumers such as lean in the carcass, lean in the loin and loin eye area, loin color, loin marbling, and drip loss. Progeny testing, extensive data collection, and computerized record keeping help breeding associations fine-tune their selection of future breeding stock.

During the period of European colonization, settlers regularly took their familiar, high-producing breeds with them to new continents and often settled in areas most conducive to the productivity and well-being of these animals, leading, for example, to the establishment of European dairy cattle in the cooler tropical highland areas in East Africa and South Asia. Set-

tlers also demonstrated significant talent in modifying and adapting introduced stock to produce animals suited to local conditions and market demands. Fine-wooled Spanish Merino sheep were imported to Australia early in the 19th century and cross-bred with local meat-type breeds to produce Australian Merinos that produced both high-quality wool for the export market as well as an improved mutton carcass for local meat consumption. Thus, Australian Merinos became a cornerstone of the expanding Australian economy. Adaptation of imported Merinos played a similar role in the developing economy of South Africa.

The introduction of high-producing breeds is still used widely as an engine for agricultural and economic progress in developing countries. Not all such endeavors have been successful, however, as there are frequently constraints related to nutrition and disease, especially in tropical regions. The genetic potential for increased production, be it of milk, egg, fiber, or meat, cannot be realized consistently unless that potential is matched by a feed supply of sufficient quality and quantity to fuel the expanded production. In many parts of the tropics, soil nutrients may be deficient, rainfall erratic, croplands limited, and the inputs and practices of crop production generally inadequate to meet the greater nutritional demands of potentially high- producing animals.

Disease is another major constraint. European breeds of dairy cattle and goats, for instance, can offer substantially increased milk production in tropical areas through cross-breeding with local stock, but these imported animals are highly susceptible to tick infestations and the numerous tropical, tick-borne diseases associated with them. In East Africa, imported Holstein cattle may need to be dipped for tick control as often as twice per week to avoid the deadly effects of East Coast fever, a hemoparasitic protozoal disease caused by *Theileria parva* and transmitted by the tick *Rhipicephalus appendiculatus*.

There are several approaches to reducing the impact of disease on efforts to introduce imported breeds with high- production potential. One strategy is to embrace the goal of producing cross-bred herds rather than creating local, purebred herds, so that valuable adaptive traits of local breeds can be retained. Another strategy is to import semen rather than livestock, so that the desired genetic traits can be introduced without the introduction of animals highly susceptible to disease, though artificial insemination does require a good supporting infrastructure for semen storage and transport to be successful. A third approach is to promote zero-grazing practices whereby valuable imported purebred animals are fed and housed in pens and not allowed to graze. This reduces exposure to ticks and other internal and external parasites and is often used with purebred dairy animals, both cattle and goats.

In any circumstance in which exotic breeds are introduced, it is essential to know what endemic diseases occur in a given region that may pose a health threat to the introduced animals. With access to such information, a suitable health management plan, including appropriate vaccinations and parasite control practices, can be devised before the animals arrive. In the future, transgenic science may allow animal breeders to develop high-producing livestock resistant to specific maladies such as tick-borne diseases and trypanosomiasis, allowing their introduction into places previously inhospitable to livestock production. Investigations into the genetic basis of resistance to important livestock diseases is likely to be an important and exciting area of veterinary research in the coming years.

Conservation of Genetic Resources

There are an estimated 4500 breeds representing 25 species of domesticated animals in the world today, and about 30% of these breeds are considered at high risk of disappearance. Most of these are local breeds of livestock that are little known out-

side their immediate geographical range but are extremely well suited to their agroecological niche. As an example, Table 4-4 lists recognized, distinct breeds of sheep and goats found in the Indian subcontinent, most of which are virtually unknown outside the region but are, nonetheless, well adapted to local conditions and useful to local livestock keepers.[6]

A major factor in the loss of breeds is the increasing reliance on only one or a few breeds that have been selected for high-input, high-output production systems. North Americans do not need to look far from home to see evidence of this trend— the Holstein cow has steadily displaced all other dairy breeds as the dominant milking cow on the continent. The high-volume milk production of the Holstein cow allows profit-conscious farmers to improve efficiency in their dairy operations by keeping fewer individual animals to achieve production targets. For large dairy operations, these high-

---

Table 4-4   Indigenous Breeds of Sheep and Goats in India[a]

Sheep and Goats of the Northwest Arid and Semiarid Zones		Sheep and Goats of the Semiarid Central to Humid Coastal Southern Peninsula	
Sheep Breeds	**Goat Breeds**	**Sheep Breeds**	**Goat Breeds**
Chokla	Sirohi	Deccani	Sangamneri
Nali	Marwari	Bellary	Malabari
Marwari	Beetal	Nellore	Osmanadabi
Magra	Jhakrana	Mandya	Kannaiadu
Jaisalmeri	Barbari	Hassan	
Pugal	Jamnapari	Mecheri	
Malpura	Mehsana	Kilakarsal	
Sonadi	Gohilwadi	Vembur	
Patanwadi	Zalawadi	Coimbatore	
Muzzafarangri	Kutchi	Nilgiri	
Jalauni	Surti	Ramnad White	
Hissardale		Madras Red	
Sheep and Goats of the Temperate Northern Region		Tiruchy Black	
		Kenguri	
Sheep Breeds	**Goat Breeds**	**Sheep and Goats of the Humid to Subtemperate Eastern Region**	
Gaddi	Baddi	**Sheep Breeds**	**Goat Breeds**
Rampur Bushair	Changthangi		
Bhakarwal	Chigu	Chottanagpuri	Ganjam
Poonchi		Shahabadi	Bengal
Karnah		Balangir	
Gurez		Ganjam	
Kashmir Merino		Tibetan	
Changthangi		Bonpala	

[a]These animals, including 40 breeds of sheep and 20 breeds of goats, show remarkable adaptation to a wide range of environments, including harsh desert conditions. In addition to showing good survival characteristics, some breeds have strong production potential. The Jamnapari goat, for example, is a very good dairy animal, well suited to tropical conditions, that has been exported to Indonesia and South America.

From: Food and Agriculture Organization of the United Nations. Sheep and Goat Breeds of India, FAO Animal Production and Health Paper no. 30. Rome: FAO, 1982.

producing animals also promote economies of scale, allowing greater increases in overall production per number of cows added during herd expansions. The net effect is that national populations of Jersey and Guernsey cattle have decreased dramatically, and populations of Brown Swiss and Milking Shorthorn cattle have all but disappeared from the rural landscapes and dairy barns of North America.

A high degree of economic and technological development supports the dominance of Holstein cattle in North American dairying. Modern agriculture on the continent readily provides the quantity and quality of protein and energy necessary to meet production potential, usually in the form of cereal-based concentrates. Environmental influences that may hamper production such as high temperature or humidity are managed by construction of well-designed, mechanically ventilated farm buildings. Losses from production-related diseases such as displaced abomasum or mastitis are minimized by access to a well-trained and well-equipped cadre of veterinarians in private practice. Overall production efficiency is supported by an extensive network of extension agents and private consultants advising on a wide array of issues including animal nutrition, reproductive performance, quality assurance, and animal health. In summary, the Holstein cow is a highly pampered and protected creature that pays back its attentive caretakers with voluminous outputs of milk.

Yet, in many developing countries, Holsteins may have a hard time of it. Inadequately fed, unprotected from prolonged drought or relentless rain, overrun with parasites, and naive to deadly infectious agents, Holstein cows may have trouble surviving, let alone realizing their production potential. In contrast, local breeds of animals will have developed remarkable adaptations that promote survival and foster productivity within the constraints of local conditions. Hence the popularity of milking buffalo in hot and humid India. Many local breeds of livestock around the world show unique or special adaptations such as disease resistance, adaptation to harsh climatic conditions, and adaptation to poor-quality or unreliable supplies of feed and water. Other desirable traits include high fertility, good maternal qualities, unique product attributes, and longevity. Such characteristics need to be better recognized and characterized, and their genetic transmission better understood. The populations that possess such traits need to be both identified, described, and protected from extinction. Their genetic potential needs to be preserved intact but at the same time be more fully exploited through both selective and cross-breeding to produce new animals that combine established adaptability with increased productivity. It should not be assumed that local indigenous breeds cannot be selected for increased production. Rather, it may be that insufficient attention has been paid to these breeds in the past by the world community of breeders and animal scientists.

There is growing interest and increased, organized effort to conserve, protect, and promote the use of rare and local domestic breeds of animals. Toward that goal, the FAO has established the Global Programme for the Management of Farm Animal Genetic Resources. The effort includes *in situ* efforts to promote the use of indigenous breeds in sustainable agriculture as well as *ex situ* efforts to collect, store, and preserve genetic material for conservation and research. The program encourages country-by-country efforts to develop inventories and collect information on the status of indigenous breeds and promotes international cooperation on conservation efforts through education, research, and policymaking. FAO also maintains the Domestic Animal Diversity Information System (DAD-IS) to manage data for the global program, available on the internet at http://www.fao.org/dad-is/. This includes the Worldwatch List for Domestic Animal Diversity, which provides regional inventories of indigenous breeds of all domestic animal species and the status of existing populations. Other organizations involved in the conservation of farm animal genetic resources are Rare Breeds International, an international nongovernmental organization, and the American Livestock Breed Conservancy, which focuses on North American breeds. Veterinarians are actively involved in these conservation efforts. For example, Pacific International Genetics, a private veterinary group in California, provides reproductive services to the American Livestock Breeds Conservancy and to other organizations, including zoos, involved in the reproduction of rare species (http://www.pacintgen.com/).

Improved Marketing of Livestock/Livestock Products

Even when farmers have the capability to produce farm goods beyond their own subsistence needs, they must have the means to market and sell those goods successfully to justify producing them. One of the major obstacles impeding the transition of subsistence farming to commercial farming in developing countries has been a lack of sufficient marketing incentives. Farmers and herders are simply unwilling to make investments for improved productivity if they believe that market access and market prices are not adequate to justify their investments.

There are a number of approaches to improving market opportunities for smallholder farmers and herders. Obviously, improved infrastructure would be an excellent catalyst, and government policymakers need to make rural road construction and road maintenance higher priorities in their overall planning. Government policies related to subsidies and price setting need to be reviewed and revised when they provide disincentives to farmers to produce. The establishment of marketing cooperatives is another important tool for empowering and encouraging farmers, giving them added control in obtaining fair prices, reducing dependence on middlemen, and favorably influencing markets for their products. The Indian effort in milk marketing, discussed elsewhere in this chapter, is an excellent example of a cooperative effort that increases income and provides incentive for expanded production to subsistence livestock owners. Another approach is to identify opportunities for farmers to develop and market value-added products. For instance, farmers with dairy animals may have trouble selling fresh milk because markets are too far away, they lack the means of transporting bulk fluid milk to market, or they are not able to keep it from spoiling (Fig. 4-16). On-farm conversion of milk to cheese or yogurt can be accomplished through simple, low-cost technologies that increase the value of the product while reducing its bulk and perishability. Similar options are available with drying meat into jerky or other products.

Vertical integration of agriculture-based industries within a country may be another way to stimulate domestic produc-

tion, as in the case of China. For decades, China exported its cashmere fiber in raw form to processors and textile manufacturers in Europe and the United States for production of finished goods. In the last 20 years, however, as part of the general industrial expansion that has occurred in that country, China has developed its own cashmere-processing industry and now manufactures and markets its own finished goods throughout the world. This economic development has been an enormous stimulus to local goat production. Chinese animal scientists have made remarkable advances in improving Chinese breeds of cashmere goats through selective breeding, resulting in dramatic per goat increases in fiber yields and fiber quality. For example, the improved Liaoning cashmere breed has average yields exceeding 500 g of cashmere down fiber per goat, whereas unimproved local goats may produce an average of 70 g of fiber. Goat numbers have also increased to meet the demands of domestic manufacture. Between 1985 and 1994, the cashmere goat population in China almost doubled from 28.5 million to 54.0 million.

Increased opportunities for exporting livestock and livestock products can also be an incentive for farmers and herders to increase production. However, many developing countries are effectively shut out of international marketing of animals and animal products because of disease constraints. Internationally established and agreed-upon regulations strictly limit the exportation of animals from countries where highly contagious diseases such as foot and mouth disease or rinderpest are known to occur. Until such diseases are reliably brought under control and the infrastructure is in place to reliably monitor and confirm that disease-free status is maintained, many countries will remain effectively excluded from participation in international trade in livestock and livestock products. The subject of livestock health and international trade is of major importance in the present era of globalization and increased free trade and is discussed further in Chapter 9.

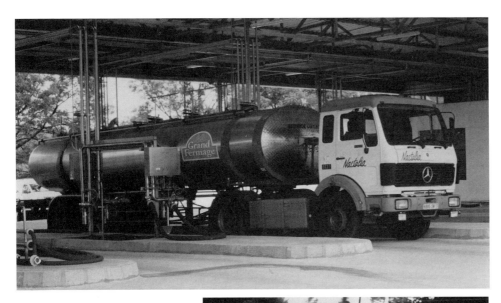

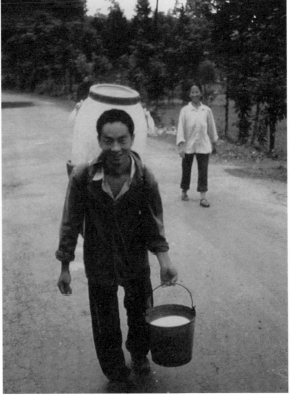

Figure 4-16. The challenge of bringing product to market faced by small-scale livestock producers in developing countries is illustrated in this pair of photographs. Top, The truck of a commercial milk hauler in France unloading milk collected from private farms at a cheese-manufacturing facility. Bottom, A Chinese dairy farmer carrying milk on his back and in an open pail to a local village market. Improved infrastructure and the development of marketing cooperatives can help small farmers like this achieve greater prosperity and well-being. (Top photo by Dr. David M. Sherman. Bottom photo courtesy of Dr. Robert Pelant, Heifer Project International, Little Rock, Arkansas)

Discussion Points

1. As presented in Table 4-1, the five domesticated livestock species with the largest population growth during the last quarter of the 20th century were geese, ducks, rabbits, chickens, and goats, all species of comparatively small size and short reproduction cycles. Discuss some of the reasons that these species are becoming more popular and the conditions under which they are raised. How well does your own veterinary curriculum prepare you to serve the people who depend on such small stock for their livelihood? What are the major disease problems of ducks?

2. Data on consumption of animal products in developing countries are often given on a per capita basis. How can this information be misleading? What factors need to be considered in interpreting such data?

3. What potential animal and public health problems might be associated with feeding different types of animal manure to livestock? How can these problems be controlled so that manure can be recycled safely as an animal feed?

4. Evaluate the potential for commercialization of energy production from the biodigestion of animal waste in your area. Are there any ongoing efforts in this regard? Discuss the pros and cons of such an effort with farmers, environmental regulators, and utility company representatives in your area.

5. What are some of the major disease problems that occur in salmon aquaculture? In prawn aquaculture? Are there other nations where veterinary medicine is farther advanced in service to aquaculture? Where can you go to find up-to-date information on veterinary issues and developments in the aquaculture industry?

6. Identify an organic livestock producer in your area and review his livestock health practices and the medications and vaccines that are used and those that are prohibited. Assess the effectiveness of the herd health program and make recommendations to improve it within the context of the farmer's organic farming framework.

References

1. Blench R. 'You Can't Go Home Again': Pastoralism in the New Millennium. London: Overseas Development Institute, 2001. (Also at http:// www.odi.org.uk/pdn/eps.pdf)

2. Brown LR. Who Will Feed China. New York: WW Norton, 1995.

3. Clutton–Brock J. A Natural History of Domesticated Mammals. 2nd Ed. Cambridge, England: Cambridge University Press, 1999.

4. Delgado C, Rosegrant M, Steinfeld H, Ehui S, Courbois C. Livestock to 2020: The Next Food Revolution. Food, Agriculture and the Environment Discussion Paper 28. Washington, DC: International Food Policy Research Institute, 1999.

5. Field CR. The camel and its place in pastoral life—a desert dairy. In: Evans JO, Piers Simpkin S, Aitkins DJ, eds. Camel Keeping in Kenya. Nairobi, Republic of Kenya: Ministry of Agriculture, Livestock Development and Marketing, 1995:1.1–1.7.

6. Food and Agriculture Organization of the United Nations. Sheep and goat breeds of India, FAO Animal Production and Health Paper no. 30. Rome: FAO, 1982

7. Harris M. Good to Eat: Riddles of Food and Culture. (Ch. 2, Meat hunger) New York: Simon & Schuster, 1985:19–46.

8. Hu FB, Willett WC. The Relationship between Consumption of Animal Products (Beef, Pork, Poultry, Eggs, Fish and Dairy Products) and Risk of Chronic Diseases: A Critical Review. A World Bank Report. Washington, DC: World Bank, 1998. (Also available through http://wbln0018.worldbank.org/rdv/animal.nsf/HotTopicsWeb?OpenView)

9. Jones RJ, Megarrity RG. Successful transfer of DHP-degrading bacteria from Hawaiian goats to Australian ruminants to overcome the toxicity of Leucaena. Aust Vet J 1986:63:259–262.

10. Lawrence PR, Lawrence K, Dijkman JT, Starkey PH, eds. Research for development of animal traction in West Africa. Proceedings of the 4th workshop of the West Africa Animal Traction Network, Kano, Nigeria, 9–13 July 1990. International Livestock Centre for Africa (ILCA), Addis Ababa, Ethiopia. 1993. 306 pp.

11. Le Sann A. A Livelihood from Fishing: Globalization and Sustainable Fisheries Policies. London: Intermediate Technology Publications, 1998.

12. Leng RA, Stambolie JH, Bell R. Duckweed—a potential high-protein feed resource for domestic animals and fish. Livestock Research for Rural Development, vol 7, October, 1995. (Also at http://www.fao.org/ag/aga/agap/frg/afris/espanol/ document/lrrd/LRRD7/1/3.HTM)

13. Marchaim U. Biogas processes for sustainable development. FAO Agricultural Services Bulletin no. 95. Rome: Food and Agriculture Organization of the United Nations, 1992.

14. Mokdad AH, Serdula MK, Dietz WH, et al. The Spread of the Obesity Epidemic in the United States, 1991–1998. JAMA 1999;282(16):1519–1522.

15. Mohr P. Power Partners. Dairy Today 2001:17(7):3.

16. National Research Council. Microlivestock. Little-Known Small Animals with a Promising Economic Future. Washington, DC: National Academy Press, 1991.

17. Novelli B. Aspects of Karimojong Ethnosociology, Museum Combonianum no. 44. Verona: Editrice Missionaria Italiana, 1988.

18. Peacock C. Improving Dairy Goat Production in the Tropics: A Manual for Development Workers. Oxford, England: Oxfam/FARM-Africa Publication, 1996.

19. Pimentel D, Dritschilo W, Krummel J, et al. Energy and Land Constraints in Food Protein Production. Science 1975;190:754–761.

20. Sere C, Steinfeld H. World livestock production systems. Current status, issues and trends. FAO Animal Production and Health Paper no. 127. Rome: Food and Agriculture Organization of the United Nations, 1996.

21. Silanikove N. The physiological basis of adaptation in goats to harsh environments. Small Ruminant Res 2000;35:181–193.

22. Smith OB, Olaloku EA. Peri-Urban Livestock Production Systems. CFP Report Series Report no. 24. Ottawa, Canada: Cities Feeding People, International Development Research Centre, 1998. (Also at http://www.idrc.ca/cfp/rep24_e.html)

23. United States Department of Agriculture. Agricultural Fact Book 1998. Washington, DC: USDA, Office of Communications, 1998. (Also at http://www.usda.gov/news/pubs/fbook98/content.htm)

Suggested Readings

Altieri MA. Agroecology. The Science of Sustainable Agriculture. 2nd Ed. London: Intermediate Technology Publications, 1995.

Banerjee A. Dairying systems in India. World Anim Rev 1994;79:8–15.

Dowling R, Alderson L. Rare Breeds. Endangered Farm Animals in Photographs. Boston: Little, Brown & Co, 1994.

Huang J, Rozelle S, Rosegrant M . China's Food Economy in the 21st Century. Discussion Paper no. 19. Washington, DC: International Food Policy Research Institute, 1997.

Nestel B, ed. Development of Animal Production Systems. World Animal Science Series, vol A2. Amsterdam: Elsevier Science Publishers, 1984.

National Research Council. The Water Buffalo: New Prospects for an Underutilized Animal. Washington, DC: National Academy Press, 1981.

Nene YL. Sustainable agriculture: Future hope for developing countries. Can J Plant Pathol 1996;18(2):133–140.

Payne WJA, Wilson RT, eds. An Introduction to Animal Husbandry in the Tropics. 5th Ed. Oxford, England: Blackwell Science, 1999.

Tarrant J, ed. Farming and Food. New York: Oxford University Press, 1991.

Wilson RT. Livestock Production Systems. The Tropical Agriculturalist Series. London: MacMillan Education Limited, 1995.

Chapter 5
Animals, Food Security, and Socioeconomic Development

OBJECTIVES FOR THIS CHAPTER

After completing this chapter, the reader should be able to

- Identify key factors contributing to food insecurity and hunger among the world's growing population

- Recognize the complex factors that constrain social and economic development in many parts of the world

- Understand different approaches to socioeconomic development in developing countries

- Appreciate the elements of sustainable development and appropriate technology transfer

- Identify the important role that livestock play in socioeconomic development and improving food security, particularly in rural areas

- Discern the factors that contribute to successful and unsuccessful livestock development projects and recognize the role that veterinarians can play in international development

Introduction

Globalization of the world economy has been a defining characteristic of our age and has been widely heralded as a powerful engine of prosperity. Certainly, the globalization of markets, trade, and finance has brought great benefits to many nations and people. Yet the process of globalization has been, and continues to be, unbalanced. The 1999 Human Development Report of the United Nations Development Programme (UNDP), *Globalization with a Human Face*, focuses on the impacts of globalization and points out some of the disparities that persist in the world, despite the successes of the burgeoning global economy.[18] Some of these disparities are sobering. Over 80 countries still have per capita incomes lower than they were a decade ago. Fifty-five countries actually have declining per capita incomes, notably in sub-Saharan Africa, Eastern Europe, and the newly independent nations that emerged from the former Soviet Union.

The divide between the rich and the poor is also growing larger. The income of the richest 20% of the world's population is 74 times that of the poorest 20%. The fifth of the world's people living in the richest countries enjoyed 82% of the world's expanding export trade, while the fifth living in the poorest countries received only 1%. The richest fifth have 74% of the world telephone lines, while the bottom fifth have only 1.5%. The 29 industrialized nations belonging to the Organization for Economic Cooperation and Development (OECD), which contain 19% of the world's population, accounted for 91% of the world's internet users in 1999. In 1998, the 200 wealthiest individuals in the world had combined assets exceeding $1 trillion, almost double the combined gross domestic product (GDP) of all 48 of the world's least developed nations, which are home to 615 million people.

While the disparities in income, material goods, telecommunications, and internet access are jarring, it is disparities in access to adequate nutrition that provide the most telling commentary on the maldistribution of wealth and the persistence of poverty in today's world. The United Nations estimates that presently, at least 1.3 billion people still live in poverty, earning less than $1 per day, and that 840 million of them are undernourished. The vast majority of the world's poor and undernourished live in the rural areas of developing countries, especially in Asia and Africa.

Worldwide, more than 5 million children die of hunger-related diseases each year, while survivors are often physically or mentally stunted, performing well below their potential at school and work. It is estimated that 17 million children born each year are underweight in *utero*. The effects are long lasting and include impaired immunity, neurological damage, and retarded physical growth. The risk of death for an infant born at two thirds of normal weight is 10 times that of a normal-weight baby. The World Health Organization estimates that for the five leading causes of child death in the developing world, 54% of cases have malnutrition as an underlying condition. The damaging effects of hunger persist into adulthood as well. A World Bank study of India found that productivity losses resulting from hunger cost the economy US$10 to 28 billion per year, an amount equal to 3 to 9% of the country's GDP in 1996.

The presence of such misery in the midst of plenty calls out for corrective action. There are numerous reasons for acting. As a matter of simple human compassion, it is natural to reach out to the less fortunate to provide them with the tools necessary to help them to help themselves. As a matter of conscience, it may seem only fair to work to encourage policies and practices that more evenly distribute the opportunities for prosperity created by economic globalization. As a matter of public policy or enlightened self-interest, it serves all the world's citizens to come to the aid of the poor. This is because poverty and hunger are breeding grounds for emergent disease, social disintegration, environmental degradation, and violent conflict, which in today's closely interconnected world can affect all the world's citizens, regardless of their social status. Many matters of global concern, such as the spread of AIDS and antibiotic-resistant tuberculosis, poaching of endangered wildlife, accelerating deforestation, and increasing urban crime or civil war, frequently have their roots in the conditions and actions of people mired in grinding poverty but quickly spill over into the environs of the affluent. Finally, as a matter of economic strategy, it makes sense to create opportunities for the world's poor so that they too can be more productive, accumulate wealth, and actively participate in global markets as producers and consumers, thus contributing further to the continued growth and development of the global economy.

Since livestock are an integral part of the daily social, economic, and cultural lives of countless rural people around the globe, veterinarians can play an important role in alleviating poverty and hunger and helping poorer nations to participate in the global economy. It is estimated that livestock actively contribute to the livelihoods of 70% of the rural poor, or over 900 million people worldwide. Some of these people are landless villagers who tether a sheep or goat by the roadside, others are pastoralists grazing large, mixed herds of livestock on open grasslands along traditional routes, while others are subsistence farmers engaged in small, mixed-farming enterprises that include a variety of crops and animals. Many of these cultivators and animal keepers are women, perhaps widowed by AIDS, violent crime, or civil war or perhaps left to tend a family farm plot by husbands who have sought wage work in mines or factories in cities far from home. All of these animal keepers can benefit from improved animal health and productivity.

As critical as livestock are to the rural poor, a good deal of the potential of livestock production remains unrealized, owing to a variety of constraints. Such constraints include, among others, limited access to grazing, inadequate land for production of forages, suboptimal animal nutrition, limited access to improved animal genetics, unfavorable pricing for livestock products, inaccessibility to markets, inadequate research on small farming and herding systems, lack of appropriate extension services targeted to the needs of small farmers and herders, the ravages of animal disease, and the lack of access to veterinary services. Inadequate animal disease control not only constrains the well-being of individual livestock owners, it also can have profound implications on national economies. Many developing nations would benefit greatly from the export of livestock products to generate much-needed foreign exchange. However, the failure to control highly contagious diseases of international concern, such as foot and mouth disease, can effectively seal off export markets, resulting in tremendous losses to the national treasury, which the country and its citizens can ill afford.

In this chapter, opportunities for the veterinary profession to improve the condition of the world's poor and the animals they depend on are presented in the context of a discussion of the demographics of hunger, the causes of poverty, the varied approaches to international development assistance, and the role of animals in poverty alleviation and socioeconomic development.

The Concept of Food Security

Since at least the 1960s, thanks in large part to the Green Revolution, the world has produced enough food to keep pace with its growing population and provide adequate nutrition for all. So why do so many people continue to be malnourished? Clearly, the production of sufficient food on a collective basis does not automatically guarantee reliable access to sufficient food on either a regional basis or an individual basis. Tremendous regional disparities exist in the capacity for food production, processing, and distribution, based on issues of geography, economics, technology, culture and public policy. Even within countries that produce adequate food on a per capita basis, marked disparities frequently exist in access to food among the nation's citizens. In this section, the concept of food security is addressed and the patterns, distribution, and underlying causes of malnutrition are discussed.

Defining Terms

Food security is the state in which people have physical and economic access at all times to sufficient food to lead a healthy and productive life. To achieve food security, three conditions must be met. The first is the availability of an adequate and reliable food supply. This food may be locally produced or even imported, as long as it is reliably available. Second is access to the food supply. Individuals must have the means to acquire their necessary food through production, barter, or purchase. Third is use. People must be able to properly store, prepare, and use foods. In this context, they must also be healthy, as some conditions, notably parasitism and chronic diarrhea, can reduce the efficiency with which people can derive nutrition from available and accessible foods.

Hunger results from *food insecurity*, the state in which food supplies are not either reliably available, accessible, and/or efficiently used. Food insecurity can be either chronic or transitory. *Chronic food insecurity* is a state in which the diet is continuously inadequate, leading to a persistent condition of undernutrition and all its associated consequences of poor growth, suboptimal development, increased susceptibility to disease, and diminished productivity. *Transitory food insecurity* is a temporary decline in access to food that can be due to instability of food prices, food availability, or purchasing power. The most extreme example of transitory food security and the most dramatic, is famine.

Traditionally, *hunger* has been synonymous with *malnutrition*, but this has changed in recent years. Obesity has emerged as a common phenomenon among the world's more affluent citizens, in both the developing and the developed world. It is becoming increasingly recognized as a public health concern, with noninfectious disease problems such as adult-onset diabetes and heart disease occurring more commonly among the overweight. Nowadays, the term *malnutrition* is generally applied to both the overfed and the underfed. As such, the state of chronic food insecurity, or hunger, is now generally referred to as *undernutrition*, while the condition of excessive food intake is referred to as *overnutrition*. These states of nutrition are related generally to either inadequate or excessive intake of food energy in the form of fat, carbohydrate, and protein. A more-specific form of malnutrition is *micronutrient deficiency*, which involves inadequate intake of necessary trace minerals and vitamins. Both the underfed and the overfed can suffer from micronutrient deficiencies. On a global basis, iron deficiency, vitamin A deficiency, and iodine deficiency are the most common and debilitating micronutrient deficiencies.

Demographics of Chronic Food Insecurity

Agricultural production has increased worldwide in recent decades. This is mainly due to rising yields for the major grains—rice, wheat, and maize. According to UNDP figures published in 1999, the per capita supply of food increased by 18% from 2129 kilocalories (kcal) to 2628 kcal in developing countries by 1996, and from 2336 kcal to 2751 kcal for the world as a whole, well beyond the average daily caloric requirement of 2500 kcal for an adult male. This per capita increase in food production occurred even in the face of rapid population growth from 4017 million in 1975 to 5743 million in 1997. This per capita increase is projected to continue at least through 2020, based on a number of econometric food-supply modeling exercises.

Yet statistical averages offer a distorted view of the actual situation. In reality, there are an estimated 800 million people, representing 15% of the world's population, that get less than 2000 calories per day, while over 165 million children under 5 years of age are clinically underweight. This means that their weight is at least 2 standard deviations below the mean weight for their age group. In reality, there are distinct differences between regions regarding the availability of calories and equally significant variations within individual countries regarding access to those calories by different segments of the population.

India is an instructive example of such internal contrasts. This south Asian nation has made impressive strides in economic development and food production in recent years. In 1998, the real growth rate of GDP in the country was 5.4%, compared with 3.9% in the United States. India has become the largest milk-producing nation in the world and in 1998 exported twice as much grain (mainly rice) than it imported (mainly wheat). The country now has a comfortable, food-secure, middle class of approximately 250 million people. However, the total population of India has recently breached the 1 billion mark, and many of the nation's citizens are not yet sharing the benefits of affluence.

According to Food and Agriculture Organization (FAO) figures reported in 1999 on data referring to 1996, the daily per capita dietary energy supply for India was 2470 calories. Nevertheless, India still had 204 million people who were undernourished. This was approximately 22% of its citizens and represented more than all the undernourished people of sub-Saharan African nations combined. Clearly, the food-secure and the food-insecure often are living side by side, with a wide variety of economic and cultural factors determining who has access to available food and who does not. This is true not only in the developing world, but in the developed world as well. In the United States, 26 million Americans, almost 1 in 10 citizens, sought emergency food assistance from the charity America's Second Harvest in 1997.

Based on FAO data, the distribution of undernourished people on a regional basis in the developing world is as follows: India, 204 million; China 164 million; other Asian and Pacific nations combined, 157 million; sub-Saharan Africa, 180 million; Latin American and the Caribbean, 53 million; and the Near East and North Africa, 33 million, for a total of 791 million people. In addition, there are an estimated 8 million chronically undernourished people in the world's industrialized nations, mainly in Europe and North America, and an additional 26 million in the transitional nations of the former Soviet Union, Eastern Europe, and Mongolia.

Looking specifically at the world's undernourished children, of whom there are an estimated 165 million, almost half, or 86 million, live in just three countries of South Asia—India, Pakistan, and Bangladesh. An additional 36 million live in East

Asia and the Pacific, 32 million in sub-Saharan Africa, 7 million in the Middle East, and 4 million in the Americas.

The prevalence of undernourishment within a country is another indicator of the scope and gravity of inadequate nutrition. Figure 5-1 presents a map of the world that identifies countries on the basis of the prevalence of undernourishment, ranging from less than 2.5% of the population to more than 35% of the population.[6] High prevalence of undernutrition suggests a generally low level of economic development in a country, indicating a high degree of poverty and/or a rapidly growing population that is outstripping a nation's capacity to produce or secure adequate food supplies.

Currently, most of the world's chronically undernourished people live in rural areas and, paradoxically, may be directly engaged in food production, albeit at a subsistence level. However, food insecurity also exists in urban areas and is likely to increase as populations in developing countries continue to shift steadily from the countryside to the cities. Whether in the cities or the country, certain groups of people can be identified as particularly vulnerable to food insecurity. These groups are listed in Table 5-1. Reviewing this list, it becomes readily apparent that poverty is the major underlying factor that puts persons at risk of food insecurity. Poverty constrains the ability of hungry people to access food, even when food is available, and also limits their ability to produce adequate food,

even when they are directly engaged in agricultural activity. In the following section, the factors that contribute to poverty in developing countries are explored, particularly in relation to rural poverty and the effect on food production and food security.

Poverty and Human Development

For a number of years, the United States Army has used a very catchy slogan in its recruitment efforts, "Be all you can be." The implied message is potent and profound. The Army is saying that within each and every one of us, there is an enormous potential for expanded capabilities and personal fulfillment. All that we lack are the opportunities and resources to fully realize our own unique potential. The Army offers to provide those opportunities and resources to its new recruits and thereby underwrite their development as fully potentiated human beings. Regrettably for the Army, recruitment figures have been declining in recent years. This is not for lack of an effective slogan. Rather, it is because American society at large, in an age of unrivaled prosperity and technological advance, offers young men and women an enormous array of opportunities for growth and fulfillment without the constraints, risks, and obligations of military service.

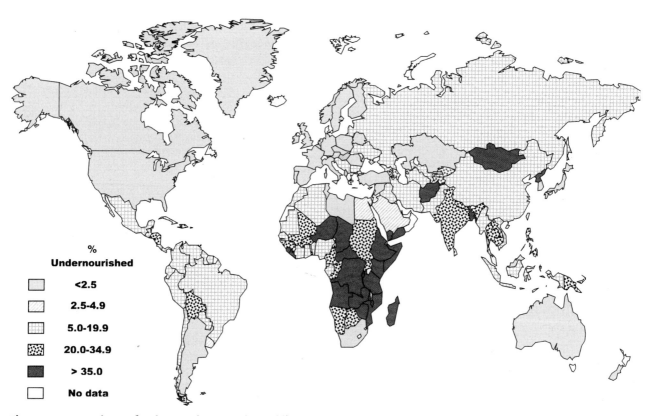

% Undernourished	
	<2.5
	2.5-4.9
	5.0-19.9
	20.0-34.9
	> 35.0
	No data

Figure 5-1. Prevalence of undernourishment in the world's countries as a percentage of population. Sub-Saharan Africa and South Asia are regions of particular concern, with many nations having a prevalence of undernutrition of 20% or more. (Adapted from Food and Agriculture Organization of the United Nations. The State of Food Insecurity in the World, 1999. Rome: FAO, 1999. Available on the world wide web at http://www.fao.org/FOCUS/E/SOFI/home-e.htm)

Table 5-1   Groups Particularly Vulnerable to Food Insecurity

Victims of Conflict
- Internally displaced persons
- Refugees
- Landless returnees
- Landmine disabled
- War invalids
- War widows and orphans

Migrant Workers and Their Families
- Migrant herders tending herds of others
- Migrant laborers seeking seasonal work
- Female-headed households left behind by migrant male laborers

Marginal Populations in Urban Areas
- School dropouts
- Unemployed
- Rickshaw and motorcycle taxi drivers
- Recently arrived migrants
- People living in slums in urban periphery
- Dock workers and porters
- Construction workers
- Workers in the informal sector
- Homeless people
- Orphans
- Street children
- Pensioners, elders without family, widows and widowers, divorcees, invalids and handicapped people
- Beggars

Persons Belonging to At-risk Social Groups
- Indigenous people
- Ethnic minorities
- Illiterate households

Persons Engaged in Vulnerable Livelihood Systems
- Subsistence or small-scale farmers
- Female-headed farming households
- Landless peasants
- Agricultural laborers
- Fishers
- Nomadic pastoralists
- Sedentary herders, small-scale livestock producers, and agropastoralists
- Forest dwellers
- Periurban small-scale agricultural producers and market gardeners
- Day or contract laborers

Dependent Persons Living Alone or in Low-Income Households with Large Family Size
- Elderly
- Women of childbearing age, especially pregnant and nursing mothers
- Children under 5 years old, especially infants
- Disabled and ill

This list was generated through the activities of the Food Insecurity and Vulnerability Information and Mapping Systems (FIVIMS), an interagency initiative mandated by the World Food Summit in 1996. From Food and Agriculture Organization of the United Nations. The State of Food Insecurity in the World, 1999. Rome: FAO, 1999. (Available on the world wide web at http://www.fao.org/FOCUS/E/SOFI/home-e.htm)

For literally hundreds of millions of people in the developing world, however, the exhortation to "be all you can be" rings hollow, as it remains largely unachievable. For the poor, the activities of each day are focused mainly on survival, not on self-improvement. Poor children are frequently robbed of their childhood, either by death or illness or by the daily grind of responsibilities that they shoulder in the quest for simple sustenance. They may be deprived of education, ill-clothed, ill-fed, and never reach their full mental, physical, or creative potential. In the most desperate circumstances, children may be sold into prostitution, be indentured workers, or even be purposely disfigured to make them more effective beggars. Abandoned, homeless children living on the street have become commonplace in various places around the world and face a daily life and death struggle. In Mongolia's capital, Ulaan Baatar, street children in recent years have been found living underground in winter among the city's subterranean heating pipes to escape death by freezing. In Rio de Janeiro, in 1993, eight Brazilian street children, regarded as a public nuisance, were murdered by off-duty policemen.

Poverty, identified as a major cause of hunger, has complex origins. Government policies, environmental degradation, expanding population, violence, discrimination, and a general lack of empowerment are just some of the factors that contribute to poverty and hunger and hinder human development. A full discussion of poverty is beyond the scope of this text. Instead, the discussion focuses on the rural poor in developing countries, as these are people who are frequently engaged in agricultural activities and often depend heavily on animals in their daily lives. First there is a brief review of how poverty is measured, particularly with regard to its effects on human development. This is followed by a discussion of how different underlying causes of poverty affect the potential of the rural poor to be self-sufficient in food production and to improve their livelihoods through agricultural activity, including animal agriculture.

Measuring Poverty

The dictionary describes poverty as the lack of resources for reasonably comfortable living. Yet surely, "reasonably comfortable" is a relative term. Would you be "reasonably comfortable" with no access to a telephone or any other form of telecommunication? How about without access to a car? Access to electric lights? A trained physician? Hot and cold running tap water? A flush toilet? A change of clothes? Soap to wash them with? A bowl of rice? Sufficient water to prepare it? Sufficient fuel to cook it with? While people in the developed world have come to accept a wide variety of conveniences and commodities as essential elements for "reasonably comfortable" living, tens of millions of people in the developing world continue to struggle daily to achieve simple survival, making do without reliable access to the most basic resources such as a bar of soap, a glass of safe drinking water, or sufficient calories to sustain them.

The scale of poverty is sufficiently large that a variety of terms have been devised to describe the different degrees of deprivation that exist in the world. The UNDP, the principal international agency concerned with matters of human development, distinguishes two main categories of poverty-income poverty and human poverty. *Income poverty* is the lack of income necessary to satisfy basic food needs, usually defined on the basis of minimum caloric requirements, as well as essential nonfood needs such as clothing, energy, and shelter. *Human poverty* is defined as a lack of basic human capabilities such as literacy, proper nutrition, normal life expectancy, and protection from preventable illness, as well as the goods, services, and infrastructure necessary to sustain those capabilities such as educational and medical facilities, safe drinking water, and sanitation services.

Indicators of Income Poverty

In the United States, the poverty level is determined as an estimate of the income necessary to purchase what society defines as a minimally acceptable standard of living. This is based on a poverty index or threshold originated by the Social Security Administration in 1964, which reflected the cost of a minimum adequate diet multiplied by three to allow for other expenses. Since then, the poverty threshold has been recalculated and reported annually by the Bureau of Census and serves as the basis for determining eligibility for federal assistance programs. In 1999, the poverty threshold for a family of two adults and two children was $16,895. This represents a daily income of $11.57 per person. Approximately 12.5% of Americans lived below this poverty threshold.

In assessing global poverty, the World Bank defines the poverty threshold at US$1 a day income. The commonly cited figure of 103 billion people living in poverty worldwide is based on this World Bank dollar-a-day figure, adjusted for purchasing power parity (PPP). Some critics suggest that the World Bank approach is arbitrary and underestimates global poverty. The 1-dollar threshold suggests that persons earning even 2 or 3 dollars a day are not struggling to meet basic needs. Given that Americans are considered to require more than $11 per day to avert poverty, this seems like a reasonable criticism, especially since persons in developing countries generally have to spend a far greater proportion of their income on food than

do those developed countries. In some developing countries, this can be as much as 80% of their income, compared with Americans who spend about 11% of their disposable income to purchase food. Furthermore, recent economic changes in many developing countries associated with the process of structural adjustment, such as the deregulation of currencies and the elimination of food subsidies, have resulted in devalued local currencies, reduced purchasing power, and increased food prices. This has made the slippery slope into poverty even more precarious for low-income people.

Indicators of Human Poverty

In 1990, the UNDP began to assemble and publish a Human Development Index (HDI) and has since produced it annually in its yearly Human Development Report. The purpose of the HDI was to measure achievements in basic human development in one simple composite index. In the annual report, countries are ranked in descending order of their HDI. This allows country comparisons to be made and progress or decline in human development to be monitored. The premise of the HDI is that a measurement of per capita income alone does not fully reflect the complexity of human development, as income is only a means to human development and not an end.

The HDI attempts to broaden the measurement of human development by assessing three main indicators for quality of life within a given country: longevity, knowledge, and standard of living. Longevity is measured as the average life expectancy at birth. Access to knowledge is measured by the adult literacy rate and the combined gross enrollment in primary, secondary, and tertiary schools. Standard of living is measured as per capita income, based on the national GDP, adjusted for purchasing-power parity. All of these parameters are combined in a calculation that represents the country's HDI. The number is reported as between 0 and 1, with a value of 1 indicating the highest attainment of human development. In 1999, Canada ranked first in the world with a HDI value of 0.932, while Sierra Leone ranked last with a score of 0.254, to give some idea of the range. In addition to individual country rankings, HDI values are presented for different regions of the world. The relative standings of different regions of the world for 1999 are shown in Figure 5-2.

While no single average measurement can capture the multitude of factors that influence quality of life for individual persons throughout the world, the HDI serves useful purposes. For anyone new to international work, it provides a useful overview of the state of the world's people on a country-by-country basis. It draws attention to the disparities that exist in human development around the world and points out where needs are greatest. There are now 10 full years of HDI data reported by the UNDP. This makes it possible to track progress or deterioration in the quality of life for citizens in different countries over the past decade and can provide a rough gauge of the impact that new policies or significant events, such as natural disasters, wars, famine, the spread of AIDS, or conversion from a collective to a free-market economy have had on the well-being of a nation's citizens.

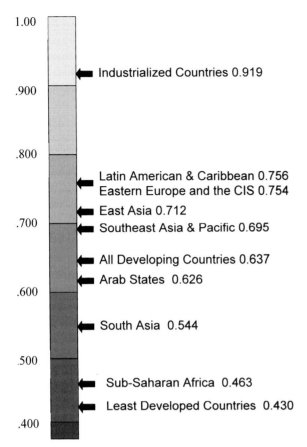

Figure 5-2. Human development index (HDI) values for various regions of the world as reported in the 1999 Human Development Report of the United Nations Development Program. See text for an explanation of how HDI values are calculated and interpreted. CIS refers to the Commonwealth of Independent States, nations that emerged from the former Soviet Union. (Reproduced with permission of the United Nations Development Programme.)

The HDI also highlights the important role that government and social policy can play in supporting human development. Countries with equivalent per capita incomes sometimes have dramatically different HDI scores. This can reflect a government's commitment and ability to implement programs for the public good in the area of health care and education, thus improving longevity and literacy even when a lack of economic opportunity keeps income relatively low.

UNDP has developed some additional indices in recent years to further refine interpretation of the data available about human development within and between countries. These include two human poverty indices (HPIs), HPI-1 for developing countries and HPI-2 for developed countries. There are also two gender-related indices, the Gender-related Development Index (GDI), and the Gender Empowerment Measurement (GEM). A summary of the factors that go into the analysis of each of the UNDP indices is presented in Table 5-2. The five highest and lowest ranking countries for each of the UNDP indices are presented in Table 5-3. The Human Development Report including the full tables for all indices discussed here is

available on the internet at http://www.undp.org/hdro/99.htm

Constraints on the Rural Poor

One of the most contemptible and slanderous stereotypes that persist in human society is that the poor are poor because they are lazy. Such a view can only be held by the untraveled. A single trip to a poor rural area of any developing country will immediately dispel the notion that poor people are lazy. On the contrary, the life of the rural poor is more aptly characterized as an exercise of relentless toil. Poor people are not poor because they are unwilling to work. Rather they are poor because the enormous work that they do does not readily translate into a higher standard of living or a better quality of life. This is due to a variety of constraints and circumstances that limit access by the poor to credit, health services, educational opportunities, property, material resources, information, markets, and employment alternatives in rural areas. Some of the main factors that constrain the rural poor and how they do so are presented in this section. These factors include population growth, lack of access to goods and services, issues of land tenure, gender inequities, economic and political constraints, violent conflicts, and environmental degradation.

Population Growth

Human population growth and the consequences of overpopulation are serious public policy concerns in the world today. These concerns are certainly justified, as the rate of human population growth in just the last 50 years has been phenomenal, reaching the landmark number of 6 billion people in 1999. It is thought that more people, 3.5 billion, have been added to the planet since 1950 than were added during the total sum of all human history up to that date. The rate at which each new billion people is added has been accelerating, and it now requires just over a decade. Currently, the population of the world is estimated to reach almost 8 billion by the year 2025. This means that about 76 million additional people are being added to the world annually. These projected numbers raise important questions about the negative impact that such population growth will have on the environment, the preservation of biodiversity, and the overall quality of life that will be possible for so many people on a planet with fixed space and finite resources. Perhaps the most fundamental question is, how will all these people obtain food?

The rate of population growth has decreased in recent years from a global high of about 2% in the early 1960s to a current average rate of less than 1.4%. While this lower average rate appears to be good news, it does not tell the whole story. The average rate of population growth in developed or industrialized countries is currently only 0.3%, and some of these countries, such as Italy, Spain, and Portugal, may actually experience population loss by the year 2025. In contrast, the annual average rate of population growth in developing countries is 1.6%, with higher-than-average rates in west and central Africa (2.5 to 2.7%), western Asia (2.2%), north Africa (2.0%), central America (1.9%), and south central Asia (1.8%). During the

Table 5-2   Factors That Go into the Analysis of Each of the UNDP Human Development Indices

Index	Longevity	Knowledge	Decent Standard of Living	Participation or Exclusion
HDI Human development index	Life expectancy at birth	Adult literacy rate Combined enrollment ratio	Adjusted per capita income in PPP$	
GDI Gender-related development index	Female and male life expectancy at birth	Female and male adult literacy rate Female and male combined enrollment ratio	Adjusted per capita income in PPP$, based on female and male earned income s hares	
HPI-1 Human poverty index for developing countries	Percentage of people not expected to survive to age 40	Adult literacy rate	Percentage of people without access to safe water Percentage of people without access to health services Percentage of under-weight children under 5 years of age	
HPI-2 Human poverty index for industrialized countries	Percentage of people not expected to survive to age 60	Adult functional illiteracy rate	Percentage of people living below the in-come poverty line (50% of median personal disposable income)	Long-term unemployment rate (12 months or more)

PPP$, purchasing power parity in US$.

Reproduced with permission from the United Nations Development Programme. Human Development Report 1999. New York: Oxford University Press, 1999.

next 30 years, the overwhelming majority of the world's population growth will occur in developing countries. This is, in large part, a function of the current age distribution within regional populations and the greater potential for child bearing among the young. Over 1 billion of the world's people are currently between the ages of 15 and 24, and one third of all people living in developing countries are under 15 years of age. As a result, expansion of global populations will remain strong in coming decades, particularly in developing countries where the potential for a decent quality of life, as measured by the HDI, is low.

In light of these statistics and trends, it is not surprising that there is a strong sense of linkage between hunger, poverty, and overpopulation in the public mind. Certainly, it is not unreasonable to perceive a connection between poverty and large family size or high population density. Nor is it unreasonable to note that regions with the worst poverty, chronic hunger, and periodic famine, also have high rates of population growth. However, the cause-and-effect relationship between poverty and hunger on the one hand and high population on the other is not as clearly defined as it might appear on first glance. While the case can be made that high population

growth contributes to poverty, a case can also be made that poverty encourages high population growth.

In economic terms, developing countries are characterized by a lack of infrastructure, investment capital, material inputs, and employment opportunities. In social terms, developing countries are frequently unable to provide adequate educational opportunities, health care delivery, or social safety nets. In rural areas, these constraints result in a number of hard realities. Survival rates of children under 5 years of age are lower than average, opportunities for income generation beyond subsistence agriculture are limited, labor remains the major input in agricultural activity, and elderly people must depend on their own children to care for them. With no clear prospects for a better economic future, having large families represents a rational coping strategy for the rural poor. High fertility rates increase the probability that at least some children will survive to adulthood. Growing children provide an added source of labor for tending animals; gathering fuel wood, manure, and fodder; caring for younger siblings; and assisting with a variety of other agricultural and household activities to sustain the family. Children who reach adulthood can provide care and support for aging and infirm parents. Clearly,

Table 5-3	Five Top- and Bottom-Ranking Countries for Each of the UNDP Indices in 1999	
Index	**Top Five**	**Bottom Five**
HDI Human development index	Canada Norway United States Japan Belgium	Burundi Burkina Faso Ethiopia Niger Sierra Leone
GDI Gender-related development index	Canada Norway United States Australia Sweden	Guinea Bissau Burundi Burkina Faso Ethiopia Niger
GEM Gender empowerment measure	Norway Sweden Denmark Canada Germany	Jordan Mauritania Togo Pakistan Niger
HPI-1 Human poverty index for developing countries	Barbados Trinidad and Tobago Uruguay Costa Rica Cuba	Central African Republic Ethiopia Sierra Leone Burkina Faso Niger
HPI-2 Human poverty index for industrialized countries	Sweden Netherlands Germany Norway Italy	New Zealand Spain United Kingdom Ireland United States

Reproduced with permission from the United Nations Development Programme, Human Development Report 1999, New York: Oxford University Press, 1999.

there are short-term advantages for the rural poor in having large families.

Nevertheless, the continued production of large families in the face of stagnant social and economic development ultimately contributes to a further destabilization of rural life and diminished prospects for a brighter future. This is particularly true in the area of food production, where fixed quantities of grazing land and arable land and limited water supplies are increasingly called upon to meet the needs of an expanding population and external inputs such as fertilizer or improved seed necessary to boost production are unobtainable. In these cases, expanding populations have some predictable, detrimental effects. Among these are the elimination of fallow periods on existing farmlands to grow additional crops, which leads to decreased soil fertility; the incursion of agricultural activity onto land not well suited for agriculture, such as steep hillsides or rainforests with poor topsoil; overgrazing and subsequent degradation of grasslands by excessive animal stocking; and in

semiarid regions, depletion of underground water supplies through drilling of deep wells for watering livestock or irrigating fields. The net result of these activities, in the face of expanding population, can be a per capita reduction in food availability. This has already been occurring in portions of sub-Saharan Africa in recent decades, and it is estimated that between 1990 and 2020, the gap between production of, and demand for, cereals in sub-Saharan Africa is likely to widen from 1 million tons to 27 million tons.

Under these conditions, a vicious cycle is established. Decreased per capita food production can lead to greater hunger, which can lead to higher rates of infant mortality. Couples may then strive to have large families to offset likely losses of children, which in turn further burdens poor families and the limited resources they depend on. On balance then, it can be said that rapid population growth and high fertility hold back development and help to perpetuate poverty.

Family-planning efforts are one important approach to slowing the rate of population growth in developing countries. Broadly speaking, these efforts include not only access to a range of contraceptive methods and improved knowledge about their use, but also improved prenatal care, child health care, and greater prevention of sexually transmitted diseases. International efforts in family planning have produced significant results. Contraceptive use has increased from less than 10% of couples in the 1960s to about 60% today. During the same period, average family size has fallen from six children to less than three.

A strong argument for promotion of family planning has been that reducing family size will increase economic opportunity and help families climb out of poverty. Increasingly, however, policy analysts have proposed that the opposite is also true, namely, that increasing economic opportunity will lead to voluntary reductions in family size. There is certainly a good deal of circumstantial evidence at regional and national levels to support this notion, since the population growth rates in highly developed countries and rapidly developing countries are much lower than those of the slowly developing and least-developed countries. Development agencies and government policymakers have begun to apply this principle at the grass-roots level within developing countries through policies and activities that facilitate new income opportunities and encourage entrepreneurship among the poor. Microcredit schemes, discussed later in this chapter, are an important tool in fostering this approach.

Lack of Access to Goods and Services

Many rural people in developing countries live in comparative isolation. They may lack access to electricity, telephone service, newspapers, or even regular mail service. Main roads with regular public bus service may be several hours' walk from farmsteads or villages. The nearest trading settlement may have a limited supply of only the most essential products. The nearest schools, hospitals, or veterinary clinics may be in the district's administrative town center, perhaps dozens of miles away. Such limited access to information, education, health care, or commercial activity, can promote social stagnation and a progressive decline in the situation of the rural poor.

Such lack of services reflects the general shortage of financial resources within the governments of developing countries. Weak overall economies, an inadequate tax base, and inefficient tax collections limit the revenues that governments have available for infrastructure development and provision of public services. In some countries, the constraints of limited revenues are further compounded by corrupt practices and mismanagement that divert significant portions of already limited funds from their intended use. Yet, even when funds are available and properly handled, rural areas may be short-changed in preference to urban areas, as legislators, generally located in capital cities, tend to be more responsive to the needs of the urban populace. This trend is likely to increase as populations continue to migrate from the countryside to the cities in developing countries. Already 75% of the population of Latin America and the Caribbean are in urban areas. In Asia and Africa, about one third of all people currently live in urban areas, but on both continents the proportion of urban dwellers is expected to exceed 50% of the total population by 2030. This means that fewer people in the rural areas, with potentially less influence on government, will be responsible for producing greater amounts of food for increasingly urban populations.

However, the lack of goods and services in rural areas places serious constraints on the potential for improved agricultural productivity by the rural poor. Perhaps most critical is a lack of available relevant information to help subsistence farmers improve farming practices and outputs. There are three interconnected reasons for this dearth of information. First, there is a lack of appropriate research on subsistence-farming systems. When developing country governments do have money to spend on agricultural research, either through national agricultural research organizations or through their university systems, the research most often focuses on improving commercial agricultural production and is frequently carried out in experimental stations rather than on privately owned farms. Similarly, research trials conducted by private agricultural corporations marketing improved seeds, fertilizers, or other external inputs, also focus on commercial farmers because that is the segment of the agricultural community with the resources to purchase their products. There is certainly nothing wrong with supporting commercial agricultural production through research, but it must be remembered that in many developing countries most food production may be derived from the activities of subsistence farmers and herders who lack the resources, tools, and information to make the transition from subsistence to commercial farming. Paradoxically, research specifically aimed at improving the productivity and income of subsistence farmers and herders is often lacking in those countries where it could yield the most benefit.

Secondly, the capacity to disseminate research information through agricultural extension efforts in developing countries is often limited. Agricultural extension has traditionally been a public function, and the burden of maintaining an adequate network of well-trained extension workers frequently is beyond the financial capacity of developing-country governments. Extension workers often are poorly paid, lack access to transportation to visit farmers, and have limited opportunities for continuing education. They are often required to serve as generalists, expected to be equally conversant in issues related to cash crop, food crop, and livestock agriculture. Contrast this to the United States, for example, where a whole cadre of livestock and crop extension specialists may exist at the state or county level, each serving a specific species or commodity in the agricultural sector.

Thirdly, even when information is available, the rural poor may be unable to use it because of illiteracy. According to the HDI in 1999, almost half (49.3%) of adults in the least-developed countries are unable to read and write. Some extension efforts attempt to overcome this by producing extension materials for radio and television, but again, the poorest of the poor often lack access to electronic media. Not only do the rural poor fail to gain information about new technologies, they also risk, through illiteracy, the improper use of existing technologies. Failure to be able to read label instructions can, in the case of fertilizers, result in wasteful overuse or insufficient application of costly inputs. At worst, as in the case of herbicides, insecticides, feed supplements, and some veterinary pharmaceuticals, it can lead to toxic overdoses with serious consequences to people, animals, and the environment.

In the context of animal agriculture, one of the most significant deficiencies of service to the rural poor is reliable access to veterinary care. People who depend directly on animals for agricultural field work, fuel, food, income, and even clothing and shelter in the form of fiber, felt, and skins often have no access at all to modern veterinary medicine and must rely solely on traditional healing practices to keep their animals healthy and productive. The constraints on veterinary service delivery to the rural poor in developing countries are discussed in more detail in Chapter 8. Opportunities to improve veterinary service delivery are also discussed in Chapter 8 and later in this chapter.

Lack of access to human health care has always been a major constraint on the rural poor, but the issue of health care service delivery has taken on a great urgency in the last decade as a result of the virtual explosion of acquired immunodeficiency syndrome, or AIDS. Progress in the control of this important human disease serves well to illustrate the contrasts in the resources and services available to people in developed and developing nations. Whereas the disease was initially considered untreatable and ultimately fatal, within a decade new drugs, drug regimens, and patient management methods had been discovered and implemented that enabled infected and clinically ill people not only to survive, but to maintain a high quality of life. However, the current availability of such treatments, which are costly and require a fair amount of patient management, is essentially limited to AIDS patients in the developed countries. In contrast, many developing countries lack the financial resources and medical infrastructure to purchase the drugs and manage the patients. Yet it is in the developing countries, mainly in Africa, and increasingly in Asia, where the vast majority of the world's AIDS cases exist (Table 5-4) and where the rate of spread of infection remains the highest. The situation has become so dire that some governments (e.g., Brazil) have declared that they feel compelled to ignore the patent restrictions on AIDS drugs and will begin to produce generic equivalents at affordable prices in their own countries.

AIDS is having a devastating impact on the quality of life in countries where it is widespread. Policymakers are now recognizing AIDS not only as a health issue, but as a crosscutting development issue affecting all aspects of social and economic life in affected countries. The disease has become a major constraint on rural development and contributes directly to poverty and food insecurity, particularly in sub-Saharan Africa. This region accounts for more than twice as many HIV-infected people and five times as many AIDS-related deaths than the rest of the world combined. By the end of 1998, 11.5 million Africans had died of AIDS, compared with 2.4 million in the rest of the world. Most of these deaths occurred in persons between the ages of 15 and 49 years, the period of maximum productivity in a typical human life. The AIDS epidemic is having a dramatic effect on life expectancy. If the epidemic is not brought under control, the life expectancy for children born between 2000 and 2015 will be reduced by decades. For example, estimates for life expectancy in Botswana are 73 years with AIDS under control and only 48.9 years without control. In Namibia, the numbers are 67.7 years with control and 41.5 without.

AIDS has direct detrimental effects on agricultural productivity and food security in sub-Saharan Africa. The sickness and death from AIDS places a severe financial burden on poor families, who may quickly exhaust meager savings and be forced to sell valuable livestock or go into debt to cover medical care and funeral expenses. The sickness and death of family members can cause serious labor shortages for the myriad, labor-intensive activities of subsistence farming and herding. Furthermore, surviving family members may not have the skills or the strength necessary to take over the specialized tasks normally carried out by the debilitated or deceased person. For example, in the case of livestock, children may be unable to handle large cattle or recognize early signs of disease leading to increased morbidity and mortality in animals. Veterinary service delivery itself may be compromised by loss of veterinary professionals to AIDS, as has occurred in a number of African countries (Fig. 5-3).

The death of a husband to AIDS can cause added complications for surviving wives and children. First of all, social custom may designate certain chores and responsibilities that belong specifically to either men or women, making it difficult for a woman to assume full responsibility for all agricultural activities even if she has the required skill. Secondly, inheritance rights in some societies may pass ownership of the farm to male relatives of the deceased husband rather than to the surviving wife. In some cases, livestock belonging to the man and his family may be taken from the surviving wife by the husband's relatives, as has been reported from Namibia.[5] The net result of all these complications can be a serious loss of agricultural

Table 5-4	Estimated Numbers of Persons Infected with HIV by World Region in 2000	
World Region	**Total No. of HIV Infections (million)**	**Adult Prevalence Rate (%)**
Sub-Saharan Africa	25.30	8.80
South & Southeast Asia	5.80	0.56
Latin America	1.40	0.50
North America	0.92	0.60
East Asia & the Pacific	0.64	0.07
Western Europe	0.54	0.24
Eastern Europe & Central Asia	0.70	0.35
Caribbean	0.39	2.30
North Africa & Middle East	0.40	0.20
Australia & New Zealand	0.01	0.13
TOTAL	**36.10**	

Data derived from UNAIDS, Epidemic Update: http://www.unaids.org/epidemic_update/index.html)

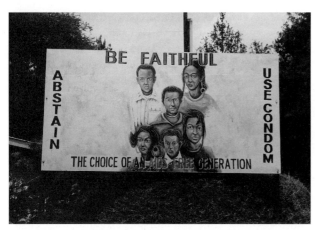

Figure 5-3. An AIDS awareness poster on the campus of the Faculty of Veterinary Medicine of Addis Ababa University, in Debre Zeit, Ethiopia. Developing countries can ill afford to lose educated professionals to the scourge of AIDS. In 1999, UNAIDS recorded that an estimated 10.6% of all adults in Ethiopia were infected with HIV. While clinical AIDS is being successfully managed with therapy in developed countries, HIV infection remains a virtual death sentence in the developing world where the cost of needed drugs makes them essentially unavailable. (Photo by Dr. David M. Sherman)

production and entry into a state of food insecurity. A bibliography of articles dealing with the impact of AIDS on agricultural production and food security, including specific studies relative to the impact on livestock production is available from FAO at http://www.fao.org/sd/wpdirect/wpre0129.htm on the world wide web.

Land Tenure Issues

The desire of peasants in agrarian societies for improved access to land and land rights has been a powerful engine for social upheaval in human history. The 20th century is well marked by such events. The Russian Revolution of 1917 was driven in large part by the objective of achieving land equity in rural areas through state seizure and collectivization of lands belonging to an entrenched landlord class unwilling to participate voluntarily in land tenure reform. Much of the civil unrest in Central America in the 1970s and 1980s was related to land reform efforts and resistance to them by powerful landowners. In the year 2000, a major disruptive battle over land rights emerged in Zimbabwe, with the government supporting efforts to confiscate white-owned farms for redistribution to black Zimbabweans.

Although considerable progress has been made in land reform in different countries in recent decades, many rural poor engaged in agriculture in developing countries still do not have the opportunity to own the land on which they grow crops or graze livestock or even to have secure rights of tenancy to that land. In Honduras, for example, it is estimated that half the nation's rural population are landless agricultural workers. Approximately 90% of the land-owning population holds less than 1 ha of land, and 66% of farmers who are involved in the production of staple food grains have access to only 8% of all cultivable land. Much of the remaining arable land is held by speculative landholders or used for extensive cattle ranching. Lack of access to land results from a variety of causes around the world, including

- The concentration of large tracts of landholdings in the hands of a wealthy minority, as has been common in much of Central and South America

- The collectivization of land, with its use mandated by government, as occurred in many countries under communism and which is now undergoing major transformation

- Laws that essentially prohibit or discourage private ownership

- Community traditions that permit use of agricultural land by families but retain communal ownership rights, as is common in many countries of Africa

- The lack of capital to purchase land, even when it is available

- The consolidation of land holdings by corporations for commercial farming activities, as has happened in recent years in Asia, Africa, and Latin America

As a result, the rural poor engaged in agriculture face limited options. They may

- Work as wage laborers on ranches, commercial farms, or plantations

- Enter into tenancy agreements with land owners, either as share croppers or by paying fixed rent, often with short-term leases

- Use land provided by the community without the right of ownership

- Become squatters and face the uncertainty and danger of occupying land not their own

- Obtain affordable land that is less than ideal for agricultural use (e.g., steep hillsides) or remain landless

Land tenancy, as opposed to land ownership, is not an inherently bad thing. For some rural poor, the opportunity to rent land serves as a stepping stone to generate sufficient income through agricultural activity to ultimately be able to buy land. The problematic aspect of tenancy is the fairness of the tenancy agreement and whether or not the terms of the agreement provide any land security to the tenant over an extended period. Either secure tenancy or outright ownership of land can offer important incentives to poor farmers. Labor productivity is likely to increase when farmers know that the fruits of their effort belong fully to them and not in part to a landlord or the state. Investment of labor or capital in long-term land improvements such as tree planting or terracing or even short-term improvements such as application of manure to soil are also more likely with ownership or secure tenancy, since as an owner or secure tenant, the farmer has a more direct stake in the productivity of the parcel of land over the long term. As a result, stewardship of land may improve with ownership or secure tenancy, as greater attention is paid to overall soil and water conservation efforts.

Also, where access to land is constrained, farmers often have to divide their parcels for adult offspring to farm, according to traditional practices. This can eventually lead to farm plots so small that economies of scale in agricultural production are not possible and overall production declines. The use of animals is affected as well, since a time may come when a family can no longer afford to maintain a draft animal for field work because the size of the farm will not support the maintenance of the animal. In some cases, farmers may seek out additional land through tenancy arrangements to have sufficient cropland for continued use of their animals or rent out their animals to neighbors for field work.

Land access issues are particularly important for societies actively engaged in pastoralism as a principal form of livelihood. Grazing land is the principal resource in pastoral systems, as discussed in Chapter 4. In semiarid areas, where much of the world's pastoralism occurs, water and grass supplies are limited, so vast tracts of land may be required to support the livestock populations required by communities for their livelihood. Under these circumstances, direct private ownership of such large land areas is impractical. Therefore, in most pastoralist societies, grazing lands are held in common, and grazing rights and privileges are worked out by consensus within communities. When left undisturbed by outside influences, this communal system of common resource management has worked reasonably well.

Pastoralists around the world, however, are experiencing increased constraints on the availability and use of common lands. These constraints include expansion of urban areas, conversion of grazing land to cropping land, establishment of ranches, exclusion from wildlife refuges, land speculation, decreasing water supplies, and greater grazing competition. As a result, pastoralists are being squeezed onto marginal lands that then quickly become degraded. This marginalization process, which threatens the pastoralist way of life and undermines the environment on which that livelihood depends, is discussed in more detail in Chapter 6.

Communal grazing also raises a number of issues related to animal health. Control of internal and external parasites, for example, becomes problematic when some herders are willing to invest in parasite control and others are not. There is little incentive to pay for anthelmintics when animals are immediately reinfected on pastures contaminated by untreated animals belonging to other herders. Infectious disease control is also a potential problem when separate herds converge at common wells or water sources, which increases the risk of direct disease transmission.

Improving access of the rural poor to land remains an important and valuable imperative for social and economic development. The explosive economic growth of China in the 1980s and the associated increase in agricultural production was fueled in large part by the policy decision to dismantle rural communes and return land to individual farmers under long-term leases. This also had a tremendous impact on poverty reduction in China, with over 100 million people moving above the poverty line between 1978 and 1998. Ongoing land reform efforts around the world involve redistribution of ownership rights, regulation of tenancy contracts, and the role of land titling. The Land Tenure Center at the University of Wisconsin-Madison is a good source of current information on issues of land tenure and is available on the internet (http://www.wisc.edu/ltc/).

Gender Inequities

Women are overrepresented among the world's poor and frequently suffer greater hardships and obstacles than men. On a worldwide basis, for instance, females have less access to education than males. At the beginning of the 21st century, two thirds of the world's 960 million illiterate adults were women, and of the 130 million children not enrolled in primary school, two thirds were girls. On the basis or either law or custom, women in many countries lack the right to own land or inherit property, obtain access to credit, attend or stay in school, earn income, or even appear in public with their faces exposed, as is currently the case in Afghanistan. Poverty also limits access by women to gender-specific health and reproductive services, placing them at greater risk to life and limb as a result of their role in child-bearing and motherhood. According to UNICEF, approximately 600,000 women worldwide die each year during pregnancy or as a result of childbirth. Great regional disparities exist, and not surprisingly, the poorest regions of the world have the highest mortality rates. A woman's lifetime risk of dying from pregnancy is 1 in 16 in Africa, 1 in 65 in Asia, 1 in 1400 in Europe, and 1 in 3700 in North America. According to the World Bank, complications of pregnancy and childbirth are the leading cause of death and disability for women aged 15 to 49 in developing countries.

It is very important in the context of rural development to recognize the central role of women in agriculture and the constraints under which they work. It is estimated that women, through their labor, are responsible for up to 50% of global food production. In some developing countries, this proportion reaches as high as 60 to 80%. The FAO states that women are the main producers of the world's staple cereal crops—wheat, maize and rice—which provide up to 90% of rural food intake. They are involved in every aspect of production including field preparation, sowing, weeding, fertilizer and pesticide application, harvesting, and threshing. They may play an even greater role in secondary crop production such as legumes and vegetables in home gardens. They are also active in animal husbandry, with responsibilities for both large and small stock. In some countries the role of women in rural agriculture, along with their household responsibilities, is increasing as men leave the rural areas to seek cash employment in urban areas, leaving the women at home to maintain the subsistence-farming operation. Rural women work extremely hard, frequently harder than men. Time studies indicate that the typical workday for women engaged in smallholder agriculture in a developing country ranges from 12 to 16 hours and includes both agricultural and household responsibilities. The workload can be even longer during periods of high production, such as harvest time (Table 5-5 and Fig. 5-4).

Despite the major economic and social contribution that women make in agriculture, they experience important inequalities. According to the FAO, for example, fewer than 10% of women farmers in India, Nepal, and Thailand own land. A study of credit schemes in five African nations found that women received less than 10% of the credit awarded to male smallholders. While women do a great deal of the physical work in agriculture, farming implements and equipment are rarely designed or constructed with women in mind, and only 15% of the world's agricultural extension agents are women. Women's efforts often remain overlooked and undervalued by politicians, planners, and policymakers when they formulate programs for economic growth and social development in the rural sector.

There is however, a growing awareness of the value of gender-based analysis during the planning stages of development programs to ensure that the status, activities, and responsibilities of women are clearly understood, their opinions heard, and their specific development priorities addressed. Furthermore, development specialists are now recognizing the added value that comes from targeting women in rural development programs. The cost-benefit ratios for investing in women's development are highly favorable. For example, it has become increasingly clear that efforts to improve access to education for women not only improve literacy, but also have a significant impact on reducing family size, as educated women are much more likely to seek out and use family planning services. Similarly, credit aimed specifically at women is more likely to improve overall family nutrition and health than credit aimed at men, because women are more likely than men to channel extra earnings from their credit-supported enterprises toward their children's welfare and household improvements.

Excellent opportunities exist to engage women directly in efforts to improve livestock productivity and veterinary service delivery in developing countries. Women, in addition to frequently having specific responsibilities for animal keeping, also frequently have specialized knowledge. For example, when women are responsible for milking ruminant animals, they often have a better understanding of mastitis and can recognize it more quickly than men. Similarly, when women are responsible for dressing out livestock carcasses after men have done the slaughtering, they may have a much greater awareness of disease occurrence as a result of closely handling and observing the animal viscera. They may be able to report with some confidence the prevalence of certain diseases that routinely show gross lesions such as pneumonia, liver flukes, or *Oesophagostamum* infestations. Aid and development agencies are increasingly using microcredit and small-scale livestock production targeted at women's groups as a means of improving income, enhancing the status of women, and empowering them with an economic and political voice. The American aid agency Heifer Project International has created a specific program, Women in Livestock Development (WiLD), to encourage direct involvement of women in rural development schemes involving animal agriculture (see http://www.heifer.org/end_hunger/women.htm).

Economic and Political Constraints

The main economic and political constraints within developing countries that block opportunities for the poor are the absence of policies specifically aimed at the alleviation of poverty; corruption; weak governance; and, inadequate representation of the poor in the political process. At the international level, the major external constraints on poor countries and the poor citizens within them are foreign debt and inequitable trading arrangements. Each of these factors is briefly addressed below.

Lack of Pro-poor Policies Surprisingly, many developing nations, even those with a high proportion of their population below the poverty line, do not have specific policies directed toward alleviation of poverty. In many cases, development policies are directed in a general way toward economic growth and expansion, based on the notion that a rising tide will lift all boats. However, lack of success in poverty alleviation suggests that this broad-based approach does not always work. Increasingly, policy analysts suggest that governments must develop and implement pro-poor policies that identify and address deficiencies and inequities within the nation's political, economic, and social structure that specifically work against the poor. The UNDP Poverty Report calculates that 77% of the world's nations have reasonable estimates of the extent of poverty within their borders, and 69% of these countries have poverty alleviation plans or specifically identify poverty in national planning efforts.[17] However, only 31% of the world's nations have concrete targets and specific timetables for poverty reduction.

Weak Governance Even when countries have poverty alleviation programs on paper, implementation may be ineffective. The UNDP identifies several problems with governance that hamper the delivery of resources and services to the poor, particularly in developing countries. These include inadequate tax collection from those who can afford to pay, lack of accountability and transparency in the use of funds earmarked for poverty programs, and lack of sufficient management experience and capacity to administrate programs properly. A major part of the crisis in governance in many developing countries is a lack of principled and selfless political leadership. President Museveni of Uganda observed in a public address in 1991 that in too many developing countries like Uganda, "people enter politics not to serve but to be served."

Table 5-5   Typical Day in the Life of Woman and a Man in the Same Family Living in a Hypothetical Place in Africa and Engaged in Producing Their Own Food and Some Cash Crops

Woman's Day	Man's Day
Rises first	Rises when breakfast is ready
Kindles the fire	Eats
Breast-feeds baby	Walks 1 km to cotton field
Fixes breakfast/eats	Works in the field
Washes and dresses the children	Eats when wife arrives with food
Walks 1 km to fetch water	Works in the field
Walks 1 km home	Walks 1 km home
Gives the livestock feed and water	Eats
Washes cooking utensils, etc.	Rests
Walks 1 km to fetch water	Walks to village to visit other men
Walks 1 km home	Walks home
Washes clothing	Goes to bed
Breast-feeds baby	
Pounds rice/cassava/maize	
Sweeps the house and compound	
Kindles the fire	
Prepares meal/eats	
Breast-feeds baby	
Walks 1 km to cotton field with food for husband	
Walks 1 km back home	
Walks 1 km to her field	
Weeds field	
Breast-feeds baby	
Gathers firewood on the way home	
Walks 1 km to fetch water	
Walks 1 km home	
Kindles the fire	
Prepares meat/eats	
Breast-feeds baby	
Puts house in order	
Goes to bed last	

Reproduced with permission from Striking a Balance, a booklet published in 1990 by the Swedish International Development Cooperation Agency (SIDA).

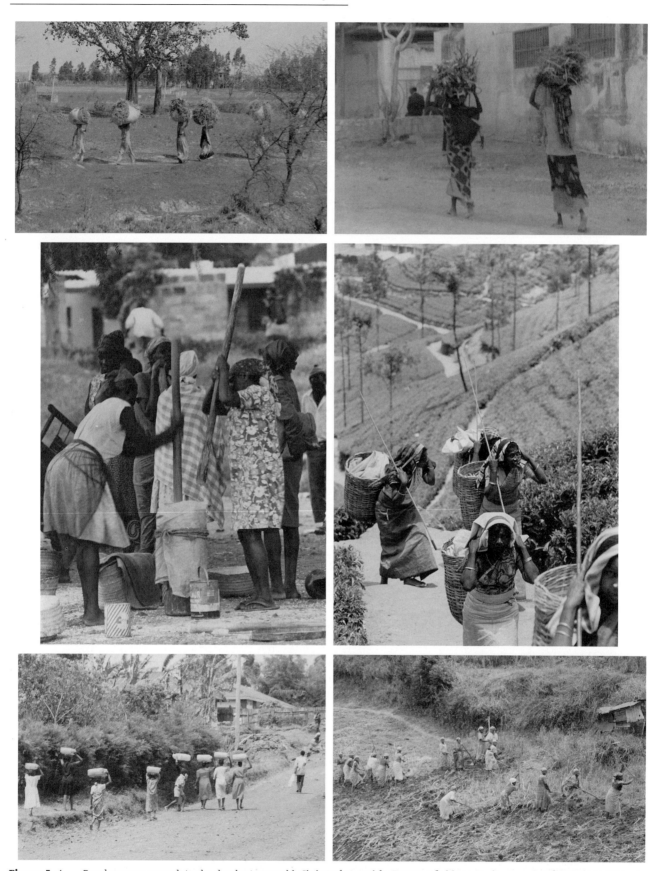

Figure 5-4. Rural women at work in the developing world. *Clockwise from top left:* Carrying fodder in India; carrying firewood in Ethiopia; picking tea in Sri Lanka; preparing a field in Uganda; carrying water in Uganda; pounding meal in Kenya. On average, 42% of rural women in developing countries, most of whom engage regularly in strenuous physical labor such as this, suffer from energy-draining iron-deficiency anemia. Iron deficiency is one of the most common forms of micronutrient malnutrition in the world and is largely correctable by inclusion of red meat in the diet. (All photos by Dr. David M. Sherman)

Official Corruption Official corruption is the misuse of pubic power for private profit or political gain. Unfortunately, corrupt practices remain widespread, especially in poorer countries in which a lack of resources, limited economic opportunities, and exceedingly low salaries and benefits for government workers all conspire to promote a culture of corruption. Government workers from trolley car conductors to policemen to postal clerks to cabinet ministers (i.e., anyone with even a scrap of authority or control) may come to consider the bribe an acceptable method of income enhancement and a justifiable surcharge for services rendered. Eventually, the population at large comes wearily to accept the bribe as a natural, everyday cost of doing business, and the culture of corruption flourishes.

However, there is an enormous social cost, as corruption severely undermines the development of a vibrant, democratic society. Corruption has a particularly severe impact on the poor, who often have inadequate access to resources even when those resources are not being shamelessly expropriated. Mobutu Sese Seko, who ruled the African country of Zaire with an iron fist for more than 30 years, is estimated to have stolen as much as 9 billion dollars in public monies during his reign, which ended in 1997 through armed revolt. Zaire, now the Democratic Republic of the Congo, remains tragically underdeveloped, despite an abundance of natural resources. In 1999, people in the Democratic Republic of the Congo had an average annual income of US$880 and a life expectancy at birth of 50.8 years. The HDI for the country was 0.479, which ranked it 141 of 174 countries assessed by the UNDP. This sorry state of affairs can be attributed in large part to corruption and a political leadership more interested in self-aggrandizement than in nation building. For three decades, corrupt government was, as one frustrated international aid worker aptly put it, "a conspiracy against the people."

One dire consequence of corruption in relation to poverty alleviation is the effect it has on the humanitarian impulse among potential donors and benefactors. Widespread corruption breeds cynicism among the citizens and governments of wealthy nations, from which much of the funding for poverty alleviation has come, in the form of foreign aid. The decrease in foreign aid in recent years is due in part to the perception that money for poverty alleviation is wasted when sent to corrupt governments. This perception has also helped to foster the emergence of numerous nongovernmental organizations (NGOs) and to expand their role in humanitarian assistance. Foreign donors are increasingly using NGOs as conduits for foreign aid funds so that the funds are more-specifically directed to targeted projects at the grassroots level rather than through government channels.

Growing disgust with corruption is also partly responsible for recent efforts to put this ugly problem under closer scrutiny. For example, there was a great deal of media attention in 1997 when the International Monetary Fund decided not to release aid funds to Kenya because of concerns about widespread corruption and mismanagement The organization Transparency International (TI) is an independent watchdog group that carries out research, tracks trends, and reports progress and abuses on matters of global corruption. This organization offers a balanced view of the corruption issue, pointing out that the willingness of corporate representatives from developed nations to pay bribes and the willingness of foreign banks to accept the ill-gotten gains of corrupt officials also contribute to the culture of corruption. The TI corruption index and other reports can be found on the internet at www.transparency.org.

Lack of Citizen Empowerment In 1986, a peaceful revolution occurred in the Philippines. The corrupt dictator, Ferdinand Marcos, fled the country following massive national demonstrations protesting his victorious outcome in what was perceived as a fraudulent election. In his place, Corazon Aquino was elected president and pledged a program of land reform, a new constitution, and establishment of a commission to regain the public wealth that had been plundered by Marcos and his family. This massive mobilization and peaceful but forceful expression of collective dissatisfaction by Filipinos was commonly referred to in the world media as "People Power." What People Power represented was the process of the nation's poor and disenfranchised people discovering the strength of their political voice and exercising it to promote positive change through the political process. The world paid attention precisely because it was so unusual for the world's poor to find their political voice and become politically empowered. In the Philippines, political mobilization by the poor has begun to pay off. In 1987, the Comprehensive Agrarian Reform Programme was established to further the goal of land reform. By 1999, more than 5 million ha of land had been distributed to almost 3 million beneficiaries under the program.

The lack of participation in political decision making among the world's poor is a major factor contributing to their plight. Without effective political organization, the poor can not gain a hearing on their needs or compete effectively for the limited resources that poor nations may have available for social and economic development. In many developing countries, priorities for governmental programs and decisions about allocation of funds at the national level may be influenced primarily by power brokers, urban constituencies, and the educated elite and often do not include considerations for the rural poor. At the local level, in rural districts, the situation may not be much better, as local government may be managed by politician appointees or civil servants drawn not from the local community, but from a distant party or group in power. The constituency of such local officials is not the people of the district, but rather the group that appointed them to positions of authority.

Many additional factors contribute to the lack of political empowerment among the poor. In rural areas, remoteness, lack of communication and transportation infrastructure, and a high level of illiteracy deprive people of information and isolate them from the political process. In some cases, a high degree of prejudice exists against some specific tribal, religious, regional, or caste group, and that community is purposely excluded from the political process. In other countries, democratic principles and institutions do not exist to provide a forum for citizen participation. In the worst cases, government is so authoritative or repressive that any form of citizen organization or collective expression of political opinion is swiftly and violently suppressed. As a result, many poor rural communities have little experience with community organization, the exercise of democratic discourse, or participation in the political process. Development projects that involve the introduction of improved livestock to poor rural communities or improved access to veterinary service delivery can serve as effective catalysts for promoting community organization, democratic institutions, and participatory processes, as discussed later in this chapter.

Foreign Debt Debt servicing by developing country governments for debts owed to foreign creditors has become a major factor in constraining the ability of these governments to address issues of poverty alleviation within their own countries. Poor, heavily indebted countries have to "rob Peter to pay Paul," drawing on limited national revenues to repay debts, thus reducing the funds available for domestic programs such as health and education. For example, in Tanzania, a whopping 46% of budget allocation goes toward debt servicing, while only 15% goes toward basic social services. The World Bank has identified 41 heavily indebted poor countries (HIPCs) in the world community. In 9 of these countries the funds allocated for debt repayment exceeds the combined expenditure on health and education annually. In 29 countries, debt-service payments exceed the amount allocated for health in national budgets. The combined debt of the 41 HIPCs amounts to approximately US$127 billion. Ninety percent of this combined debt is owed to individual governments, the World Bank, and the International Monetary Fund. Of the 41 HIPCs, 33 are in Africa, 4 in Latin America, 3 in Asia, and 1 in the Middle East.

The origins and development of the debt crisis are complex. In general terms, the situation became problematic in the 1980s when world market prices dropped sharply for basic raw materials and commodities such as copper, iron ore, timber, sugar, cotton, and coffee. Most poor nations are nonindustrialized and depend mainly on raw material and commodity exports as their primary sources of foreign currency to purchase needed imports. Many of these nations also depended on foreign hard currency loans to meet national needs. Suddenly they found themselves with greatly diminished export revenues available for paying off loans. Though debts were sometimes refinanced or rescheduled by lender nations and institutions, many poor countries fell seriously behind in payments and have been unable to catch up to this day. This has resulted in a vicious cycle of indebtedness. Without sufficient funds for nation building, productivity remains static or declines, and the ability to pay off mounting debts becomes even more improbable.

High foreign debt load can have a direct adverse impact on agriculture and food security and can add to the plight of the rural poor engaged in subsistence farming. In their efforts to pay off foreign debt, governments may set policies to encourage the use of agricultural land for cultivation of cash crops for export to increase foreign exchange earnings. Land most suit-

able for growing food for domestic consumption may be lost to commercial cash crop enterprises, and subsistence farmers may be marginalized to less suitable lands on which farming leads to environmental degradation and reduced yields.

There has been a growing movement, fueled largely by church groups, NGOs, and some policymakers in industrialized nations to forgive debt for the poorest, most heavily indebted nations. This is, of course, a controversial subject, but it is seen by some as both a moral imperative and an economic necessity if the poorest countries are to break out of the downward spiral of indebtedness and decline. Some critics have been reassured by efforts to link debt relief with commitments by governments to use the freed-up funds for health, education, and other programs specifically aimed at poverty reduction. The World Bank initiated a debt-reduction program for HIPC nations in 1996. By the end of 1999, the World Bank had reached agreements with 14 HIPC nations to reduce debt by a total of US$23 billion.

Trade Imbalances Proponents of global free trade insist that the liberalization of trade directly benefits poor countries through increased productivity and prosperity. However, many critics contend that agreements negotiated by the World Trade Organization (WTO) are unfavorable to developing countries and may have unintended deleterious effects in poorer nations. Writing in the *Financial Times* on June 19, 2000, even the director general of the WTO, Mr. Mike Moore, was obliged to acknowledge that free trade carries special risks for poor farmers, although he vigorously defended free trade overall as a powerful tool for poverty alleviation.

There is particular concern about the WTO Agreement on Agriculture (AOA), which became operative in 1995. Critics contend that it contains provisions that favor the developed nations over the developing ones in agricultural trade and may even produce risks for maintaining food security in developing nations.

The greatest concern voiced by critics is that if developing countries abide by the open-market trade policies embodied in the AOA, then industrialized nations with highly developed commercial agricultural production could flood the developing country markets with low-priced food. This could have several damaging effects. First, it could have a dampening effect on domestic agriculture. Farmers will not grow food for domestic markets if they are consistently undersold by imports. This could increase rural poverty through the loss of livelihood by marginal farmers. Secondly, increased importation of food from abroad means greater expenditure of foreign currency reserves, potentially aggravating the debt situation and channeling further scant government resources away from social programs. Finally, food security could be threatened if domestic food production falls and poor nations become dependent on food imports. Under such circumstances, any unexpected rise in food prices in global markets could make imported food suddenly inaccessible to poorer segments of the population, with dire consequences for those affected.

Many observers also feel that the developing nations are disadvantaged in their bargaining with developed nations in the WTO because they lack the resources to research, prepare, and present their positions thoroughly during negotiation sessions. UNDP and other international agencies have implemented technical training and support programs to assist developing nations in preparing for meetings on trade policy issues and are also encouraging regionalization efforts so that neighboring countries with similar economic conditions and concerns can have a more effective voice in negotiation. Much of the ongoing protest and demonstration at WTO meetings, which began in Seattle in 1999, is aimed at calling attention to the need for fairer representation of developing countries in WTO negotiating processes and greater sensitivity to their needs.

Violent Conflicts

Major transitions in the pattern of human conflict occurred during the 20th century. The first half of the century was characterized by global wars of high intensity in which groups of nations formed alliances to fight each other on multiple fronts. In the second half of the 20th century, no such world wars occurred, probably, in large part, because of the threat of global destruction associated with nuclear weapons. However, conflict still existed between the two major power blocs of the communist world and the free world. These conflicts assumed the form of proxy wars, in which the major Cold War adversaries, the United States, the USSR, and China, supported one side or the other in what otherwise would have been considered internal conflicts within a single country, such as in Vietnam, Nicaragua, Angola, and Afghanistan.

Following, the collapse of the Soviet Union and the end of the Cold War at the close of the 20th century, human conflict assumed yet another form, the genuinely localized conflict. This latest manifestation of hostility includes insurgencies, civil wars, and conflicts between neighboring countries. From a political point of view, many of the conflicts that persist today, have their roots in either colonial history or the breakup of the Soviet bloc. Many African and some Asian nations, for example, have boundaries that were created by occupying colonial administrations in the late 19th and early 20th centuries. These boundaries often did not reflect the distribution of distinct indigenous groups of peoples, often dividing some groups while joining others together under a single administrative authority when it served the political and economic goals of a foreign power to create imbalance among these indigenous groups. These colonial boundaries were, by and large, retained upon independence and have emerged as a source of conflict as different indigenous groups seek autonomy, as in Eritrea, or claim rights of ownership or management to local resources, as in Nigeria. In the Soviet bloc countries, different ethnic and religious groups were brought together under state control, and traditional tensions between those groups were suppressed by authoritarian rule. Now, as in the former Yugoslavia and Russia, these ethnic and religious tensions have once again boiled over into violent conflict.

While political history can explain a good deal of current conflict, there are two new theories on war that help to explain why today's conflicts are found in primarily poorer nations. The first theory is framed in the context of behavioral ecology and sociobiology. It suggests a strong correlation between the outbreak of collective aggression and a rapid population growth that results in a high proportion of young males between the ages of 15 and 29 relative to older males.[12] The second theory links poor agricultural production to the emergence of conflicts, proposing that when people are unable to meet their food requirements, survival strategies often lead them to join rebellions or engage in criminal activity.[4] In the period between 1989 and 1997 there were 40 wars recorded, war being defined as conflicts with more than 1000 battlefield deaths. Over half of these wars, 22 in all, occurred just in sub-Saharan Africa and southeast Asia, two of the poorest regions of the world. It is not surprising then, that theories are emerging that link poverty, population growth, low agricultural production, and competition for natural resources as interrelated causes of war.

Wars, in turn, contribute further to the loss of agricultural production, disrupt lives, destroy infrastructure, and widen the circle of poverty and food insecurity. While drought remains an important underlying cause of famine in the Sahel region of Africa, armed conflicts have been directly identified as exacerbating causes of famine in Ethiopia and Sudan in past years. In Afghanistan, it is estimated that there are over 10 million land mines and other pieces of unexploded ordinance. Many land mines were purposely placed in inhabited and agricultural areas to terrorize the population. Land mines not only prevent access to land, thus reducing food production and contributing to malnutrition, they also maim and cripple both humans and the livestock they depend on (Fig. 5-5). Drought coupled with war is doubly disastrous. Afghanistan was affected by the severe drought that hit south Asia in 1999. The FAO reported that in the Afghan cities of Kandahar and Herat, livestock were being sold for only 10% of what they had brought the previous year, as countless desperate rural livestock herders, unable to find sufficient feed for their flocks, depressed prices by flooding the market with animals in the hope of obtaining cash to purchase food for themselves.

War also greatly increases the risk that people will lose the livestock on which they depend. Livestock are frequently commandeered without compensation to feed armies or rebels on the move. Seizing or killing of livestock may also be used as a political weapon to undermine the security of opposing groups who depend on animals for their livelihood.

Large refugee populations are another consequence of war. When poor rural people are forced to move by fear of violent conflict or have the opportunity to return home when conflict ends, their livestock often move with them. This can create various problems, including the spread of contagious diseases and environmental degradation. For example, a large number of Rwandan Tutsi exiles who had fled their own country for neighboring Uganda and Tanzania in the 1960s chose to return to Rwanda after the bloody civil war of 1994, which led to the restoration of a Tutsi-dominated government. By the beginning of 1995, these exiles had brought several hundred

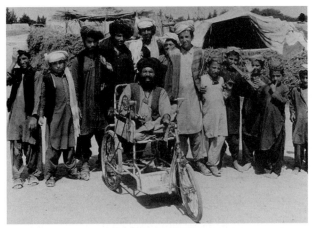

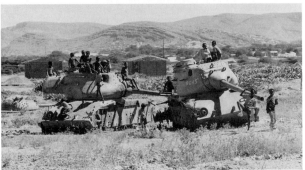

Figure 5–5.   Faces of war: Ethiopia and Afghanistan. Top: A paraplegic Afghan landmine victim with Afghan youths in a refugee camp in Pakistan. Afghanistan closed out the 20th century with 20 years of continuous warfare that is still ongoing. Bottom: Young Ethiopian boys play on damaged tanks left over from the war of Eritrean independence. Five years after this picture was taken in 1995, Eritrea and Ethiopia were again at war. Some theorists suggest that conditions of low-yield, low-input agriculture coupled with high population growth rates and a disproportionately high percentage of young men in the general population predispose to civil unrest and open warfare. These conditions describe both Ethiopia and Afghanistan. (Photos by Dr. David M. Sherman)

thousand head of cattle back to Rwanda with them and concentrated them primarily in northeastern Rwanda, which was the only part of the country with expanses of open grassland suitable for cattle grazing. This region also happened to be the home of Akagera National Park, an important wildlife refuge and historic source of tourist revenue for the country. Within a year, severe overcrowding, overgrazing, degradation of grasslands, and outbreaks of contagious bovine pleuropneumonia (CBPP) and foot and mouth disease (FMD) had resulted in widespread cattle loss due to starvation and disease. At the same time, Akagera National Park suffered extreme degradation, with its grasslands decimated, settlements established within park boundaries, trees cut for buildings and fuel, and much of the wildlife either killed or driven away. The park was home to 50 mammalian species and 180 reptile species, with over 525 bird species recorded. Some conservationists doubt that the park can recover.

Veterinary service delivery can be greatly disrupted by war, resulting in serious declines in livestock health and productivity as well as increased risk to public health. Detailed studies of such effects are not widely reported, but one such study exists for Zimbabwe. Lawrence et al. reported on the effects of the 7-year civil war between 1972 and 1979 that resulted in the creation of Zimbabwe from the former Rhodesia.[9] The disruption of veterinary services during that period resulted in serious disease epidemics. The termination of tick-dipping resulted in the deaths of over 1 million cattle from tick-borne diseases. Over 300,000 head of cattle died from trypanosomiasis after prophylactic therapy of cattle and tsetse fly control efforts were disrupted. Control of FMD outbreaks was hampered by inability to vaccinate at-risk herds in adjacent areas because of hostile actions and risk of death or injury. Anthrax outbreaks, previously limited to specific areas of the country became widespread as the ability to enforce control of cattle movements was lost because of collapse of the rule of law. Rabies, which had been restricted to the border regions with Mozambique and Botswana, became widespread throughout the country, and many human deaths due to rabies and anthrax occurred. The financial losses associated with the deaths of more than 1.3 million cattle from previously controlled diseases is difficult to calculate. Not only were revenues for export beef lost to commercial farmers, but subsistence farmers and their families were harmed as well by the loss of wealth, draft power, and household milk supplies.

Environmental Degradation

Environmental degradation is closely interconnected with many of the contributing causes of poverty already discussed. Lack of access to land coupled with high population growth pushes poor rural people onto lands unsuitable for agriculture, which contributes to deforestation, overgrazing, and other forms of land degradation. Lack of access to goods and services means that farmers may not learn about or implement practices that can prevent soil erosion, soil nutrient depletion, or water wastage. Civil wars result in the creation of refugee camps, which may become semipermanent settlements, for which the carrying capacity of surrounding land and water supplies are inadequate, leading to severe environmental degradation. Eventually, environmental degradation itself becomes a contributing factor to poverty and hunger as the depleted landscape leads to decreased agricultural production and diminished food security. The relationship of agriculture and the environment is discussed further in Chapter 6.

Development and Development Assistance

Development can be defined as the process of improving the living conditions of the whole population of a given culture, region, or nation to a level that allows all individuals to meet their basic needs and to live with dignity through recognition and protection of their basic human rights. Basic needs include the minimum requirement for food, housing, and clothing as well as access to vital public services, including safe drinking water, sanitary facilities, health services, schools, and public transportation.

Poverty and hunger persist in all nations, and from that perspective, all nations are still engaged, to a greater or lesser extent, in a process of development. In the so-called developed countries, with high average per capita incomes, poverty does not persist because of a deficiency of wealth and resources, but rather from inequities in access to wealth and the opportunities to achieve it. In developing countries, however, where average per capita incomes are low, poverty and hunger persist not only because of inequities in the distribution of wealth, but also because of inadequate production of wealth. In developed countries, poverty alleviation depends primarily on the implementation of social policies that directly overcome the barriers that prevent the poor from entering the economic mainstream. In developing countries, poverty alleviation first requires the creation of the economic mainstream itself and the political will to develop policies and practices that ensure that all citizens participate in, and can benefit from, the fruits of economic expansion.

Development assistance, or foreign assistance, has become a major enterprise in the last 60 years. A great body of theory and research has evolved on the subject, and development has become a legitimate focus for academic study at a number of universities around the world. A very large and multifaceted network of organizations, agencies, and institutions exist worldwide that are engaged in the business of development assistance, representing a variety of roles and approaches to its implementation. In the following discussion, a brief overview of development assistance is presented, leading ultimately to the subjects of rural development, the role of livestock in socioeconomic development, and the participation of veterinarians in livestock-based development projects aimed at reduction of poverty and hunger.

Brief History of Development Assistance

Most of human political history has been characterized by rich and powerful nation-states invading, plundering, and exploiting poorer and weaker nation-states. The relatively modern concept of foreign assistance, whereby rich and powerful nations actually help poorer and weaker nations to develop and prosper, was catalyzed, in large part, by the widespread devastation and human suffering of World War II. This new concept of cooperation was embodied in the United Nations Charter in 1945, which committed the world community to "employ international machinery for the promotion of the economic and social advancement of all peoples." The United States was the first to act on this principle in any major way, primarily through implementation of the Marshall Plan, an aid program aimed at rebuilding western European nations whose economies and infrastructures were destroyed during the war. Between 1947 and 1952, the United States allocated $13 billion to this European Recovery Program. This successful program, as magnanimous as it seems, was not entirely altruistic.

The very real political goal of the United States, through the Marshall Plan, was to stabilize Europe quickly to limit the spread of Communism in this strategically important region.

The Cold War rivalry between the West and the Soviet bloc continued to drive much of the world's foreign assistance activity until the Soviet Union ceased to exist on January 1, 1992. In the United States, President Kennedy had an important influence on foreign assistance, creating the independent United States Agency for International Development in 1961 to replace the earlier foreign assistance apparatus controlled by the State Department. Kennedy also launched the Alliance for Progress, an economic and social development assistance program for Latin American countries. Again, concerns about the spreading influence of communist Cuba provided the political motivation for this program. American foreign aid activities in Asia and Africa were also driven largely by Cold War strategies. This sometimes led to foreign assistance being channeled to inept and dictatorial governments whose practices were abhorrent, but whose purchased allegiance helped to maintaining the balance of power in different regions of the world. Much of the foreign aid provided to these unsavory and frequently corrupt governments resulted in serious misuse or outright theft of aid funds, fueling a negative perception of development assistance among the American public, which to a large extent persists to this day.

Another important stimulus for foreign assistance was the abrupt decline of colonialism and the emergence of a large crop of newly independent nations, mainly in the 1960s. The former colonial powers, particularly England, France, and the Netherlands, committed significant development assistance to their former colonies to help with the process of nation building, partly out of a sense of obligation, but also to maintain and foster cultural, economic, and trade ties in their historical spheres of influence. The emergence of so many new and potentially impressionable nations also stimulated the contribution of considerable foreign aid from both the free world and the Soviet bloc in an effort to attract new allies in the Cold War. Many of these new nations joined the ranks of the so-called nonaligned nations and became rather adroit at extracting foreign assistance from both sides in this power struggle.

Since the collapse of the Soviet Union, foreign assistance in the United States and Western Europe has taken on a new geographical focus, namely Eastern Europe and the newly independent states of the former USSR. There is considerable concern about the potential for economic stagnation, ethnic violence, border conflicts, political instability, and the rise of new forms of authoritarianism in either political or religious guise. Development assistance to these countries focuses not only on the traditional area of supporting economic growth, but increasingly on the building of democratic institutions, adapting to privatization, and creating a civil society as well. The end of the Cold War also created the opportunity for large donors of aid to make more discriminating decisions about who receives foreign assistance and why, since the importance of aid as a tool for promoting strategic alliances had largely been eliminated. This has allowed aid to be more specifically targeted at the poor in developing nations and has allowed donors to place more conditions on the use of donated funds to be sure that they are used as intended.

Now, at the beginning of the 21st century, a large and complex machinery of foreign assistance is in place. Yet, throughout the 1990s, there was a steady decline in *official development assistance* (ODA), defined as aid given to recipient governments by donor governments or government-supported multinational agencies. World Bank figures indicate a decline of over one third in ODA between 1991 and 1997, from approximately $74 billion to $47 billion. There are a number of reasons for this. One is disaffection with the foreign assistance machinery itself. The causes of this disaffection are clearly spelled out in the highly critical book *Lords of Poverty* by journalist Graham Hancock.[7] Hancock charges that much of the money earmarked for development assistance is wasted through bureaucratic inefficiency, wrong-headed policies, outright corruption, and the excessive administrative overheads and salaries of official aid agencies and their employees. The United Nations in particular was taken to task, and Hancock's documentation of errors and excesses at various UN agencies may be partly responsible for some the reform efforts that are currently under way within that institution.

Another reason is that many critical observers believe that aid, even when it does reach intended recipients, does not reliably produce the intended results. As discussed later in this chapter, there certainly have been some highly visible and highly unsuccessful development efforts that support this criticism. However, there have also been some innovations in the field of development assistance that are helping to reduce the occurrence of such failures, notably the greater involvement of NGOs in the implementation of development projects, greater participation of target communities in the design of development projects, and the use of direct, small loans to poor citizens, commonly referred to as microcredit.

A third reason for the decline in foreign assistance is that over the last decade, private investment and expansion of free trade have led many to believe that free markets will accomplish the job of economic growth in developing countries, thus making foreign assistance irrelevant. However, current evidence does not support this position. Expansion of free markets and private investment, while it has been remarkably successful in selected countries as an engine of economic growth, is not a panacea. The main reason is that private investment is unevenly distributed. The greatest cash flow goes to countries showing the greatest economic growth potential and, therefore, the greatest return on investment. In fact, in 1997, well over half of the $400 billion of foreign direct investment went into the 29 highly developed member countries of the OECD, while less than 5% went to countries in the poorer regions of south Asia and sub-Saharan Africa combined. Many of the poorest and neediest nations have been virtually ignored by private investors, and these countries continue to require the commitment of, and effective use of, development assistance.

Institutions Involved in Development

Several different types of organizations are involved in development assistance, serving different primary functions. For the sake of this discussion, three main functional types of organizations are identified. These are donor organizations, which provide the funds for development assistance; implementing organizations, which carry out the development projects or activities that are being funded; and supporting organizations, which are involved in various activities such as research, training, data analysis, and policy advising that inform and strengthen overall development efforts.

Many institutions carry out multiple activities and are discussed here in the context of their primary function. For example, the primary function of the World Bank in the context of development assistance is as a donor agency. However, the World Bank also maintains extensive databases of information relevant to development assistance activities. It also supports a good deal of policy analysis on various issues relating to development and development assistance and makes available a wide range of publications on the these subjects (see the World Bank website at www.worldbank.org). The list of organizations discussed here is by no means exhaustive. One directory of development organizations available on the internet, lists over 18,500 individual organizational contacts worldwide with some relation to the field of development assistance (see http://www.devdir.org/index.html). The organizations selected for this discussion were chosen because they are widely recognized as major development assistance organizations; they are of particular relevance to the issues of rural development, agriculture, livestock production, and animal health; and they may offer opportunities for veterinarians to become involved in various aspects of development assistance. A sampling of these organizations is presented in Table 5-6 along with the mission or goals of each organization as articulated by the organization itself.

Donor Organizations

In the area of official development assistance, funds for development activities are provided to the governments of the countries in which the development activity is going to take place. The agreement can be with a multinational organization or can be a bilateral agreement between a single donor government and the recipient government.

Multinational Donors   Multinational donor organizations are essentially international-membership organizations that are mandated by their member nations to provide loans or grants to individual governments to support development projects. The World Bank, with 181 member nations, is the largest, and probably the best known of the multinational donor institutions. The World Bank is actually a group of 5 institutions, each with a particular mandate. The International Development Association (IDA) of the World Bank provides long-term loans at zero interest to the poorest of the developing countries, those with a per capita income in 1998 of less than $895. The

Table 5-6 Mission and Goals of Various Organizations Involved in Development Assistance[a]

Institution Name and Internet Address	Institution Type	Mission or Goal Statement As Presented on the Institution Website
International Rescue Committee (IRC) www.theirc.org	International relief NGO	The IRC helps people fleeing racial, religious and ethnic persecution, as well as those uprooted by war and violence.
World Bank www.worldbank.org	Multinational funding agency	The Bank uses its financial resources, its highly trained staff, and its extensive knowledge base to individually help each developing country onto a path of stable, sustainable, and equitable growth.
African Development Bank (ADB) www.afdb.org	Multinational funding agency for Africa	To assist Regional Member Countries (RMCs) to break the vicious cycle of poverty in which they are entrapped. Working towards this goal, the Bank would endeavor to facilitate and mobilize the flow of external and domestic resources, public and private, promote investment, and provide technical assistance and policy advice to RMCs.
CARE www.care.org	International relief and development NGO	CARE . . . believe(s) that each family should enjoy a basic level of livelihood security. This means that every family should have: Food; Health care; A place to live; Education; A safe and healthy environment; and, The ability to participate in decisions affecting their family, community and country.
United Nations Development Programme (UNDP) www.undp.org	Multinational development agency of the UN	UNDP's mission is to help countries in their efforts to achieve sustainable human development by assisting them to build their capacity to design and carry out development programs in poverty eradication, employment creation and sustainable livelihoods, the empowerment of women and the protection and regeneration of the environment, giving first priority to poverty eradication.
International Committee of the Red Cross (ICRC) www.icrc.org	International relief NGO	To protect the lives and dignity of victims of war and internal violence and to provide them with assistance.
World Vision www.wvi.org/	International faith-based relief and development NGO	World Vision is an international partnership of Christians whose mission is to follow our Lord and Savior Jesus Christ in working with the poor and oppressed to promote human transformation, seek justice, and bear witness to the good news of the Kingdom of God.
Overseas Development Institute (ODI) www.odi.org.uk	British development policy institute	Our mission is to inspire and inform policy and practice which lead to the reduction of poverty, the alleviation of suffering and the achievement of sustainable livelihoods in developing countries. We do this by locking together high-quality applied research, practical policy advice, and policy-focused dissemination and debate.
Food and Agricultural Organization of the United Nations (FAO) www.fao.org	Multinational technical assistance and agricultural development agency of the UN	The FAO works . . . to alleviate poverty and hunger by promoting agricultural development, improved nutrition and the pursuit of food security—the access of all people at all times to the food they need for an active and healthy life. The Organization offers direct development assistance, collects, analyses and disseminates information, provides policy and planning advice to governments and acts as an international forum for debate on food and agriculture issues. FAO is active in land and water development, plant and animal production, forestry, fisheries, economic and social policy, investment, nutrition, food standards and commodities and trade. It also plays a major role in dealing with food and agricultural emergencies.

(continued)

Table 5-6	Mission and Goals of Various Organizations Involved in Development Assistance[a] *(Continued)*	
Institution Name and Internet Address	**Institution Type**	**Mission or Goal Statement As Presented on the Institution Website**
Swedish International Development Cooperation Agency (SIDA) www.sida.se	Foreign aid funding agency of the Swedish government	A world without poverty and oppression will be better for everybody. In order to solve the major challenges of our era—poverty, environmental degradation, and conflicts—great co-operative efforts are necessary. International development co-operation is an investment in ensuring people a better life, in environmental conservation and peace, in democracy and equality. It should pave the way for equal relations and make itself redundant.
United States Agency for International Development (USAID) www.usaid.gov	Foreign aid funding agency of the US government	The agency works in six principle areas crucial to achieving both sustainable development and advancing U.S. foreign policy objectives: Economic growth and agricultural development Population, health and nutrition; Environment; Democracy and governance; Education and training, and; Humanitarian assistance.
Norwegian Agency for Development Cooperation (NORAD) www.norad.no	Foreign aid funding agency of the Norwegian government	NORAD's purpose is to assist developing countries in their efforts to achieve lasting improvements in political, economic and social conditions for the entire population within the limits imposed by the natural environment and the natural resource base.
VETAID www.vetaid.org	British livestock-oriented development NGO	VETAID is a non-profit, overseas development organization working for poverty reduction and food security of people dependant on livestock. VETAID's remit is to improve livelihoods of small-scale farmers and pastoralists by improving access to livestock health and husbandry resources, building on traditional livestock practices where possible.

[a]Organizational types represented include donor agencies, implementing agencies, technical assistance agencies, research organizations, and policy "think tanks." Descriptive information for each organization is taken from that organization's web site to reflect how the organization describes itself.

mission of the IDA is to support efficient and effective programs to reduce poverty and improve the quality of life in its poorest member countries. Currently, 78 countries are eligible to borrow from the IDA.

Regional multinational development banks akin to the World Bank also exist, notably the African Development Bank and the Asian Development Bank. The African Development Bank, with headquarters in Abidjan, Cote d'Ivoire, has 76 member nations, 53 from the Africa region and 23 from outside Africa, mostly industrialized nations of Europe and the Americas. The Asian Development Bank, with headquarters in Manila, the Philippines, has 58 member countries, 42 within the region and 16 outside. Its primary mission is to extend loans and equity investments to its developing member countries for their economic and social development. The European Union (EU), through its European Investment Bank and the European Commission, provides 10% of the worldwide total of official development assistance (Fig. 5-6.)

The United Nations is also an organization of member nations who contribute toward the UN operating budget. As such, those United Nations agencies that have development goals in their mandate (e.g., the UNDP), have funds budgeted for development assistance. The UNDP, established in 1965, receives

approximately $1 billion annually from member nations to support its programs. Each UNDP country mission has its own operating budget to support development activities under grant agreements with host-country governments. Other UN agencies, such as the FAO, have an intermediate status as donors. The FAO also has country-specific missions and has budgets to support some development activities within the host country. However, FAO is also expected to seek funding from other donor agencies in support of its country and regional programs. For example, about 22% of its budget for field program activities comes from the UNDP.

The International Fund for Agricultural Development (IFAD) is a member-supported specialized agency of the United Nations, established in 1977 as an outgrowth of the World Food Conference of 1974, which was convened in response to the serious Sahelian drought and food crisis of the early 1970s. The IFAD was created with a specific mandate to combat rural hunger and poverty in developing countries through direct funding of programs specifically designed to promote economic advancement of the rural poor. As such, IFAD activities are directed at small farmers, the rural landless, pastoralists, artisanal fisherfolk, indigenous peoples, and poor rural women. According to information available at the organization's website (http://www.ifad.org/), IFAD has, since its establishment,

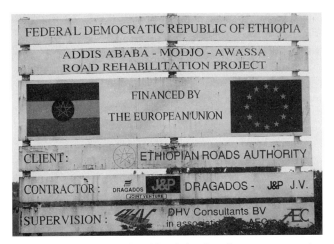

Figure 5-6. Sign outside Addis Ababa identifying a major road rehabilitation project in Ethiopia funded by the European Union. Road building and road maintenance can be important to rural development, as passable, all-weather roads can improve marketing opportunities for rural farmers to get their produce to urban centers. (Photo by Dr. David M. Sherman)

financed 584 projects in 115 countries, to which it has committed US$7.0 billion in grants and loans. Recipient governments have contributed US$ 7.4 billion, and multilateral and bilateral donors have provided US$6.2 billion in cofinancing. These projects have aimed at assisting 44 million poor rural households, equivalent to approximately 240 million people.

Bilateral Donors *Bilateral donors* are individual donor nations that enter into bilateral agreements with a developing country to provide foreign assistance. Bilateral donors are, by and large, the highly industrialized nations of the world. Though there is variation in how foreign assistance is administered by donor nations, each usually has a specific agency or government department responsible for administering foreign assistance, frequently within a ministry of foreign affairs. For example, Canada has the Canadian International Development Agency (CIDA); Denmark, the Danish International Development Assistance Agency (DANIDA); Germany, the German Agency for Technical Cooperation (GTZ): Japan, the Japan International Cooperation Agency (JICA) and other agencies within the Ministry of Foreign Affairs; Norway, the Norwegian Agency for Development Cooperation (NORAD); Sweden, the Swedish International Development Cooperation Agency (SIDA); the United Kingdom, the Department for International Development (DFID); and the United States, the United States Agency for International Development (USAID). For the reader unfamiliar with the universe of development assistance, it is useful to visit the websites of each of these agencies to gain a better understanding of their structure, function, goals, and activities, particularly the scope and nature of projects in which they are involved in developing countries around the world.

The United States, through the Marshall Plan, showed tremendous generosity and leadership in the realm of foreign assistance following World War II. More recently, however, that generosity has been increasingly constrained. Morrison and Weiner of the Overseas Development Council reported that the expenditures for U.S. economic assistance included in President Clinton's federal budget request for FY2001 were at the lowest level relative to the size of the U.S. economy since the end of World War II.[13] Aid spending as a percentage of the overall U.S. economy is just half of what it was in the 1980s and has been in decline since the 1960s. The United States ranks last among the 21 donor countries in the OECD when the percentage of the gross national product (GNP) devoted to foreign economic assistance is used as the yardstick. U.S. spending on agricultural development programs declined from US$900 million in 1990 to just US$300 million in 1999.

A survey carried out in 1995 by the Program on International Policy Attitudes at the University of Maryland (see http://www.pipa.org) revealed that many Americans are misinformed about their country's commitment to foreign aid, believing that the government spends 15% or more of the annual federal budget on foreign assistance. In fact, the government spends less than 1% of the budget on foreign aid. When informed about the actual percentage, most Americans surveyed believed that the amount should be maintained or increased, and more than 70% opposed cuts to community-based programs including child survival, the Peace Corps, humanitarian relief, environmental aid, and family planning.

Private Donors Whether a donor country provides funds for development assistance through its own bilateral donor agency or by contributing funds to a multinational donor as a member state, it is ultimately taxpayer dollars that are the source of these funds. In addition, however, many citizens actively choose to donate money to organizations involved in development, from Ted Turner, who pledged $1 billion to the United Nations in 1998, to the neighborhood children who collectively have raised $63 million since 1955 by trick or treating for UNICEF at Halloween time. Private citizens can choose to donate money or time to a wide range of organizations involved in development assistance, which reflect their own principles, beliefs, concerns, or interests. In addition, corporate and family foundations are becoming an important source of private funds for development.

Implementing Organizations

Once a commitment of funds has been made by a donor for specific development projects or services, three main types of organizations may be involved in project implementation and service delivery. These are governments and their respective agencies, contracting/consulting firms, and NGOs. Increasingly, development assistance involves participation of multiple organizations drawn from the three main types.

Government Agencies Traditionally, multilateral donors and bilateral donors enter into direct agreements with the governments of countries receiving development-assistance funds either as grants or loans. For example, funds for large-scale projects related to infrastructure development, such as road building, would be transferred to the recipient government, which would then administrate the program through the Ministry of Public Works or some other, similarly named government agency responsible for infrastructure. In many cases, however, the recipient country does not have the in-country technical capacity to carry out the project, so competitive bids are invited by the government in the form of tenders to outside organizations with the capacity to undertake the actual work of the project. Once the outside contracting/consulting firm is selected, they work in cooperation with ministry staff assigned to projects. Typically, senior staff within the contracting group each work with a specific "counterpart" individual designated by government from the ministry staff.

Contracting/Consulting Firms These are for-profit businesses that possess a particular area or areas of expertise in some technical or disciplinary field, and specialize in delivering technical or management services in a development context. Their range of expertise is varied. Some may be engineering firms, with strong capability in the area of road building or irrigation and a good track record of successfully implementing projects under difficult conditions in developing countries. Others may have a disciplinary specialty, such as education or communication, and have a good reputation for project implementation and innovation. Others may emphasize a multidisciplinary approach to project management and implementation, with a focus on rural development There are even consulting firms that deal specifically with livestock production and veterinary matters, for example, RDP Livestock Services in the Netherlands. Many donors, such as the EU and USAID, frequently use consulting firms for project implementation and management. As a result, many U.S. consulting firms involved in development assistance have their offices in the Washington, D.C., metropolitan area, where it is easier to stay abreast of new opportunities. For their part, many European consulting firms have offices or representatives in Brussels, the EU headquarters.

Nongovernmental Organizations The NGO is a private, non-profit organization that is independent of government affiliation. As the community of NGOs is very diverse in its varied missions and goals, it is hard to provide a single definition for NGOs. Even the term *nongovernmental organization* itself is not used consistently. In the United States, for example, it is not unusual for NGOs to be referred to as private voluntary organizations, or PVOs. They are also loosely referred to as private development organizations (PDOs), charitable organizations, nonprofits, and humanitarian agencies.

NGOs may raise their operating funds and their project funds from a number of sources, including individual donations by private citizens, church groups, service organizations, corporations, and foundations. Increasingly and importantly, NGOs also receive funds from governmental aid agencies and multilateral donor organizations when their organizational philosophy permits it. Some NGOs eschew government funding because they feel it places excessive bureaucratic burdens on them and that donor priorities may distort their own clarity of purpose. Many American-based NGOs, however, do receive

funds for their field projects abroad from USAID. USAID for its part has steadily increased the amount of development assistance that is channeled through NGOs. During the Clinton administration, the percentage of foreign aid delivered through private groups increased from 17% to an expected 40% by the year 2000.

Incredibly, estimates of the number of NGOs operating around the world are in the range of 250,00 to over a million distinct agencies, depending on how an NGO is defined and the source of the estimate. Several broad categories of NGOs are generally recognized, based on their location (Fig. 5-7). International NGOs have branches in at least three countries, for example, Save the Children Alliance. The different country branches of such international NGOs have shared goals and vision but likely have separate administrative and fund-raising operations. Northern NGOs are those based in developed countries but that work internationally, with project offices in various countries around the world. Heifer Project International (www.heifer.org), with headquarters in Little Rock, Arkansas, is an example. Southern NGOs, or indigenous NGOs, are based in developing countries and most often operate only within their country of origin. Egypt alone has over 20,000 NGOs registered with the government to operate within the country. Many indigenous NGOs are grassroots organizations formed to address a specific community need for a well-defined constituency anywhere from the village to the national

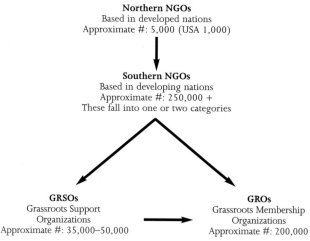

Figure 5-7. The distribution and approximate number of NGOs around the world is represented in this figure adapted from the April 1995 edition of *Connections*, published by the Alliance for a Global Community, a program within InterAction. InterAction, a coalition of over 160 American member NGOs, exists to enhance the effectiveness and professional capacities of its members engaged in international humanitarian efforts (www.interaction.org). *Arrows* represent the flow of funds and other assistance.

level. In Bangladesh, for instance, the Directory of Development identifies 126 different NGOs, most of which are local NGOs. Their names reflect a diverse list of constituencies and functions, for example, the Rehabilitation and Development Organization for the Landless, the Muslim Women's Welfare Organization, Shakti Foundation for Disadvantaged Women, the Bangladesh Rural Advancement Committee, and the Bogra Metal Enterprises Development Project. Throughout the countries of the developing world, there are similar types of indigenous NGOs trying to empower local communities, stimulate economic growth, promote sustainable development, protect natural resources, and/or achieve social justice.

It is difficult to categorize NGOs according to function, as their objectives and activities are so diverse, but some effort at categorization is useful in trying to understand the expanding NGO universe. A World Bank analysis suggests six main types:

- *Relief and welfare agencies* provide aid and other forms of disaster relief or ongoing assistance during and following emergencies, e.g., International Rescue Committee, Catholic Relief Services.
- *Technical innovation organizations* develop new or improved approaches to problem solving and are involved in transferring such innovative technologies to targeted constituencies, such as subsistence farmers. Appropriate Technology International is an example of such an NGO. They have been involved in innovative approaches to veterinary service delivery in East Africa and elsewhere.
- *Public service contractors* are contracted to handle certain aspects of official aid programs that they can perform more effectively than governments because of special logistical and management expertise. Such organizations are usually funded by developed-country governments and work with developing-country governments and official aid agencies. CARE is an example of such a public service contractor.
- *Popular development agencies* are groups that usually work to support efforts for social and economic development, self-help, and promotion of democratic participation in society. Such groups may be indigenous Southern NGOs, or Northern NGOs working within a developing country. Examples include Heifer Project International, FARM Africa, and Oxfam.
- *Grassroots development organizations* are indigenous NGOs in developing countries whose members themselves are poor and who work for local empowerment and development. Examples include some of the Bangladeshi NGOs already mentioned.
- *Advocacy groups and networks* focus on public education, information dissemination, and lobbying to encourage awareness and support for issues in which they believe, such as poverty alleviation, human rights, or environmental protection. Examples include Bread for the World, Amnesty International, and the Rainforest Action Network.

There are several likely reasons why NGOs have proliferated so widely in the last decades of the 20th century and why bilateral and multilateral donor agencies are increasingly inclined to fund development projects through, or with the participation of, NGOs:

- Corruption, inefficiency, mismanagement, and a perception of poor results have fostered a negative view of official donor assistance that is channeled directly to the governments of developing countries. In contrast, there is a perception of greater transparency, accountability, and effectiveness of NGOs involved in development.
- Many of the poorer developing nations are no longer able to provide basic social services because of weak economies, limited tax revenues, debt obligations, and structural adjustments imposed by lender agencies that resulted in scaling back of government agencies, staff, and budgets. Similarly, the nations that have emerged from the former Soviet bloc are no longer able to provide the extensive social services that were available under the collectivist state. In all these cases, citizens have organized their own NGOs to lobby for better services, protect what is available, or create new mechanisms for providing social welfare outside of government.
- The modus operandi of the typical development NGO generally fosters citizen involvement, self-help and local problem solving and promotes democratic decision making within targeted groups. Many development policy analysts and the donor institutions they advise see improved governance as a major avenue to facilitating greater social and economic development. They also see NGOs as a good way to instruct people and involve them in good governance through empowerment and participation. For example, up until 1988, only about 6% of development projects funded by loans from the World Bank involved NGOs. Currently, over 50% of World Bank loans involve NGOs in project implementation.

- Because of the downsizing of governments that has occurred under structural adjustment, many university graduates in developing countries can no longer depend on government employment, nor can they be confident of emigration to developed countries with greater employment prospects. Many of these educated persons are finding meaningful work within their own countries through establishment of, or employment with, NGOs. The global communications revolution, with access to email and the internet, has also allowed people in remote regions and underdeveloped countries to access information, develop alliances, and cultivate international support for their local efforts.

While NGOs are generally considered to have provided innovation, energy, and accomplishment to the world of development assistance, NGOs are not without their critics as well. White and Eicher of Michigan State University wrote a provocative assessment of NGOs performance, entitled "NGOs and the African Farmer: A Skeptical Perspective."[19] A key point in their analysis is that while NGOs enjoy a favorable reputation relative to developing country governments with regard to the effectiveness of their project efficiency and productivity, there is, in fact, very little objective research to confirm that NGO performance is, in fact, superior. The authors point to a number of constraints under which NGOs must work that may actually result in less than optimal effectiveness and that may make NGOs less able to handle complex tasks associated with agricultural development than national governments, the private sector, or public/private partnerships. The authors also note that few, if any, studies have been undertaken to specifically compare the performance of these different organizations or combinations of organization in carrying out development functions, for example, providing farmer-support services in Africa.

Supporting Organizations

Some organizations are not directly involved in project implementation associated with development assistance but provide valuable support functions to the development community at large. Key areas of support include research, policy analysis, advocacy, and training. Agencies involved in these support functions may be NGOs themselves, while others may be affiliated with governments, foundations, corporations, or universities.

Research and Education Organizations A number of universities and institutes provide training and conduct research relevant to issues of rural and agricultural development. Three examples are Wageningen University in the Netherlands, which offers a doctoral degree program in rural development studies (www.wau.nl), the Institute for Development Studies at the University of Sussex in the U.K. (www.ids.ac.uk/ids/), and the Institute of Rural Development at the University of Gottingen in Germany (www.gwdg.de/~uare/). In the area of veterinary medicine, the Veterinary Economics and Epidemi-

ology Research Unit (VEERU) at the University of Reading in the U.K. offers graduate degree programs oriented toward veterinarians interested in livestock production and disease control issues in a developing country context (www.veeru.reading.ac.uk/veeruweb2000/).

An important source of agricultural research targeted specifically to the needs of developing countries is the global network of research institutions belonging to the Consultative Group on International Agricultural Research (CGIAR) (www.cgiar.org). The CGIAR is funded by a consortium of foundations and governments. There are 16 research centers in the CGIAR network, each focusing on a particular farming system or important agricultural commodity and located in an area of the world where that particular farming system or commodity is relevant. Research foci include forests (Indonesia), tropical agriculture (Colombia), drylands production (Syria), potatoes (Peru), rice (the Philippines and Cote d'Ivoire), aquatic resources (Malaysia), and wheat and maize (Mexico). Research in animal agriculture and veterinary medicine are addressed through the CGIAR system at the International Livestock Research Institute (ILRI), with facilities in Nairobi, Kenya, and Addis Ababa. More information about the CGIAR system is provided in Chapter 10.

Policy and Advocacy Organizations A number of "think tanks" exist that focus primarily on issues of international development and its theories and practices. These organizations do considerable research and analysis, publish extensively, and advise government officials and other policymakers on matters of development policy. Two examples of such think tanks are the Overseas Development Institute in London (www.odi.org.uk/index.html) and the International Food Policy Research Institute in Washington, D.C. (www.ifpri.org). A visit to the websites of these organizations will give the reader a good introduction to the scope of development issues addressed and the range of publications available.

Other organizations may provide advocacy and lobbying efforts for their constituencies. InterAction, for example, is an umbrella organization that serves more than 160 NGO member organizations in the United States (www.interaction.org). Based in Washington, DC, InterAction has its ear to government to monitor issues related to international development and the role of NGOs. In 1995, when the U.S. Congress was considering major cutbacks in foreign aid budgets and a reorganization of USAID that would place it in the State Department and limit its independence, InterAction mounted a strong and effective media and lobbying campaign to create greater public awareness about the importance of foreign assistance and the role of NGOs in development assistance.

Foreign Assistance and Livestock in Development

For veterinarians interested in rural development in an international context, the entry point for participation is most likely to be with development projects involving animal agriculture.

Approaches to improving livestock health and productivity have changed considerably over the years, reflecting the general changes in development strategies that have emerged for specifically addressing the needs of the rural poor. In the succeeding sections, a brief history of the evolution of livestock development strategies is presented, followed by a discussion of the role of livestock in poverty-focused development and the various tools available to veterinarians and other development workers to improve the conditions of people who depend on animals. Finally, specific opportunities for veterinarians to work in a development context are presented.

The Evolution of Livestock Development Practices

In his book *Africa: Dispatches from a Fragile Continent*, author Blaine Harden relates an incredible story from the 1970s of well-intentioned, but misguided and inappropriate rural development project involving the pastoralist, livestock herding Turkana people of northern Kenya and the Norwegian Aid Agency, NORAD.[8] At that time, many western observers and policymakers held the largely unsupported view that pastoralist livestock keeping was the principal cause for the degradation of the thin soils and vegetation of the dry Sahelian zone of Africa and thus undermined the pastoralists' own livelihoods through irreversible environmental damage. Highly publicized episodes of drought associated with barren grasslands, widespread losses of livestock, and dramatic human suffering among pastoralists in the Sahel reinforced this perception. The pastoralist way of life was also under attack from some government leaders and politicians in the newly independent African nations who perceived traditional nomadic herders as backward and unproductive. These attitudes and perceptions fed a general attitude that the life of pastoralist herders must somehow be "fixed."

In dry northwestern Kenya, where the Turkana live and graze their cattle, there is a lake, appropriately named Lake Turkana, which is fed from the Omo river in Ethiopia. The lake contains Nile perch and tilapia, both excellent food fish with considerable commercial potential. Local fisherfolk, who were not Turkana people, made a reasonable living by catching, drying, and marketing the fish. The Norwegians, themselves a fishing culture, proposed an ambitious scheme to recruit the Turkana away from livestock keeping and transform them into fishermen, providing them with an alternative source of food and increased opportunities for cash income. The *piece de resistance* of this scheme was the construction of a massive frozen fish-processing plant on the shore of Lake Turkana at Ferguson's Gulf, the site on the lake where tilapia catches had been most abundant in the recent past. In 1971, Norwegian volunteers arrived to build boats, train fishermen, and carry out fishing tests. The following year technical consultants arrived, along with 20 fiberglass fishing boats, 4 motor boats, and a 36-foot fishing research vessel. Norwegian fishing industry experts were brought in to develop a business plan aimed at optimizing profits. They concluded that the processing of frozen fish fillets offered the greatest profit potential. As such, the construction of an ice-making, freezing, and cold-storage plant was proposed by Norway and accepted by the Government of Kenya. The plant was built, as was an improved road connecting the plant to the capital city, Nairobi, at a combined cost of $22 million. As many as 20,000 Turkana were enticed to become fishermen, receiving training, nets, and boats.

Unfortunately for the Turkana, things did not turn out quite as planned. By the time the processing plant was completed in 1981, it became evident that the energy costs for operating the diesel-powered cooling equipment in the torrid heat of northwestern Kenya made the processing of frozen fillets unprofitable. Furthermore, local clean water supplies were inadequate for proper plant operation and sanitation. The plant operated only a few days before it was shut down. Soon after, a drought in Ethiopia reduced the flow of the Omo River into Lake Turkana, and portions of the lake began to dry up, including the Ferguson's Gulf region where the plant had been situated and the harvests of tilapia had been so rich in previous years. Suddenly, Turkana people who had been induced to settle near the lake shore and fish had no source of income. In the meantime, their livestock, which were now concentrated around the lake shore, quickly overgrazed the sparse grass supply and began to die. Many of the Turkana who participated in the fishing scheme were forced to seek food aid from charitable agencies or face starvation. In the end, rather than helping the Turkana, the NORAD scheme actually contributed to their pauperization and the debasement of their traditional way of life.

This Lake Turkana fishing project, as preposterous as it seems in retrospect, was not atypical of an approach to foreign assistance that prevailed during the 1960s and 1970s. Some key elements that characterized this approach include

- A project that was donor-driven rather than demand-driven
- A project that featured large capital investments in physical facilities with prestige value
- A wholesale transference of developed country technology to a developing country, with little or no adaptation to local conditions
- A heavy dependence on external inputs and expertise to achieve development goals
- Inadequate assessment of project feasibility, appropriateness, and sustainability
- Inadequate local infrastructure, resources, and technical capacity to support the project
- A top-down implementation approach that failed to seek out or consider the ideas, needs, priorities, or local experience of supposed project beneficiaries
- A project that provided substantial financial benefits to citizens and corporations in the donor nation who provided consulting support, management, materials, and equipment for project implementation

The Turkana fishing project was, in a large sense, an "antilive-stock" project in that it tried to lure traditional livestock keepers away from livestock keeping for "their own good" and ostensibly for the good of the local environment. However, many "prolivestock" projects of the era, intended to improve livestock health and production, also suffered from similar flaws in design and implementation, resulting in outright failure. To understand these failures, one must recognize that a major goal of donor nations in undertaking development assistance was to stimulate economic activity within the donor country. Hence, many inappropriate development schemes were promoted by bilateral donors because they offered the potential to increase exports of animals, equipment, and expertise from breeders, manufacturers, and contractors in the donor country without due consideration of the ability of the developing country to use or support the offered improvements.

As a result, sophisticated veterinary diagnostic laboratories were built and outfitted in countries without a reliable supply of electrical power to dependably operate centrifuges, refrigerators, and incubators. Artificial insemination was promoted and frozen semen was sold to countries without a reliable source of liquid nitrogen to preserve the semen, adequate telecommunications for farmers to notify inseminators when animals were in heat, or sufficient transportation infrastructure for inseminators to get to farms reliably. Intensive dairy operations were constructed in unsuitable agroecological zones that had neither sufficient forage and grain supplies available to adequately feed high-producing dairy cattle to meet their production potential nor a well-developed veterinary service available to keep imported animals healthy and protect them from local, tropical diseases.

The Holstein cow, through no fault of its own, has become a symbol of the type of inappropriate livestock development intervention that primarily benefits the exporting nation. This large, black-and-white dairy breed is indisputably a marvel of selective animal breeding, with a milk production capacity that is nothing short of astonishing. However, the Holstein cow is the product of a particular environment. It is a European creation that was bred to reflect the agroclimatic conditions, farming systems, feed base, and market demands of that particular temperate, industrialized region of the world. Therefore, the superior use of the Holstein cow is, to a great extent, contextual. Its production potential can only be fully realized when a broad array of necessary inputs are available to support it. These inputs are successfully duplicated in other temperate industrialized regions, such as North America, with relative ease. Tropical regions, however, are more problematical.

If a picture is worth a thousand words, then the photos of Holstein cows in E. R. Orskov's book *Reality in Rural Development Aid* speak volumes about their frequently inappropriate use as a tool for rural development.[14] In his very informative text on approaches to improving livestock production in developing countries, Orskov has included a series of pictures of unhappy, underfed, heat-stressed, and heavily parasitized Holstein cows

struggling to survive in developing countries around the world, including Laos, Mongolia, Chile, Iran, Indonesia, Brazil, and Mexico. The cattle in these pictures either are poorly adapted to climatic conditions in the local agroecological zone, lack adequate resistance to local internal and external parasites, or are inadequately managed by livestock keepers with insufficient experience or adequate resources to provide the necessary nutritional and veterinary inputs required to maintain the health and productivity of these highly bred cattle. This is not to say that Holsteins cannot be successfully raised in these countries. Rather it points out the high level of intervention in terms of management expertise, feed resources, and veterinary care that must accompany introduction of such animals to realize their production potential. Yet, in many cases, providing the necessary inputs to maximize production is not profitable, because so much of the necessary feed, medicine, and supplies must be imported, often at a cost that strips all profitability from the dairy enterprise.

Orskov points out that in many of these situations, the Holsteins are in such dire straits that they end up producing little more milk than the local, indigenous cows that they were intended to replace or supersede. Given the fact that local breeds are usually better adapted to local climatic conditions, possess demonstrable resistance to local diseases, and are better able to use locally available feedstuffs, Orskov concludes that if the real goal of development assistance is to improve local livestock production rather than to provide economic benefits within the donor country, it is far more logical to invest time and energy in efforts to improve the productivity of local cattle through selective breeding and enhanced use of locally available feedstuffs than to import so-called high-producing breeds that will not produce highly under local conditions.

Happily, donor nations have gradually come to understand these constraints and to reorient their development strategies. The Netherlands, for example, has a highly developed, intensive dairy cattle industry, and for many years, the nation's foreign assistance programs served largely to create export opportunities for Dutch cattle breeders. In 1987, the Dutch government undertook a critical self-appraisal of its foreign assistance programs involving cattle export and concluded that the importation by developing countries of dairy cattle originating from the Netherlands to improve livestock production was not often as successful as anticipated. The findings of this self-evaluation have been summarized by de Smit.[3] He identifies five phases in the evolution of Dutch foreign assistance involving cattle export:

- Phase 1. *Widespread distribution of cattle to small-scale or subsistence farmers.* This effort was largely unsuccessful because of poor adaptation of imported cattle to local conditions due to marked differences in climate, feed, and management. Of particular note was the fact that subsistence farmers depend on their livestock for multiple uses, including draft power as well as milk production and that the imported cattle were poorly suited to draft purposes, making them less attractive to subsistence farmers. They frequently suffered from disease, stress, leg problems, and infertility.

- Phase 2. *Promotion of large-scale modern dairy farming.* When it became apparent that imported cattle were a poor fit for subsistence farmers, the Dutch government decided to promote the establishment of large-scale dairy farms. This too was largely unsuccessful as there was insufficient local expertise to manage such farms successfully, and the imported equipment was not well adapted to local demands and circumstances.

- Phase 3. *Support to small-scale farming activities.* In this phase it was recognized that in many developing countries, local conditions favored the practice of small-scale farming rather than large commercial farming. The Dutch therefore began to refocus their development efforts on small-scale farmers by providing a broader package of development assistance interventions beyond simple provision of imported cattle. In this context, it is useful to recall the history of dairy development in India, which has now become the largest milk-producing nation in the world. This was accomplished largely through the creation of improved marketing opportunities for small-scale, subsistence farmers rather than by developing large, commercial, intensive dairy enterprises (see sidebar "People Power: The Success of Cooperative Dairying In India," in Chapter 4).

- Phase 4. *The integrated approach.* Dutch development officials, through their efforts in phase 3, became increasingly sensitized to the needs and priorities of small-scale, subsistence farmers, particularly with regard to their requirements and desire for multipurpose cattle. Efforts increased to carry out more thorough technological and economic analyses prior to project implementation and to solicit inputs from farmers about their husbandry practices and activities for incorporation into project design.

- Phase 5. *The comprehensive approach.* At this phase, there is acknowledgment not only that development interventions should be demand-driven and tailored to suit the needs and priorities of local farmers, but also that development efforts need to consider the broader social, ecological, and macroeconomic context of the nation or region where development assistance is being provided. This means directing additional development efforts toward the resolution of large-scale problems that affect the small farmer. Such efforts may require targeted policy reform or infrastructure development to address issues such as agricultural pricing and marketing structures, taxation systems, road and irrigation networks, land tenure policies, agricultural research efforts, and the management of degraded or depleted natural resources. Only through such a comprehensive approach can appropriate livestock interventions be conceived and implemented to full positive advantage and be an effective tool for poverty-focused development.

Clearly, as the Dutch example illustrates, many lessons have been learned over the past decades concerning effective approaches to foreign assistance in general and poverty-focused rural development involving livestock in particular. In dealing directly with poor farmers and herders, a new paradigm for foreign assistance has gradually emerged, whose essence can be captured in the dual notions of participation and sustainability. In the following section, the concept of participatory, sustainable development is explored, with particular reference to animal health and production in poverty-focused development.

Livestock and Poverty-Focused Development

As is made very clear in the book *When Aid is No Help* by John Madeley, large-scale, top-down, technology-driven, foreign-assistance projects often fail to reach the poorest and neediest, even when they are intended to do so.[11] This is especially tragic when such projects involve livestock, since livestock play such an important role in the daily lives of the rural poor and offer great opportunities to improve agricultural productivity, enhance family nutrition, raise income, create employment, reduce risk, and secure better livelihoods.

Failure to reach poor livestock owners often results primarily from the failure to include them in the initial stages of project definition and design. As a result, their specific needs and constraints are neither understood nor taken into account. In some cases, this may be intentional, as when donors and governments are seeking to modify traditional livestock practices that they deem harmful or inappropriate, for example, discouraging communal grazing by pastoralists by promoting ranching schemes. In other cases, the projects may be designed to increase animal production in countries receiving aid, independent of any specific consideration for aiding poor farmers, for instance, the promotion of periurban, intensive, commercial dairy operations intended to increase milk supplies to urban centers. Still other projects may ostensibly be targeted specifically at the poor but still miss their mark because of flaws in the project design. Madeley offers several examples of projects that included either minimal income requirements to qualify for credit or literacy requirements to receive inputs or training. These obstacles effectively excluded the poorest of the poor from participation in the project, though their needs and potential to benefit were the greatest.

Even when development organizations do specifically identify the poor as their clients, projects may still fail. Ronald Bunch, in his excellent guide to people-centered agricultural development, *Two Ears of Corn*, emphasizes that a key element in any project's success is to first properly and carefully identify the needs and constraints of the client as the client perceives them.[1] In any given agricultural system, there are usually one or two main factors that limit productivity. In providing development assistance, the goal should be to work with the client, who usually understands the local farming system and its constraints better than the outside consultant, to identify those limiting factors and then work together to design, test, and implement the appropriate interventions to overcome the existing bottlenecks to enhanced productivity and improved livelihood.

Past project failures involving distribution of Holstein cows to the rural poor in tropical countries are not an indictment of the Holstein cow. Rather they reflect a failure to properly identify constraints to animal production in a local context. In many cases, the limitations on productivity of indigenous breeds of cattle are more related to lack of feed resources and access to veterinary care than to genetic potential. Therefore,

the improved genetic potential possibly available from Holstein cows is wasted if nutrition and health issues are not first addressed. To help identify constraints in the planning stages of a livestock development project that targets the poor, the research and policy group Livestock in Development has developed a very useful decision tree.[10] By working through the decision tree, development practitioners can determine the suitability of livestock projects for a group of prospective beneficiaries. The decision tree helps the project planners identify the specific constraints limiting livestock production in that community and offers a pathway for developing appropriate interventions, programs, and policies that will help overcome the identified constraints, to achieve the necessary and desired outcomes. The initial portion of this decision tree is presented in Figure 5-8.

Useful Tools and Principles

Development practitioners generally have come to recognize several important elements that must be included in their development efforts to reach the poor effectively and to develop program interventions that are both beneficial and sustainable. These useful tools and principles include community participation, community organization, the use of appropriate technology, microcredit, and stewardship of natural resources. Each of these elements is discussed below.

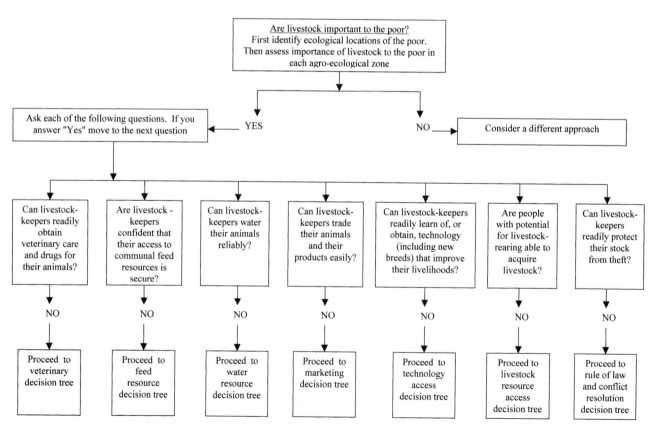

Figure 5-8. Entry-point decision tree for planning poverty-focused interventions involving livestock. Each of the bottom boxes leads to a separate additional decision tree. (Reproduced with permission from Livestock in Development. Livestock in Poverty-Focused Development. Crewkerne, UK: Livestock in Development, 1999.)

Community Participation

Imagine that you decide you needed a sturdy new pickup truck to improve your livelihood as a large animal practitioner at the "Extreme Poverty Veterinary Practice." You go to the large auto dealership nearby, "Magnanimous Donor Vehicle Supply." A salesman, Ernest Consultant, comes to greet you. He seems genuinely polite and friendly, and your initial feeling is that he is sincerely interested in helping you. But then, something strange and unexplainable happens. Instead of asking you what you need and questioning you about the specific requirements of the vehicle you are looking for, he promptly steers you past the pickup trucks to the sports car section of the display lot and begins a heartfelt and enthusiastic pitch for a small, red, two-seater sports car, the *Inappropria 2000*. Although the shiny little red car is undeniably attractive, it is clearly not what you need. Despite your obvious lack of interest, Ernest persists in his praise of the two-seater and even offers to give it to you free. Clearly there is something wrong here. The salesman seems incapable of asking you what you need but is prepared to give you something you don't need. You begin to develop a sense of deep distrust of Ernest. You suspect he has ulterior motives. You feel insulted that he has not bothered to solicit your opinions. You start to wonder if there is not actually something seriously wrong with the little two-seater and the dealership. You begin to withdraw, first emotionally and then physically. You walk away from Ernest Consultant and you leave Magnanimous Donor, filled with strong feelings of anger, disappointment, suspicion, and maybe even betrayal.

How could the salesman and the dealer possibly address your needs if you were never invited to articulate them? Obviously, they could not, except by sheer chance. Yet, this is essentially how much development assistance to the poor was carried out over several decades. Eventually, it became clear to astute development practitioners that too many development projects were failing to alleviate poverty, mainly because the poor themselves were not consulted about their lives and their needs. Formal recognition of this fact by governments, donor agencies, and international organizations occurred at the World Conference on Agrarian Reform and Rural Development held in Rome in 1979, which more or less marks the point that poverty-focused development efforts shifted toward a more participatory approach.

Participatory approaches in poverty-focused development are based on recognition that the poor themselves have a wealth of useful and relevant knowledge about their own situation and circumstances. Unless they are recently arrived refugees, most farmers, herders, and landless villagers have considerable experience with their own agroecology. They know the rainfall patterns and the soil characteristics. Through generations of trial and error they have made crop selections and developed farming practices that suit local conditions. They have observed patterns of disease in their livestock and can relate them to certain changes in season, food supply, watering sources, or even movements of wildlife. They can tell you how tree cover in the region has changed over the last 10, 20, or 30 years and what effect that has had on soil erosion. They can show you local plants with medicinal value. They can tell who in their community is rich and who is poor and by what standards wealth is measured. They can tell you who does what work and how it is valued. They can identify the constraints that they recognize in their daily lives that hamper improved crop or livestock production or more successful marketing of their products. Most of all, they can inform you, from their own perspective, what they recognize as the major impediments to a better quality of life as defined by their own values and experience.

The prospects for project success are greatly improved by soliciting community participation from the beginning and then continuing throughout the development process. First, there is the obvious benefit of improved project definition and design that derives from gathering relevant data from potential beneficiaries about local knowledge, needs, practices, and experience in the early stages of project planning. But there are also intangible benefits from directly engaging the poor in active participation. In everyday life, the poor often remain invisible to the powerful, and their opinions are rarely sought. Seeking input from the poor and being willing to listen, confirms the value of their ideas and experience, thereby showing them respect Through this act of inclusion, the poor become genuine stakeholders in the project and more likely to remain committed to its successful outcome.

Coming to fully understand all the various aspects of an unfamiliar culture and its practices is no trivial task. Anthropologists may spend years studying a particular group of people to understand their social structure and their relationship to place. Yet in the context of development project implementation and execution, studying people and their customs for extended periods is often not possible. This is because much development is carried out with funds from donor agencies that put contractual limitations on project lifetimes. If funding is available for a 2-year period to implement a project, it is not practical to spend the first year learning about the community of targeted beneficiaries. However, social scientists have developed a set of approaches, techniques, and methodologies, often referred to collectively as participatory rural appraisal, which can be used to gather useful and meaningful information about a community and its practices in a relatively short period. A useful introduction to participatory rural appraisal is *Rural Appraisal: Rapid, Relaxed and Participatory*, by Robert Chambers.[2]

Rapid rural appraisal techniques include open-ended interviews and the use of visual depictions of community life created by the community members. Such visual depictions may include graphic calendars of seasonal farming activities; timelines of daily chores or seasonal labor distributions; and maps of natural resource distribution around the village, such as communal pastures, woodlands, croplands, and water sources. Participatory group discussions are also used to gather a wide variety of information including, but not limited to, wealth rankings in the community, disease rankings in livestock, or identifying commonly perceived constraints on agricultural production. Increasingly, gender analysis has been included in rapid rural appraisals to specifically determine the role of women in agricultural life, solicit their inputs, and determine their particular needs.

Rapid rural appraisal techniques can be useful in veterinary programs as well. For example, the author was invited to Ethiopia to provide intensive technical training on dairy goat health and management to veterinarians from four regions in Ethiopia who were to provide veterinary support services to a Dairy Goat Development Project being carried out by the NGO Farm Africa (see sidebar "FARM Africa's Dairy Goat Development Project in Ethiopia"). To make the 5-day training as relevant as possible to local practitioners, trainees were asked the first morning to break up into groups according to their geographic region and to work together within each group to develop (1) a ranking of the five most important diseases of goats in their area and (2) a graphic representation of the farming system in their area, including seasonal rainfall patterns, temperature variations, the major crops with their time of planting and harvesting, and the time of year that the most common diseases were most often seen in local goats. The graphic calendar developed by the group of veterinarians from Amhara region along with the seasonal distribution of their five most important goat diseases is shown in Figure 5-9. From this information it was possible to adjust the training to reflect the diseases of importance to local veterinarians, identify the relationship of animal disease to seasonal changes and availability of food supplies, and develop a timetable for strategic interventions to control internal and external parasites and reduce losses in newborn animals.

Another area in which participation can pay great dividends is agricultural research. When subsistence farmers participate directly in farm trials, the results are directly applicable to their own experience and can lead to significant improvements in productivity and resource management. Small, on-farm demonstration trials often can be devised and integrated directly into an overall development project at little additional cost. For example, if improved, crossbred dairy goats are introduced into a community under zero-grazing conditions to reduce disease risk, then goat keepers will have to cut and carry available forages to feed the confined animals. Through participation, grasses and shrubs traditionally consumed along roadsides and field edges by local grazing animals can be identified, and a controlled feeding trial can be devised to determine the relative palatability and nutrient value of these forages to the newly introduced goats, thereby identifying an optimal ration using local feed resources. Similarly, farmers may have traditional medicines that they use to treat animals for parasites which can be evaluated under controlled conditions to establish their

true efficacy. Such participatory research demonstrates respect for the poor through solicitation of their ideas and can lead to innovations that are locally relevant and clearly productive. Furthermore, when such successful innovations are identified from within the community, they are more likely to be disseminated and adapted throughout that community because there is a pride of ownership and a trust that the innovation is appropriate.

Community Organization

Closely linked to community participation as an effective tool of poverty-focused development is community organization through the building of local institutions such as community self-help groups, agricultural cooperatives, credit societies, and women's associations. Community organizations such as these are a key element in facilitating sustainable progress in rural development. Such organizations may be formed to address an immediate technical function such as managing a local well,

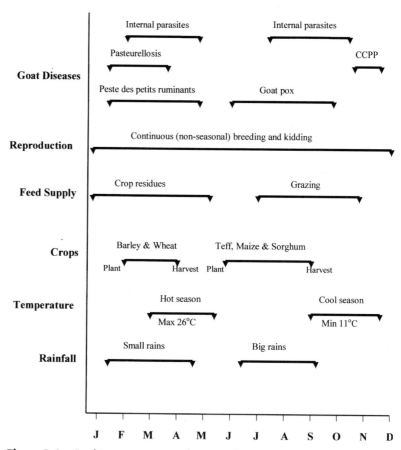

Figure 5-9. Graphic representation of a seasonal agricultural calendar for the farming system of North Shoa zone, Amhara Region, Ethiopia, with special reference to goat production and health. The graph was created by veterinarians from North Shoa attending a training seminar on dairy goat management. Note the biphasic rainy season and the increase in internal parasitism associated with each period of rainfall. Also notice the convergence of high temperatures, lack of rainfall, and feed shortages from mid-May through June. A high mortality in newborn kids would be expected at this time. Using the information presented here, consider some recommendations for strategic deworming and vaccination and for breeding management to improve kid survival.

irrigation pump, or cattle tick-dipping station; a marketing function such as negotiating prices for farm products with middlemen or sharing the transportation costs for marketing produce outside the immediate vicinity; or a financial function such as lending money to women to buy livestock. Beyond their immediate function however, participation in groups empowers the poor both socially and politically. Community organizations provide the poor with an effective instrument for participation in local decision-making, help them to cooperate more fully in the development of their communities, and give them a collective voice to exert pressure on local politicians, where necessary, to improve their conditions.

Eventually every foreign assistance project ends, and the foreign advisors and consultants go home. If the project has been any good at all and with a bit of luck, the poor may be left with a particular technological innovation or material input that improves their immediate situation. More importantly though, if the poor have been helped to develop and manage self-governing organizations, then the community is also left with new-found strength to look after its own affairs confidently and to create new opportunities for itself well into the future. Finally, strong local organizations that represent the interests of the poor can begin to influence the existing institutional frameworks that determine or control the social and economic practices of the culture at large. Through this process, institutional priorities can change, and public policies that are more pro-poor can emerge.

Appropriate Technology

In the context of poverty-focused rural development, *appropriate technology* is technology that is suited to the skills, income, environmental conditions, and resource base of the people by whom it is to be used. Implicit in that definition is the notion that use of the technology can be sustained once it is introduced. It is not uncommon for inappropriate technologies introduced during a development project to fall into disuse once the project is over and the technical support and capital subsidies provided by the donor agency are withdrawn. Several examples of inappropriate technology were identified above in this chapter, including the frozen fish-processing plant at Lake Turkana, the distribution of Holstein cows to subsistence farmers in the tropics without provision for adequate nutrition or health care, and the introduction of frozen semen for artificial insemination where liquid nitrogen supplies are unreliably available.

Even simple technologies that might be taken for granted in a western context may be inappropriate in a developing country context. Take the example of collecting blood samples in the field for veterinary diagnostic testing or disease surveillance. In the temperate, developed world, blood is now routinely drawn into vacuum-filled tubes and kept on ice in a cooler box or in a refrigerator on the mobile veterinary unit. The field veterinarian then drives on well-paved roads back to the veterinary clinic where there is a reliable source of electricity and a properly serviced and well-maintained centrifuge to spin the blood. The serum can then be either tested imme-

diately or frozen for later use. In remote regions of Ethiopia, Afghanistan, Mongolia, or any other underdeveloped country whose economic life depends heavily on livestock, animal disease surveillance is of critical importance. Yet often there may be no sources of ice or refrigeration, no paved roads, no reliable source of electricity, no trained service technicians to maintain the operation of centrifuges, and no freezers to store samples. In that context, the simple vacuum-tube blood-collection system so familiar and appropriate in the developed world becomes an example of inappropriate technology.

Veterinarians and physicians with field experience in developing countries have recognized this and have worked to develop more-appropriate technologies. Such innovations have included a hand-cranked centrifuge and even adaptation of a vehicle's radiator fan to serve as a centrifuge. While clever, these adaptations still don't address the issue of maintaining the harvested serum under extreme ambient temperatures on long trips back to a central laboratory. The simplest and most elegant solution to this overall problem has been to collect blood with a regular syringe and needle and place a few drops of blood on a strip of filter paper and allow it to dry. The filter papers are then dropped into eluting solution when the field team returns to the laboratory, and antibodies are detected from the eluate by appropriate diagnostic tests. This technique has been evaluated for diagnosis of a number of diseases, and diagnostic test results were found to be equivalent to those from tests run on serum from centrifuged blood samples. Diseases for which the technique has been evaluated include trypanosomiasis, hydatidosis, toxoplasmosis, and schistosomiasis in humans; infectious bursal disease and Newcastle disease in poultry; and anaplasmosis in cattle. Ramadass and colleagues reported the use of a dried-blood filter paper-based ELISA test for diagnosis of bovine rinderpest in 1993.[15]

Bunch, in *Two Ears of Corn*, offers an excellent analysis of the criteria to be considered in identifying appropriate technology and ensuring its adoption by targeted beneficiaries.[1] In summary, Bunch advises that the technology under consideration should

- Address a felt need articulated by the beneficiaries
- Offer financial advantages to the user
- Produce recognizable returns quickly
- Fit local farming or husbandry practices
- Use resources already available to the poor
- Be relatively free from risk to the intended beneficiaries
- Be culturally acceptable
- Be labor intensive rather than capital intensive
- Be simple to understand
- Be easy to teach and require minimal supervision or oversight
- Be aimed at increasing outputs for which ready markets exist that are not quickly saturated

FARM Africa's Dairy Goat Development Project in Ethiopia

FARM Africa is a British NGO established in 1985 with the goal of reducing poverty in Africa by enabling marginal African farmers and herders to make sustainable improvements to their well-being through more effective management of their human and natural resources. In 1988, FARM initiated the Dairy Goat Development Project in Ethiopia, with initial funding from Band Aid, the musical charity created in 1984 to raise money for African development in response to the dire Sahelian drought occurring that year. In contrast to the many agencies offering short-term relief aid to the drought stricken, FARM Africa focuses its efforts on long-term development assistance.

The goal of the Dairy Goat Development Project was to provide poor rural women farmers in the central highlands region of Ethiopia with a means of improving their families' livelihood. The highlands region is a desperately poor area beset by a number of problems. Population density in the region is very high, average family size is six members, rural infrastructure is poorly developed, and the average size of family farm plots ranges only between 0.25 and 0.6 ha (0.6 to 1.5 acres). The crops produced are mainly sorghum, maize, root crops, and some legumes under a rain-fed subsistence farming system. Yields are generally low, and crop failures are common. The region is subject to periodic drought and the associated risk of famine. Soils are sandy or clay loam with shallow depth. The vegetation cover has been depleted by years of intense cultivation, overgrazing, and tree cutting for fuel wood, which has contributed to high levels of soil erosion.

FARM Africa sought to focus their development effort on the poorest women in this region. They selected project sites where poverty levels were high and rural infrastructure, such as schools, health clinics, and roads, was limited. Then, through a community interview process and wealth-ranking techniques, project staff identified the poorest families in these communities, who generally owned no livestock and depended solely on their subsistence crop agriculture for survival. Participants were given the opportunity first to acquire indigenous goats through a credit scheme and later to acquire crossbred goats with higher milk production potential. Acquisition of a crossbred goat by village women was linked to a package of interventions to ensure that the goats would be properly cared for and produce according to their improved potential. The package included training in goat management and nutrition, an agreement to keep the crossbred goats under zero-grazing conditions, and a demonstrated effort to integrate forage crops into the farming enterprise, usually in the form of leguminous shrubs in backyard plantings, alley cropping, or living fences. FARM Africa helped to develop seedling nurseries for the preferred forage crops. The crossbred animals available to village women were produced as part of the overall project by crossing local Somali goats with imported Anglo-Nubian bucks at two University-based breeding stations (Alemaya University shown). Later on, crossbred breeding bucks were distributed to designated buck keepers at the village level to provide breeding services to goats owned by other project participants. Efforts were also made to identify commercial farmers or business people who would take over management and breeding of the purebred bucks as a commercial enterprise.

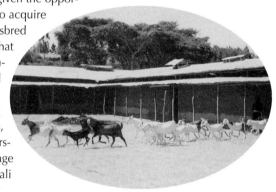

Nucleus breeding herd for the project at Alemaya University. (Photo by Dr. David M. Sherman)

FARM Africa's strategy was to use the introduction of goats as a catalyst to achieve multiple development goals. At the most basic level, FARM sought to provide goats to poor farm women to broaden their agricultural activity by integrating livestock into their subsistence farming activity, diversify their risk beyond crop production, provide the potential for additional income, improve family nutrition, and reduce the threat of famine in the event of drought. However, in addition to direct material assistance to participating women and their families, FARM also used the goat distribution scheme to promote community organizations, encourage democratic participation, empower women, and expand the access of poor communities to services normally not available to them such as education, credit, and veterinary services. A key element in this community thrust was the formation of women's groups at the village level for project oversight. These local groups were responsible for management and repayment of project credit, development of a savings and credit fund, and participation in decision making along with FARM Africa staff about various aspects of the goat project, such as the election of officers for the women's groups, the selection of group members for training as community-based animal health workers (CBAHWs), evaluation of CBAHW performance, and selection of local women to function as buck keepers for the village breeding program, such as the woman pictured below left with neighbors and the FARM project veterinarian. FARM provided training in literacy and numeracy for women's group leaders. The women's groups demonstrated their independence, empowerment, and authority in a variety of ways, including the dismissal of officers who were deemed ineffective and the replacement of CBAHWs who were not adequately serving their communities.

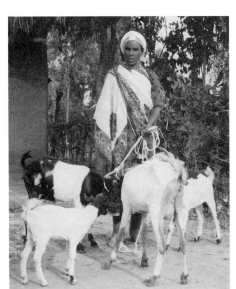

Village woman selected as breeding buck manager with project veterinarian. (Photo by Dr. David M. Sherman)

FARM also used the goat project to strengthen rural veterinary services in a number of ways, including training and outfitting CBAHWs; generating interest among local government veterinarians by recruiting them as CBAHW trainers and monitors; establishing veterinarian-operated drug shops to improve the supply of locally available drugs; and providing continuing-education opportunities to veterinary professionals through training workshops on goat medicine and production as well as by supporting advanced-degree studies for selected individuals. The picture below right shows a woman CBAHW candidate receiving training on goat examination from local veterinarians, surrounded by interested community members.

The Dairy Goat Development Project received external funding from 1988 through 1997, initially from Band Aid, but mainly from the foreign assistance agency of the British government, the Department for International Development (DFID). During the life of the project, over 1600 families received local goats, repaid their credit, planted forage, and received training in improved goat management. Five hundred families obtained crossbred goats. Crossbred goat owners saw milk production increase from 200 to 300 mL per day from local goats to as much as 2 L per day from crossbred goats. This provided additional milk for children and also for sale, allowing women to earn discretionary cash income. One hundred women were trained as CBAHWs, and 100 women's groups were established. Some 475 extension staff were trained in goat production techniques, and 9 government or FARM staff received advanced-degree training.

While numbers provide some indication of achievement, less-quantifiable measures speak of broader success. The Dairy Goat Development Project helped to transform the status of women in the areas in which it operated. The women's groups gave women a voice in community affairs. Their training as CBAHWs and their responsibility for breeding animals and forage nurseries demonstrated

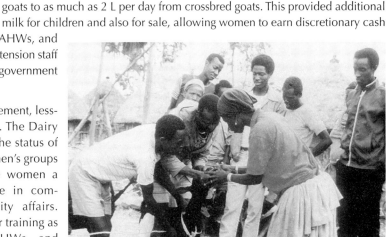

Village woman being trained as a CBAHW. (Photo courtesy of FARM Africa-UK)

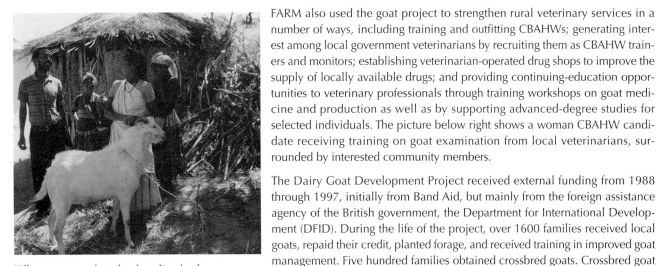

Proud recipient of project goats. (Photo courtesy of FARM Africa-UK)

their capacity to perform outside the traditional sphere of "women's work." The ability to serve their communities produced a sense of pride and accomplishment among participating women and earned them heightened respect from village men. A heightened role for women in community affairs and greater respect from politicians and government authorities are likely to persist wherever FARM Africa's Dairy Goat Development project was active. FARM has since initiated similar goat projects elsewhere in Ethiopia as well as in Kenya and Tanzania and has stimulated great interest in the development potential of goats through initiation and support of an East African Goat Development Network (EAGODEN) with participation at periodic workshops of representatives from Kenya, Tanzania, Uganda, Ethiopia, Malawi, Zambia, and the United Kingdom.

- Not produce adverse environmental effects
- Be widely applicable to regional farmers beyond the original target beneficiaries

The terms *appropriate technology* and *inappropriate technology* differ from the terms *high technology* and *low technology*. High technology interventions can be appropriate interventions under the right circumstances. At present, biotechnological innovations are receiving relatively bad publicity in the world media, particularly with regard to the introduction of genetically modified food crops. Objections to the introduction of such technology include issues of environmental safety, public health, and perceived exploitation of poor farmers by large corporations who are seeking to require farmers to purchase seed annually rather than allowing them to save back seed from previous harvests as is traditionally done. Despite these valid objections, there are tremendous potential opportunities for agricultural development, improved human health, and poverty alleviation to be derived from genetically engineered crops.

Take for instance the reported development in 1999 of "golden rice" plants that have been transgenically altered with genes from a daffodil and a bacterium to produce high levels of beta carotene, a precursor of vitamin A, in the rice endosperm, or grain. Milled rice, which is low in vitamin A, is the dietary staple for billions of the world's people. Vitamin A deficiency is one of the three main nutrient deficiencies occurring in the world's poorest people, many of whom can afford to eat little else but milled rice and have little or no access to commercial vitamin supplements. An estimated 200 million children suffer from vitamin A deficiency worldwide, 500,000 go blind each year, and over 3 million exhibit eye damage. Incorporating beta carotene-producing genes into rice plants to increase the vitamin A content in the diet of hundreds of millions of the world's poorest people is clearly a beneficial development. Since rice is already grown by poor farmers under local conditions and the mechanics of rice farming are therefore familiar to them, the genetically engineered rice represents a potentially appropriate and valuable intervention. For it to be accepted, however, genetically engineered strains must remain suitable for local growing conditions, seed supplies must be readily available and not prohibitively expensive, and the safety of the genetically altered crops for human consumption and the environment must be proved.

In the implementation of veterinary programs in developing countries, there are countless decisions to be made about appropriate technological interventions. Veterinarians must make choices based on the local availability of products and their efficacy and safety, familiarity to local livestock owners, ease of use, and potential environmental impact. It is not appropriate to introduce a new drug, no matter how well it works, if the supply of that drug can not be reliably ensured or its proper use adequately maintained. It may do more harm than good to create short-term expectations and long-term disappointments. For example, large-scale livestock projects that pro-moted the building of tick-dipping stations to control tick-borne diseases in cattle sometimes had unintended detrimental outcomes. As long as dipping stations were properly maintained and insecticides were reliably available, tick control was effective in reducing tick-borne disease and improving cattle health and productivity. But when project support was withdrawn, local communities sometimes failed to maintain the dipping stations properly, and local authorities failed to supply insecticide reliably. In such cases, cattle subsequently suffered even greater damage from tick-borne disease because, during the interim period of regular dipping, resistance to tick-borne diseases diminished in cattle populations as a result of the temporary reduction to tick exposure. Nowadays, the availability of pour-on or spot-on tick control medications may obviate the need for maintaining tick-dipping stations. This is particularly advantageous in very hot climates with low rainfall, where finding water supplies to maintain tick dips and keep them at proper dilutions may be difficult. However, the use of these new products must be approached cautiously, as their cost may exceed the means of many poor farmers, and the potential for insecticide resistance can also emerge.

Veterinary interventions need to fit into existing husbandry practices and accommodate logistical constraints. For example, in places where extensive grazing of sheep and goats is practiced, there is often the need for an effective antibiotic to control predictable outbreaks of pneumonia, keratoconjunctivitis, contagious abortion, and other infectious diseases. In small ruminants, common causes of infectious disease include not only bacteria, but *Chlamydia* and *Mycoplasma* spp. as well. In these situations, if a single effective antibiotic is going to be introduced to animal health workers serving the needs of extensive herders, then oxytetracycline represents a good choice of antibiotic, as its spectrum of activity includes *Chlamydia* and *Mycoplasma* spp. as well as many bacteria. Yet given the difficulty of reliably reaching herders who are extensively grazing sheep and goats, the decision to use oxytetracycline can be extended a step further. Long-acting oxytetracycline that provides therapeutic concentrations of drug for up to 72 hours with a single injection would be much preferred to tetracycline formulations lasting only 24 hours, because it is logistically difficult to administer daily injections to animals that are extensively grazed and moving regularly, especially when veterinary personnel may not have reliable access to transportation. Even with this level of detailed consideration, the choice of antibiotic may still be problematic. If the animals are lactating and milk is consumed by the herder or family, then milk discard times also become an issue.

Another important aspect of appropriate technology and its application is to seek out indigenous knowledge. Veterinarians working in development have become increasingly open to seeking out local information concerning traditional medicines and treatments. This willingness to listen and consider alternative solutions is a healthy development and has resulted in the expanding field of ethnoveterinary medicine. Ethnoveterinary medicine and resources related to it are discussed in more detail in Chapter 8. An example of the potential role of indigenous knowledge in solving veterinary problems in relation to the control of external parasites in sheep and goats is also given in that chapter in the sidebar "Ethnoveterinary Medicine: To Spray or Not to Spray? That is the Question."

Microcredit

Improving access to agricultural credit by small farmers has long been recognized by development specialists as an important tool for eliminating poverty. However, providing credit to the poorest of the poor has, until recently, proved difficult. Traditionally, typical lending institutions normally insist on having the applicant put up some form of reliable collateral as a condition of making the loan, and the poorest of the poor usually have no collateral to offer. So they are left without credit or forced to borrow from local moneylenders, frequently at usurious rates that may drive them deeper into poverty. This situation began to change dramatically in 1976, when Mohammed Yunus, an economics professor in Bangladesh, founded the small-scale lending program that led to formation of the Grameen Bank.

The preceding year, Yunus had carried out a survey on the lives of poor women and concluded that there would be a much greater chance for the poor to benefit from their own labor if they had access to even small amounts of financial capital. The Grameen Bank was founded in Bangladesh specifically to make small loans to the poor without the requirement of collateral. Instead, loan applicants in a village or area had to form into small groups of five. The groups met regularly to discuss their aspirations and investment ideas with each other and a bank representative, and eventually two group members were selected by mutual consent to submit their requests for the initial loans of up to US$250. The remaining group members could not receive their loans if the initial two loan recipients defaulted on their loan repayment. Using this approach of peer pressure and shared responsibility in lieu of collateral and by bringing bank representatives to the village rather than making villagers go to the bank, Yunus demonstrated that the poor were, on average, even more responsible about loan repayment than wealthier borrowers who put up collateral for traditional loans, but who defaulted at higher rates.

Grameen bank was conceived as a rural bank rather than simply an agricultural bank, based on the recognition that all the rural poor are not directly involved in agriculture and that women and the landless especially may have other income-generating ideas and skills beyond farming that can improve their own livelihoods and strengthen the overall economic and social life of the rural community. The idea has basically been proved correct. Loan recipients have used their loans for a variety of purposes, including shop keeping or other trading activities, processing value-added goods from local commodities such as cheese making or basket making, providing transportation services with draft animals or rickshaws, storing agricultural produce to take advantage of off-season prices, and establishing various types of service-oriented businesses, such as bicycle repair or tailoring. Once initial capital has been obtained, with average loans of about US$70, many of the poor

have shown remarkable entrepreneurial skill, continually trading up their initial investments and returns to expand or diversify their activities. It is not unusual for family incomes to triple or quadruple when loans are used to advantage.

Since its inception 24 years ago, Grameen Bank has established over 1100 rural branches serving almost 40,000 villages. More than 2.2 million women have received loans, and more than 123,000 men. The total amount loaned has now exceeded US$3 billion. More information about the Grameen Bank is available on the internet at http://www.grameen-info.org/.

Among its many accomplishments, the activities of the Grameen Bank have demonstrated one important fact that should be of interest to advocates of livestock in development. The poor, especially poor women, recognize livestock as a valuable and critical investment to improve their livelihoods. The purchase of cattle, goats, and poultry is one of the highest preferences for women seeking loans from the Grameen Bank (Fig. 5-10). Through the purchase of livestock, many women realize increased income and improved nutritional status for their children. It is common for women to start with poultry or goats to sell birds, eggs, kids, or milk and then trade up to the purchase of a cow for milk production or fattening. They are then able to generate sufficient income to send children to school, improve their housing, or make other purchases to improve the quality of their family's lives that were previously unimaginable.

The power of microcredit to change the lives of the poor has been dramatically demonstrated by the Grameen Bank. That experience has now been studied, adapted, and refined by numerous organizations, from multilateral donors such as IFAD, to local NGOs that now provide microcredit to poor people throughout the world, including inner city communities

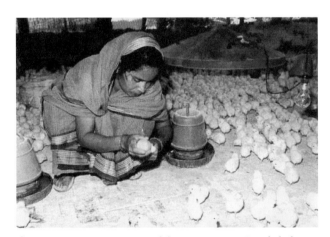

Figure 5-10. A Grameen Bank loan recipient in Bangladesh tending chicks in her poultry enterprise. The value of livestock and livestock-based activities to the rural poor as a tool for improving livelihoods is underscored by the high frequency with which microcredit is sought for investment in livestock by poor women around the world. (Courtesy of the Grameen Bank. For additional photos see http://www.grameen-info.org/)

within the United States. An international Microcredit Summit was held in 1997 in Washington, DC. Presentations from that Summit as well as updated information about new developments in microcredit are available on the internet at http://www.microcreditsummit.org/.

Stewardship of Natural Resources

The rural poor have limited access to external inputs in their daily lives. Much of what they depend on for their livelihood derives from the local natural resource base of soil, water, sunshine, vegetation, and animal life, both domestic and wild. Several factors are placing increased pressure on the natural resource base of the rural poor. These include high population growth rates, and the dislocation of the poor into marginal agroecological zones through urbanization, by the expansion of commercial agriculture, or by civil unrest leading to refugee movements. Serious problems such as deforestation, soil erosion, land degradation, and the loss of biodiversity are due, at least in part, to the desperate actions of poor people pushed to the margins of existence.

To be sustainable, therefore, poverty-focused development must foster practices that promote stewardship of natural resources. This can be accomplished through efforts to restore damaged environments, such as reforestation, or by efforts to minimize further losses, such as terracing hillsides to reduce soil erosion. It also can be accomplished through the development and introduction of appropriate technologies that reduce dependence on limited local resources (e.g., solar cookers that would reduce dependence on scarce fuel wood or drip irrigation practices to reduce water use).

Existing resources also can be used more efficiently, resulting in greater overall productivity and better resource management. Better integration of animals into smallholder farming systems offers such an opportunity. Livestock can convert crop residues and kitchen wastes into animal protein. Their manure can be turned back onto croplands to enrich the soil and improve crop production or used as a substrate in farm ponds to produce fish for sale or consumption. It can also be used to produce methane in biodigesters, which can substitute for wood as a cooking fuel and provide heat and light. Draft animals can provide needed power for agricultural work without greater dependence on nonrenewable resources such as the fossil fuels needed to power tractors or rototillers. For animals to serve effectively in the stewardship of natural resources, they must remain healthy, which requires greater access to veterinary services for the rural poor.

Opportunities for Veterinarians in Development Work

Given the important role of animals in the daily lives of the poor and the constraints that exist on animal health and productivity in many developing countries, there are clearly opportunities for veterinarians from developed countries to become involved in development work. That such a need exists is confirmed by the number of veterinary-focused NGOs

that have arisen in recent years. These include Vetaid (www.vetaid.org) and Vetwork (www.vetwork.org.uk) in the U.K.; Volunteers in International Veterinary Assistance (VIVA) and Christian Veterinary Mission (www.vetmission.org/) in the United States; and Veterinaires Sans Frontieres (VSF), with independent chapters based in France (www.vsf-france.org/), Belgium, Spain (www.pangea.org/vetsf/) and other European nations. In addition, there are a number of NGOs that focus more broadly on issues of rural development but recognize the importance of livestock in sustainable development. These NGOs, such as Heifer Project International (www.heifer.org) and FARM Africa (www.farmafrica.org.uk/), increasingly incorporate veterinary components into their overall development programs and use veterinarians as staff, consultants, or volunteers.

These veterinary and development NGOs are involved in a variety of activities aimed at assisting the world's poor who depend on animals for their livelihood. They may work in a relief context, providing short-term veterinary support for the animals of refugees and displaced persons during times of war, drought, and other natural and man-made disasters, or they may be involved in long-term development projects aimed at improving the health and productivity of livestock owned by small farmers and herders through education and training programs, community organization, or the introduction of new management techniques and small-scale livestock enterprises. They may also focus on improving reliable access to veterinary services for the rural poor. Toward this end, many projects in recent years have involved the training of paraprofessional, community-based animal health workers (CBAHWs) who can help provide basic veterinary assistance to villagers and herders in remote areas that are served by neither government veterinarians nor private veterinary practitioners. An example of a community-based animal health program is provided in this chapter in the sidebar on Ethiopia and also in Chapter 8 in the sidebar on Afghanistan.

Another important development in the last decade has been the movement in many developing countries to privatize veterinary services by downsizing the ranks of government veterinarians and moving them into the private sector. As there is little experience with veterinary private practice in many of these countries, a number of aid agencies are bringing veterinarians from developed countries to lend their experience and expertise as private practitioners to veterinarians in developing countries who face the unfamiliar and daunting prospect of making a living from private practice (see sidebar "Hard Times in Mongolia: American Veterinarians Help with a Difficult Transition to Private Veterinary Practice"). The general trend toward privatization of veterinary services in developing countries and the reasons behind it are discussed further in Chapter 8.

Animal health issues affecting the poor extend beyond the village level. The capacity for nations to diagnose and control infectious diseases is critical to maintaining a healthy national livestock resource, a strong agricultural economy, and a thriving

Hard Times in Mongolia: American Veterinarians Help with a Difficult Transition to Private Veterinary Practice

Mongolia is a landlocked country in Central Asia, characterized by vast open grasslands, the rugged Altay mountains, and the Gobi desert. It is more than twice the size of Texas but has a total population of only 2.6 million people. About half of Mongolians live in urban areas, primarily in the capital city of Ulaan Baatar, while the other half live in rural areas. With only 1% of the land suitable for crop production, the vast majority of rural people are pastoralist herders, engaged primarily in livestock keeping. The basic pattern of rural life in Mongolia has changed little since the time of Genghis Kahn, the great Mon-

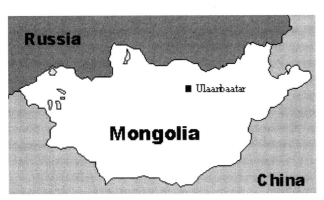

golian hero who conquered much of Asia and Europe in the 13th century. Herders still live in portable gers, the circular dwellings made of felted wool hung on a wooden frame, whose only door always faces south. While some herders use motorcycles, most still move about the plains on horseback, tending mixed flocks of sheep, goats, and cattle, regularly moving their stock in search of adequate water and forage. In the colder, more mountainous north, cattle may be replaced by the heartier, more cold-adapted yak, and in the drier Gobi region to the south, by the two-humped, or Bactrian, camel, but in all regions, sheep and goats prevail. Most of the herders' basic needs, including food, clothing, shelter, and cash income are derived from the animals they keep. Overall, agriculture contributes about 31% of the GDP of Mongolia, primarily through livestock.

For much of the 20th century, Mongolia was an autonomous, communist republic with strong economic and political ties to the Soviet Union. Under the Mongolian communist system, herders did not own their own animals, but rather, managed them for the state. Quotas for wool, meat, and milk production were set by government, and herders were responsible for producing the set quotas. The Soviet Union was the major purchaser of animal products and, essentially underwrote the entire economic life of Mongolia. Under the socialist system, herders fared reasonably well. They had an assured market for their animal products and received a regular salary for their herding work. They also received numerous social welfare benefits from the state, including reasonable access to health care, education for their children, a retirement pension, and free veterinary service for their livestock from a state veterinary service. Mongolia even had its own veterinary faculty in Ulaan Baatar, established in 1942.

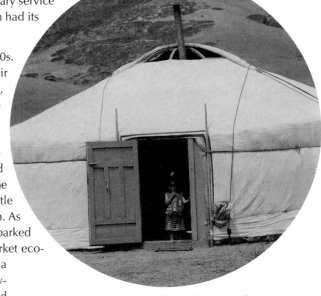

Significant changes began to occur in Mongolia in the early 1990s. Despite the relative prosperity Mongolians enjoyed under their communist regime, they bristled at the overall authoritarianism, abuse of human rights, and lack of religious freedoms. A democracy movement developed, and in 1990, the communists were obliged to give up their constitutional powers and free elections were held. In 1992, the Soviet Union was dissolved, and the economic support provided by the Soviets in the form of subsidies and reliable markets for Mongolian livestock products disappeared. The weak economy of the emergent Russian Federation offered little hope that significant sales to Russia would resume anytime soon. As a result, Mongolia faced serious financial obstacles just as it embarked on its new experiment in democratic government and free-market economics. The loss of trade with the former Soviet Union meant a dramatically shrunken economy and reduced government revenues. As a result, many government entitlements were eliminated or reduced, and many Mongolians experienced a reduction in their standard of living. Many formerly collectivized industrial enter-

A Mongolian ger, the traditional portable home of Mongolian herders. (Photo by Dr. David M. Sherman)

prises were privatized, and considerable numbers of urban workers became unemployed. Many returned to the countryside to take up the activity that has supported Mongolians through the ages, namely, herding.

(*continued*)

Hard Times in Mongolia: American Veterinarians Help with a Difficult Transition to Private Veterinary Practice *(Continued)*

One important casualty of the shrinking economy in Mongolia has been veterinary service delivery, a vital activity in a country in which most citizens depend directly on livestock production. Under the communist system, veterinarians were employed by government and used drugs, supplies, and vaccines that were either produced or procured and distributed by government. Services to livestock owners were provided free of charge. Abruptly in 1999, however, the government announced that it was privatizing the government veterinary service. It produced a list of district veterinary clinics around the country that had been operated by government and staffed by government-employed veterinarians. These clinics would now auctioned off to veterinarians or veterinary assistants through a competitive bidding process that gave no special consideration to the veterinarians who had been staffing the clinics. At the same time, however, the government retained control over the procurement and distribution of vaccines and drugs and let it be known that vaccines and deworming medicines were being made available to the newly privatized veterinarians for free, even though the vets would now have to charge their clients for the drugs to make a living.

It would not be an exaggeration to say that the delivery of animal health services to herders in Mongolia is currently in crisis. It remains to be seen if the current privatization effort can result in effective delivery of clinical veterinary services in the private sector. A number of constraints are readily identifiable, including

- A reluctance by herders to pay for veterinary services that for decades were provided for free under the communist system,

- Difficulty of herders to pay, because of limited access to cash in a subsistence herder economy,

- A lack of understanding by herders of the range of services that trained veterinarians can offer and how such services can improve livestock health and productivity,

- A lack of appreciation by herders of the highly favorable benefit-cost ratio of certain veterinary interventions in terms of decreased morbidity and mortality and improved growth and production,

- Logistical problems such as low population density, extensive distribution of livestock, and poor communication and transportation infrastructure, which make it difficult for veterinarians to deliver timely and economical service and be financially successful at the same time,

- A lack of confidence among veterinarians themselves about their professional abilities and the ability to run a private veterinary practice successfully,

- A lack of access to professional information about contemporary developments in clinical veterinary practice,

- The absence of a veterinary practice act to provide a clear legal framework for private veterinary practice,

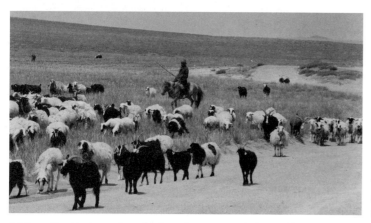

A Mongolian herder on horseback tending goats and sheep. (Photo by Dr. David M. Sherman)

- A government-controlled system of vaccine and drug procurement and distribution that keeps the private veterinarian's "means of production" under strict government control, that does not reliably deliver adequate supplies of needed materials in a timely fashion, and which is unresponsive to changing patterns of demand.

Several American NGOs have been actively involved in rural development activities in Mongolia in recent years and have focused a significant portion of their efforts on the issue of veterinary service delivery. Agriculture Cooperation Development International/Volunteers in Overseas Cooperative Assistance (ACDI/VOCA) is one such agency, with funding from the USAID, with programs in both agronomy and livestock development, including veterinary medicine. ACDI/VOCA employs a full-time American veterinarian on staff in Mongolia but also has had nine American veterinary volunteers and consultants come to Mongolia to assist in their effort to support the successful privatization of veterinary services. These veterinarians represented a wide range of professional experience, including private large animal practitioners, academicspecialists, and former officers of the American Veterinary Medical Association (AVMA). Consulting activities included evaluations of the constraints on private practice, epidemiological investigations of gastrointestinal parasitism with development of recommendations on strategic worming, and assistance in the organization of the Mongolian Private Veterinary Association, including the drafting of a constitution and bylaws. ACDI/VOCA is also involved in providing credit for the purchase of basic supplies, medicines, and equipment to Mongolian veterinarians seeking to establish private practices in ACDI/VOCA's project districts. Veterinarians who qualify for credit are also supported with business and technical training.

Christian Veterinary Mission, a faith-based American NGO is also active in Mongolia through the umbrella organization Joint Christian Services (JCS) International. There are two full-time American veterinarians in Mongolia with JCS, and up to 50 additional short- and long-term veterinary volunteer/consultants have visited Mongolia since 1994 in support of the veterinary effort there. JCS has worked closely, one on one, with Mongolian veterinarians in their project districts, providing technical assistance, small business management, and loans to equip and outfit veterinary practices. In addition, they have been actively involved with the Faculty of Veterinary Medicine in Ulaan Baatar, participating in veterinary training and providing financial inputs to upgrade laboratory teaching facilities.

A third American NGO, Mercy Corps International, is the implementing agency for the USAID-funded Gobi Regional Economic Development Initiative. The goals of the Gobi Initiative are to improve agricultural practices in the Gobi region, particularly with regard to herding and cashmere production; to enhance business practices; to increase the quality and quantity of market information available to producers; to improve the capacity of local government to support economic growth; and to help civil society organizations function more effectively in promoting beneficial rural policies. Though veterinary medicine was not specifically identified as a program focus, staff came to realize that veterinary service delivery was a critical aspect in promoting improved herding practices and cashmere production. As a result, the Gobi Initiative invited two American veterinary consultants to Mongolia in 1999-2000 to evaluate the state of veterinary services in their project districts and to make recommendations on how improved veterinary service can be integrated into the overall Gobi Initiative programs

In addition to American involvement in Mongolian veterinary medicine, other nations are also involved. The technical assistance agency of the German government, GTZ, is also involved in veterinary privatization efforts in the districts where they work. They are organizing private veterinarians into buying cooperatives to help them obtain the drugs and equipment they need at prices that allow them to provide services to subsistence herders at affordable prices. The Japanese government is also involved through the Japan International Cooperation Agency, working with the Mongolian government to improve the technical capacity of the national veterinary diagnostic laboratory facilities and thereby improve national disease surveillance activities.

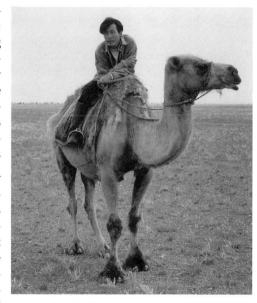

A Mongolian herder mounted on a Bactrian camel. (Photo by Dr. David M. Sherman)

The importance of veterinary medicine to Mongolia can not be overemphasized. As much as 50% of the Mongolian population depend directly on healthy and productive livestock for their subsistence and livelihood. In addition, the economic future of the country depends heavily on the renewed capacity to export high-quality and wholesome livestock products to global markets. A breakdown in veterinary services delivery presents a serious obstacle to achieving this economic recovery. The urgency of the situation was brought home in March of 2000 when an outbreak of foot and mouth disease occurred in Mongolia, effectively shutting down export markets until the country could demonstrate that the outbreak had been effectively contained.

export market. Effective control of diseases such as rinderpest, East Coast fever, contagious bovine pleuropneumonia, or foot and mouth disease require suitable diagnostic tests, effective disease surveillance programs, reliable vaccines, and well-organized vaccination campaigns. Finding solutions to these problems also requires a strong commitment to animal health research in the developing country context. A number of agencies use veterinary specialists to provide technical assistance to governments in developing countries to address such issues. These organizations include the International Livestock Research Institute (ILRI), the FAO of the United Nations, and numerous developed-country governments through their respective foreign assistance agencies. USAID, for example, has funded a number of large-scale foreign assistance projects that focused on development of veterinary infrastructure, disease control research, vaccine production, and/or veterinary service delivery. The review by Turk of animal health projects carried out by USAID between 1960 and 1993 provides a useful overview of the types of issues which need to be addressed, and some of the problems encountered in the implementation of large scale aid projects.[16]

More information about agencies and organizations involved in different aspects of development work is available in Chapter 10. A visit to the website of any of the organizations mentioned in the preceding paragraphs or in Chapter 10 will give the reader a better flavor of the scope and variety of the work that they do in the context of livestock in development and the range of opportunities available to interested veterinarians.

Discussion Points

1. Over the years, scientists, relief workers, and aid agencies have sought signs that would give early indications of impending severe drought so as to better avert major famines. As such, famine early-warning systems have been developed. What are the agroclimatic, social, and economic indicators that help to anticipate famine? What can be done to minimize the effects on livestock keepers and improve their prospects for recovery?

2. Identify a country from the former Soviet bloc and attempt an analysis of the impact of the transition from a socialist command economy to a private, free-market economy on veterinary service delivery in the country. What sorts of assistance might be useful to assist in the transition?

3. Poultry-raising schemes for poor village women are increasingly popular with NGOs working in poverty-focused rural development. Imagine you are consulting with an NGO on a village poultry-introduction scheme and are responsible for developing training materials related to health. What diseases and disease-control practices would you recommend? You can make the exercise country specific to reflect local conditions.

4. Practice rapid rural appraisal techniques. Visit a local farm family and have them develop a seasonal calendar of agricultural and livestock activities and a timetable of labor expenditures for each family member relative to the farm operation. Develop a rough map of the farm inventory and natural resource distribution. Identify and discuss with the farmer any constraints that the farmer faces with respect to improving the productivity and profitability of the farm operation.

5. There is increasing interest in the development community of linking village- or family-level livestock improvement projects directly to micronutrient nutrition for children in that village or family. What are the opportunities to exploit improved micronutrient nutrition through the introduction of animals or through increased animal production. What micronutrient requirements cannot be met through increased intake of animal products in the diet?

6. Many NGOs, on their websites, describe their specific field projects in poverty-focused development around the world. Review some of these projects, select one, preferably involving livestock, and evaluate it in the context of sustainability. Will the project offer lasting benefits to targeted beneficiaries? If you think not, what elements of project design are lacking that might otherwise promote sustainability? What questions might you want to ask the NGO project manager?

7. Many analysts believe that it is in the best self-interest of the United States to increase foreign assistance to the poorest countries of the developing world. Identify some of the potential benefits to the United States of increasing economic and development assistance to specific countries in Asia or Africa.

References

1. Bunch R. Two Ears of Corn. A Guide to People-Centered Agricultural Development. Oklahoma City: World Neighbors, 1982.

2. Chambers R. Rural Appraisal: Rapid, Relaxed and Participatory. IDS Discussion Paper no. 311. University of Sussex, Brighton, England: Institute of Development Studies, 1992.

3. de Smit H. Assisting livestock development in the Third World: the role of cattle export. Equator 1992;4(2):4–6.

4. De Soysa I, Gleditsch NP. To Cultivate Peace: Agriculture in a World of Conflict. Report 1/99. Oslo, Norway: International Peace Research Institute, 1999. (Also at http://www.futureharvest.org/peace/PRIOReport.shtml)

5. Engh I-E, Stloukal L, duGuerny J. HIV/AIDS in Namibia: The Impact on the Livestock Sector. Rome: FAO, 2000. (Also at http://www.fao.org/WAICENT/FAOINFO/ SUSTDEV/WPdirect/WPan0046.htm)

6. Food and Agriculture Organization of the United Nations. The State of Food Insecurity in the World, 1999. 1st Ed. Rome: FAO, 1999. (Also at http://www.fao.org/FOCUS/E/ SOFI/home-e.htm)

7. Hancock G. Lords of poverty. The power, prestige, and corruption of the international aid business. New York: Atlantic Monthly Press, 1989.

8. Harden B. Africa: Dispatches from a Fragile Continent. New York: WW Norton, 1990.

9. Lawrence JA, Foggin CM, Norval RAI. The effects of war on the control of diseases of livestock in Rhodesia, (Zimbabwe). Vet Rec 1980;107:82–85.

10. Livestock in Development. Livestock in Poverty-Focused Development. Crewkerne, UK: Livestock in Development, 1999.

11. Madeley J. When Aid is No Help. How Projects Fail and How They Could Succeed. London: Intermediate Technology Publications, 1991.

12. Mesquida CG, Wiener NI. Human collective aggression: a behavioral ecology perspective. Ethol Sociobiol 1996;17(4):247–262.

13. Morrison KM, Weiner D. Declining Aid Spending Harms U.S. Interests. ODC Policy Paper. Washington, DC: Overseas Development Council, 2000. (Available on the internet at http://www.odc.org/commentary/cbpprpt.html)

14. Orskov RE. Reality in Rural Development Aid with Emphasis on Livestock. Aberdeen, Scotland: Rowett Research Services Ltd., 1993.

15. Ramadass P, Ganesan PI, Meerarani S, et al. Usefulness of filter paper ELISA for detection of rinderpest antibodies. Ind Vet J 1993; 70(9):795–797.

16. Turk JM. An assessment of animal health projects: U.S. Agency for International Development, 1960-93. Agriculture and Human Values, Spring, 1995:81–89.

17. United Nations Development Programme. Overcoming Human Poverty. Poverty Report 2000. New York: UNDP, 2000. (Also at http://www.undp.org/povertyreport/)

18. United Nations Development Programme. Globalization with a Human Face. Human Development Report, 1999. New York: UNDP, 1999. (Also at http://www.undp.org/hdro/99.htm)

19. White R, Eicher CK. NGOs and the African farmer: a skeptical perspective. Michigan State University, Department of Agricultural Economics, Staff Paper no. 99–01, East Lansing, 1999.

Suggested Readings

Cohen JE. How Many People Can the Earth Support? New York: WW Norton, 1995.

Food and Agriculture Organization of the United Nations. Strategies for sustainable animal agriculture in developing countries. Mack S, ed. FAO Animal Production and Health Paper no. 107. Rome: FAO, 1993

Food and Agriculture Organization of the United Nations. Participation in practice. Lessons from the FAO People's Participation Programme. Rome: FAO, 1997. (Also at http://www.fao.org/WAICENT/FAOINFO/SUSTDEV/PPdirect/PPre0044.htm)

Gardner G, Halweil B. Underfed and overfed. The global epidemic of malnutrition. Worldwatch Paper no.150. Washington, DC: Worldwatch Institute, 2000.

Heifer Project International. Symposium on human nutrition and livestock in the developing world. Miller BA, ed. Little Rock, AK: Heifer Project International, 1998.

Lastaria-Cornhiel S, Melmed-Sanjak J. Land tenancy in Asia, Africa and Latin America, a look at the past and a view to the future. Working Paper no. 29. Madison, WI: Land Tenure Center, 1999.

Latham MC. Human nutrition in the developing world. Food and Nutrition Series no. 29. Rome: FAO, 1997. (Also at http://www.fao.org/DOCREP/W0073e/w0073e00.htm)

Leisinger KM. Development assistance at the threshold of the 21st century. Basel, Switzerland: Novartis Foundation for Sustainable Development, 2000. (Available on the world wide web at http://foundation.novartis.com/development_assistance.htm)

Peacock C. Improving Goat Production in the Tropics. A Manual for Development Workers. Oxford, England: Oxfam/FARM-Africa Publication, 1996.

Pinstrup-Andersen P, Pandya-Lorch R, Rosegrant MW. The world food situation: recent developments, emerging issues, and long-term prospects. 2020 Vision Food Policy Report. Washington, DC: International Food Policy Research Institute, 1997.

Wilson RT, Ehui S, Mack S, eds. Livestock Development Strategies for Low Income Countries. Proceedings of the Joint FAO/ILRI Roundtable on Livestock Development Strategies for Low Income Countries, ILRI, Addis Ababa, Ethiopia, 27 February-02 March, 1995. Food and Agriculture Organization/International Livestock Research Institute, Nairobi, Kenya, 1995.

Chapter 6
Animals and
the Environment

OBJECTIVES FOR THIS CHAPTER

After completing this chapter, the reader should be able to

- Identify major global environmental problems that are associated with animal health and production

- Understand how animal production systems can sometimes exacerbate environmental problems

- Understand how animal production systems can be managed to reduce or alleviate environmental problems

- Understand how animal health can be directly and indirectly affected by various environmental problems

- Appreciate the potential long-range effects of global environmental perturbations

- Recognize the role that veterinarians can play in maintaining the balance of animal health and environmental health

Introduction

From the moment that our human ancestors discovered the use of fire, human activities have carried environmental consequences. However, when the human population was small and technology was limited, Earth generally accommodated human influences, being possessed of an inherent resiliency and a strong capacity for regeneration. Today, the situation is markedly different. Enormous increases in human population along with powerful technological advancements now allow human beings to transform the earth in profound and potentially irreversible ways, including alterations in atmosphere and climate, depletion of nonrenewable resources, accelerating rates of biological extinction, and persistent contamination of air, water, soil, and living organisms with manufactured chemicals and radioactive isotopes. Such profound, global environmental change may actually undermine the capacity of the earth to maintain the health and sustenance of the planet's biological community, including humankind.

While science and technology have provided society with the tools for serious environmental perturbation, they have also allowed us to better understand how the global ecosystem functions and to better assess and monitor the environmental effects of human activity. As scientific evidence of long-term environmental degradation continues to mount and the consequences of this degradation are better understood by the public, there is an increased willingness among politicians and policymakers to understand and address the environmental costs of social and economic progress.

Virtually every aspect of human activity is now being recognized for its potential impact on the environment. Animal agriculture is no exception. In fact, both traditional and contemporary livestock production systems have come under criticism for their perceived negative consequences on the environment. Pastoralism and ranching, for instance, have been implicated in the processes of desertification, land degradation, deforestation, and loss of biodiversity, while intensive, industrial livestock production has been associated with chemical pollution, excessive natural resource consumption, contamination of groundwater, and even global warming.

Animal agriculture can contribute to these environmental problems, but the extent to which it does is sometimes misunderstood or overstated. In other cases, a full understanding of the role of livestock production is yet to be fully elucidated. In this chapter, current knowledge concerning the environmental costs of animal agriculture is discussed, with emphasis on the relative role of livestock production in environmental degradation, compared with that of other human activities.

Livestock can, in some circumstances, contribute to environmental problems, but environmental problems can also impinge on the health and productivity of animals. As global demand for animal products continues to steadily increase, it is essential for veterinarians to understand the constraints that environmental degradation can place on meeting that demand

now and in the future. Therefore, this chapter also identifies and discusses global environmental problems that can adversely affect the health and productivity of animals. Such problems include global warming, climate change, ozone depletion, nuclear radiation, and persistent chemical pollutants that can disrupt normal endocrine function in domestic animals as well as humans and wildlife.

Agriculturists and environmentalists have often been on opposing sides of issues. However, as the notion of sustainable agriculture gains acceptance, there is increasing recognition of common ground. This is true also in the area of animal agriculture. Veterinarians have a unique opportunity to show leadership in bringing these two communities together in constructive and mutually beneficial ways and in promoting policies and perspectives that integrate environmental stewardship with livestock production. Livestock can and should be managed in ways that balance their usefulness and productivity with environmental health and a sustainable future. As such, veterinarians must to be aware of global environmental problems and recognize their role as scientists to contribute to a better understanding of the relationship of animal agriculture and the environment.

Issues of Land Transformation

Land is our most fundamental and finite natural resource. It is the principal limiting factor mitigating against continued human population growth. Approximately 65% of our planetary surface is water, about 5% is ice, and only 30% is land. Of the land, just 11% is considered arable, or suitable for agriculture. Another 60% is grassland and rangelands suitable for livestock grazing, and the remainder is composed of forest, wetlands, desert, high mountains, and other lands unsuitable for food production.

Human population growth and the accompanying demand for land to support basic human needs has put intense pressure on existing land resources and has resulted in considerable transformation of the landscape. This transformation is often associated with degradation of the land and its productivity. The World Resources Institute reports that by the early 1990s, almost 40% of the earth's land surface had been converted to cropland and permanent pasture, largely at the expense of grassland and forest.

Three categories of terrestrial decline are discussed in this section of the chapter. These are land degradation, desertification, and deforestation. Livestock keeping has been associated with all three of these types of land deterioration. However, livestock are by no means the only cause of these problems or even the principal cause. In fact, most land degradation is associated with the planting of crops, either by clearing of new lands or the overuse or improper management of existing lands. The forces that dictate land use and land stewardship are complex. Nevertheless, veterinarians working in a global context need to understand these processes of land deterioration and be able to assess the role of livestock from an informed perspective. This is especially important, as the perception that livestock are responsible for widespread land degradation has become pervasive among policymakers in recent decades and has led to a retreat from international aid efforts that focus on livestock development activities in developing countries.

As human activity continues to degrade land, society looks increasingly to the lakes, oceans, and seas to support the human demand for food. In so doing, the process of habitat destruction has been extended to aquatic environments as well. The last portion of this section looks briefly at the implications of aquaculture and fisheries on the health of natural aquatic ecosystems.

Land Degradation

Land degradation is an environmental and societal problem of global dimensions. The loss of productivity of land used for food production raises serious questions about the world's capacity to adequately feed expanding human populations in the future. At the same time, the continuing transformation of natural landscapes for human use, to compensate for the decreased productivity of existing land, has serious, negative impacts on ecological health and biodiversity, which in turn can undermine the well-being of human society.

The Scope of Land Degradation

To say that land is degraded implies a value judgment. It means that there is a human expectation concerning what outputs that land can produce and that the expected outputs of the land are no longer being achieved. The cultural values and economic status that prevail in any society strongly influence perceptions regarding the inherent value and intended use of land, and these perceptions change over time.

For example, a square mile of forest in New England provided Native Americans with significant benefits consistent with their culture in terms of hunting and foraging, and there is evidence that a certain level of woodland management was practiced to encourage greater yields of game from the forest. At that time, the land was most valued as woodland. Subsequently, European colonists, with their agricultural tradition, perceived a different value for the woodlands. They cleared the forests to produce lumber for the construction of permanent dwellings and to create open fields for the cultivation of crops and pastures for domestic animals. Today, with commercial agriculture having shifted westward in the United States, the value of former cropland in New England is now most often measured by its potential for the development of suburban housing, industrial parks, or shopping malls. Once so developed, the agricultural value of such land is essentially lost forever, while its newly perceived value as real estate continues to appreciate. An excellent reflection on the evolving relationship of land and its inhabitants can be found in the book *Ceremonial Time: Fifteen Thousand Years on One Square Mile*.[30]

At present, most of the world's human population is still based in rural areas, and these people are directly involved in their own food production. For most rural inhabitants, the primary value of land remains, first and foremost, its agricultural potential. In the agricultural context, land degradation can be defined as the process of depleting or destroying the soil by using its nutrients and minerals faster than natural processes can restore them, resulting in a loss of productivity, or offtake.

The problem of land degradation is widespread. Table 6-1 shows the percentage of arable land on each continent that has been degraded over the 45-year period following the end of World War II.[21] Globally, this represents 38% of the world's total cultivated area, or 552 million ha of degraded land. It is further estimated that 15% of this land, or 86 million acres, is degraded to the point that it is beyond restoration or would require significant engineering inputs to revitalize it.

Both natural and social forces are at work in land degradation. The transformation of landscape is a natural physical process that has been going on as long as Earth has existed. Alterations of soil due to leaching, erosion, and compaction as well as alterations in plant cover are always occurring somewhere on Earth in response to climate, weather, and other physical factors, independent of human intervention. For example, upland rivers, swollen by rain, have always carried soil and soil nutrients downstream and deposited them in alluvial plains, thus enriching the soil downstream while depleting it upstream.

However, human interventions in the landscape can amplify these natural processes, often with negative consequences. Take the river example just mentioned. When forests are cut on mountains or hillsides near the river's source, the water-retaining capacity of the mountain soil is diminished, the force of the water's impact on the land is increased, and the stability of the soil itself is undermined. In such situations, heavy rains can have catastrophic effects, causing deadly mudslides and severely destructive flooding, as water previously retained

Table 6-1	Share of Agricultural Land with Degraded Soils, by Region, Occurring over the Period 1945–1990
Region	**Amount Degraded (%)**
Australia	16
Europe	25
North America	26
Asia	38
South America	45
Africa	65
Central America	74

From Gardner G. Shrinking Fields: Cropland Loss in a World of Eight Billion. Worldwatch Paper no. 131. Washington, DC: Worldwatch Institute, 1996:27.

by mountain forests, rapidly swells the river. Soil erosion under such circumstances is extensive. While widespread deforestation leading to sporadic mudslides and flooding are a dramatic example of human-induced land destruction, there are other human activities that contribute to a steady degradation of land. Crop agriculture is the process most associated with soil erosion, but livestock grazing and forest clearing are also recognized as important causes.

Land Degradation and Crop Agriculture

Agricultural cultivation of land can predispose to soil erosion by exposing the soil to the action of wind and rain. Excessive plowing or tilling mobilizes soil for potential loss. Removal of vegetative cover allows soil to remain exposed, and failure to provide adequate moisture allows soil to dry, making it more susceptible to removal. Once these conditions are in place, soil erosion becomes more likely because of the action of wind and rain.

Soil erosion is costly for several reasons. Not only does it lead to decreased fertility of land and lost crop production, there are serious off-site costs as well. Soil blown by wind or moved by rain finds its way into waterways, carrying with it chemical fertilizers, pesticides, and herbicides. Silting and obstruction of waterways interferes with power generation, water flow, and recreational uses. It diminishes flood control and water storage capacities of dams and reservoirs and slows replenishment of underground springs. The consequences of soil

erosion and other causes of land degradation are summarized in Table 6-2.

While the severe gullying that occurs with flash floods is strongly associated with the process of soil erosion in the public mind, most serious erosion occurs in a more steady and insidious manner, through the process known as sheet erosion. *Sheet erosion* is the even removal of thin layers of soil over time by the steady action of wind or water. Even the slightest grade in so-called flat lands contributes to sheet erosion. In sheet erosion, the organic matter and finer grains of mineral soil are preferentially lost because of their lightness, while the heavier sand and bits of rock stay behind.

Water and wind can conspire in other ways to degrade land. In hot, dry regions, irrigation is often used to bring otherwise nonarable land under cultivation. While irrigation has proved to be an excellent tool for improving global food production, certain problems are associated with it when sites are not carefully selected and irrigation systems are not properly designed or managed. In some circumstances, soluble salts and minerals in the soil readily enter the water introduced by irrigation. Hot winds playing over the surface of the wet soil induce a constant evaporative action that wicks the soil moisture to the surface, allowing the water to dissipate, while the soluble salts precipitate out on the soil surface forming a white, chalky crust and creating concentrated salinity in the upper soil layers that is essentially toxic to most plant growth. Salinization is one of the earliest known causes of widespread land degra-

Table 6-2 Consequences of Soil Erosion and Other Causes of Land Degradation
Loss of topsoil
Gullying of land surfaces
Reduced area of cultivable land
Silting of waterways from soil runoff, with impairment of water supplies
Contamination of water supplies with fertilizers, pesticides, and herbicides
Loss of soil organic matter, with diminished water and mineral retention
Leaching of soil minerals, with loss of soil fertility
Soil compaction, with diminished seed germination
Decreased productivity of cultivated land
Increased need for costly external inputs to restore or replenish soil nutrients
Waterlogging of soils from improper irrigation, leading to root rot
Salinization of soils from improper irrigation, leading to salt toxicity for plants
Loss or alteration of natural vegetative cover
Loss of biodiversity
Drying and dusting of soils with wind blowing, leading to desertification

dation. Archeologists studying early agriculture in the Near East have documented the gradual degradation of the irrigated farmlands between the Tigris and Euphrates Rivers in ancient Mesopotamia, based on records of wheat and barley planting. Barley is a much more salt-tolerant crop than wheat. About 3500 years ago, wheat and barley each accounted for about half the cereal crop in the region. Within 1000 years, barley accounted for five sixths of the cereal crop, and by 1700 BC, wheat cultivation had essentially ceased.[36] Today, this area, now in southern Iraq, is largely a wasteland.

In modern times, the process of salinization accounts for large-scale land degradation in many areas of the world, notably Australia, China, and the south Asian countries of India and Pakistan, where, respectively, 13 and 22% of irrigated land is now unusable due to salinity. Salinization is not the only potential adverse consequence of irrigation. Waterlogging of soils, with subsequent damage to plant roots, is another important constraint in irrigation systems that are not properly drained. In addition, bringing too much land under irrigation can have serious effects on water supplies. Underground aquifers can be lowered or exhausted by overpumping, and above-ground water sources can be depleted or diverted to the detriment of other uses. A startling and dramatic example is the ecological devastation of the Aral Sea and the collapse of its fishing industry due to the virtual draining of that inland sea to provide irrigation water for widespread rice and cotton cultivation in Uzbekistan and Tajikistan.

Soil must be viewed as a finite resource of great value. The average depth of topsoil in the United States is about 18 to 20 cm. Wind alone can remove a thin layer of 0.4 cm, each year from the surface of tilled land. This wind action removes more mineral nutrients per acre than would be taken away in a 35-bu crop of oats or one and a quarter tons of hay. The Dustbowl, which occurred in the United States in the 1930s, is a well-known example of the seriousness of soil erosion on a massive scale. The stage was set for the Dustbowl in the 1920s, when the southern plains areas of Kansas, Nebraska, Colorado, Texas, Oklahoma, and New Mexico were brought under cultivation mostly for wheat production, spurred by the boom economy that followed World War I. These areas had inadequate rainfall, which made them inappropriate for dryland farming. When wheat prices subsequently fell early in the Depression, much of the wheat land was abandoned or returned to grazing, thus leaving it exposed to the elements. During the prolonged drought that occurred in the early 1930s in the American Midwest, enormous amounts of topsoil were lost to wind erosion as blowing dust. An area of over 65,000 km² was affected. Clouds of black dust literally darkened the skies as far east as Chicago.

Out of this experience grew a greater awareness of the need for soil conservation, supported by both greater research and regulatory efforts. As a result, many soil conservation practices are now identified and encouraged, including no-till farming, reduced-till farming, terracing of steeply graded land, contour plowing against the grade of the land, crop rotation, the use of sod-based crops to bind soil, and the use of cover crops, grass

strips, and wind breaks to reduce the effects of wind and rain. Today, in North America, advances in soil conservation practices are showing some success. Since 1992, U.S. farmers have reduced soil erosion on croplands by about 1 billion tons through the Conservation Reserve Program, technical assistance, and regulatory compliance. The greater risk for loss of prime agricultural land in the United States has become suburban expansion around major metropolitan areas.

Worldwide, land degradation persists as a major problem. The United Nations Environmental Programme (UNEP) finds land degradation to be increasing in Africa, Asia and the Pacific, and Latin America. They consider the situation stable in Europe and improving in North America.[44] Some examples of the extent and character of land degradation problems as they occur in different parts of the world are presented in Table 6-3.

Broadly speaking, the human-induced degradation of land used for agriculture occurs under three sets of circumstances. The first is when inappropriate types of land are brought into use. The second is when useful land is improperly managed, and the third is when there is conflict over the best use of the land.

Inappropriate Types of Land Are Brought into Use   Farmers have two basic choices with regard to increasing agricultural productivity. They can increase the output from existing farmland or they can bring new land under cultivation. An increase of agricultural output on existing farmland usually requires the addition of external inputs such as fertilizers, pesticides, irrigation systems, or mechanized equipment, which are commonly beyond the economic grasp of subsistence farmers in many parts of the world. Therefore, cash-poor farmers often turn to the cultivation of marginal lands or to the conversion of existing natural habitats into cropland. As a result, steep hillsides, grasslands, flood-prone bottomlands, land with poorly drained soils, tropical forestlands, and other lands not primarily suitable for sustained crop production are brought under cultivation. In many poor, developing countries with large rural populations and high population growth rates, expansion of agriculture into marginal lands and wilderness areas remains the short-term option for increasing food production.

Politics and history can also push poor farmers into the cultivation of marginal lands. In Africa, for instance, European colonists in the 19th and early 20th centuries systematically identified and appropriated the most productive agricultural lands to establish commercial farming operations. Indigenous people were displaced, and sometimes confined, to marginal lands where efforts at subsistence agriculture were poorly rewarded and mainly served to exacerbate problems of land degradation. Today, nations such as Zimbabwe and South Africa are faced with major political and economic problems as they attempt to right historic inequities through land restitution and redistribution programs. At the same time they must address the physical problem of rehabilitating degraded lands.

Sometimes, citizens are offered incentives to move to inappropriate lands under politically motivated land reform, land tenure, or land distribution schemes aimed at placating the

Table 6-3	Selected Examples of Soil Degradation in Different Countries
China	Erosion affects more than a third of China's territory—some 3.67 million square kilometers. In Guangxi province, more than a fifth of irrigation systems are destroyed or completely silted up by eroded soils; salinization has lowered crop yields on 7 million hectares, use of untreated urban sewage has seriously damaged some 2.5 million hectares, and nearly 7 million hectares are polluted by industrial wastes
Russia	Eroded area increases by 400,000–500,000 ha each year and now affects two thirds of Russia's arable land; water erosion has created some 400,000 gullies covering more than 500,000 ha
Iran	Nearly all—94%—of Iran's agricultural land is estimated to be degraded, the bulk of it moderately or strongly; salinization affects some 16 million hectares of farmland and has forced at least 8 million hectares from production
Pakistan	Gullies occupy some 60% of the 1.8 million hectare Pothwar Plateau; more than 16% of agricultural land suffers from salinization; in all, more than 61% of agricultural land is degraded
India	Degradation affects one quarter of India's agricultural land; erosion associated with shifting cultivation has denuded approximately 27,000 square kilometers of land east of Bihar; at least 2 million hectares of salinized land have been abandoned
Haiti	32% of land is suitable for farming, but 61% is farmed; severe erosion eliminated 6000 ha of cropland per year in the mid-1980s
Australia	More than 4.5 million hectares of drylands—10% of all cropland—and more than 8% of irrigated area are affected by salting; area affected by dryland salting doubled in size between 1975 and 1989

From Gardner G. Shrinking Fields: Cropland Loss in a World of Eight Billion. Worldwatch Paper no. 131. Washington, DC: Worldwatch Institute, 1996:28-29.

landless poor or establishing political control of specific regions. Such schemes may be associated with ill-conceived policies that encourage land degradation, such as the clearing of tropical forests or a requirement for continuous cultivation as a condition of taking title to the land.

Land That Is Useful Is Not Properly Managed   Not all arable land or grazing land is properly managed for extended productivity. Rangelands may be overgrazed by livestock, leading to alterations in vegetative cover with reductions in nutritive value of plants and increased risk of soil erosion. On croplands, irrigation systems may be inappropriately applied or improperly managed, leading to salinization or waterlogging. Sloping fields may be improperly terraced, contributing to soil erosion. Grass strips and shelter belts around fields, which protect against erosion, may be removed to make way for more crop planting.

For various reasons, soils may become depleted of nutrients. Farmers may not have adequate capital resources to buy chemical fertilizers, and animal manure may be burned as fuel instead of applied to fields to enrich the soil. Cash crops that are particularly exhaustive of soil nutrients, such as cotton, may be planted to provide additional income.

In many poorer countries, technical and financial support for small farmers is lacking, and this can contribute to the persistence of practices that lead to land degradation. There may be no credit schemes for farmer inputs. Extension services may be lacking or geared toward large-scale or commercial farmers rather than traditional, smallholder, subsistence farmers.

Conflicts over the Best Use of Land   Determining how land will be used is an increasingly complex issue. The intentions or aspirations of local farmers and herders are often overridden by more-powerful external interests or by events difficult to control, as in the following examples:

- Industrialization and urbanization have been, and continue to be, important consumers of prime farmland as countries develop economically. In industrialized Asian countries such as Japan and, more recently, China, cropland is lost at the approximate rate of 1.4% per year as a result of expanding cities and factories.

- Some developing nations with significant international loan repayments to make may offer incentives to encourage the production of exportable cash crops rather than locally consumable food crops, so that the nation can earn much-needed foreign exchange. Repetitive planting of some cash crops can seriously deplete soil nutrients.

- National policies may encourage the settlement or sedentarization of pastoralists for a variety of social, economic, and cultural reasons and promote the conversion of rangelands to irrigated farmlands or cattle ranches. These alternate uses, if not carefully conceived and managed, can lead to land degradation.

- Absentee landlords are a growing phenomenon in developing countries with an expanding affluent urban middle class that frequently looks to land purchase and speculation as a means of investment. Such lands may sit idle, be put to inappropriate uses, or be managed improperly.

The Role of Livestock in Land Degradation

While crop agriculture is a major cause of land degradation, livestock production also contributes to this global problem. The situation in which land degradation is most strongly associated with livestock is the grazing of rangelands. Rangelands are grasslands unsuitable for crop production due to inadequate moisture, difficult terrain, unsuitable soils, or a short growing season. Approximately 37% of the earth's habitable land is classified as rangelands, and livestock grazing is an important activity on much of this rangeland. Rangelands account for 9% of the world's beef and 30% of sheep and goat meat production. Broadly speaking, livestock grazing is carried out for commercial purposes, as in ranching, or for subsistence purposes, as in pastoralism. Livestock grazing is the only means of livelihood for about 100 million people in semiarid and arid grazing zones and perhaps an equal number in sub-humid and humid zones.

To understand how extensive grazing of livestock can be detrimental to rangelands, it is useful to compare it with the natural grazing systems of wild ungulates. Wild herbivores evolved as integral components of grassland ecosystems. They play key roles in normal ecosystem function such as spreading seed; promoting germination of seed; aerating soil with their hooves; returning nutrients to the soil through manure, urine, and degrading carcasses; and generally participating in energy flow through the ecosystem as solar energy is converted to various forms of biomass, both plant and animal.

In natural rangeland ecosystems, multiple species of ungulates with different adaptive feeding strategies are present. For example, in the vast grasslands of East Africa, various mixtures of gazelles and antelopes, buffalo, zebra, and giraffe may be seen together at a particular site, each group selecting different plants for consumption, eating different portions of plants, or consuming plants at different heights. These adaptations reduce competition but also promote grassland health. Certain browsing animals clear shrubs and trees, thus reducing their shading effect and allowing more penetration of sunlight to promote grass growth. This, in turn, allows more grazing animals to be present and to replenish soil with their manure and urine. A recent experiment in the Serengeti National Park in Tanzania demonstrated that large herbivores played a critical role in nutrient recycling in that grassland ecosystem.[29] In areas of the park where large herbivores were seen to graze heavily, nitrogen and sodium in the soil were present in forms more readily available for uptake by plants growing in those areas. Similar soils in nearby areas where animal density was sparse and grazing limited, had nitrogen and sodium present in forms less available for uptake by plants. It was concluded

that grazing animals select grazing sites of higher sodium availability and, in turn, enhance that availability.

Predators also play a role in the management of the grassland ecosystem. They keep herbivores moving through the landscape. This helps to minimize the risk of overgrazing of specific areas and reduces the risk of soil compaction which occurs when large herds remain too long in a single place. Predators also help to control herbivore populations, keeping them in balance with the available nutrient supply. Herbivore populations are also controlled by fires and droughts, so that animal numbers will rise and decline in response to changes in food and water supplies. Fire also plays a role in maintaining the grassland itself. Periodic fires, fueled by the energy contained in abundant grass, serve to control shrubs and brush, keeping their encroachment on grassland in check.

Domestic animal-grazing systems approximate, but do not replicate, natural herbivore-grazing systems. When properly managed, livestock grazing can promote rangeland health (Table 6-4). However, when improperly managed, the grazing of domestic animals can distort some of the natural processes of the grassland ecosystem, frequently with deleterious effects on the land (Table 6-5). In most ranching enterprises, mixed wild animal populations on grazing land are replaced by a single domestic animal species, usually cattle, and their movement is restricted by fencing. Predator species are systematically eliminated to reduce losses of livestock. As a result, ranched cattle, unlike wild ungulates, neither migrate nor are stimulated to move by fear of predators. They may often stay in one place too long. They also graze preferentially, selecting certain grasses over others. If preferred grasses are taken repeatedly during periods of flowering, nutrient storage, or root expansion, plant vitality and growth suffer. As grass growth is reduced, shrubs and brush gain an advantage, and this woody growth further contributes to reduction of grass growth by competition for water and by shading. Eventually, the presence too many cattle for too long a time (overstocking) or an ex-

Table 6-4	**Positive Effects of Properly Managed Livestock on Rangeland Health**

- Removes excessive biomass, which reduces risk of wildfires; goats are particularly useful in removing brush understory from woodlands and forests
- Reduces shrub growth, which favors grass growth by allowing more sunlight penetration to ground
- Promotes a favorable mix of plant species on rangeland
- Disperses plant seeds via hooves, hair coat, and manure
- Promotes seed germination with hoof penetration of soil
- Breaks dried soil crusts with hoof penetration
- Promotes grass tillering (upward growth of shoots)
- Enriches soil with manure

Table 6-5	Negative Effects of Livestock on Rangeland through Overstocking and/or Overgrazing

- Reduced presence of palatable species of grasses
- Encroachment of herbaceous plants and bushes
- Soil compaction with creation of "hardpan"
- Soil erosion
- Decreased soil fertility and water infiltration
- Loss of organic matter
- Loss of water retention capacity
- Degradation of river and stream banks at watering sites

cessive intensity of grazing relative to the forage available (overgrazing) can convert an extensive grassland to a scrubland of patchy brush interspersed with bare ground. Once the ground becomes exposed, without the root system of grass to anchor it, the soil becomes especially vulnerable to erosion and gullying through the impact of wind and rain. Changes to the landscape may become irreversible.

Clearly, rangelands are a natural resource that must be properly managed to remain healthy and productive. In response to the challenge of understanding the inherent ecology of rangeland ecosystems and how they respond to various forms of human exploitation, the science of range management has evolved. The Society for Range Management (SRM) is the professional scientific organization concerned with studying, conserving, managing and sustaining the varied rangeland resources of the world. Established in 1948, SRM has over 4000 members in 48 countries, including many developing nations. The organizational mission is to promote and enhance the stewardship of rangelands to meet human needs based on science and sound policy. The SRM journal is available on the internet at (http://srm.org).

It is beyond the scope of this book to review in detail the principles and practices of range management with regard to livestock grazing. Traditional assessments made by range scientists include calculations of stocking rates and carrying capacities for specific rangelands, the types of livestock to be used, and the specific production goals for the grazing system being managed. In recent years, greater emphasis has been placed on patterns of movement and the feeding behavior of grazing livestock in recognition of the fact that the key element of damage to rangeland by cattle may be the repeated consumption of preferred grasses without allowing an adequate interval for regeneration and growth of those grasses. Certain management practices are being promoted in recognition of that fact. These management practices include rotational grazing, which involves the periodic movement of livestock to fresh, restricted areas of grazing, and timed grazing, which limits the time that livestock can spend grazing in one place and coordinates the grazing periods with critical stages in plant growth cycles.[38]

There is no one single prescription for using rangeland resources properly, since there is considerable diversity of terrain, climate, soil, and vegetation in different rangelands around the world. There are also distinct cultural and economic expectations for the exploitation of these rangelands. Failure to recognize these differences can lead to inappropriate policies and even disastrous interventions. For example, many recommendations by western advisors to encourage fenced ranching in Africa in place of extensive livestock grazing met with failure because they did not take into account the extreme seasonal, interannual, and spatial variability of rainfall in Africa and did not recognize the traditional practice of herders to use dry season or wet season grazing areas well outside the limits of fenced ranches.

Cultural values and economic intentions of the people are very important in defining land degradation. On cattle ranches, for example, shrub encroachment is perceived as an important indicator of land degradation. In the context of commercial cattle ranching, where the rancher is primarily interested in maximizing offtake as measured by overall meat production or calf crop, this is understandable. By nature, cattle are grazers, not browsers, and if shrubs increase and grass supplies diminish, ranchers will either have to reduce stocking rates, which reduces offtake, or provide supplemental feed, which increases costs. In either case, shrub encroachment at the expense of grass is clearly an indicator of degraded land from the commercial rancher's point of view.

The situation is different when the focus is shifted from the American West to the African Sahel, where extensive livestock grazing is the traditional way of life. For many of the pastoralists in this arid, fragile, rangeland ecosystem, the objective of livestock keeping is often subsistence or survival, not commercial production or trade. These pastoralists generally keep mixed herds of livestock, including not only cattle, but sheep, goats, and camels as well. In the Sahel, even though there is a well-defined wet season from late May to October, rainfall during that wet season can be highly unpredictable, and drought is an ever-present possibility, so mixed herds of livestock represent a survival strategy based on risk reduction. In fact, pastoralists may adjust the mix of various species within their herds to reflect patterns of available vegetation in different seasons or years.

During prolonged drought, when grasses wither and die, the pastoralists' grazing animals, namely cattle and sheep, may also die, while their browsing animals, goats and camels, are more likely to survive by eating the remaining woody plants. Browsing goats and camels can continue to provide milk, meat, and other products to the pastoralists during the drought period to ensure their survival until the next rains, when they can restock their cattle. For these pastoralists, the presence of woody plants in rangeland does not represent land degradation. On the contrary, such plants represent a vital food supply for the camels and goats on which the pastoralists may depend for their own survival.

In this context, the concept of overstocking also must be considered carefully. Pastoralists have frequently been criticized by outside observers for "keeping too many livestock," and this has been identified as a cause of degradation of plant communities on Sahelian rangelands. However, the case can be made that it is the variability of rainfall, not the number of animals, that determines the composition and health of the plant community on rangeland. Keeping what appears to be too many livestock during periods of relatively lush vegetation is part of a flexible overall survival strategy that pastoralists adopt to make it through unpredictable and difficult periods of low rainfall and sparse vegetation in anticipation of potentially high levels of mortality.

The use of grasslands for ruminant livestock grazing is the most sustainable and productive use of such land with respect to food production. While the potential for land degradation always exists in rangeland livestock systems, the alternatives, with regard to food production, may be even more destructive. When good grazing land is coopted for crop production, it restricts the grazing options of traditional herders. As a result, overstocking and overgrazing on the remaining grazing areas of reduced size accelerates the process of land degradation through poorly managed grazing. Time and again throughout the world, grazing lands traditionally used by pastoralists as dry season grazing have been annexed for irrigation schemes as a result of government policy or private entrepreneurial initiatives. Ironically, pastoralists are then frequently blamed for the resulting land degradation that occurs.

Impacts of Inappropriate Livestock Introductions

While livestock grazing can contribute to rangeland degradation, appropriate husbandry and informed management can minimize its environmental impact. Unfortunately, some of the most egregious cases of environmental degradation by domestic animals have been associated with animals turned loose to fend for themselves without any human management or husbandry at all. These situations have become so well known that they have contributed to a general bias against livestock with respect to the environment.

The age of European maritime exploration and mercantilism that began in the late 15th century created global opportunities for the dissemination of alien plant and animal species into new environments, either intentionally or unintentionally. The maintenance of adequate food supplies on extended ocean voyages was a logistical challenge for seafarers, and one partial solution to the problem was to set livestock free on island way stations where the animals could possibly fend for themselves, multiply, and be subsequently harvested for meat when ships passed by on future voyages. Goats and pigs were often the animals of choice, in recognition of their superior adaptability and prolificacy. The problem of course was that without natu-

ral predators and under favorable conditions of climate and vegetation, populations of these animals quickly expanded, and they overran the islands, wreaking ecological destruction by denuding the islands of vegetation and crowding out indigenous species of animals. This scenario was repeated in various venues for almost 350 years. The Portuguese released a small herd of goats on St. Helena Island in 1513; Captain Cook released goats at numerous locations in New Zealand and the Sandwich Islands (Hawaii) in the 1770s; and Admiral Perry released goats onto the Bonin Islands off Japan in 1853.

Yet even in these seemingly obvious cases of livestock destroying the environment, the situation was perhaps more complex than it first appears. Dunbar has critically assessed the putative role of goats in ecological destruction.[19] Among other examples, Dunbar examines the history of St. Helena island, an important way station in the south Atlantic for ships moving between Europe and the Far East around the Cape of Good Hope. Originally, the island was heavily forested when the Portuguese first deposited goats there. However, the trees on the island were quickly recognized as a valuable resource by mariners stopping for ship repairs and fuel on their long voyages. The cutting of trees on the island by sailors became commonplace, and eventually the island was denuded. Goats surely contributed to the deforestation by consuming new seedlings that sprouted before the young trees could establish themselves. Goats, however, did not destroy the forest. Their contribution was to prevent the regrowth of forests that had been decimated by human activity.

The goat is often cast as scapegoat when environmental degradation is observed and goats are present. However, goats are famous for their adaptability for surviving under harsh conditions. Often goats remain in degraded environments after the people and other animals primarily responsible for that degradation have abandoned the premises. The casual observer, arriving late on the scene, may draw the false conclusion that the goats are at fault, based on the simple circumstantial evidence that they are present. The eastern Mediterranean region, or Levant of ancient times, is an important example. After millennia of deforestation and continuous cultivation without fertilization, land in the region became so degraded that most types of cropping and the grazing of cattle became impossible. Peasants turned to goat herding because goats represented one of the few agricultural enterprises that such a degraded landscape would support. Goats are not primarily responsible for the degraded condition of the landscape observable today. Rather, goats are helping local people to eke out a livelihood on a landscape severely degraded by the careless management and shortsightedness of their ancestors. This is not to say that goats cannot contribute to further degradation if not properly managed. However, they are not primarily responsible for it.

Desertification

Desertification is the most extreme form of land degradation and occurs mainly in arid and semiarid environments, especially in regions adjacent to true deserts. Whereas less-extreme forms of land degradation are considered reversible through proper land management or corrective interventions, desertification implies irreversible damage to soil, rendering the landscape unusable for productive purposes. The terms *sandization* and *desertization* have also been used to describe the process of desertification. While desertification is often thought of as the process of deserts expanding by pushing outward, it may be more appropriate to think of deserts as being drawn outward beyond existing boundaries by mismanagement of adjacent lands.

The causes of desertification are usually multiple and complex. Direct causes can be "biotic," such as overgrazing and inappropriate agricultural practices, or "abiotic," as in the case of prolonged drought or climate change. The adverse effects of these direct causes are frequently exacerbated by misguided economic and development policies, lack of understanding of dry ecosystems and their use by local people, political expediency, and management practices aimed at short-term gains rather than sustainable use.

The Implications of Desertification

Desertification is an important global issue. It is estimated that the security and livelihoods of up to 650 million people living on desert margins are threatened by the process of desertification. In the context of food production, desertification, as the endpoint of land degradation, contributes permanently to the loss of land available for food production, either by livestock grazing or through crop cultivation. At present, cropland availability and cropland productivity are declining on a per capita basis worldwide. On a regional basis, this trend is particularly apparent in places where a large percentage of the available land is in arid and semiarid regions and population growth rates are high, notably in Africa and south Asia. Desertification is also costly from an environmental perspective, as complex ecosystems in arid and semiarid regions are destabilized and transformed, with a resultant loss of biodiversity.

The Scope of Desertification

Over the millennia, many places on the planet have been transformed from grassland or forest to desert, mostly as a result of climate change, sometimes as a result of the actions of human beings. The discovery of cave paintings in Algeria depicting pastoralists with their cattle, in what is now the heart of the Sahara desert, bear witness to the changes in landscape that have occurred over long periods. The paintings of pastoralists at Tassili-n-Ajjer date back approximately 7000 years. Also present at the site are paintings of hippopotami, suggesting a previous abundance of water in the region. These images reflect what was possible after the last Ice Age waned and brought a moist climate to North Africa.

In our own times, there are renewed concerns about the desertification process and its rate of advance. There is recognition that we are living in a period of notable climatic change, characterized by global warming and severe El Niño activity. These processes can destabilize existing rainfall patterns and

may increase aridity in already dry areas, particularly inland continental areas. In addition to concerns about climate change, the role of human agency in desertification has emerged as an equal or greater concern. Human population growth has proceeded at alarming rates in many areas at risk for desertification such as the African Sahel and the Rajasthan region of India. This has subjected arid and semiarid lands to excessive pressure and inappropriate use. Furthermore, the technological power of modern human society to transform such landscape in destructive ways has also increased. The use of extensive irrigation and mechanized tillage to convert semiarid grasslands into croplands, for instance, can speed the degradation of soils and lead to desertification if not properly managed.

The map in Figure 6-1 shows those areas of the world considered susceptible to desertification, based on geophysical and climatic factors usually associated with proximity to true deserts. This map also factors in human population density as a potential cause of desertification. The actual rate and risk of desertification in these areas will vary considerably depending on a number of social factors such as government policies, agricultural practices, and level of economic development in different countries and regions. Approximately 30% of the land surface area of the earth is in arid zones, including true desert. Some estimates suggest that up to an additional 6 to 15% of the earth's land surface may already be affected, to some degree, by the irreversible process of desertification. Areas considered to be most at risk for advancing desertification today include northwest China, Central and South Asia, and the African Sahel.

While desertification is a real concern, there has been considerable debate in recent years on just how severe or extensive the problem really is. A growing number of responsible scientists and policymakers believe that the problem has been exaggerated. This is due in part to the historic difficulty of obtaining and critically evaluating scientific data on a widely distributed global problem that occurs at multiple sites under very different and complex circumstances. Another reason has been an imprecise definition of the term *desertification* itself. For a long time, the definitions used failed to differentiate adequately between drought-induced changes in vegetative cover that are reversible with the return of rains and more-severe changes in landscape that are essentially irreversible. What is now identified and discussed as potentially reversible land degradation was, for much of the 1970s and 1980s, identified as desertification, which is now more specifically and restrictively defined as irreversible change.

The Role of Livestock in Desertification

For veterinarians interested in global issues of livestock production, this debate on the scope of desertification is of more than rhetorical concern. Livestock grazing, the predominant and traditional form of livelihood in arid and semiarid areas, is often identified, rightly or wrongly, as a major contributing factor to widespread desertification. Veterinarians should

Risk of Human Induced Desertification

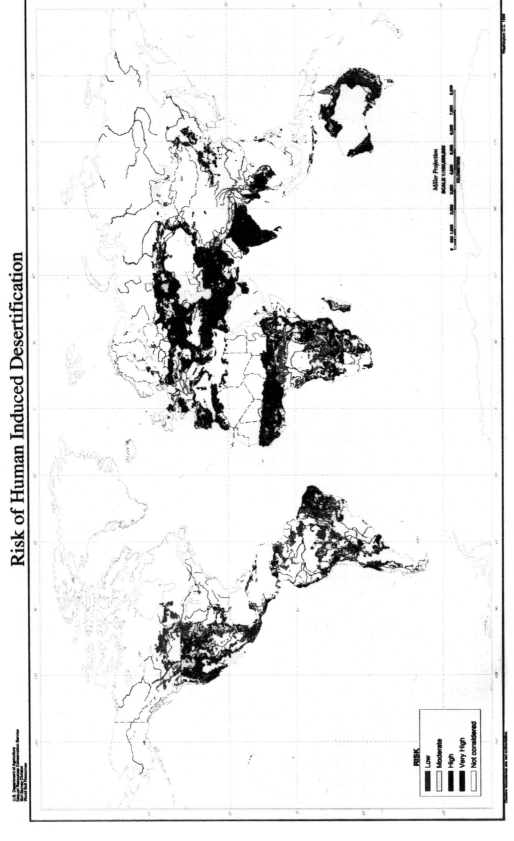

Figure 6–1 Regions of the world at risk for desertification. The map was prepared by determining the risk of desertification on the basis of soil characteristics and climate in combination with patterns of human population density. Where landscapes are fragile, increased population pressure can exacerbate the risk of desertification. Note the regions of high risk in the African Sahel, the Indian subcontinent, the Middle East, and the Mediterranean. (Map prepared by and provided courtesy of USDA Natural Resources Conservation Service, Soil Survey Division, World Soil Resources.)

be aware of some of the prevailing attitudes about livestock grazing in areas susceptible to desertification, the source of these attitudes, their appropriateness, and the challenges they present. It is instructive to look at livestock grazing in the African Sahel to better appreciate the situation.

The Sahel is the margin of arid and semiarid grassland that roughly defines the southern border of the Sahara desert. It stretches across the continent from Mauritania and Senegal in the west to Ethiopia and Somalia in the east. Historically, this has been a region of pastoralist herders, with livestock grazing being the most suitably productive use of this land, given the climate, rainfall, and vegetation. Even livestock grazing, however, is a risky proposition. The Sahel is characterized by extreme year-to-year fluctuation in rainfall that can cause enormous changes in the character of the environment, with marked change in the amount of vegetative cover, as shown in the series of photographs in Figure 6-2.

The desert margin is not defined by a fixed, sharp-edged border, but rather, by a dynamically shifting front. While vegetation recedes along that front during periods of drought, the vegetation is resilient, and the loss of vegetation is not permanent. During subsequent periods of rainfall, vegetation returns, and the leading front of the desert recedes. This pattern is clearly shown in Figure 6-3. During the first interval, between 1982 and 1984, the desert edge appears to have advanced southward approximately 240 km (150 miles) across the width of the continent. However, by 1985 after only 1 year of rain, the desert edge had essentially retreated back to its original position, renewing approximately 724,000 km² of plant cover.[41]

These extensive and dramatic changes in vegetation occur in response to abiotic stimuli, namely variable rainfall or long-term climate change, largely independent of the influence of human activity. Paleoclimatological data suggest that there long have been highly variable cyclical fluctuations in climate in the Sahel, with intermittent wet and dry periods ranging from 20 to 270 years in length. In the face of this climatic uncertainty, indigenous people in the Sahel evolved livestock production strategies based on long experience with unpredictable rainfall, variable vegetation, and the risk of prolonged drought that have allowed them to survive. Extensive grazing of mixed herds emerged as the most rational productive use of grasslands under semiarid and arid conditions. The ability of pastoral cultures to adapt successfully to the harsh environment of the Sahel through mixed livestock grazing is testimony to their understanding of the complexity, limits, and potential of that ecosystem.

Social transformations in the Sahel in the last 40 years have, in many ways, caused more lasting and dramatic perturbations for pastoralists than has climate change and have contributed to the perception that livestock grazing is a major cause of desertification. The modern period of drought, beginning in the mid-1960s, roughly coincides with the end of colonialism and the emergence of independent African states. Many emerging nations embraced the concept of modernization and wel-

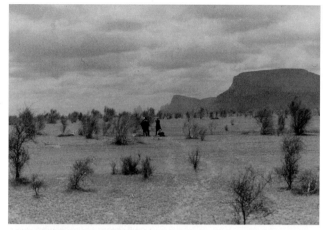

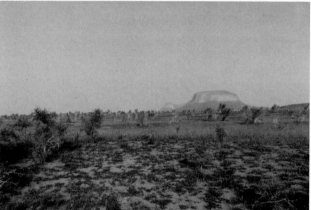

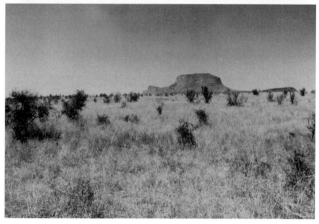

Figure 6-2. There is inherent resiliency in dry land vegetation. This series of photos shows a steady increase in vegetative cover over the period 1986 (*top*), 1987 (*middle*), and 1988 (*bottom*) at a site 3 km north of the town of Hombori, in Mali. All photos were taken in October of their respective years. The 1986 photo shows the vegetative barrenness that persisted for some time after the severe drought of 1984. However, by 1988, dense grass cover is evident. The casual observer visiting once in 1986 might erroneously assume that desertification had occurred. Total annual rainfall at this site in the drought year of 1984 was 152 mm. In 1986 it was 232 mm; in 1987 it was 218 mm; and in 1988, 302 mm. (Photos courtesy of Dr. Pierre H. Y. Hiernaux, International Livestock Research Institute, Niamey, Republic of Niger)

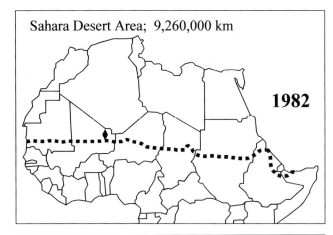

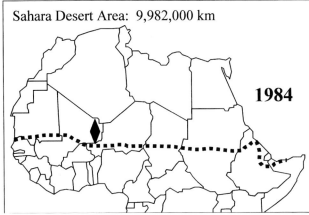

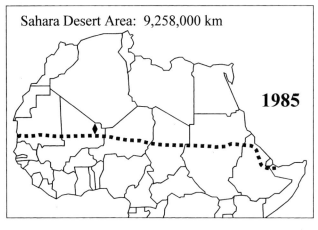

Figure 6-3. These schematic maps illustrate the dramatic shifts that occur in the Sahelian region as a result of rainfall, indicating the dynamic nature of the desert border. The *dotted line* on each map represents the northern boundary of vegetation for each year shown, which is also the southern boundary of the Sahara desert. El Niño-associated drought was severe in the Sahel region in 1984 and was associated with a marked recession southward of vegetation, compared with the situation in 1982. However, as the 1985 photo shows, subsequent rain supported a substantial northward return of the vegetation cover. The southern border of Algeria is used as a reference point to visualize the south/north movement of the vegetation zone, denoted by the *diamond-shaped marker*. The shift represented between 1984 and 1985 is 110 km. This shift of the vegetation zone northward reduced the area of the Sahara desert by 724,000 km². (From data in Tucker CJ, Dregne HE, Newcomb WW. Expansion and contraction of the Sahara desert from 1980 to 1990. Science 1991;253:299-302.).

comed foreign aid and technical input to support it. Many new governments began to look at grasslands with an eye toward their agricultural potential, misperceiving the appropriateness and high productivity of traditional livestock grazing. Regrettably, pastoralism and pastoralists were identified as the antithesis of modernity. Schemes to settle pastoralists and have them take up crop cultivation became popular, and when pastoralists resisted, it reinforced the perception that they were backward thinking and uncooperative.

Newly elected governments favored agricultural schemes over livestock for a number of reasons. Cash crops for export could earn these young and cash-poor countries much-needed foreign currency. Expanding urban populations required increasing amounts of food in the form of grain and, western donors, impressed by the success of the Green Revolution in Asia, encouraged the development of new agricultural schemes using irrigation and improved seeds and offered foreign aid for implementation.

Agricultural development causes dislocation of traditional herders and contributes to the perception that livestock are degrading the environment. Rangelands converted to cropland become unavailable to livestock, and pastoralists are thus limited to decreased grazing areas. The risk of overgrazing on reduced land areas is then increased. Frequently, the rangelands that are converted to crop production are the same rangelands that pastoral cultures depend on in dry periods for emergency feed supplies for their livestock. This represents a double jeopardy. When dry periods do come, people are deprived of food on two counts-the crops fail, and the animals that previously survived by accessing the land are no longer available either.

Settlement schemes may have adverse consequences as well. By encouraging pastoralists to become agropastoralists and establish sedentary bases, traditional grazing patterns can be disrupted. Herders may move their livestock over a reduced range in the periphery of settled villages, once again contributing to focal overgrazing detrimental to vegetation and soil. A similar phenomenon can occur when governments or aid agencies drill wells or boreholes to provide water for people and livestock in semiarid regions during dry periods. Herders may respond to the new water supply by increasing stock numbers and restricting their range of movement, leading in some cases to overstocking and overgrazing in the vicinity of boreholes. From a veterinary perspective, these wells can also serve as point sources for disease spread, as cattle increasingly concentrate in the area around the well and augment the risk of transmitting infectious agents through saliva, feces, or direct contact.

Thus, it would appear that livestock can potentially contribute to the desertification process but do so primarily when traditional patterns of livestock management are disrupted by the introduction of nontraditional uses of dry rangelands, a modern phenomenon driven largely by expanding human populations and the impetus for economic development. Dodd has reviewed the literature concerning animal impact on different types of rangeland in Africa.[18] He observes that very few studies effectively separate the impact of domestic grazing from weather impacts in their analyses. Similarly, few studies convincingly distinguish short-term and long-term effects. He concluded that there was no scientific evidence that nomadic or even commercial use of domestic livestock causes irreversible changes in range vegetation away from watering points and habitations.

Clearly, there is a need for further, well-defined research to accurately assess the complex relationship of livestock grazing on the viability and productivity of dry lands and to better understand pastoral grazing systems themselves. From a policy perspective, the appropriateness of traditional grazing practices in many dryland regions must receive greater acknowledgment, and the complex threats that distort those traditional practices must be recognized. According to de Haan et al.,[17] several objectives need to be achieved to ensure a future role for pastoralists in the stewardship and productive use of drylands through livestock grazing:

- Halt the buildup of further human pressure in arid zones

- Ensure that external interventions take into account the nonequilibrium status of pastoral systems in arid zones and enhance, rather than restrict, flexibility and mobility in those systems

- Strengthen traditional pastoral institutions and resource management practices by encouraging pastoralist associations, devolving more administrative responsibility to local groups, clarifying resource user rights, and creating reliable mechanisms for conflict resolution

- Identify effective drought management policies that encourage and facilitate early destocking in the face of drought, such as credit and savings schemes and improvements in marketing of livestock

- Develop incentives for sustainable rangeland use such as grazing fees, full cost recovery for water supply improvements and animal health care, and the removal of price supports and subsidies for competing agricultural activities that encroach on grazing land

Deforestation

The clearing of forests as a human activity is not new. There is evidence that inhabitants of New Guinea removed trees by fire, felling, and the ringing of bark to facilitate growth of yams, taro, and bananas as long as 30,000 years ago. In Britain, following the last Ice Age 12,000 years ago, people cleared small areas of forest by fire to promote secondary forage growth to attract red deer for hunting.[36] Most of the original forest in Europe, North Africa, and the Middle East was cleared centuries ago. Some Caribbean islands, such as Cuba, Haiti, and Barbados, were completely deforested to clear land for sugar cane

plantations during colonial times. The early history of the United States is closely tied to deforestation. Up to 85% of original New England forest was cut by European settlers for agricultural and timbering purposes by the mid-19th century. So why has deforestation become such a critical social and environmental issue in our own lifetime?

Importance of Forests

There are important and valid reasons why the loss of forests is currently perceived as a crisis. In our scientific age, we have a greater awareness and understanding of the many important roles that intact forests play in maintaining the stability of the global ecosystem, in supporting diversity of life on Earth, and in providing goods and services for human use. These varied roles include

- Conversion of solar energy into biomass. Forests act as a sink or reservoir for much of the planet's cycling carbon. The world's tropical forests store 46% of the world's living terrestrial carbon supply, while their soils store 11%.

- Buffering against global warming. Forests withdraw the greenhouse gas carbon dioxide from the atmosphere for production of sugars through the photosynthetic process. Photosynthesis converts water and carbon dioxide to carbohydrates and returns oxygen to the atmosphere.

- Regulation of climate. Forests help to maintain regional rainfall patterns by cycling moisture from vegetation to the air through transpiration.

- Water conservation. Forests control runoff and promote the recharging of aquifers. Forest vegetation structure has evolved to minimize the deleterious effects of intense rainfall, facilitating the diffusion, dispersion, trapping, and resorption of water.

- Soil conservation. Forests bind soil with roots, and by diffusion and absorption of heavy rainfall, they reduce flooding and subsequent soil erosion. In a study in Ghana, conversion of savanna forest to agricultural use increased soil erosion rates from 1 ton per hectare to 100 tons per hectare

- Support of biodiversity. It is estimated that tropical rainforests contain 50% of the earth's plant and animal species, known and yet to be known.

- Storehouse of useful resources. Forests contain numerous and diverse extractable and renewable materials for use by human society, including rubber, chicle, myriad fruits and nuts, oils, traditional medicines, and building materials, including timber and vegetable fibers, to name but a few.

- Source of hidden treasures. Forests contain yet-to-be-discovered chemicals and compounds with potential application in medicine and industry including among others, antibacterial agents, antiprotozoal agents, antineoplastic agents, analgesics, and various resins, gums, and oils.

Furthermore, society has awakened to the fact that the rate and scope of forest destruction have increased dramatically in our own time, particularly in the last half of the 20th century. This realization has been aided by modern satellite technology that allows global surveillance and visual representation of specific vegetation patterns over time. Due to differences in the various assessment technologies used, as well as to differences in definition of forest by various agencies and governments carrying out studies, there is still a lack of quantitative precision regarding the exact extent of forest loss. Nevertheless, the trends are indisputably and alarmingly clear. Forests are disappearing at an unprecedented rate. This is especially, but not exclusively, true for tropical rainforests in developing countries.

It is estimated that in prehistoric times, the tropical forest belt, including both moist and dry forest types, covered about 25 million km^2 of Earth. Currently, the tropical forest belt has been reduced to approximately 18 million km^2, and the estimate of moist, tropical rainforest cover is between 7.5 and 8 million km^2. About half of all remaining tropical rainforest is contained within only four countries—Brazil, Peru, the Democratic Republic of Congo, and Indonesia, none of which has historically identified forest conservation as a high national priority.

Rates of forest loss vary between regions. From 1980 and 1990, worldwide loss of woodlands, was 2% of the world's wooded land area. However, the loss in developed countries, where mostly temperate forests prevail, averaged only 0.04%, while in developing countries, where moist tropical rainforest prevails, the average was 3.6%. When the analysis is limited to natural forests only, excluding plantations and other non-forest woodlands, the average total loss in developing countries, located mainly in Asia, Africa, and Latin America, was 8% of total forest area.[45] As shown in Figure 6-4, the rates of forest loss for each continent vary considerably, but all share the unfortunate pattern of steadily increasing from 1960 to 1990. It is estimated that tropical deforestation probably exceeded 130,000 km^2 a year in 2000.

At current rates of tropical rainforest removal, it is projected that 90% of the remaining forest could be lost in less than 40 years, well within the lifetime of many readers of this book. Temperate forests continue to remain susceptible to threats from air pollution, acid rain, uncontrolled fire, and careless commercial exploitation. However, it is the breakneck speed of tropical rainforest devastation and the potential biological, environmental, and economic losses associated with rainforest destruction that have made rainforests the principal focus of forest conservation awareness in our time.

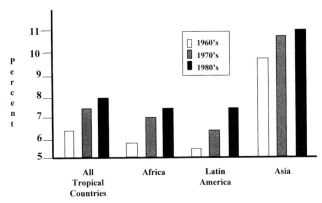

Figure 6-4.   Estimated rate of tropical deforestation by continent and decade between 1960 and 1990. (Adapted from World Resources Institute. World Resources 1996-97. London: Oxford University Press, 1997.)

Causes of Deforestation

Temperate forests are, in general, not currently being subjected to the same deforestation pressures that are occurring in the tropical regions. However, they are not immune from exploitation in the future, particularly when one considers the rate at which tropical forests are currently being consumed. The current financial crisis in Russia, for example, could stimulate a major increase in cutting of the vast Siberian forest reserves, as the authorities look for ways to generate foreign exchange income to meet their international debt obligations. Meanwhile, extensive forest fires in far eastern Siberia in 1998 have destroyed up to 11,700 km^2 of valuable forest. The government was unable to control them for months because of lack of financial resources to mount an effective fire-fighting effort. Fires, either intentionally set to clearing agricultural land or occurring naturally due to lightning, have become a growing concern in recent years, as the number and size of such fires increases. In addition to the direct, adverse effects on the forest and its inhabitants, large fires, as occurred in Indonesia in 1998, produce serious air pollution, contribute to global warming, and can have a detrimental effect on human health.

Temperate forests are also subject to destructive forces other than direct cutting. Most notably, there has been serious forest degradation in recent years in northern coniferous forests across North America, Europe, and Asia, strongly associated with air pollution. Acid rain and increased ozone levels have been strongly linked to declining forest health. Widespread yellowing and loss of needles on coniferous trees was first noticed in Germany in the 1970s. By the 1980s the pattern was widespread in central Europe, and similar debilitation was noted in the spruce trees of New England. Trees weakened by the effects of acid rain and ozone have increased susceptibility to pests and disease, and degradation of temperate forests has been widespread in the last two decades.

As the rainforests are located primarily in developing countries in tropical regions, they are subject to a set of demographic, economic and political forces that exert much greater influence on forest use than is currently occurring in the developed countries of the temperate regions. These forces include rapidly growing human populations, limited economic opportunity, sizable foreign debts, oligarchic traditions of political power and economic control, and lapses in the rule of law, which, through corruption and cronyism, allow unregulated destruction of forest resources. For instance, in the face of the political instability that has confronted Indonesia since the fall of Suharto in 1998, forest profiteering is running rampant in that country, with brazen illegal logging now commonplace in the country's national parks.[32] Under such conditions, tropical rainforests are too often perceived as a commodity to be exploited for political advantage and short-term financial gain, rather than as a valuable resource to be managed for long-term sustainability and continued prosperity.

Ultimately, the underlying causes of contemporary tropical deforestation are poor stewardship, inappropriate policies, and inattention to significant social and economic problems whose roots are outside the forest sector. How these various factors affect forest loss can be appreciated by examining different categories of forest use.

Forest As an Instrument of Social Policy Forests have been used by governments to address a number of social problems. These include various efforts to

- Relieve regional overpopulation, especially in urban areas, by encouraging rural migration

- Encourage settlement of underpopulated areas of a nation for security or development purposes, as has occurred in Indonesia

- Respond to calls for land ownership by the rural poor by opening up forest land for settlement rather than appropriating agricultural land held by a powerful and influential elite, as frequently happens in Latin America

- Compensate for lack of employment opportunities in the economy at large

To accomplish these objectives, forest land is offered by government for settlement and agricultural development, including cattle ranching. This has rarely turned out to be an adequate or even appropriate policy solution for the problems that are intended to be addressed. The main obstacle to small-scale agricultural development and cattle ranching in most rainforest areas is that it is not sustainable. The soils will not support it. About 70% of moist tropical rainforests sit on old, weathered, acidic, and infertile soils from which minerals have been leached. Rainforest vegetation compensates for nutrient-deficient soil by various adaptations, including a high percentage of above-ground root system networks or root mats that draw nutrients from the forest floor humus litter with the aid of mycorrhizal fungi. Whereas in temperate zone forests, minerals are more evenly distributed between the vegetation and the soil bank, in the tropics, minerals are mostly in the

plants. In a Venezuelan study, for example, an assessment of calcium found 3.3% in leaves, 62.2% in wood, 14% in roots, 3.1% in litter, and only 17.4% in soil.

Indigenous people in rainforest regions understand this constraint of soil infertility with regard to agricultural productivity. This knowledge helps to explain the traditional slash-and-burn, or swidden, form of agriculture that has prevailed in tropical forest systems. Land for cultivation is prepared in the dry season. Rather than removing the forest vegetation from the cleared land, it is cut and burned in situ, so that the minerals stored in the vegetation are returned to the soil in the form of ash. Even with this fundamental effort at soil enrichment, cultivation on a given plot of land falls off dramatically by the second or third year, and the plots are often abandoned for new ones by about the fifth year of cultivation.

When human populations are low and pressures on the forest from human encroachment are not excessive, slash-and-burn agriculture, practiced on small, frequently shifted plots, produces little long-lasting ecological damage. Clearance and abandonment of small agricultural plots mimics small-scale natural forest disturbances such as the falling of a mature tree during a severe rainstorm. The event is followed by a healthy ecological succession of flora through the advancing regeneration of preexisting seedlings and saplings and by vegetative sprouting of stem bases and roots. Furthermore, in traditional swidden agriculture, plots are usually cultivated with multiple root, vegetable, and tree crops. This polyculture system is more forgiving to soil than crop monoculture. It reduces weeds and reduces pests by creating habitat for pest predators.

The point of most government-sponsored settlement schemes, however, is not shifting cultivation, but permanent settlement. On the thin, nutrient-poor soils of the rainforest, this is a difficult challenge. Early settlement initiatives in the Amazon basin of Brazil are instructive in this regard. Not long after the Transamazon highway was begun, the government, hoping to encourage poor families from the northeast to resettle in the interior, offered incentives for settlers to establish small farms and plant upland rice in the Amazon Basin. The project turned out to be ill conceived and was plagued by difficulties. Rice production required too many external inputs in the form of fertilizer, herbicide, and insecticide that farmers could not afford or obtain. The rice seed distributed was not appropriate, as the stalks collapsed under heavy tropical rain prior to harvest. Ground doves, rats, soil erosion, and fungal rot plagued farmers and reduced yields. Farms were placed near the roadside, and the roadside plantings facilitated rapid spread of agricultural pests, the road serving as a pest corridor. As farms failed, they were often bought up by land consolidators who would convert the cleared land to cattle ranching or simply hold the land for speculation.

Forest As a Source of Foreign Exchange and Investment With the world economy expanding as it has in the past two decades, demand for wood products on world markets has been high, and developed countries have increasingly looked to the developing world as a source of lumber for construction and pulp for plywood and paper products. The developing countries on their part, often strapped with high debt from foreign loans, have welcomed foreign investment and corporate participation in logging and have promoted the sale of logs and timber in foreign markets as a means of earning much-needed foreign exchange. As much of the tropical rainforest in developing countries is owned by governments, they have been able to offer it for sale. With money to be made and government controlling the resources, the situation has lent itself to considerable graft and cronyism in the distribution of logging rights. Many retired politicians and generals in numerous countries have been awarded logging concessions. These people often have little knowledge or interest in proper forestry management and are motivated primarily by realization of a quick profit. Under such circumstances, management of forest resources for sustainable production has not been a high priority. Furthermore, being influential with government they are able to avoid numerous taxes and duties on forest products, thus depriving the government of the full value of their forest resources. For example, in the Philippines, in 1987, the government received only one sixth of the full resource value of the 3 million cubic meters of timber harvested that year, a harvest valued in excess of $250 million.

Often, there is insufficient technical expertise within government to properly manage and regulate forests. There may be few properly trained foresters, and they may lack sufficient resources and transportation to monitor and manage logging operations properly. Wasteful logging practices are well documented. Loggers may select and cut only 10% of the timber in an area, focusing on mature trees. Yet in the process, they may inadvertently destroy up to 50% of the remaining trees, including younger stock of the very species they are selectively logging. In addition, many developing countries, in an effort to promote employment and economic activity within the country, have established policies that require processing raw timber into lumber at domestic sawmills before export. Unfortunately, this frequently adds to the wastage of the timber resource, as the sawmill technology for maximizing yields from raw timber during cutting is not often available in local sawmills. Foreign buyers actually prefer to receive raw timber to be processed after delivery.

Mining is another activity with considerable foreign exchange earning potential. The Amazon Basin contains deposits of copper, tin, nickel, bauxite, manganese, iron, and, notably, gold, and the Amazon rainforest has become a major center of mining activity in recent years. The environmental and health consequences of this activity are significant. For example, crude or pig iron is extracted from ore at the site of iron mining through a smelting process that requires enormous amounts of fuel wood, producing heavy pressure for deforestation around mining sites. Gold mining has an even more pervasive impact. Metallic mercury is used to aggregate gold particles for extraction from the crude ore. At various stages of ore processing, the mercury is released into either the air, soil or water. Through oxidative processes, it reacts to become methylated mercury, which is bioactive and toxic and becomes in-

creasingly concentrated in living tissues as it progresses up the food chain, including, ultimately, humans. Concentrations of mercury in human urine samples taken from people in and around gold mines in Amazonia have reached as high as 840 parts per billion, when 10 ppb is considered normal. People are exposed primarily through inhalation or by eating contaminated fish or other tainted animals. Mercury is present in wood, so forest burning for any reason, if extensive, can contribute significant amounts to the atmosphere.

Mercury pollution has emerged as a major public health and pollution issue in Brazil. Organic mercurials are teratogenic and carcinogenic and also produce neurological disturbances. In January 1998, medical investigators reported the first cases of Minamata disease among human inhabitants of the Amazonian Basin, linking the cases to chronic consumption of fish taken from the rivers. Minamata disease, a neurological form of mercury poisoning, is named after Minamata Bay in Japan, where, in the 1950s and 1960s, thousands of people, mostly fishermen, became ill because of contamination of the bay and its fish as a result of mercury dumping by a large, local plastics-manufacturing plant. Animals are at risk as well. One of the first indications of Minamata disease in Japan was abnormal behavior in domestic cats, which danced weirdly and threw themselves into the bay.

Forest As a Resource for the Poor Forests are a critical asset for human survival in developing countries, where many people live in rural areas and have low incomes and few economic prospects. Many such people depend on subsistence agriculture and gleaning natural resources for survival. In addition to the clearing of forest land for cropping, an important pressure on forests by the rural poor is the harvesting of fuel wood for cooking and, in cooler, high altitude regions, for heating. For people in developed countries, who have immediate access to energy for cooking or heating by the flick of a switch, the extent to which the world's rural poor depend on fuel wood, the intensity of the effort they expend to procure it, and the scope of the environmental impact of fuel wood gathering, are largely unrecognized. Only 1% of total energy consumption in developed countries comes from fuel wood, whereas the average share of total energy provided by fuel wood in developing countries is 26%. This varies considerably by region, with Africa deriving 52% of its energy from fuel wood, Asia, 22%, and Latin America 20%.

Fuel wood supplies are becoming scarce in certain regions, particularly dry woodland regions where vegetation is less dense to begin with. Villagers, particularly women and children, spend increasing portions of each day ranging farther from their homes in search of fuel wood, often at the expense of other important daily tasks and responsibilities (Fig. 6-5). In some countries, it takes up to 300 person-days of work to supply the annual fuel wood needs of a single family. The pressures on existing woodlands are enormous, and the risk of woodland degradation high. Based on projections developed in 1987, it was estimated that by the year 2000, more than 1871 million people in Asia, 512 million in Latin America, 535

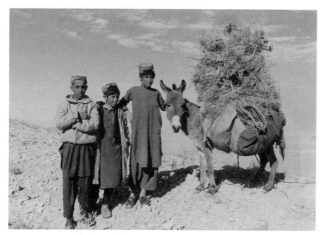

Figure 6-5. School-aged boys spend their days collecting and transporting fuel wood by donkey in a virtually treeless region of western Pakistan. In arid and semiarid regions of the world, people, especially women and children, spend ever-increasing amounts of time collecting fuel wood for cooking. As fuel wood resources grow scarcer and gatherers have to range farther afield, the proportion of the day spent in this activity increases at the expense of other important and more rewarding human endeavors. (Photo by Dr. David M. Sherman)

million in sub-Saharan Africa, and 268 million in the Near East and North Africa would be affected by fuel wood shortages. The implications for forest and woodland conservation are enormous.

Cattle Ranching and Forest Loss

In recent years, there has been much public outcry concerning the destruction of tropical rainforest for the purpose of raising cattle. Sometimes the criticism is so strident that one is left with the impression that cattle ranching is the principal cause of forest loss worldwide. This is far from the case. Cattle ranching is but one factor in the story of global deforestation. Cattle raising has been an important cause of forest loss on a regional basis, primarily in Latin America, where, in particular countries such as Costa Rica and Brazil, it has had significant social and environmental impact. However, elsewhere in the world, other primary causes of forest loss predominate, notably commercial logging and crop agriculture. The relative significance of different causes of tropical deforestation in South America, Asia, and Africa is given in Table 6-6.

The Spanish brought cattle to the New World in the 16th century, so cattle ranching per se is not a new phenomenon in Latin America. However, early efforts took advantage of existing grasslands and brushlands for grazing. Some forest clearing took place in colonial times, but it was usually dry forest. The clearing of rainforest for cattle ranching in Latin America began in earnest in the mid-20th century, stimulated by the interest of foreign investors, the support of bilateral aid agencies, and the aspirations for economic development of national governments.

The results have been dramatic in terms of the transformation of landscape. In Central America since 1950, about 100,000 km² of tropical forest has been cleared, or 35% of the total forested area of 290,000 km². Between 1950 and 1980, about 60% of lowland forests had been felled for agriculture and pasture. Between 1950 and 1992, cattle pastures increased from 30,000 to 95,000 km², and cattle numbers doubled from 4.2 to 9.6 million head. In the Amazon Basin of Brazil, overall loss of Amazon forest since the 1960s is about 10%, with an annual ongoing rate of loss of 0.4%, though this varies from state to state.

Despite initial expectations, beef cattle ranching in cleared rainforests has not been a great economic success, largely because most rainforest soils will not support pastures for long enough periods to make cattle ranching profitable. In addition, policies that were established to encourage cattle ranching were often ill conceived and economically short-sighted or put political considerations before planning objectives. The situations in Brazil and Costa Rica are illustrative.

Cattle Ranching in Brazil The construction of the futuristic capital city of Brasilia in the late 1950s symbolized Brazil's commitment to modernization and economic development. In its efforts to stimulate such development, the government also initiated construction of the Transamazonian Highway in 1958, to provide a vital link for transportation and commerce in the physically vast nation. The road has become the defin-

Table 6-6 Differences in Rates and Causes of Deforestation on Different Continents, 1980–1990						
Region	**Annual Loss of Forest Area (km²)**	**Annual Rate of Change (%)**	**Remaining Forest Area (km²)**	**Causes of Deforestation (% of total)**		
				Cropping	**Livestock ᵃ**	**Logging**
Latin America	19,000	0.4	4,540,000	25	44-70	10
Africa	5,000	0.5	860,000	55-60	Negligible	20
Asia	22,000	1.1	1,770,000	70	Negligible	20

ᵃCattle ranching is a significant cause of deforestation only in Latin America.

Adapted from de Haan C, Steinfeld H, Blackburn H. Livestock and the Environment: Finding a Balance. Commission of the European Communities, 1997.

ing force in the transformation of the rainforest landscape. During the first 20 years of the existence of the highway, about 2 million people entered previously forested regions of Brazil, and in the same period, 5 million cattle were introduced.

Starting about 1966, the Brazilian government offered owners of large cattle ranches generous tax breaks and subsidies, encouraging a small number of wealthy individuals to establish vast cattle ranches within Amazonia. As a result, more than 600 cattle ranches, each in excess of 20,000 ha (49,420 acres) were subsidized by government in the form of long-term loans, tax credits against investment costs, tax holidays, and write-offs. Yet, despite this largesse, the ranches were uneconomical, losing more than half their invested capital within 15 years. The beef derived from these subsidized ranches averaged only 9% of the projected offtake. Rather than serving as productive elements in the Brazilian economy, most ranches served as tax shelters for a privileged, well-to-do few. The Brazilian government has since suspended incentives for new cattle ranches in Amazonian forests, but not before the initial subsidy program cost the treasury more than $2.5 billion in lost income.[37]

Cattle ranching attracted not only the wealthy elite. Many factors favored cattle ranching, even when it was economically unsound in the long term. The building of roads into the rainforest raised the value of land and fueled land speculation. A high rate of inflation, which was an important factor in the Brazilian economy in the 1980s, also made real estate investment attractive. Forestland clearing to indicate productive use was required as a condition of title in Brazil, and many speculators and investors turned to ranching as an attractive startup venture because it is not labor intensive and requires few inputs once the land was cleared. Clearing the land for ranching also discouraged squatters, mainly the landless poor looking to establish cultivation plots, and who were more likely to invade forested areas. In Brazil, about 70% of deforested areas are converted to ranching, at least initially. Currently, about 10 million hectares or 100,000 km^2 of what was formerly Amazon rainforest has been occupied by cattle ranches.

Despite this extensive conversion of forestland to cattle ranches, the Amazon region has never produced more than 5% of total beef output in Brazil, and this has not been destined for export. The grasslands of the Mato Grosso, the traditional site of cattle production in Brazil, continue to provide most of the beef produced in the country for both domestic consumption and export. While there has been much talk of the so-called Hamburger Connection, in which U.S. interests promote cattle production in Latin America to ensure cheap ground beef prices in the United States, involvement of Brazil in such a connection has been marginal. There is no importation of fresh, frozen or chilled beef from Brazil into the United States because Brazil is not free of foot and mouth disease, and therefore, such imports are prohibited by the U.S. Department of Agriculture (USDA). There is a limited amount of canned and other processed beef products from Brazil, but these are trivial, as Brazil is not included in the USDA list of the top 35 beef importers into the United States.

Cattle ranching in the Amazon rainforest has not served the goal of economic development well. That the Brazilian government has slowed its schedule for development of the Amazon Basin in the 1990s and removed new subsidies for large-scale cattle ranching bear testimony to this view. Ranching has not been sustainable or profitable and, in some cases, has actually displaced more profitable and sustainable uses of forest. Studies in the state of Acre demonstrated that because of poor pasture quality and low carrying capacity, revenue from uncut forest could yield four times more revenue from wild rubber and Brazil nuts on a per hectare basis than from cattle ranching.[37]

Cattle Ranching in Costa Rica   Costa Rica is a small Central American nation of dazzling natural beauty. Packed into a country about four-fifths the size of West Virginia are beautiful coastlines on two oceans, mist-covered mountains, active volcanoes, lush rainforests, rushing rivers punctuated by waterfalls, colorfully bloomed dry forests, fertile valleys, and enormous biological diversity. More species of land birds breed in tiny Costa Rica than in all the United States and Canada combined, and it is estimated that as much as 5% of all the world's plant and animal species reside in this small country.

Costa Rica was part of the Spanish colonial kingdom of Guatemala and became an independent republic in 1831. Today, the country is a constitutionally based, participatory democracy with strong social institutions. It is distinguished by the absence of a standing army and, in recent years, by its recognition of the intrinsic value of its natural resources and their ecological significance, a recognition expressed through environmental and conservation policies being implemented at the national level. Nevertheless, the Spanish colonial experience has left its legacy in Costa Rica in important ways, including a strong identification with cattle raising and the existence of a small, wealthy, land-owning elite that holds title to much of the nation's agricultural land. The top 1% of farm owners own one quarter of the nation's agricultural land, while the bottom 50% of landowners own about 3% of the land. Approximately 70% of the country's rural population is landless.

In the 1960s and 1970s, when beef prices were high, Costa Rica, with strong support and encouragement from U.S. agribusiness interests, embarked on a large-scale program to increase beef production for export. This was the most direct example of the so-called Hamburger Connection, in which Latin American cattle production was promoted for the U.S. consumer market. The offer of low-interest loans stimulated a rush to cattle ranching. Traditionally limited to the dry, northwestern province of Guanacaste since colonial times, land clearing for pasture began in earnest in other parts of the country, notably the Atlantic lowlands and the Pacific southwest. Forest clearing on the steep slopes of the Pacific southwest for cattle pasture has caused serious flooding problems in the adjacent lowlands. The cattle ranching mania continued into the 1980s. Between 1981 and 1985 Costa Rica felled forest at the rate of 3.9%. By 1983 about 83% of its forest had been felled, much of it to make way for export beef production, and today, about 70% of the deforested land in Costa Rica is cattle pasture.

Cattle ranching in Costa Rica has had environmental and social costs. In addition to the flooding problems already mentioned, the clearing of rainforest in Costa Rica represents a serious loss of biodiversity. This includes the potential loss of plant and animal species of tremendous commercial potential including, for example, fungi in forest leaf litter with pharmaceutical potential as antiprotozoal agents or poison dart frogs whose poison structure serves as the basis for analgesics more potent than morphine but without the side effects. On the social side, consolidation of land for cattle ranches owned by a handful of landowners has displaced many landless peasants in rural areas. Ranching offers few employment opportunities, and subsistence farming or extraction of forest resources become unavailable to the rural poor when the land is cleared and fenced for cattle.

Even though Costa Rica has become the largest cattle exporter in Latin America, cattle export has never accounted for more than 9% of Costa Rica's total export earnings, always running behind coffee and bananas, the main crop exports. While Costa Rica remains an agriculturally based economy, revenue from tourism has been steadily increasing in recent years, and ecotourism has become a cornerstone of Costa Rica's economic future. The government and, to a great extent, the citizens have come to recognize the tremendous economic potential of the country's natural beauty and its biological richness. A new conservation ethic is building in the nation, evidenced in the attitudes of the schoolchildren, who speak proudly about their forests, and the government, which has been actively developing a nationwide system of parks, preserves, and protected lands. Most telling perhaps, is the situation in Guanacaste, the traditional home of cattle ranching, where dry forests were cleared centuries past to make way for cattle ranches. Some landowners whose families have been ranching in Guanacaste for generations, are selling their cattle and converting their ranches to ecotourism sites. There is even a large-scale effort at restoration ecology, to reconvert cattle pasture back to dry tropical forest (see sidebar "Restoration Ecology in Action")

Restoration Ecology in Action: Guanacaste Conservation Area, Costa Rica

In prehistoric times, approximately half the forest cover in Central America was dry tropical forest and half was moist tropical rainforest. When the Spaniards came to the New World five centuries ago and began colonization, dry forest areas were prime targets for land clearance. The dry forests, which predominated on the lower Pacific coastal plains of Mesoamerica, were less dense and more accessible than the inland, elevated, mountain rainforests and were composed mostly of deciduous trees. Furthermore, the Pacific coastal climate included a long dry season of up to 6 months, which made it particularly easy to clear the deciduous forests by burning. By the end of the 20th century, dry forests of Central America, which once covered more than 552,110 km², were reduced to about 2% of that area.

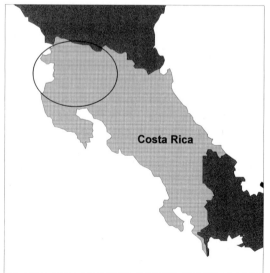

Costa Rica

In the 1970s and early 1980s, Costa Rica depended heavily on cash crops and cattle for foreign exchange earnings to settle international debts. However, in the 1990s, Costa Rica recognized that its natural beauty and biological richness are its greatest economic assets. The country has embarked on an extensive and much heralded program of national conservation that firmly links environmentalism with economic development. The program focuses on protection of habitat in a national system of parks and reserves, preservation of biodiversity, and encouragement of ecotourism. This innovative program has been implemented through a series of strong legislative initiatives and the cultivation of public/private partnerships that include national and foreign governments, university consortia such as the Organization for Tropical Studies (http://www.ots.duke.edu/), and international wildlife organizations such as the Nature Conservancy (http://www.tnc.org/). A good example of what has been accomplished is embodied in the Guanacaste National Park Project, a landmark effort in restoration ecology.

Guanacaste Province of northwestern Costa Rica was a dry forest region that had been cleared for crop agriculture in colonial times and then seeded with African pasture grasses for cattle ranching. Many small cattle ranches have been abandoned in recent years,

Compatible Livestock/Forest Use

The experience of Brazil and Costa Rica illustrates that clearing tropical rainforest for the express purpose of cattle grazing is difficult to justify on either economic or environmental grounds. Policymakers and funding agencies have recognized this, and governments have backed away from the subsidies and incentives for cattle ranching that were offered in decades past. Market forces may be dampening enthusiasm for expanded beef production as well, since the worldwide growth in consumer demand for meat has largely favored pork and poultry over beef.

The clearing of rainforest for cattle ranching aside, there are numerous opportunities for the compatible use of animals and trees that represent less-invasive and more-sustainable activities. These opportunities have received far less attention. There is significant potential for expanding these alternative uses of livestock and trees and improving their efficiency. There are opportunities for veterinarians to be involved in the development, promotion, and implementation of such activities. Categories of compatible livestock/forest use include the use of trees as fodder, the use of animals for sustainable extraction of forest products, the integration of livestock raising into tree plantation systems, and the rearing of some forest animals for food production. These are discussed separately below.

Trees As Fodder   Rather than cutting down trees to make way for livestock, a more sustainable approach is to harvest tree leaves, branches, and seeds and bring them to confined livestock. Increasingly, community development projects involving the rural poor in tropical countries have promoted zero-grazing livestock-production systems. In such systems, a small number of animals with high production potential, such as a milk cow or several milk goats, are kept in total confinement on a farmstead, and fodder is cut and carried to the animal. Trees, especially leguminous trees, are a potentially valuable asset in zero-grazing systems. Legumes are plants that fix nitrogen. As such, they are attractive livestock fodder because

but the incursion of adjacent forest onto abandoned pastures by natural succession, which characterizes tropical rainforest regeneration, has not occurred. There are two important reasons for this. First is the high frequency of grass fires that occur regularly during the dry season. These wildfires destroy the seeds and saplings of canopy tree species, blocking their establishment. Secondly, many seeds of desired successional species are disseminated by birds and small mammals whose presence in the region has diminished due to loss of habitat.

The Guanacaste Conservation Area (GCA) (circled on map) was established in 1988 with the goal of reforesting the region and linking the dry forest habitat to adjacent wet forests and marine habitats to ensure the survival of its biodiversity for the future. Tropical biologist Dr. Daniel Janzen of the University of Pennsylvania has played a key role in marshalling this cooperative effort. Today the GCA covers about 131,000 ha, built up from the original Santa Rosa National Park area of roughly 30,000 ha through the purchase of unused or abandoned ranchland.

The management plan consists of purchasing land adjacent to core areas of original remnant dry forest and encouraging the spread of the original forest onto that adjacent land. This is done through the use of controlled burning to create fire breaks that prevent the extensive grass wildfires that historically have inhibited establishment of forest trees species. Fire lanes are created in strategic locations by first mowing and then burning. Subsequently, controlled grazing of cattle on the lanes keeps the grass down during fire season. Without the threat of fire, seeds and saplings of desired forest tree species can become established on the former ranchland. However, not all species of trees have their seeds dispersed by wind. To encourage the return of birds that play a role in seed dispersal, large trees and hedgerows have been planted on pasture edges to provide protective habitat for birds.

Community participation is an extremely important component of the overall program, as constant local surveillance for unexpected fires and community effort to put them out are critical elements in the success of the program. As such, conservation education has been introduced into elementary schools in the region, and many former ranch and agricultural workers are being retrained and offered employment in the overall conservation effort as park guards, research assistants, and guides. In addition, some cattle ranchers have seen the economic opportunity offered by the restoration of wild habitat and have converted their ranch haciendas to ecotourism lodges, offering forest walks, bird watching, horseback riding and other nature-oriented recreational activities.

they usually have considerably higher protein content that nonleguminous plants. Legumes occur as grasses, shrubs, and trees. Leaves, stems, and seed pods are all potentially usable as fodder.

Tropical rainforests typically contain more leguminous plant species than any other plant family, so there is tremendous opportunity to exploit this resource for animal feed in cut-and-carry systems. Additional research is required to determine the feed value of different leguminous trees as livestock fodder and to identify any detrimental or adverse effects that might be associated with certain plants, for example the action of mimosine in the leguminous tree *Leucana leucocephala*, discussed in Chapter 4.

Reforestation plans should also factor in the importance of livestock in rural societies. For decades, international agencies promoted the importation and planting of eucalyptus trees for use in reforestation projects in Africa and Asia, especially around villages. While the eucalyptus is attractive because it is fast growing and valuable as timber, it has a number of adverse characteristics. Eucalyptus rapidly depletes soil moisture and nutrients, thus inhibiting plant growth adjacent to the trees. In addition, *Eucalyptus* spp. may contain aromatic oils and cyanogenic glycosides that make them unsuitable as fodder. Numerous alternatives to eucalyptus can be used in reforestation that not only protect against soil erosion, but also provide animal feed, fuel wood for local use, and even fruit, nut, or pod crops that can be sold for cash. A number of leguminous tree species, notably leucaena, pigeon pea, calliandra, sesbania, and tree lucerne, have been promoted in recent years for planting around villages for their value as fodder trees and fuel wood.

Livestock for Sustainable Extraction of Forest Products

Many proponents of rainforest conservation emphasize the economic advantage of sustained harvesting of forest products from intact forest as opposed to clear-cutting with subsequent introduction of cropping or ranching. They advocate for establishing "extractive reserves" in which deforestation is discouraged in favor of the continued extraction of forest products with notable economic value such as rubber, chicle, Brazil nuts, and timber taken by selective logging.

Animals can play an important role in supporting economic activity based on forest product extraction. Elephants, for instance, have been used traditionally in logging operations in Asia to bring logs from the forest interior to collection stations near logging roads. Elephants produced minimal ancillary damage to forests during the logging process. In contrast, large, modern mechanized log haulers and skidders require additional trail clearance into forests and damage many young, standing trees during hauling. The pace and destruction of mechanized logging has become so severe in recent years that Thailand introduced a complete ban on logging in natural forests in 1989. Elephants have an important role to play in low-impact harvesting of selectively logged trees such as teak in Asia, and their use should be encouraged.

In the Peten region of Guatemala, many local residents derive a substantial portion of their income from harvesting forest products, including chicle, the latex of the chicle tree (*Manilkara zapota*) used in chewing gum; xate, the fronds of a common palm tree used in construction; and the berry of the *Pimenta dioica* tree, which produces the kitchen seasoning allspice. These local people depend on burros and horses to transport the forest products back to market. The animals provide reliable transport and draft power with minimum impact on forest ecology. There is a considerable need for improved veterinary services for the animals used for forest harvesting, particularly with regard to parasite control and traumatic injury associated with ill-fitting pack frames.

Integration of Livestock into Agroforestry Systems While there may be some opportunities to integrate livestock production into natural forests without detrimental effect to forest ecology and biodiversity, there are a considerable number of opportunities to integrate livestock production into systems of commercial silviculture, or tree farming. Tree plantations for production of commercial products are an important agricultural activity in many countries. In tropical regions, palm oil, coconuts, rubber, sago, cocoa, and tropical fruits are important tree crops. In drier countries, dates are grown in tree plantations. In a world where cultivable land is at a premium, maximizing outputs from available land should always be a high priority. Inclusion of livestock and other vegetable crops into tree plantation systems helps to achieve this goal.

For example, the grazing of beef cattle under coconut palms reduces grass cover beneath the trees and increases the harvest yield, as fewer fallen coconuts are lost in tall grass. In addition, the cattle reduce weeds, improve soil fertility with manure and urine, and, when sold as beef, provide an additional cash commodity for the commercial operation. Such multiple-use schemes of course require proper management. Animals introduced too soon will damage young trees, while mature plantations may have a complete canopy that shades out the sun and reduces grass growth beneath trees. However, there are numerous examples of agroforestry efforts around the world that successfully integrate livestock. These include the use of draft and milking buffalo in oil palm plantations in Malaysia; sheep grazing under apple trees in Pakistan; poultry, rabbit, and ruminant grazing in fruit and nut orchards in Chile[2]; sheep and cattle grazing in radiata pine forests in New Zealand[42]; and the integration of pine planting into beef cattle pastures in south Georgia, USA.[26] Furthermore, many tree plantation crops, when processed, produce wastes or byproducts with potential value as livestock feeds. There is considerable untapped potential for development of livestock-production systems in close proximity to tree product-processing facilities to maximize use of byproducts and increase profitability of the overall enterprise.

Veterinarians should be involved in the development of new agroforestry initiatives that involve livestock, as unanticipated health problems may develop in animals. For example, in New Zealand, abortions were noted in pregnant cows that grazed among radiata pine or were fed wilted foliage or lopped branches. It turned out that the pine contained a phytoestrogen that disturbed reproductive function.

Forests As a Source of Alternative Livestock In many forest regions, local people have traditionally hunted certain forest animals as a source of animal protein in their diet. In their incursions into the forest to hunt, using snares and other techniques, many additional animals are often disturbed, trapped, or killed. In some cases, populations of the desired animals are diminished to the point of endangerment. One alternative, which veterinarians can become actively involved in, is the captive rearing and production of animal species that are currently hunted. Two examples of this approach involve forest rodents in different parts of the world-the grasscutter or cane rat of western Africa and the paca of Central America. This topic is discussed in further detail in Chapter 7.

Challenges for the Future

The accelerated loss of forests worldwide is a major problem, with important implications for global health and the environment. While much attention has been focused in the media on deforestation for the purpose of cattle ranching, this is but one cause of deforestation, and it is primarily of regional importance in Latin America. Effective efforts to reverse the trend of deforestation must recognize and embrace the wider dimensions of deforestation, acknowledging the underlying political, economic, and demographic factors that have, in recent years, favored forest exploitation for short-term gain. The World Resources Institute, which tracks global deforestation and is actively involved in promoting sustainable forest use policies, has identified a number of key objectives that must be realized to reverse the current trend of deforestation (see http://www.wri.org/rio-5/rio5frst.html). These key objectives include

- Building the capacity of forested nations to manage forest resources sustainably and to respond effectively to the rapidly changing global timber market, including pressures from outside logging interests

- Enacting legislation that revamps forest concession policies

- Providing economic incentives for industry to manage forests more sustainably

- Establishing programs for valuing forests for carbon sequestration, biodiversity prospecting, and the nontimber products they provide

- Establishing mechanisms for joint management of forests by national governments and local communities

- Establishing key forest parks and reserves that protect critical areas of biodiversity and the cultures of indigenous forest-dwelling peoples

For veterinarians, there are numerous opportunities in research, education, and extension to participate in the development, promotion, and implementation of more environmentally sound approaches to livestock production that are better integrated with the sustainable use of forest resources.

Aquatic Environmental Degradation

The world's oceans, seas, lakes, and rivers are subject to a wide array of assaults and injuries that degrade aquatic habitat, reduce water quality, and diminish the value and availability of resources that human society traditionally has derived from aquatic environments. A wide range of activities result in harm to water resources. Pollution, for instance, is a major threat to the health of aquatic environments, with pollutants derived from a variety of sources including acid rain from industrial emissions, untreated sewage from urban centers, oil spills from tankers, or chemical runoff from factories and farms, to name but a few.

The focus of the present discussion, however, is on the impact of fishing and aquaculture on the health of marine environments. Since prehistoric times, human beings have looked to Earth's waters as a source of sustenance. Whole cultures have evolved around the pursuit of a particular fish or marine mammal as a source of food. There are numerous examples in North America of Native American tribes that focused on whaling, seal hunting, or salmon fishing as their principle means of livelihood.

Millions of people around the world continue to depend on fishing as their primary source of food and income. Today, however, in addition to traditional, small-scale fishing activity, large-scale commercial fishing has become a major global enterprise. Changes in consumer demand and global marketing along with the increased size and advanced technology of fishing vessels have resulted in the harvesting of enormous amounts of fish. The size of the global commercial catch and the methods used to achieve it have become issues of major concern to environmentalists and policymakers, as there is growing evidence that fisheries are being irreversibly depleted and that some modern fishing methods are seriously damaging aquatic habitats.

Aquaculture, or mariculture, if carried out in salt water, is the cultivation of aquatic flora or fauna under controlled conditions for human use or consumption. Aquaculture practice has grown dramatically in the last four decades, largely in response to consumer demand for fish and shellfish products and to advances in aquaculture-related technology. Proponents of aquaculture often cite the industry as an important new source of animal protein to feed the world's people in the face of decreasing stocks of wild caught fish. Generally speaking, this is a valid position. However, certain forms of intensified aquaculture, notably shrimp production and the raising of carnivorous fish such as salmon, may themselves contribute to accelerated depletion of wild fish stocks and also contribute to environmental degradation. The impacts of modern commercial fisheries and certain forms of aquaculture on aquatic environmental health are presented in the following sections.

General Condition of the World's Fisheries

Since the end of World War II, commercial fishing has shown a strong, steady expansion, growing from 17.5 million tons in 1945 to 92 million tons in 1995. On a per capita basis, though, fish production worldwide has leveled off in relation to rapid population growth. Per capita consumption jumped from 9.5 kg per person in 1955 to 14.7 kg in 1965 but has only increased to 15.9 kg per person between 1965 and 1995.

The steady increase in fish catches, however, belies some serious problems in commercial fishing. Yields remain high for a number of reasons. Modern fishing techniques and equipment allow more-efficient location and capture of fish stocks. Sonar and global-positioning systems allow large fishing vessels to locate fertile fishing grounds accurately and return precisely to those grounds repeatedly. Newer, larger vessels using larger nets also can capture more fish. In addition, new fishing grounds are being identified and aggressively harvested. Most significant, perhaps, is the taking of large numbers of fish species that in the past were considered to have little or no commercial value. This practice is increasing as the more highly valued species are systematically overfished.

Overfishing is a major challenge of our time. The Food and Agriculture Organization of the United Nations (FAO) estimates that up to 70% of the world's marine fish species that they monitor are currently overfished or fished beyond the limits of sustainability. Furthermore, FAO analysts suggest that 11 of the world's 15 major fishing grounds are seriously depleted of fish stocks, and that by the year 2010, global demand for fish will exceed supply by as much as 40 million tons annually. In the United States, the National Marine Fisheries Service has reported that in U.S. waters, 96 of 279 fish species surveyed are essentially overfished.

An important example of the impact of overfishing is the Atlantic Cod, *Gadus morhua*, which for centuries served as the economic foundation of coastal fishing communities in northeastern Canada and the United States from Massachusetts to Newfoundland. It is believed that Basque fisherman were catching, salting, and drying cod off North America for European markets as early as the 1300s, long before Columbus ostensibly discovered the New World. The abundance of these bottom-dwelling fish on Georges Bank in New England and the Grand Bank of Canada was legendary for centuries. In the *Cyclopedia of Commerce and Commercial Navigation*, published in New York in 1858, it was observed that cod is "too well known to require any description. It is amazingly prolific. Leewenhoek counted 9,384,000 eggs in a cod-fish of a middling size-a number that will baffle all the efforts of man to exterminate." Yet, by 1992, the Canadian government was obliged to close Newfoundland waters, the Grand Banks, and most of the Gulf of St. Lawrence to fishing for cod and other bottom-dwelling fish. Similarly, restrictive catch quotas and reduced fishing periods have been established in New England for cod and other groundfish on the Georges Bank. Though once unimaginable, fierce competition and the ruthless efficiency of modern trawlers had depleted the multitudes of cod.[25]

A major contributing factor to overfishing is an excess of capacity. There are an estimated 89,000 trawling vessels operating around the world, capable of taking 100 million tons of fish annually. The FAO estimates that world fishing fleets currently have about 30% excess capacity. Some conservation groups put that overall estimate as high as 155% and up to 250% for those nations with the largest fishing fleets. Acknowledging the seriousness of this problem, member nations of the FAO, in February 1999, agreed to assess the size and capacity of their fleets and to develop national plans for reduction of oversized fleets. The agreement, known as the International Plan of Action for the Management of Fishing Capacity, also requires countries to reduce government subsidies to the commercial fishing industry. Such subsidies have been an important stimulus for creating overcapacity. Worldwide, governments were spending US$15 to 20 billion annually in support of vessel construction and modernization and other industry supports.

Environmental Impacts of Commercial Fishing

Traditional, or artisanal, fishing, which occurs on a small scale and is largely nonmechanized is minimally damaging to the environment. As the scale of operation increases along with the degree of mechanization, the environmental impact of commercial fishing increases. A number of issues related to modern fishing methods are of environmental concern. These include overfishing, wastage of marine resources associated with by-catch, threats to endangered species, and damage to marine habitats.

Overfishing Overfishing itself can cause ecological distortion. Many commercial fish species are at the top of their food chains or are a major source of food for other animals. Their depletion alters the balance of other fish species and marine mammals. For example, the reduction of cod in the Georges Bank area of the North Atlantic is associated with an increased number of pelagic, or midwater, species, such as herring, mackerel, and menhaden. The implications of such unintended manipulation of fish populations are not always clear, though sometimes direct relationships can be identified. Off Nantucket, Massachusetts, there is a hook-and-line fishery for tautog, a desirable food fish of the wrasse family. Tautog feed on the green crab, which in turn are known to feed on small bay scallop larvae. When fishermen overfished the tautog several years ago, there was a population explosion of the green crab. The green crab then fed on the incoming scallop spat, leading to a collapse of the local scallop fishery. Another example, on the west coast of the United States, involves the pollock fishery. In 1998, U.S. federal officials placed stricter limits on trawling for pollock in Alaskan waters because of concerns that the Steller sea lion, an endangered species that feeds on pollock, was being deprived of adequate food supplies.

Given the efficiency of modern fishing practices, fish species can be seriously depleted before their biology is even understood. This is the case with the orange roughy, a fish found in the deep waters around Australia and New Zealand. When

North Atlantic whitefish stocks such as cod began to decline in the 1980s, commercial interests began to look for other types of nonoily whitefish. The orange roughy was targeted and heavily fished before it was recognized that the fish can live for 100 years and do not spawn until about 20 years of age. As a result, breeding stock were depleted, and some orange roughy populations declined dramatically within a decade of the start of intensive fishing.

Wastage Through By-Catch *By-catch* is the untargeted portion of a commercial catch that is subsequently discarded as unwanted. The reasons for discarding by-catch include low economic value or limited marketability of the by-catch, quota limitations on a particular species, regulations restricting size or age of catch, or prohibition of taking or keeping threatened or endangered species. By-catches can be enormous. As much as 25% of the entire global fish catch, or 27 million metric tons of marine life, are tossed or shoveled back into the sea from ships' decks annually. Many of these fish, shellfish, and mammals are already dead or dying when returned to the sea, so their commercial value is lost. Furthermore, small, immature fish are lost to the breeding population, thus further reducing the potential to replenish overall fish stocks. Different types of fisheries are associated with varying levels of by-catch. Shrimp trawling, for example, generates considerable by-catch. For each pound of shrimp retrieved around the world, 2 to 8 pounds of other marine life are discarded.

The wastage of by-catch is particularly anomalous in light of the fact that up to 30 million tons a year of schooling fish are caught specifically to be processed as fishmeal and fish oil for livestock feeds. This includes feed both for terrestrial livestock, such as cattle, pigs, and poultry, and for intensively raised fish and crustaceans, such as salmon and shrimp, as discussed in the later section on aquaculture. It would represent a tremendous efficiency in the commercial fishing industry if the by-catch presently wasted could be channeled into fishmeal and fish oil production to reduce wastage of the by-catch and to reduce fishing pressure on pelagic school fish.

Threatened and Endangered Species A number of threatened and endangered marine mammals, fishes, and reptiles are subject to increased losses through commercial fishing. Several different modern fishing techniques are each associated with direct losses. Drift netting as practiced widely in the 1980s by the Pacific tuna fishery was associated with the inadvertent capture and drowning of large numbers of dolphins. Shrimp trawling is a major source of mortality for endangered sea turtles, which become caught in nets. Longline fishing as practiced for catching swordfish results in the taking of many young sharks, turtles, and some marine mammals. Gill nets used in the shark fishery snag turtles and marine mammals.

Increased awareness and public outcry has led to some efforts to reduce such losses, but not all of these adverse consequences are easily corrected. Net sizes have been modified in some cases to allow unwanted species to pass through, but even then, a full net often has its openings effectively blocked by densely packed fish and losses, albeit reduced, still occur.

Destruction of Marine Habitat Different fishing techniques vary in their potential for degrading marine habitat. In recent years, trawling and dredging of the ocean bottom have been sharply criticized for their destructive effect on the ocean environment. Not only do these commercial fishing practices result in considerable by-catch, they also have the potential to disrupt or obliterate the structural components and organization of the ocean floor ecology. Some of the more vociferous critics have likened bottom trawling of the oceans to clear-cutting of the rainforest.

Bottom trawling is a fishing technique associated with taking bottom-dwelling groundfish, such as cod, haddock, pollock, scrod, and flounder, as well as shrimp. Dredging, a similar process, is used in taking scallops. Bottom trawling involves dragging a large net along the sea floor behind one or two ships. Open mouthed nets are often as much as 200 feet wide, with 500-pound weights or doors, at each end. The "upper lip" of the net is held open by floats. The "lower lip" of the net, known as the sweep chain, drags along the bottom surface. Comparison of undersea photographs of areas subjected to trawling with those of nearby areas free of trawling demonstrate that the sweep chain indeed scours the ocean floor (Fig. 6-6). On gravelly ocean bottom, such as occurs in Georges Bank, all manner of marine life appears to be obliterated, and it may take as long as 2.5 years for the normal flora and fauna to be restored, presuming that the area is not trawled again in the interim. The disturbance of the benthic community of the sea bottom can seriously diminish its function as a nursery ground for many aquatic species and as a source of food for commercial fish. For many years, trawling was limited to flat areas of the ocean floor because protrusions such as coral reefs or rock formations would snag the sweep chain and disrupt the trawling. However, more recently, wheellike rollers, or "rockhoppers," have been added to trawling nets, enabling their use in more-irregular ocean floor terrain, with attendant risk of damage to coral structures.

While most environmentalists and marine scientists decry the practice of large-scale, repeated bottom trawling, its deleterious effects are not fully documented. Some industry defenders suggest that the practice may have some positive influences. For example, in the case of scallops, periodic disturbances from dredging may actually improve scallop habitat and increase yields over time.

In tropical seas, particularly in the Pacific, there are several fishing practices strongly associated with widespread destruction of coral reefs. The most common and destructive is cyanide fishing, associated with the taking of live reef fish. The live catching of colorful, tropical reef fish is aimed at two distinct markets. One is the hobby aquarium trade, and the second, newer, rapidly expanding market is the specialty restaurant fish trade. The demand for live tropical fish is strong in south China, especially in Guangdong Province and Hong Kong where economic prosperity has spurred consumption. Reef fish such as groupers and parrotfish can be seen in restaurant aquariums, awaiting selection by patrons. This is an extremely lucrative market, with high demand driving the capture of live fish. A serving of Napoleon wrasse lips is reported to cost $250.

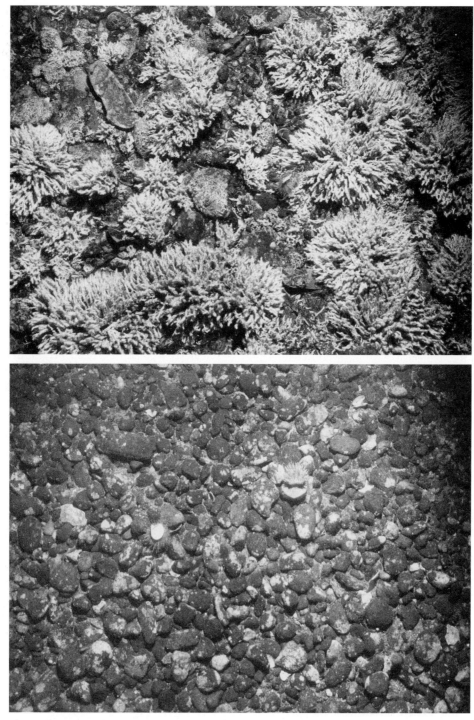

Figure 6-6.   U.S. Geological Survey photos of the seabed on eastern Georges Bank, off New England and Nova Scotia. *Top,* The seabed at a depth of 89 m in an area not fished with bottom trawls and dredges. Fragile calcerous worm tubes are plentiful on the seabed. *Bottom,* The seabed at a depth of 80 m at a nearby site on eastern Georges Bank that is fished with bottom trawls and dredges. The seabed floor shows only clean gravel, with scant evidence of life forms. (Photos courtesy of Dr. Page Valentine, U.S. Geological Survey, Woods Hole, MA)

As a result of this growing market, there has been enormous fishing pressure on coral reefs in the Indo-Pacific region, particularly around the Philippines and Indonesia. The method of choice for taking live fish in recent years has become cyanide fishing. Divers, armed with spray bottles containing potassium cyanide, systematically work the reefs. They chase fish into nooks and crannies in the reef and then spray them with a cloud of cyanide. When the poisoned fish struggle out of their hiding places they are seized by the diver and held in nets to be transported to the surface. When fish do not struggle out of hiding, the divers will break or tear away the coral to reach their prey. However, it is not the physical damage to the coral that is most destructive. The cyanide itself is lethal to the coral polyps. Within weeks of being sprayed, the affected corals are bleached white and become covered with algae. Cyanide fishing has become a major industry, and the death of coral reefs is widespread. It began in earnest in the Philippines in the mid-1970s and by the late 1980s had spread to Indonesia. It is now estimated that in Indonesia, only 7% of the nation's coral reefs remain in a healthy state. Thirty percent of the reefs have been essentially destroyed by cyanide fishing, and the remaining two thirds are seriously threatened. As the demand for live fish has increased, cyanide fishing and its attendant destruction of coral reefs has spread to south Pacific islands such as Papua New Guinea and westward to the Maldives in the Indian Ocean.

Fishing with explosives, commonly referred to as dynamite fishing, is another negligent fishing practice that is especially damaging to coral reefs. The practice is particularly widespread in the south Pacific. It represents a lazy, but dangerous, method of collecting large numbers of fish rapidly with a minimum investment in equipment. The explosive is dropped into the water, and the dead and dying fish float to the surface for collection. In the process, coral reefs are damaged.

Environmental Impacts of Aquaculture

Aquaculture had its origins in China at least 3000 years ago, with the development of carp cultivation in freshwater ponds; however, in the last three decades aquaculture has experienced enormous growth as a global industry. This growth has been stimulated in large part by the recognition that commercial overfishing has reduced the stocks of wild-caught fish at the same time that demand for fish and seafood products is increasing. Between 1986 and 1996 the value and weight of aquaculture production doubled worldwide, and the aquaculture industry now accounts for 25% of the world's food fish supply. Overall, aquacultural output grew at a rate of 11% per year during the 1990s and may soon overtake beef cattle production as a global source of animal protein.

The vast majority of aquaculture enterprises are carried out with little or no harm to the environment. In fact, many fish-farming schemes actually contribute to sustainable agricultural production by recycling waste materials into food. Manure and other biodegradable wastes are added to freshwater fish ponds, where they stimulate the growth of algae and plankton that serve as a source of feed for farmed fish such as carp, tilapia, and catfish. Shellfish farming, too, has little adverse environmental impact. Cultivators set out immature shellfish, or spat, in appropriate marine environments where, as filter feeders, the spat grow by extracting their nutrients from the surrounding water and are subsequently harvested at maturity. Increasingly, oysters, clams, scallops, and mussels are being raised through such cultivation.

Environmental problems arise in aquaculture particularly with regard to the cultivation of salmon and shrimp, two of the faster-growing sectors of the overall aquaculture industry.[33] While these two sectors make up only 5% of all farmed fish by weight, they account for over 20% by value. Currently, a quarter of world shrimp production comes from farmed shrimp, with a market value of over $6 billion. The world market value of farmed salmon in 1997 was over $2 billion.

Salmon Farming   Salmon farming began in Norway in the 1960s and has since spread to other, mostly industrialized nations with abundant coastline and suitably cool water temperatures. The major producers of farmed salmon today include Norway, the U.K., Canada, the United States, and Chile. Farmed salmon spend their first year in freshwater ponds. Then they are transferred to large net pens or floating sea cages anchored in coastal bays, where the fish grow to market size over a period of 1 to 2 years. Salmon are carnivorous fish. As such, commercial production requires feeding a diet that contains 45% fishmeal and 25% fish oil. To prepare this ration, enormous numbers of schooling fish, such as mackerel, caplin, anchovies, and sardines, are caught and processed as feed for salmon.

The farming of carnivorous fish such as salmon represents one of the major concerns of environmentalists and social critics, who question the large-scale harvesting of fish that can be eaten directly by humans to serve instead as feed for another fish species that produces only about 1 pound of salmon for each 2.8 pounds of school fish provided as feed. This may put additional pressure on natural fisheries that are already under intense pressure from overfishing. It also may deprive local human populations of animal protein derived from locally caught fish, as school fish are diverted to salmon feed. It has been estimated that the European salmon farming industry alone requires an amount of fish equivalent to about 90% of the primary production of the fishing area of the North Sea. As a result, the industry depends heavily on importation of fishmeal derived from South American fisheries.

Other environmental and ecological concerns are associated with salmon farming as well. The concentration of farmed fish in coastal bays can lead to pollution problems associated with uneaten feed and the production of large volumes of feces. Salmon farms in Scandinavia produce feces with a nitrogen content equivalent to the sewage produced by a city of 3.9 million people and a phosphorus content equal to that of a city of 1.7 million people. These pollutants can adversely affect water quality and the varied forms of marine life present near fish-farming areas. The escape of farmed fish and subsequent interbreeding with native salmon species is also a concern, as it may lead to genetic degradation of wild salmon populations whose genetic makeup is often related to the specific river habitats where they spawn. Such concerns have been heightened by the development of transgenic salmon with enhanced growth potential. Fish farms also attract predators that must be controlled. To deter sea lions and seals from raiding caged salmon, noise deterrents have been used, which, in addition to deterring the pinnipeds, have discouraged whales and other fishes from entering traditional feeding grounds.

In addition, as with any other food animal species, the intensive management of high concentrations of farmed fish under confinement conditions increases the risk of disease transmission. This, in turn, leads to increased use of antibiotics and pesticides that may end up in local waters. The diseases themselves, if not controlled, may adversely affect native species as well, with ecological as well as economic implications. (See sidebar "Salmon Fishing vs. Salmon Farming in Scotland.") There are significant opportunities for veterinarians to become increasingly involved in the development of management systems and strategies for farmed-fish production that reduce the risk of disease and minimize the use the drugs.

The salmon farming industry has expanded and matured sufficiently in recent years to have supported the development of an effective range of vaccines to replace the use of antimicrobial agents for most bacterial diseases of salmonids that occur in Europe and North America. However, there continue to be research opportunities for the development of vaccines for bacterial diseases of salmonids raised elsewhere in the world as well as for bacterial, viral, and parasitic diseases of other farmed fish. Some current, oil-adjuvanted, intraperi-

toneal vaccines of salmonids produce significant side effects and merit refinement. Others have questionable efficacy. There are also opportunities for research into the application of biotechnology to develop new strains of salmonids and other fish that are inherently disease resistant. Development of improved diagnostic techniques for screening eggs and fry prior to importation is also an important goal of disease control. As the conditions for salmon maturation differ from those for brood stock, the latter are often raised elsewhere and imported, with an attendant risk of introducing disease.

Shrimp Farming Farmed shrimp production has increased at least sevenfold since the 1980s. The explosive growth of shrimp farming in the last two decades reflects the general economic growth and increasing affluence of the period. Once perceived as a luxury food reserved for special occasions, shrimp now have become standard menu fare at franchise restaurants. Shrimp consumption has increased primarily in the developed world, especially in the United States, Japan, and the European Union countries. Together, these developed nations account for about 90% of world shrimp consumption. The United States is the leading consumer, eating about

Salmon Fishing vs. Salmon Farming in Scotland

It is not difficult to conjure up an idyllic, rustic vision of salmon fishing in Scotland-pristine mountain streams, pink-purple fields of heather, tweed caps and wicker creels, hand-tied flies, stone castles, and a single-malt whiskey, fireside, at the end of the day. The power of this image is not lost on the Scots themselves, who managed for decades to market this piscatorial vision effectively to wealthy anglers who came to Scotland for the cachet, and the catch, of salmon fishing. Nowadays, however, there is a slight problem. The salmon are disappearing from Scotland's rivers, and the wealthy fisherman are heading instead to Iceland and Argentina. Scottish conservationists, along with tourism industry leaders, think they know the reason why the wild river salmon and the tourists are in decline. That reason, they believe, is the development of a salmon-farming industry along the northwestern coast of Scotland.

Coastal salmon farming along the Scottish Highlands was supported by government as a means of generating jobs and income for the economically disadvantaged region. At present there are 340 active fish farms, mostly in the northwest. Initially, angling associations viewed the development favorably, on the assumption that the availability of cheaper, farm-raised salmon would reduce the poaching of wild salmon, leaving more for the sportsmen. Salmon has indeed become cheaper, but contrary to expectations, the

wild river salmon have become scarcer. Anglers believe that the fish farms directly harm wild salmon, as well as sea trout, in a number of ways. Wild salmon returning from the sea to spawn in Scotland's rivers must swim through estuaries polluted with the concentrated feces of intensively reared, caged fish. In addition, they are exposed to the diseases of the caged fish, most notably, sea lice. The sea lice, *Lepeophtheirus salmonis* and *Caligus elongatus* are parasitic copepods particularly troublesome

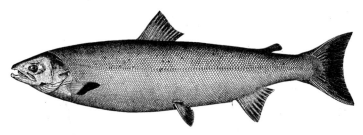

360,000 tons of processed shrimp per year. Between one half to two thirds of the shrimp consumed annually are imported, farmed shrimp. Shrimp imports into the United States in 2000 were valued at US$3.76 billion.

While most farmed-shrimp consumption occurs in developed countries of the temperate zones, most shrimp farm production occurs in developing countries of the tropical zones, especially in Asia and Latin America. Thailand and Ecuador together produce 45% of the world's farmed shrimp, while Indonesia, China, India, Vietnam, Bangladesh, Mexico, Colombia, and Honduras together produce another 45%.

Tropical warm-water shrimp farming is carried out in ponds created near estuaries or coastlines to provide a ready source of brackish or saltwater for regular flushing of the shrimp beds for aeration and cleansing. Cultivation ponds are frequently created near tropical coastline at the expense of coastal mangrove forests, which are clear-cut and then excavated to create the ponds. The loss of mangrove forest in Asia and Latin America as a result of shrimp farming has not been trivial. In fact, it represents a serious environmental and social loss.

Mangrove forests represent a unique coastal ecology. The mangrove trees themselves are unique in their reproduction and growth in brackish water. Their complex water-based root system acts as a trap for organic matter and silt, and over time, mangrove forests add land mass to islands and coastal areas. Mature mangrove forests serve multiple functions. They act as a buffer against severe tropical storms, reducing windfalls and soil erosion. The forests provide habitat for a wide range of terrestrial and aquatic flora and fauna. The decaying, dropped leaves of the trees are an important source of nutrients for marine life. Furthermore, the relatively calm waters of the intertidal mangrove swamps provide a safe nursery for a multitude of fry and larvae of marine species that ultimately populate the adjacent seas and estuaries, promoting biodiversity and providing bountiful harvests for local fisheries. Finally, when properly managed, the mangrove forest provides a sustainable supply of important products for local people including fuel wood, charcoal, tannins, and food.

The inherent value of mangrove forests has been overlooked in the rush to cash in on the expanded global market for farmed shrimp. In Thailand, for example, about 253,000 of the country's

to cage-reared Atlantic salmon, *Salmo salar*. They attach to the skin and feed on tissue, produce hemorrhage and anemia, and create a portal of entry for other pathogens. Critics also believe that chemicals used to treat sea lice, such as dichlorvos, are also harmful to the wild fish.

Leaders of the salmon-farming industry disagree. They point out that the decline in river salmon is well documented, going back to the early 1950s, while commercial salmon farming did not begin in earnest until the 1980s. Industry supporters believe that the reasons for the decline are more complex and far reaching and include commercial overfishing at sea, a major increase in

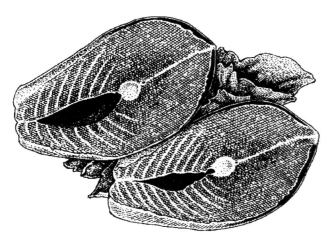

fish-eating seal populations in the Atlantic Ocean and North Sea, and general increase in the types and intensity of ocean pollution. Furthermore, fish farmers believe that it is just as likely for wild salmon to introduce new diseases into farmed fish as it is for disease transmission to occur in the other direction. In the meantime, the farm-fish salmon industry has created thousands of jobs.

No one disputes that disease can be transmitted to local fish by fish stocks introduced from other locations. In 1937, Great Britain passed the Diseases of Fish Act, the first such legislation in the world, to prohibit importation of live salmonids or eggs after an outbreak of furunculosis (*Aeromonas salmonicida* infection) occurred in wild salmon in England, Wales, and Scotland following importation of live rainbow trout from Germany. Clearly, the question of disease transmission between farmed and wild fish is a major source of conflict, competition, and confusion. The opportunities for veterinarians to make a meaningful professional contribution in this arena are enormous. Participation of veterinarians can help improve farm management; improve disease recognition, treatment, and control; clarify patterns of disease transmission; enhance diagnostic capabilities; develop more-sophisticated epidemiological surveillance; provide informed and balanced regulatory oversight; and offer leadership for effective community participation in conflict resolution.

380,000 ha of mangrove forests already have been obliterated to make way for shrimp farms. Yet the short-term economic gain of shrimp farming may not equal the long-term losses of the mangrove ecosystem. Intensively managed shrimp ponds often have a productive life limit of only 5 to 10 years because of degradation of soil and water quality and the occurrence of disease in the densely populated shrimp beds. In the meantime, the sustainable harvest of mangrove forest products is lost, along with significant reductions in local marine life and fish harvests as a result of nursery grounds being destroyed. The land under abandoned shrimp ponds often cannot be reclaimed for agricultural purposes because of intense salinization that inhibits crop growth. In addition, there is reduced economic opportunity for local people. Like most forms of intensive, land-based agriculture, shrimp farming is capital intensive, not labor intensive. As traditional forms of fishing and agriculture are displaced by shrimp monoculture, livelihoods may be disrupted and communities weakened.

Other issues arise with regard to shrimp farming. As the shrimp beds are often located in or near estuaries, they are often downstream from agricultural lands to which pesticides and herbicides have been applied. Runoff contaminates shrimp beds and represents a potential health hazard for the consumer market. Intensively managed shrimp ponds are densely stocked to maximize production. A hectare of natural mangrove swamp might yield 25 to 100 kg of shrimp (among other things), and a traditional, extensively managed shrimp pond might be stocked with up to 20,000 postlarvae, yielding up to 1000 kg of shrimp in a year. In contrast, an intensively managed hectare of shrimp pond will be stocked with as many as 600,000 postlarvae and yield as much as 10 to 16 tons of shrimp, at least while it can be maintained in a productive state. These densely packed ponds are self-polluting and require massive and frequent flushing with fresh and brackish water to dilute and expunge effluent. This sometimes depletes local water tables, as has happened in instances in India and Taiwan. Effluent is often pumped into adjacent coastal waters, where it has a polluting effect.

As might be expected in a management system with such high stocking densities, disease outbreaks are common, and their control requires considerable input of antibiotics and pesticides. Even with these efforts, massive disease outbreaks occur that can result in the permanent closure of shrimp ponds. A World Bank analysis of the shrimp industry in 1996 estimated that global losses due to shrimp disease are around $3 billion annually and recommended an investment of $275 million over 15 years in support of shrimp disease research. Like farmed salmon, intensively farmed shrimp require considerable input of fishmeal and fish oil in their diet and produce protein at a net loss. Similarly, ponds are frequently stocked with nonindigenous species of shrimp that can dilute the genetic stock of native species. Disease problems may also spread to native species.

Despite all the problems with shrimp farming, some governments have turned a blind eye to their destructive aspects. Many countries where shrimp farming occurs are in dire need of foreign exchange to pay off international debts, and the lucrative shrimp export market offers ready access to foreign currency. However, other governments are beginning to take stock of the long-term deleterious consequences. In December 1996, the Supreme Court of India ordered the shutdown of approximately 40,000 ha of commercial shrimp farms and established precedents for compensation to people adversely affected by shrimp farming. The Court also ruled that no new shrimp aquaculture operations can be sited in prime agricultural land, wetlands, mangroves, estuaries, saltpans, or public land or be located within 500 m of the coast. Shrimp farms also were prohibited from causing salinity or chemical pollution of fresh water.

Issues of Climate Change

Climate is the prevailing set of weather conditions for a place or region as determined by temperature patterns and meteorological changes over a period of years. A number of distinct and differentiable climatic categories exist in the world. The five major categories are: humid tropical climates, dry climates, subtropical climates, continental climates, and polar climates. Within these major categories there are numerous subcategories. These climatic subdivisions are conditioned by a number of factors, for example, topography, area of land mass, and nearness to oceans. The prevailing factor in defining the climate of a region, at least with regard to temperature, is its latitude, or distance from the equator. The climatic pattern in any given region of the world plays a dominant role in shaping both the ecology of that region and its human cultural geography.

Climate is not a static phenomenon. In fact, climate change has been, and continues to be, one of the most dynamic forces that define the patterns of life on earth. For example, just 10,000 years ago, a fleeting moment in geological time, much of North America and Europe were covered by glacial ice and unsuitable for habitation. All of the human activity, physical infrastructure, and economic development apparent today in Canada, much of the United States, and most of northern Europe are possible only because of a mild and gradual warming of the Earth's atmosphere that caused the glaciers to recede and opened huge areas of land for human habitation.

There is considerable evidence that today, we are once again in a period of significant climate change. What distinguishes the current situation from previous periods, however, is that human activity appears to be a driving force in this current period of climate change. A number of climatic, meteorological, and atmospheric changes, such as global warming, acid rain, and ozone depletion are increasingly associated with human activities such as burning fossil fuels, industrial production, agricultural practices and such physical transformation of the landscape as the widespread cutting of rainforests.

The implications of global climate change can be profound. History tells us that whole civilizations have come and gone under the influence of climate.[36] The overall impact of current trends in climate change remain unknown, and the timetable of change uncertain. However, computer modeling of some possible outcomes for different rates and severity of global warming offer disturbing scenarios for the welfare of human society and the biosphere in general.

Depending on the continued rate and volume of production of greenhouse gases, computer models suggest that average atmospheric temperatures may rise from 1.0 to 4.5°C over the next 100 years. Even at the more conservative end of the spectrum, dramatic changes in the natural environment are possible. They include polar ice melts, elevated sea levels, submersion of coastlines and islands, alterations in the hydrological cycle, and modifications of ecosystems and vegetation. The social costs of these changes will be felt in the occurrence of large, environmentally induced migrations of human populations, changing patterns of agricultural production, shifts in economic activity, and new patterns of disease occurrence.

It is beyond the scope of this volume to discuss all aspects of climate change and their potential effects on the biosphere and human society. The following discussions focus on aspects of global climate change that should be of professional interest to veterinarians, particularly with regard to the health and productivity of domestic animals. Topics include global warming, El Niño and related phenomena, and ozone depletion.

Global Warming

Earth's atmosphere is made up of gases. Some of these gases, notably water vapor, carbon dioxide, nitrous oxide, and methane, exert a "greenhouse" effect that helps to maintain the temperature of the Earth's atmosphere at levels compatible with life. Like glass in a greenhouse, these gases allow most wavelengths of solar radiation to pass through the atmosphere and reach Earth to warm it. However, when infrared radiation is subsequently reflected back into the atmosphere from Earth's surface, these gases trap up to 90% of that infrared energy as heat, which facilitates the stabilization of atmospheric temperatures at a level much higher than that outside the atmosphere. Life on Earth as we know it depends on this greenhouse effect. Without it, average temperatures near Earth's surface would be more than 30°C lower.

Global warming is the progressive increase in mean temperature of Earth's atmosphere. The process is linked to increases in the historical concentrations of various greenhouse gases, because increases in concentrations of these gases augment the overall trapping effect of infrared energy in the atmosphere.

Different atmospheric gases have different radiative indices, or capacities for trapping infrared energy. The trapping effect of a molecule of methane, for example, is thirty times that of a molecule of carbon dioxide. The contribution of an atmospheric gas to the greenhouse effect is therefore a function not only of its concentration, but also of its radiative index. Even gases in low concentrations, such as chlorofluorocarbons, can exert a profound greenhouse effect because of their high ra-

diative indices. Some greenhouse gases, such as carbon dioxide, occur naturally but also enter the atmosphere as a result of human activity. Others, such as chlorofluorocarbons, are being contributed primarily by human industrial activity. Further information on the characteristics of various important greenhouse gases and their contribution to global warming is given in Table 6-7.

Science and Policy

Serious scientific inquiry into the process of global warming and its implications began in 1979 when the World Meteorological Organization of the United Nations (WMO) sponsored the World Climate Conference and launched the World Climate Program. The main activities of this program were to gather and analyze data on climate change, share the data with individual nations for planning purposes, carry out impact studies based on available data and computerized models, and carry out research to better understand and predict future climate change.

In 1988, in conjunction with the UNEP, the WMO established the Intergovernmental Panel on Climate Change (IPCC). This international, multidisciplinary body of scientists was brought together with a number of objectives: to carry out and evaluate research on the greenhouse effect, global warming, and climate change; to assess the potential impacts of global warming on human society and natural ecosystems; and to recommend potential courses of action to policymakers for ameliorating the effects of climate change.

In 1990, the IPCC issued its first "Scientific Assessment of Climate Change," which summarized for the world what was known about global warming. The IPCC documented that a contemporary warming trend was in fact under way. Global mean surface air temperature had increased by 0.3 to 0.6°C over the preceding 100 years, and mean sea level had increased by 10 to 20 cm over that same period. Since that report, several other indicators have been identified that further support the occurrence of global warming: the 14 warmest years on record since record keeping began in 1866 have all occurred since 1980, the rate of ice cap melting in the Andes mountains of South American has increased since the 1970s, the volume of glaciers in the European Alps has reduced by half since the 1850s, the north Greenland ice cap has been thinning by 2.5 cm per year, and there has been up to a 25% reduction in the volume of sea ice around Antarctica

In its first scientific assessment, the IPCC also offered several scenarios concerning the effects of global warming, based on whether or not there is any appreciable change in the future rate of greenhouse gas production on the planet. Under the "business-as-usual" scenario, which assumed no foreseeable reduction in the rate of production of greenhouse gas emissions, it was projected that atmospheric carbon dioxide concentrations would double over present levels by 2080 and that average global temperature would increase by approximately 0.3°C per decade. This would result in a temperature rise of about 1°C by 2025 and of 3°C by 2100. Under this same sce-

Table 6-7   Characteristics of Various Atmospheric Greenhouse Gases Relative to the Phenomenon of Global Warming

Greenhouse Gas	Radiative Index [a]	Preindustrial Concentration[b] (ppm)[c]	Present Concentration (ppm)[c]	Current Annual Increase in Atmosphere (%)	Total Contribution to Global Warming (%)	Sources and Contribution to Global Warming (%)	Lifespan in Atmosphere (years)
Carbon dioxide (CO$_2$)	1	280	350	0.4	50	Fossil fuels (35) Deforestation (10) Agriculture (3) Industry (2)	500
Methane (CH$_4$)	30	0.7	1.7	1.1	16	Fossil fuels (4) Deforestation (4) Agriculture (8)	7-10
Nitrous oxide(N$_2$O)	150	0.28	0.3	0.3	6	Fossil fuels (4) Agriculture (2)	140-190
Ozone (O$_3$)	2000	0	0.1	0.25	8	Fossil fuels (6) Industry (2)	Hours to days
Chlorofluorocarbons (CFCs)	10000	0	0.0006	6.0	20	Industry (20)	65-110

[a]Potential for a molecule of the substance to trap infrared energy relative to CO2, which is assigned a radiative index of 1.

[b]Prior to the Industrial Revolution.(before AD 1750).

[c]Atmospheric concentration in parts per million by volume.

nario, sea levels would rise by about 65 cm (25.6 in.) by 2100, with the potential to cause extensive coastal submersion and catastrophic social and economic disruptions.

Public awareness was increased by the first IPCC assessment. Subsequently, several international conferences have been held for scientists, government leaders, and policymakers to address the issue of global warming and develop plans and agreements on how to curb greenhouse emissions. In Rio de Janeiro, Brazil, in 1992, the United Nations Framework Convention on Climate Change (UNFCCC) was developed. The convention created an international framework for action to limit or reduce greenhouse gas emissions. In 1995, the IPCC issued its second scientific assessment, which concluded that "the balance of evidence suggests that there is a discernible human influence on global climate." The IPCC findings led to the drafting of the Kyoto Protocol in Japan, in 1997. It committed industrialized countries to quantified targets for abating their emissions of greenhouse gases. Further discussions and refinements of the convention and the Kyoto Protocol were made in Buenos Aires, Argentina, in 1998. Full texts of the UNFCCC and the Kyoto Protocol are available on the Internet at http://www.unfccc.de/.

By March 1999, 176 nations, including the United States, had ratified the UNFCCC, and 84 nations had signed the Kyoto Protocol. Under the Kyoto Protocol, the United States would have been required to reduce greenhouse emissions to 7% below 1990 levels by the year 2012. This would require the elimination of approximately 500 million metric tons of carbon pollution each year. In January of 2001, the IPPC issued a draft summary of its third scientific assessment with upwardly revised projections on the rate of global warming and concluding that the Earth's average surface temperature would rise 1.4° to 5.8°C between 1990 and 2100. However, in March of 2001, U.S. President George W. Bush said that the United States would not ratify the Kyoto Protocol, citing economic harm to the United States and insufficient obligations by developing nations to reduce greenhouse emissions under the protocol. The United States is responsible for producing one third of all carbon dioxide emissions produced by the world's industrialized nations.

Implications for Agriculture

Global warming has the potential to alter temperature and rainfall patterns over much of the world, creating new regional climates with profound impact on agricultural patterns and productivity. Global warming could produce both positive and negative effects on agriculture, depending on the intensity of climatic alteration and the regions involved. The watchword, in either case, is change. Agriculturists will have to be aware of the changes that are occurring and, when possible, respond appropriately. Some of the potential positive effects of global warming on agriculture are as follows:

- In the high latitudes, potentially cultivable regions will be extended northward: A 1°C increase in mean temperature is projected to move cultivation northward in North America by 175 km.

- Growing season will be extended in cooler areas. In the Canadian prairies, growing season would be extended by 10 days for every 1°C increase in mean temperature.

- Increased atmospheric carbon dioxide will increase the growth rate of some crops. Experimentally, a doubling of carbon dioxide increased wheat, rice, and soybean yields up to 50% and maize, sorghum, sugarcane. and millet crops by up to 10%.

On the other hand, detrimental changes for agriculture are foreseen with regard to global warming, as follows:

- An increase in the number of extremely hot days can suppress growth of heat-intolerant crops. In northern India, a doubling of atmospheric carbon dioxide would result in mean temperatures high enough to exceed the heat tolerance of wheat and eliminate its production.

- A reduction in rainfall and soil moisture can make some regions noncultivable or seriously increase demands for irrigation: Areas most likely to be affected are northern, midlatitude, midcontinental regions. These would include the U.S. Great Plains, the Canadian prairies, southern Europe, and Ukraine, all major production sites of cereal grains.

- Accelerated crop development can lead to premature ripening: This would lead to lower yields of some cereal crops.

- Warmer temperatures can result in increases in weeds, pests, and diseases: A 1°C increase in mean temperature would increase the range of the European corn borer northward from 165 to 500 km, depending on other conditions.

- Rising sea levels and serious flooding can result in losses of arable land: In Bangladesh, where most of the population farms in the Ganges flood plain, a 1-m rise in sea level would flood 17% of the country and displace millions of people.

Animal agriculture, as well as crop agriculture, will be affected by global warming. In the following sections, the potential effects on animal health and production and the implications for veterinarians are discussed. In closing the section on global warming, the contributory role of ruminant livestock to greenhouse gases through production of methane is addressed.

Impacts on Livestock Health

In analyzing global warming models on the future impact of greenhouse gas emissions, the various agencies and scientific bodies have examined the potential impact on a wide range of environmental, social, and economic parameters. The subjects of animal health and production, however, have received relatively little attention in these exercises, and the veterinary profession has been underrepresented in the ongoing study of climate change. On the IPCC, for example, there has been only one veterinarian among the 50 or so health professionals involved in assessment of health issues.

Yet the potential alterations in temperature, humidity, soil moisture, growing season, vegetation patterns, arthropod survival, and pest dispersion being studied by health professionals and scientists in other disciplines surely have application to the future health and productivity of livestock and, therefore, should be of considerable professional interest to veterinarians. Currently, insufficient data exist to draw specific conclusions about the future effects of global warming on animal health and production. However the tools of climate modeling coupled with our general knowledge of animal management practices and the natural history of infectious and parasitic diseases permit some reasonable speculation about possible effects, as discussed in the following sections.

Extensively Managed Animals Global warming will likely alter the distribution of livestock grazing in different regions of the world, reducing grazing activity in some areas while creating new opportunities in others. Global warming will increase the risk of drought wherever temperatures increase with little attendant increase in rainfall. In arid and semiarid. zones, such as the Sahel, increased temperatures may lead to an overall reduction in soil moisture and reduced vegetation cover. As grass cover and water supply are the limiting factors in cattle grazing, many pastoralists who keep cattle in mixed herds with smaller stock may find their opportunities to herd cattle drastically restricted. Camels and goats, better adapted to dry conditions, will become increasingly important to arid-zone people who depend on livestock for survival. The cultural implications for traditional cattle herders and the negative economic impact in the region would be profound.

In temperate regions, particularly in more northerly latitudes, there may be increased opportunities for grazing. Warmer temperatures will mean longer growing seasons. Also, it is believed that increases in atmospheric carbon dioxide concentrations will encourage leaf expansion and preferential growth of vegetative crops and pastures over cereal crops. In addition, grazing lands at higher altitudes, or upland pastures, are likely to be more lush, allowing higher stocking rates.

Longer growing seasons and warmer temperatures will affect the management of grazing animals. Aitken, in Scotland, has described some of the hypothetical changes in herd health and management that are likely to occur in association with increased temperatures in the United Kingdom.[1] Some of the possible implications for grazing animals are as follows:

- A longer grazing season, with greater dependency on grass as feed, could lead to unanticipated nutritional disorders. Earlier availability and use of grass could lead to an increased incidence of hypomagnesemic tetany in the spring, while extension of the grazing season into the fall could increase the occurrence of cobalt and selenium deficiencies in lambs.

- Patterns of gastrointestinal parasitic disease may alter significantly. Warmer winters would allow greater overwintering of some nematode ova and larvae and encourage earlier and more rapid development to infective stages in the early spring. For example, a 2°C rise in mean temperature would shift the peak hatch of the sheep nematode, *Nematodirus battus*, 4 to 6 weeks earlier than it currently occurs in April and May. This could be beneficial, as peak larval infectivity may be in decline by the time spring-born lambs are consuming large amounts of grass. On the other hand, a 2°C rise in temperature would extend the range of the gastric nematode, *Haemonchus contortus*, northward and increase its overwintering survival on pastures. This would lead to heavier year-round burdens, increased use of anthelmintics, and greater risk of development of anthelmintic resistance.

- Tick-borne diseases may become more widespread: The tick-borne, hemoparasitic disease babesiosis, caused by *Babesia divergens*, occurs in cattle primarily in the western U.K., where a milder, wetter climate favors the survival and multiplication of the tick vector, *Ixodes ricinus*. Increased temperature and moisture in the British Isles could extend the range of the vector, exposing immunologically naive populations of cattle to babesiosis. In addition, warmer, wetter weather would accelerate the rate of development of immature stages of the tick, leading to higher overall rates of disease transmission. Warmer temperatures also increase the risk that cattle infected with babesiosis will suffer clinical disease, with a 2°C rise in temperature potentially doubling the number of clinical cases. Zoonotic disease patterns of tick-borne infections could also change. Lyme disease occurrence could increase, for example, as tick populations increased around urban areas.

- New vector-borne diseases may be introduced: While the U.K. does not currently experience bluetongue of sheep or African horse sickness, these conditions are present in the Iberian peninsula. While midges capable of transmitting both causative viruses are present in the U.K., climatic conditions do not permit the infection to become established. In the case of bluetongue, for example, an overwintering generation is critical for the persistence of midges. A rise in winter temperatures might permit such overwintering and allow the establishment and persistence of the bluetongue virus in Britain after introduction from the south. The spread of arthropod disease vectors to expanded ranges and their enhanced potential to cause disease in humans and animals as a result of climate change are major concerns of public health officials around the world.

- Microbial infections with wild mammal reservoirs might increase. Bovine tuberculosis occurs in badgers in the U.K. Warmer winter temperatures with more available winter food supplies could increase badger populations and thereby increase contact with grazing cattle and free-living deer, thus promoting transmission of the disease. Similarly, increases in rodent populations could potentially increase the risk of leptospirosis and salmonellosis in domestic animals through contamination of pastures and water supplies.

- Reproductive management of herds and flocks may have to be altered in response to changes in parasite risk and pasture availability. With seasonal changes in feed availability and parasite infectivity, breeding and birthing schedules for various species of grazing livestock may require alteration to avoid the occurrence of nutritional deficiencies and parasitic infections associated with climate-induced alterations in pasture as discussed in the preceding bulleted items.

Intensively Managed Animals Animals managed under confinement conditions may be more protected from the direct effects of climate change because their environment and nutrition are more controlled. However, intensively reared livestock such as swine and poultry are fed large amounts of grain, and the economics of confinement production could be greatly affected by changes in the market availability of cereal crops, which may be influenced by global warming. Water intake will be increased as mean temperatures rise, and in some areas, water cost and availability could become a production constraint because of excessive demands on local water supplies brought about by global warming. Excessive heat can reduce feed intake in livestock and thereby decrease rates of gain and extend production schedules. Efforts to counteract this effect by use of air conditioning will increase fuel consumption and raise production costs.

Serious adverse consequences may occur in poultry production facilities as a result of increased temperatures, with im-

plications for both productivity and health. Heat stress is a major management problem in intensive poultry operations. In 1986, for instance, when average daily temperatures in Georgia and North Carolina reached 37.8°C (100°F), some producers were losing up to 500 birds a day from heat-related problems. Heat stress in poultry has public health implications as well. Salmonellosis transmitted to people from poultry products is an important contemporary issue in food safety, as discussed further in Chapter 9. Poultry frequently carry subclinical *Salmonella* infections, but can begin to actively shed the organism under stresses such as heat stress. *Salmonella enteritides* shed by stressed chickens can be passed into eggs before the shell is formed, thus creating a potential source of human infection. Such occurrences could increase with elevated mean temperatures in warmer regions such as the southern United States, where intensive poultry rearing is an important industry.

Contribution of Livestock to Global Warming

Methane is a major end product of ruminant digestion, representing about 25% of the gas produced when rumen microorganisms break down complex carbohydrates, including cellulose. Depending on size, species, and diet, ruminant animals can produce between 250 and 500 L of methane per day, which is released into the atmosphere by eructation as part of normal rumination. With approximately 1.3 billion cattle on the planet and 1.7 billion sheep and goats, this represents a considerable volume of methane.

Methane also happens to be an important atmospheric greenhouse gas. While it only constitutes about 3% of total greenhouse gases, it contributes significantly to the greenhouse effect because of its higher radiative index. It is considered responsible for approximately 20% of the total greenhouse gas effect of global warming. Concerns about methane in the atmosphere are heightened by the fact that methane concentrations have increased five times faster than carbon dioxide concentrations since the Industrial Revolution.

The contribution of cattle to atmospheric methane is estimated to be about 20% of the total atmospheric concentration of that gas. Other sources of methane include wetlands, coal mining, natural gas exploration, biomass burning, and rice paddy production. Additional production of methane from livestock is associated with storage of animal wastes in tanks or pools, which, under anaerobic degradation, produces methane. Manure spread on fields does not contribute significantly to methane production, as the breakdown of such manure involves oxygen.

Livestock owners and veterinarians may feel defensive about media reports that trumpet the contributory role of cattle to global warming. After all, the role of cattle seems insignificant compared with the contribution of fossil fuel burning and industrial activity leading to carbon dioxide production. Yet every cloud has a silver lining. Concerns about methane emissions from livestock can provide opportunities for improving the nutrition, productivity, and profitability of ruminant animals around the world, especially in developing countries. The rate of methane production in cattle is influenced by a number of factors, including types of carbohydrate in the diet, level of feed intake, physical characteristics of the feed, and alterations in rumen microflora. Of particular importance is the amount of available nitrogen in the diet. When nitrogen is readily available, rumen microflora can build amino acids from carbohydrate sources by the addition of nitrogen. When nitrogen is limiting, much additional carbon from carbohydrate is lost in rumen gas as eructated methane.

In developing countries, dietary protein is often the limiting factor in ruminant nutrition because of high cost and limited availability. In temperate regions of Asia, for example, winter feed is often limited to straw left from grain harvests. Such a diet often barely supports maintenance and survival of the animal, with little opportunity for growth or production. Interventions that provide cheap dietary sources of available nitrogen, for example, urea, as a supplement to straw diets, provide a double benefit. They improve the nutritive value of the ration, with attendant improvements in productivity, and reduce the overall volume of methane produced by cattle. This represents an opportunity to help the farmer and the environment simultaneously.

El Niño/Southern Oscillation (ENSO) and La Niña

El Niño was the name given decades ago, by Spanish-speaking inhabitants of Peru, to the noticeable warming of the Pacific Ocean that periodically occurs along the west coast of South America and that brings heavy rains and a sharp reduction in catches for local fishermen. The association of this phenomenon with El Niño, or the Christ child, was that this periodic warming occurred most commonly around Christmastime. In recent years, meteorologists, oceanographers, and other scientists have improved their understanding of El Niño and now recognize that the phenomenon is part of a recurring pattern of cyclic variations in atmospheric pressure and ocean currents that can dramatically affect weather patterns around the globe. Taken together this global cyclic pattern is now known as the El Niño/southern oscillation, or ENSO. La Niña is a second, distinct alteration of normal equatorial Pacific oceanic and atmospheric conditions, with the potential to affect global weather, though usually less dramatically than ENSO. La Niña tends to accentuate normal weather patterns, making dry areas drier, wet areas wetter, and cold areas colder. On a regional basis, La Niña effects are roughly opposite to those of ENSO.

In contemporary times, major ENSO events have occurred in 1972, 1976, 1982–1983, 1991–1994, and 1997–1998. Based on records kept for about the last 130 years, the 1991–1994 event was the longest ENSO on record, while the 1997–1998 episode was the strongest, with ocean temperatures exceeding those set in 1982–1983. Some observers believe that the frequency and severity of ENSO events increased through the 20th century on the basis of available historical data. Others disagree, suggesting that the events are being more carefully observed or recorded and that a century is too short a period of observation to draw any firm conclusions about increased occurrences of ENSO.

Similarly, there is disagreement about the role of global warming in the genesis of ENSO. Some scientists believe that higher mean atmospheric temperatures are fueling the generation of ENSO events, while others believe that the two phenomena are independent. In 1999, German meteorologists suggested that if global warming continues at the current pace, by 2050 the eastern Pacific would become warm enough that the conditions currently associated with intermittent El Niño events would become more-or-less constant. While the association of ENSO with global warming remains a subject of debate, there is no dispute concerning the fact that ENSO events do occur and that they can seriously affect many aspects of daily life. Whatever their professional interests, veterinarians are likely to encounter the influence of ENSO events in the course of their professional activities, be they in the area of livestock agriculture, pet practice, wildlife conservation, or public health, as discussed below.

Genesis of ENSO

The influence of ENSO on global weather patterns originates in the equatorial Pacific. Normally, equatorial Pacific climate is primarily influenced by the so-called Walker circulation, which begins when the equatorial sun warms the waters of the western Pacific around Australia and Indonesia so that large volumes of warm, moist air rise high into the atmosphere, creating a low-pressure system. As the air proceeds to cool in the higher atmosphere, it dumps its moisture as rain, and the cooler, drier air is pushed eastward by winds in the upper atmosphere. By the time this air reaches the west coast of the Americas, it is cold and dense enough to begin to sink, creating a high-pressure system near the ocean's surface. This dense mass of descended air then begins to move westward again, pushed by east-to-west trade winds heading back toward Australia and Indonesia. As the trade winds move westward, they push the top layer of warm ocean water westward as well, drawing it away from the west coast of South America. In response, colder, deeper ocean water, rich in nutrients, is drawn to the surface, which accounts for the normally bountiful fishing along the Peruvian coast.

In ENSO years, for reasons not fully understood, the east-to-west phase of the Walker circulation is disrupted. Atmospheric pressure becomes higher near Australia than near South America, a change referred to as the southern oscillation, and the east-to-west trade winds decrease or fail. As a result, the warmer surface waters of the eastern Pacific are not pushed westward. Instead they generate large volumes of warm, moist air that rise high into the atmosphere over the western coast of equatorial South America, producing torrential rains there and depriving the western Pacific region of the atmospheric moisture required to produce the seasonal monsoons of south Asia. The equatorial ocean waters off the Americas stay warm, so that the normal convection of nutrient-rich, cold bottom waters does not occur, thus disrupting the marine ecosystem and reducing commercial fish catches.

Other atmospheric events may be linked to ENSO, extending its impact on global weather patterns well beyond the equatorial Pacific zone where the phenomenon originates. For example, in ENSO years, the polar jet stream tends to remain in the higher latitudes instead of sweeping southward. This produces milder winters in much of Canada and the northern United States. High-altitude winds in the tropics tend to disrupt cyclone cloud formation and thereby reduce the number of hurricanes originating in the mid-Atlantic. Cooling in the Indian Ocean creates high-pressure fronts that potentially block rains from reaching southern Africa.

As with ENSO, the development of La Niña reaches its peak in the months of December through March, and it may exert its influence for several months thereafter. However the genesis of La Niña and its effects are roughly opposite to those of ENSO. La Niña events are associated with stronger than normal east-to-west trade winds, abnormal cooling in the eastern Pacific, and the movement of warm sea water toward the western Pacific. This leads to increased rainfall from Australia, through India, as far west as South Africa. The polar jet stream moves farther south than normal, causing colder winter temperatures in Canada and the northern United States. Caribbean hurricanes, encountering no strong western wind resistance, are more frequent during La Niña periods. The 1997–1998 ENSO was followed by a La Niña in 1998 that resulted in some of the deadliest hurricanes in history, notably Georges and Mitch. In the past 100 years, there have been, depending on the definitions of the reporting agency, 23 ENSO events and 15 La Niña events.

The practical effects of these meteorological cycles on everyday life can be extraordinary, as the recent ENSO of 1997–1998 clearly demonstrated. Warm Pacific waters began to accumulate off of Australia in March 1997 and by September 1997 had reached the Peruvian coast. Over the following 9 months, until about June 1998, dramatic weather-related events around the globe were being linked to ENSO. Many were associated with catastrophic outcomes. Severe droughts associated with raging forest fires occurred in Indonesia, Malaysia, northeastern Brazil, and Florida. Drought and crop failures were felt in Texas, Pakistan, northern India, the Philippines, and parts of Australia. Severe flooding with loss of lives, crops, and property occurred in Peru, California, Sudan, and Kenya.

Some consequences of the 1997–1998 ENSO were more benign. Milder winters in the northern United States and Canada led to drastic reductions in winter heating costs and fuel consumption. Tropical storms in the Caribbean were less frequent, and sport fisherman from northern California to Alaska were catching tuna and marlin, usually confined to more southern waters. Nevertheless, the 1997–1998 ENSO is estimated to have produced over US$33 billion in property damage and resulted in the loss of several thousand human lives.

Impacts on Animal Health and Production

The impact of ENSO events on animals can be direct or indirect and will vary from region to region, based on the type of weather changes induced in a specific area. The ENSO of 1997–1998 as well as the El Niño of 1982–1983 was replete with examples of how the health, productivity, and survival of domestic and wild animals may be affected.

Wildlife Recent ENSO events have posed notable dangers for wildlife. Their impact on wildlife have underscored the fragility of certain unique natural habitats and highlighted the tenuous hold on survival of some endangered species whose total populations are small or who have a restricted geographical distribution.

In 1997–1998, raging forest fires associated with the ENSO-induced drought in Indonesia created severe stresses for forest-dwelling animals. The orangutans of Kalimantan, the Indonesian portion of the island of Borneo, especially suffered, facing mass starvation due to the destruction of their forest habitat by fire. With vast expanses of forest blackened, there was little to eat or drink. Infants too weak to cling to their mothers were falling to their deaths from trees. Orangutans that fled the forest into areas of human inhabitation were sometimes killed by villagers. Dozens of young orangutans were rescued and brought to the Wanariset Samboja primate refuge for treatment and recuperation, though their future prospects in the wild remain uncertain. Orangutans on Borneo were already under extreme pressure from hunting and forest clearing, and some conservation specialists express concern that the fires of 1997–1998 may hasten the extinction of orangutans on that island.

Coral reefs and the multitude of marine animals that depend on them have been adversely affected by ENSO events throughout the Pacific, from the Great Barrier Reef off Queensland in Australia eastward to various reefs on the Pacific coast of Costa Rica, Mexico, and the Galapagos Islands. Higher ocean temperatures associated with ENSO events cause coral polyps to expel their symbiotic algae, which under normal circumstances capture many of the nutrients, including calcium that the coral needs to grow. In 1997–1998, ocean temperatures in the Great Barrier Reef reached 31.1°C (88°F), causing widespread algal expulsion and contributing to the coral bleaching that is occurring in that world-famous ecosystem. The effects of ENSO continue even after water temperatures begin to cool, hampering coral recovery. Cooling of the water from such high temperatures brings coastal upwelling, with an influx of deeper, nutrient-rich cold water that favors the proliferation of some important coral predators, notably starfish (*Ananthaster* sp.) and sea urchins (*Diadema* and *Eucidaris* spp.). These predators can consume ENSO-damaged coral at a rate faster than the coral can rebuild. Scientific studies carried out on coral reefs following the ENSO of 1982–1983 indicate that while recovery is possible, it may be slow, and some coral mortality will occur.

Coral bleaching is only one of many impacts of ENSO on the unique ecosystem of the Galapagos Islands and its wildlife inhabitants. During the ENSO of 1982–1983, the islands experienced over six times their normal rainfall, and sea temperatures averaged 3°C warmer than normal. The normally abundant ocean fish stocks that supported the islands' pelagic birds left the area for cooler seas, and the bird populations suffered. Populations of the flightless cormorants (*Nannopterum harrisi*) were reduced by 45%, and 78% of the rare Galapagos penguins (*Spheniscus mendiculus*) died. There was widespread breeding failure among waved albatrosses (*Diomedea irrorata*). Up to 70% of marine iguanas (*Amblyrhyncus cristatus*) starved when green sea algae, the normal diet of these creatures, was replaced by inedible red algae.

The normally dry and sparsely vegetated islands experienced a spurt of abundant vegetative growth that facilitated an increase in the famous finch populations but also supported the proliferation of fire ants and rats, alien species previously introduced to the island with the potential to spread disease and compete with indigenous species in specialized ecological niches. As the Galapagos Islands are home to the entire world populations of many unique, endemic species, these ENSO-related losses threaten the survival of some species.

Elsewhere in the eastern Pacific, the warmer ocean temperatures of 1997–1998 were creating difficulties for other populations of marine fauna. Hundreds of nursing sea lions starved to death off San Miguel Island in California when their mothers were unable to find the squid and small fish that usually compose their diet. The usual prey had moved to deeper, cooler waters beyond the diving range of the sea lions. Pup mortality rates, usually about 25%, reached 70% in the 1997 season. Warmer waters on the other hand, were attractive to large schools of predatory mackerel, which moved much farther north up the Pacific coast of North America than usual. The mackerel arrived off the coast of British Columbia just about the time that juvenile Chinook salmon were migrating out to sea. The mackerel consumed the young Chinook at alarming rates, adding yet another pressure to an already endangered species. Large-scale predation of sockeye salmon by mackerel also occurred in the ENSO of 1992, leading to a very poor salmon run in 1996.

Livestock   ENSO events are characterized by drought in some regions and excessive rainfall in others. Both situations can affect the health, management, productivity, and economics of livestock production. The severity of ENSO effects on livestock, however, is modulated by numerous other factors associated with local resource bases and the capacity to plan for, and respond to, crises. Areas with well-developed transportation infrastructure, veterinary services, and feed reserves, for example, will fare much better during periods of extended drought or flooding than will areas without such resources.

Under conditions of drought, livestock may die acutely from lack of water or subacutely from lack of feed. Adaptability of various species of livestock to drought is an important determining factor in survival. In arid and semiarid regions, such as the Sahel in Africa, cattle, sheep, and donkeys are generally less drought resistant and will succumb before goats and camels, which are better adapted to store water internally and, as browsers, to consume a wider range of potential feed

sources. Indigenous breeds of cattle usually fare better than exotic, imported breeds.

Range animals everywhere show choice in diet selection and under normal conditions will shun unpalatable weeds and shrubs, many of which are potentially toxic. Under drought conditions, however, they are far more likely to consume such plants and develop specific plant-related toxicities. In the southwestern United States, for instance, several plants are associated with disease in livestock during periods of drought, as they may be the dominant plants available on drought-affected rangelands and will be consumed in large quantities. These plants include bitterweed (*Hymenoxys odorata*), carpetweed (*Kallstroemia hirsutissima*), guajillo (*Acacia berlandieri*), coyotillo (*Karwinskia humboldtiana*), and the bitter-tasting selenium-accumulator plants such as locoweeds (*Astagalus* spp.) In addition, producers may be obliged to feed poorer quality stored feed to livestock during periods of drought than they might otherwise, thus increasing the risk of aflatoxicosis from moldy corn or silage.

Suboptimal feed intakes for extended periods by livestock can adversely affect reproductive performance through reduced fertility, increased predisposition to abortion, and reduced offspring survival through decreased milk production in the dam. There may also be reductions in immunity, with increased predisposition to infectious disease. Prolonged drought may force pastoralists to move stressed and susceptible livestock long distances in search of food, whereby the animals may come into contact with other livestock or vectors carrying disease. As droughts are frequently associated with abnormally high temperatures, heat stress and hyperthermia are also likely to increase.

In commercial operations, slower growth rates, decreased weight gains, and lower production outputs such as milk are to be expected. The Ministry of Agriculture and Fisheries in New Zealand has analyzed the national cost of the 1997–1998 ENSO in that country, where drought conditions prevailed. Overall losses for horticulture and livestock were estimated at $256 million, $170 million of which was livestock related in the beef, sheep, dairy, and deer sectors. Centers of loss included lower lamb and cattle slaughter weights, lower cull ewe weights, decreased fleece weights, a 20,000 tonne shortfall in projected milk production, and in deer, lower velvet, fawn, and meat outputs. In addition, another projected loss of $169 million was anticipated for 1998–1999 due to the carryover of reduced lambing rates, the need to rebuild herds, reduced productive life of surviving ewes because of excessive tooth wear during drought grazing, and other recovery costs.

Heavy rains also affect livestock production. Flooding may lead to acute death losses by drowning. Suboptimal feed intake may also result because grazing lands and forage or grain crops intended for livestock consumption may be damaged. Commercial operations will be directly affected by poorer performance and increased costs of production as feed costs rise.

Increases of certain disease problems can also be expected with heavy, extended rainfall. Foot rot is associated with persistently wet pastures and grazing lands, and widespread foot rot had a devastating effect on sheep and goats in the Horn of Africa during the heavy ENSO-associated rains in late 1997 and early 1998. Foot rot is deadly for extensively managed animals that must move over large areas of land in search of feed. Diseases caused by spore-forming organisms also generally increase following flooding of lowlands, as spores deep in the soil are brought to the surface and subsequently consumed. Anthrax and clostridial diseases such as blackleg and are notable examples.

Perhaps the greatest potential impact of heavy rains on livestock health is a rise in vector-borne disease. Insect vectors, such as mosquitoes, which require standing water to complete their life cycle, proliferate during ENSO-related periods of prolonged, wet weather. In 1997–1998, a dramatic and deadly outbreak of Rift Valley fever, a mosquito-borne viral disease, occurred in East Africa, causing serious morbidity and mortality in livestock and humans (see sidebar "Kenya and El Niño 1997–1998: A Challenge for Veterinarians"). Heavy rain may also increase feed supplies that lead to expanded populations of intermediate hosts, such as rodents, involved in the transmission of vector-borne diseases. This may have more direct consequences on humans and pet animals than on livestock as discussed below.

Companion Animals During the winter of 1997–1998, atypical, heavy rainfall inundated much of the American Southwest. The desert bloomed with an abundant array of wildflowers and other plants rarely seen in the region, to the delight of visitors and residents. Along with the rains came an explosion of grasshoppers and other insects, whose numbers became so dense that people had to take care sometimes not to skid on them while walking on pavement. Less obvious and more ominous was an explosion in rodent populations, including deer mice and piñon mice that found abundant food in the increased insect and seed supply. In New Mexico, trapping studies indicated that rodent populations had increased from an average of 5 per hectare to 50 per hectare. With the increase in rodent populations came an increase in flea populations, which led to an outbreak of plague in domestic animals and humans.

In January 1998, the first case of plague in the epizootic was diagnosed in a domestic cat in New Mexico. By mid-July 1998, there were 20 cat, 3 dog, and 2 human plague cases confirmed in the northern part of the state, stretching over a distance of 160 km. Plague is caused by the bacterium *Yersinia pestis* and is transmitted primarily by the bite of fleas. It is believed that in the periods between epizootics, deer mice, possibly other rodents, and their fleas may act as maintenance hosts for the infection. Heavy rains facilitate the expansion of rodent populations by increasing food supplies but also lead to increased death and injury or rodents because heavy rains will flood rodent shelters and burrows and force them out. This leads to increased contact between rodents and outdoor pets who may become infected with *Y. pestis* when they ingest rodents or become unwitting hosts to fleas abandoning the dead or dying

rodents. People may become infected by flea bites, by contact with infected pets, and through discharges from erupted lymph nodes in animals with bubonic plague or respiratory aerosols from animals with pneumonic plague.

Zoonotic Disease and Public Health

Climate is a key factor in defining the geographic distribution of vector-borne zoonotic disease. Climate essentially sets the limits of spatial distribution of disease vectors whose life cycles and natural history are constrained by climatic parameters such as seasonal temperature ranges and rainfall patterns. Based on field observations and computer models, there is both evidence and concern that global warming can contribute to significant alterations in the geographic distribution of serious human diseases that are transmitted by arthropod vectors such as mosquitoes. These diseases include, among others, malaria, dengue fever, yellow fever, and viral encephalitides.

Weather, in contrast to climate, plays a significant role in determining the frequency and severity of vector-borne or zoonotic disease outbreaks within the existing geographic range of a specific vector or animal host. ENSO events, with their power to significantly alter local weather patterns, are being recognized as important elements in vector-borne zoonotic disease occurrence. Diseases that are endemic in an area, meaning that the local ecology supports the persistence of disease at very low levels, can become epidemic, or widespread in susceptible local populations as a result of changes in weather associated with ENSO events. The 1993 outbreak of human hantavirus infections in the Four Corners region of the southwestern United States—where the borders of New Mexico, Arizona, Colorado, and Utah all meet—is a well-studied example, with parallels to the 1997–1998 plague outbreak among domestic animals and humans in the same locale. In the case of hantavirus, the viral disease is transmitted primarily by contact with rodent carriers of the virus or their droppings.

Hantaviruses, in the family *Bunyaviridae*, include human pathogens responsible for hemorrhagic fevers and nephropathy. The most notable outbreak of hantavirus-associated disease was in UN and American troops in Korea during the Korean War of the early 1950s, in which thousands were affected. The hantaviruses are associated with rodents, which are normally asymptomatic carriers that shed the virus in saliva and excretions. In the United States, the "Sin Nombre" strain of hantavirus has been associated with deer mice (*Peromyscus maniculatus*) in the southwestern United States but until 1993 had not been linked to outbreaks of human disease.

The Four Corners region had experienced almost 6 years of drought leading up to 1992. Rodent populations and rodent-predator populations, such as owls, were severely depressed during that drought period. Subsequently, heavy, above-average rainfall associated with ENSO occurred from November 1992 through March 1993, creating opportunities for marked increases in rodent populations, particularly deer mice populations at elevations between 1800 and 2500 m and in piñon pine/juniper forests. As predator populations take longer

Kenya and El Niño 1997-1998: A Challenge for Veterinarians

The relentless rains El Niño brought to East Africa between October 1997 and February 1998 would have impressed even Noah. In some parts of the region, rainfall for the period was eight times normal, producing floods of biblical proportion. Particularly hard hit was Kenya, where El Niño took a heavy toll. Economic damage was extensive. Wildlife tourism, a key element of the economy was disrupted when the dirt tracks in many of the National Parks became impassable because of persistent mud. Traffic on the principal commercial roadway in the region, A109, from the port of Mombasa to the capital, Nairobi, was repeatedly delayed because of flooding, washouts, and collapsed bridges, causing serious disruption to the flow of essential goods, with major economic losses. Heavy rains hampered the harvest of coffee and tea, major export crops that are critical sources of foreign exchange earnings for Kenya. Food crops such as maize and beans, ordinarily planted in October to take advantage of the normal seasonal rains, were instead lost to waterlogging from the unexpected deluge that occurred.

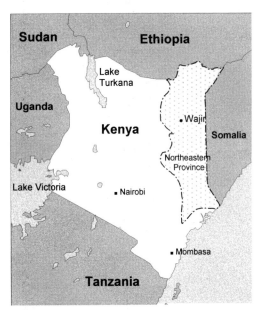

Map of Kenya.

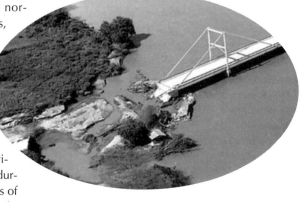

Washed out bridge on Kenya's main highway. (Photo courtesy of the United States Marine Corps/ U.S. Joint Task Force, Kenya)

While much of the country experienced difficulties during these 5 months of heavy rain, the most seriously affected region of the country was the northeast, where excessive precipitation and flooding set the stage for devastating disease outbreaks that resulted in the loss of much human and animal life and threatened famine in the region. Northeastern Province is one of the more remote regions of Kenya. It is an area of flat semiarid grazing lands populated largely by tribes of pastoralists with ethnic and linguistic links to the Somalis, who graze mixed herds of cattle, sheep, and goats. There are swamplands in the region, with seasonal rivers that feed into the perennial Tana River, which flows into the Indian Ocean. There are no large cities, few large towns, some airstrips, and limited road access.

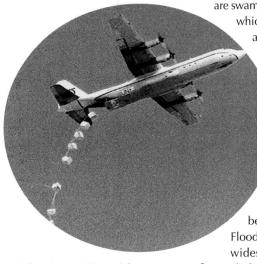

Relief air drop in Kenya. (Photo courtesy of World Food Programme/Kenya/ B. Barton)

Drought conditions during the previous 2 years had already caused serious hardship in the region. Livestock numbers were reduced, and pastoralists had limited cash to purchase cereal grains. With the nutritional status of both humans and animals already diminished and disease resistance compromised, the persistent El Niño rains that began in October 1997 catalyzed a number of serious human and animal health problems. Under the wet conditions that prevailed, insect populations exploded, and vector-borne disease became widespread. Human malaria, transmitted by mosquitoes, reached epidemic proportions. By February 1998, in Wajir District of Northeastern Province alone, over 1500 malaria deaths had been reported, and new human cases were occurring at the rate of 45 per day. Flooding also overwhelmed limited sanitation systems, and enteric diseases became widespread. Provincewide, dozens of people were dying daily from malaria, cholera, starvation, or some combination of the three. With roads impassable and airstrips flooded, international relief agencies such as the World Food Programme of the United Nations (WFP) and even the United States Marine Corps were participating in airdrops of food into the area to provide emergency assistance for an estimated 500,000 people in peril.

Another serious mosquito-borne disease that affected both humans and livestock in the province was Rift Valley fever (RVF). The virus is widely distributed in Africa, but major outbreaks are infrequent, occurring in 5- to 20-year cycles. Clinical disease can quickly reach epidemic proportions, however, when weather patterns produce conditions that are favorable to the rapid proliferation of mosquito vectors, particularly those such as *Aedes mcintoshi*, which can lay infected, drought-resistant eggs that remain dormant in shallow land depressions and then hatch synchronously when the depressions, or dambos, fill with rain or flood water. In people, RVF has historically produced flu-like signs with low mortality. More recently, though, a more severe hemorrhagic form of the disease has occurred. This form, with bleeding from body orifices, occurred in Northeastern Province in 1997-1978. Before the epidemic subsided in March 1998, an estimated 89,000 human cases of RVF occurred, with approximately 450 deaths.

Mosquito-borne RVF also affected cattle, sheep, goats, and camels in the region. Mortality was highest in young animals, while abortions were very common in adult females. Rains and flooding brought out other animal diseases as well. Infectious foot rot became a serious problem in sheep and goats with chronically wet feet and led to widespread mortality when it became too painful for animals to move in search of food. Starvation killed some animals outright, while malnutrition predisposed many small ruminants to respiratory diseases such as contagious caprine pleuropneumonia and pneumonic pasteurellosis, which further increased mortality. Increased soil moisture also favored the survival and maturation of infective nematode larvae, and haemonchosis became prevalent in sheep and goats. Similarly, wet fleeces and haircoats predisposed animals to debilitating mange. While most of these conditions are treatable or even preventable with vaccination, the delivery of animal health care services to pastoralists in remote regions is difficult even in the best of times, let alone during severe crises. Strategies for delivery of veterinary services in remote regions under difficult conditions is discussed in Chapter 8 of this book.

By the end of February 1998, when rains ended and flooding subsided, the pastoralist communities of Northeastern Province were reeling. Many herders were sick and malnourished themselves, had lost family members and animals during the crisis, and faced an unsure future. The loss of animals, their main source of livelihood, was extensive and severe. Government surveys in March

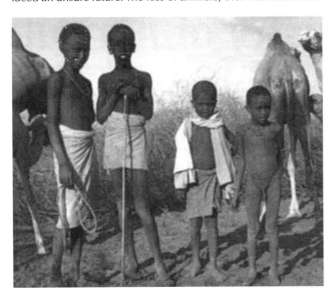

Pastoralist children in Kenya. (Photo courtesy of Farm Africa, London, UK)

1998 indicated that 200,000 sheep and 520,000 goats, or 53% of the small stock in the province, had died since the rains began in October 1997. Herders were left with depleted herds, few animals to sell, and little cash to purchase maize or other feedstuffs, which were selling at increased prices because of transportation difficulties and crop shortfalls. By March 1999, international health experts declared that the risk of RVF in the Horn of Africa had returned to negligible levels. Yet this was small consolation for the pastoralists of Northeastern Province. By mid-1998, the rains of El Niño had been replaced by a La Niña-induced drought and there were serious concerns about food security for hundreds of thousands of people and their animals in the region.

Pastoralist cultures face a number of important threats to their survival. Many of these problems are political, cultural, and economic, as discussed in Chapter 4. However, there is increasing concern that the natural resource base on which pastoralists depend is increasingly at risk because of events linked to global climate change. The ENSO is one such example. The effects of atmospheric and oceanic events originating thousands of miles away in the equatorial Pacific off the coast of Indonesia are adding significantly to the array of man-made problems that threaten the survival of traditional, livestock-based pastoralist cultures in the Horn of Africa. In addition, El Niño events are challenging veterinary and human health service providers to devise more-effective ways of addressing weather-related situations that affect health before, during, and after those situations develop.

to rebound, there were no effective controls on the expanded deer mouse population, which in some places was 20 times normal. This population explosion was presumed to bring people into more frequent contact with rodents outdoors. By June 1993, below-normal rainfall had returned to the region, creating serious food shortages for the expanded rodent population. At this point, rodent invasions of homes in the region noticeably increased, particularly in rural homes distant from surface water supplies. This led to greater rodent-human contact. By 1995, the rodent numbers in Four Corners had essentially returned to normal, but from 1993 until 1995 when the epidemic subsided, 53 human cases of human hantavirus occurred in the region.

Predicting ENSO Events

During the ENSO of 1997–1998, there was a notable tendency for the media to attribute every quirky or dramatic weather-related event during the period directly to El Niño. Yet local and regional weather patterns and events are influenced by a wide range of variables besides the ENSO phenomenon. The predictable occurrence of ENSO events and their impact on daily life varies from region to region. In some places the occurrence and impact are more consistent than in others, with coastal regions demonstrating less-variable patterns than regions farther inland. This is of particular relevance with regard to agriculture. For grain farmers in the American Midwest, the impact of ENSO on weather is quite variable, as local weather is influenced by other factors as well. The rainfall and temperature data from Illinois presented in Table 6-8 indicate the relatively unpredictability of the effect of ENSO events in the state. On the other hand, wheat farmers in coastal Queensland, the northeastern state of Australia, have come to consistently expect drought conditions in association with ENSO events, leading to serious, sometimes devastating reductions in wheat production because of failure of summer monsoon rains that would ordinarily begin in December. The 1994 wheat crop, in the midst of the longest ENSO event on record (1991–1995) was only 12% of normal.

In some parts of the world, Peru and Australia, for instance, the ability to predict ENSO events would allow planning to reduce loss of life and property destruction associated with acute catastrophic events such as flooding and allow informed decision making in economic sectors such as agriculture and tourism, which are particularly affected by climatic and seasonal variations. Fortunately, the ability of scientists to track and predict ENSO events has improved considerably in recent years.

By 1994, the U.S. National Oceanic and Atmospheric Administration (NOAA) had set up an informative surveillance system to measure critical oceanic and atmospheric indicators that would herald a developing El Niño. The tropical atmosphere/ocean array (TOA) is a series of 70 monitoring buoys spread across the equatorial Pacific linked to mobile research ships, polar-orbit satellites, and NOAA data-analysis stations (see http://www.pmel.noaa.gov/tao/). Through its World Cli-

Table 6-8 Departures from Normal for Temperature and Precipitation in Illinois during Strong El Niño years, 1951–1992[a]

Summer (June, July, and August)

Year	Temperature (°F)	Precipitation (%)
1951	+1.9	+21
1957	+0.2	+7
1963	-0.2	-10
1965	-1.7	-1
1969	-1.1	+9
1972	-1.7	+4
1976	-0.5	-24
1982	-2.4	+6
1987	+1.4	+7
1991	+1.4	-21

Winter (December, January, and February)

Year	Temperature (°F)	Precipitation (%)
1951-52	+1.9	+13
1957-58	+0.4	-15
1963-64	-1.2	-44
1965-66	-0.4	0
1969-70	-3.5	-34
1972-73	0.0	15
1976-77	-6.8	-47
1982-83	+5.1	+14
1986-87	+4.2	-37
1987-88	-1.0	+16
1991-92	+5.2	-12

[a] No consistent effect of ENSO is observed on either temperature or precipitation despite the documentation of ENSO events in the years listed. The variation indicates that while El Niño events may influence weather patterns, local conditions in some regions can mask or modulate El Niño effects.

Data derived from the Internet site of the Illinois State Climatologist Office at http://www.sws.uiuc.edu/atmos/statecli/ElNino/elnino.htm

Copyright (c)1999 Illinois State Water Survey

mate Program, the World Meteorological Organization has also set up a tracking program, the Climate Information and Prediction Services (CLIPS), which collects and coordinates weather information from national meteorological services around the globe.

Using the TOA system, NOAA, in April 1997, was able to foretell the impending ENSO event that began to build off Indonesia and Australia a month later. This allowed time for proactive planning to ameliorate the negative effects of altered weather and to capitalize on potential opportunities. For example, in Peru, storm drains and channels were systematically repaired and cleared of debris so that when the torrential rains subsequently arrived, the damaging effects of flooding were considerably lessened, with little loss of life.

New surveillance technology and better understanding of the relationship of ENSO events to disease patterns can also help to forecast disease outbreaks, thus providing public health officials with valuable time to increase public awareness and institute prophylactic measures. The Southern Oscillation Index has been used to predict the probability of epidemics of vector-borne diseases in Australia, for example, Murray Valley encephalitis. Satellite remote sensing, which can detect areas of abnormal precipitation via increases in vegetation, identified exactly those areas subsequently hit by the Rift Valley fever outbreak in East Africa in late 1997 and early 1998. Remote sensing is also being used to predict cholera outbreaks, which have now been associated with oceanic plankton blooms that harbor the causative organism, *Vibrio cholerae*.[27] Such plankton blooms have been linked to ENSO-associated increases in ocean temperatures and subsequent outbreaks of cholera, thus establishing cholera as a global pandemic disease whose occurrence is tied to climate.[15]

Implications for Veterinarians

That weather can affect patterns of disease occurrence is not a new concept in veterinary medicine. Yet the notion that ENSO events can influence weather on a regional basis and that these patterns likely will be predicted with increasing reliability in the future increases opportunities for improvement of veterinary services.

In the areas of clinical practice, for example, advanced knowledge about potential plague outbreaks in New Mexico would allow implementation of client-awareness campaigns, vaccination of humans at high risk, such as veterinarians and veterinary technicians, and initiation of aggressive flea control in local pet populations.

In the area of epidemiology and public health, there are research opportunities to better understand the ecology of important animal and zoonotic diseases, particularly in relation to weather and climate. There are also research opportunities to improve disease prediction and field opportunities worldwide for better conception and implementation of disease-control strategies such as regional vaccination campaigns for conditions such as anthrax, blackleg, or Rift Valley fever.

In the area of emergency and disaster medicine, there are challenges for veterinarians to develop appropriate veterinary knowledge of, and critical-care interventions for, threatened and endangered species across a wide taxonomic spectrum, from iguanas to orangutans. In addition, there are opportunities to improve international emergency response procedures and to develop strategies and techniques for working effectively and safely with animals in unfamiliar and potentially dangerous environments under emergency conditions induced by weather and climate change.[22]

Ozone Depletion and Ultraviolet Radiation

Ozone, when present in the air we breathe, is considered a pollutant. It is generated in the lower atmosphere from oxygen by various chemical and electrical processes and is recognized as a common constituent of polluted air in industrialized societies, particularly in urban areas. When present in inspired air, ozone can produce inflammation of the lungs of humans and animals. Plants, including some important agricultural crops, such as alfalfa, potatoes, tomatoes, wheat, spinach, and tobacco, are very sensitive to ozone, and low levels of ozone can result in lower yields and premature senescence of affected crops. In the United States, an estimated \$2 billion in losses due to crop damage are incurred annually as a result of the action of ozone and other photochemical oxidants.

When ozone is present in the stratosphere, however, it plays a critically important role in sustaining life on the planet, as it is primarily responsible for removing harmful ultraviolet radiation from sunlight before it reaches Earth. Ozone's beneficial role in the stratosphere and the dangers associated with depletion of stratospheric ozone are discussed in the following sections.

Genesis of Ozone Depletion

Ultraviolet (UV) radiation is part of the spectrum of electromagnetic radiation emitted by the sun and transmitted to the earth. UV radiation has higher energy and shorter wavelength than visible light. Three categories of UV radiation are recognized, according to their physical properties and photochemical effects. These are UVA, with wavelengths of 315 to 400 nm; UVB, with wavelengths from 280 to 315 nm; and UVC, with wavelengths of 200 to 280 nm.

UV radiation has harmful biological potential. It can disrupt the replicative and metabolic processes of single-cell organisms or unprotected cells in higher organisms and ultimately kill them. It is unlikely that the complex, terrestrial life forms we recognize today on earth could have evolved successfully if the full load of UV radiation reaching the outer limits of Earth's atmosphere actually penetrated to Earth's surface. Fortunately, during the course of development of the planetary biosphere, a protective mechanism evolved that filters out most UV radiation in the stratosphere, 10 to 50 km above Earth's surface. The key element in that filtering process is stratospheric ozone.

Ozone (O_3), or triatomic oxygen, is the most chemically active form of oxygen, but is also an unstable molecule. Oxygen (O_2) itself can absorb shorter-wave UV radiation. It is the absorption of incoming solar UVC radiation by oxygen in the stratosphere that results in the generation of ozone. In turn, ozone can absorb UV radiation of longer wavelengths, up to about 310 nm, and is responsible for filtering most of the UVB radiation entering the stratosphere. Ozone, being unstable, is also broken down by a variety of natural chemical processes. As a result, a normal equilibrium of stratospheric ozone concentration is achieved. The distribution of ozone above the earth, however, is not uniform. The ozone layer is normally thicker over the polar regions than at the equator, so that in general, less UV radiation reaches Earth at high latitudes than at lower latitudes. Moving in a direction from the poles toward the equator, there is about a 4% increase in UVB radiation reaching the earth per degree of latitude change. UVB radiation also increases in intensity at higher altitudes.

The phenomenon of ozone generation from oxygen in the stratosphere was first explained in 1930. In 1957, atmospheric scientists began regular monitoring of ozone concentrations in the ozone layer. It was recognized that the distribution of ozone in the ozone layer has a natural variability based on solar intensity and atmospheric circulation, with concentrations varying seasonally as much as ±20%. By the late 1970s, cumulative monitoring data had identified some disturbing developments in normal ozone distribution and concentrations. Average global concentrations of ozone were down by 5%, and scientists observed that at the beginning of spring in the southern hemisphere, stratospheric ozone over Antarctica was about 35 to 40% lower than the average for data from the 1960s. By 1984, it was reported that this so-called ozone hole formed over Antarctica in the spring, remained there for about 2 months and then moved over Australia and New Zealand. The event recurred annually, though the cause of the ozone depletion was unknown. The explanation, however, was not long in coming. It involved the appearance of synthetic organic compounds in the stratosphere.

Chlorofluorocarbons, or CFCs, are synthetically derived organic compounds that were developed in the 1930s primarily as refrigerants to replace ammonia. The CFCs were chemically stable, nonflammable and nontoxic and found widespread commercial and industrial use as coolants, in plastics manufacturing, and as propellants in aerosol sprays. By the early 1970s about 1 million tons of CFCs per year were produced for industrial use. Because of their relatively high stability, CFCs released into the air were able to gradually accumulate in the earth's atmosphere without degradation by sunlight, water, or oxidation. However, existing natural patterns of global atmospheric circulation drew CFCs high into the stratosphere and concentrated them over Antarctica. High in the stratosphere, the chemical stability of CFCs was compromised. At altitudes above 28.8 km (18 mi) the high-energy UV radiation of the sun can breakdown CFCs and release highly reactive chlorine atoms. When chlorine reacts with two molecule of ozone it breaks down the ozone to oxygen and

generates the free radical, chlorine oxide. Chlorine oxide in turn catalyzes a repetitive chain reaction in which a single chlorine atom released from CFC can remove up to 100,000 molecules of ozone from the stratosphere. Researchers have identified other compounds that can contribute to ozone depletion, notably carbon tetrachloride, methylchloroform, nitrous oxides, and the pesticide, methyl bromide. However, based on detection of increased levels of stratospheric fluorine as well as chlorine, CFCs have been confirmed the major culprit in ozone depletion.

Projections derived from the accumulating data on ozone depletion suggested that during the 1990s, a maximum 6 to 7% reduction in normal ozone concentration would occur at midlatitudes in the northern hemisphere during summer and fall. At this reduced ozone level, the average annual dose of harmful UV radiation reaching Earth would increase by 6 to 12%. Epidemiological data suggested that for every 1% drop in ozone concentration at midlatitudes in summertime, there would be a 0.5% increase in the incidence of ocular cataracts, and a 2% increase in the incidence of nonmelanomic skin cancer in humans.

Widespread public acceptance of the information linking CFCs to ozone depletion and its implications for human health was surprisingly swift. Politicians and policymakers, working with scientists, were quick to develop and adopt international agreements to meaningfully reduce the dangers of ozone depletion. The Montreal Protocol on Substances that Deplete the Ozone Layer was drafted in 1987, only 2 years after the ozone hole over the Antarctic was definitively confirmed by satellite. The Montreal Protocol, ultimately ratified by 180 nations, established policies that would reduce the release of CFCs into the atmosphere to a level half that of 1986. That treaty was subsequently made stronger by approval of various amendments in London in 1990, Copenhagen in 1992, and again in Montreal in 1997. These amendments resulted in agreement for a complete ban on the manufacture, importation, and use of CFCs in industrial countries by 1996 and in developing countries by 2010. Current information on the status of implementation of the Montreal Protocol and its various amendments, as well as their full texts, can be obtained at the website of the Ozone Secretariat of the UNEP (http://www.unep.ch/ozone/index.shtml).

International cooperation on ozone depletion through the Montreal protocol is a triumph of global environmental diplomacy, with great potential benefit for the protection of human, animal, and environmental health. For example, computer modeling has indicated that in a "business as usual" scenario, with no reduction in the use or manufacture of CFCs, human skin cancer rates in the United States and northwestern Europe due to increased UV radiation from ozone depletion would increase by approximately 325% by the year 2100. This would represent an additional 1.5 million cases in the United States and 440,000 in Europe. With phased reduction of CFC use as originally agreed in the Montreal Protocol, the increase in skin cancer rates would be reduced to about 98%.

With implementation of the total ban on CFC use agreed upon in the Copenhagen Amendments, the increase in skin cancer cases by the year 2100 for the same regions would be only 2%.

Unfortunately, ratification of the Montreal Protocol and its amendments does not mean that all risks of harmful biological effects associated with UV radiation have been eliminated. Several factors suggest that problems of UV radiation exposure associated with ozone depletion will persist for decades. Some of the factors contributing to this persistence are as follows:

- CFCs currently in the lower atmosphere will remain there for a long time. As CFCs are highly stable in the atmosphere, accumulated concentrations remain high. These CFCs in the lower atmosphere will continue to move up to the stratosphere for years to come, and there they will ultimately be degraded to produce ozone-depleting chlorine.

- Some skin cancers are triggered by childhood exposure to UV radiation but are not expressed until adulthood. The risk of basal cell carcinomas of the skin, for example, increases with age but is strongly determined by UV exposure during childhood. Today's children may still be manifesting basal cell carcinomas 60 years from now even if ozone depletion is slowed.

- Global warming may contribute to ozone depletion even in the face of reduced atmospheric CFCs. In 1998, new atmospheric research suggested that increasing concentrations of greenhouse gases may be leading to colder, more-stable vortex circulations in winter that accelerate the removal of ozone at high latitudes. This effect may continue even after stratospheric chlorine levels begin to decline.

- Some continued use of CFCs can be expected into the future. The Montreal Protocol permits total phaseout of CFCs in developing countries to be complete in 2010. Furthermore, in an imperfect world, total compliance with the CFC ban cannot be expected. Already there is a considerable illegal, black-market trade in CFCs smuggled into the United States where demand remains high in automobile repair shops and refrigeration companies for restoration of older cooling systems that used CFCs. In Miami alone, federal agents seized over 1 million pounds of contraband CFCs in an undercover operation designated "Cool Breeze."

As a result, environmentalists and health professionals, including veterinarians, must continue to be able to recognize and respond to the known potential harmful effects of UV radiation and to be alert to any as-yet unrecognized impacts on health and the environment.

Biological Effects of UV Radiation

Conjugated bonds in organic molecules effectively absorb UV radiation. The radiant energy of absorbed UVB leads to photochemical reactions that can produce molecular damage. In living systems, this molecular damage can lead to functional disruptions or death of cells. In the conjugated bonds of aromatic rings, as are found in DNA base pairs, the absorption of UV radiation is greatest in the UVB range. Damage to molecular DNA from UVB radiation is significant. It is estimated that a single epithelial cell in the epidermis of a light-skinned person spending a sunny summer day at the beach can develop 100,000 to 1,000,000 damaged sites in its DNA. While living cells possess the capacity to repair DNA, some damage may persist and result in faulty replication of DNA, leading to mutation and possibly oncogenesis.

Complex organisms have evolved a variety of protective adaptations to minimize the potentially deleterious effects of normal levels of solar UV radiation. However, increased levels of UV radiation can overcome these defenses and pose additional danger for simpler, less well adapted organisms, for example marine plankton. While UV radiation striking a person will not penetrate beyond the depth of the dermal layer of the skin, UV radiation striking the ocean can penetrate tens of meters into clear water. Plankton serves as the foundation of the global marine food chain. Proliferation of plankton can be depressed by UV radiation, and rates of phytoplankton production measured in waters around Antarctica, under the ozone hole, are reduced. The potential effects of plankton reductions on marine biodiversity in general and commercial fisheries in particular should be of concern to human society. Furthermore, phytoplankton contain chlorophyll and act as a sink for carbon dioxide, so reduction of phytoplankton in the world's oceans may also contribute to global warming.

In addition, the eggs and developing larvae of various fish, amphibians, and other aquatic species that develop in shallow water may experience mutation that leads to either death or developmental anomaly when exposed to excessive UV radiation. In recent years there has been a global alarm bell sounding with regard to a widespread decline in amphibian populations and a growing incidence of freakish amphibian malformations, such as frogs with multiple extra legs. Though the causes of this worldwide phenomenon are not fully understood and indeed may vary among locations, there is evidence that increased UV radiation associated with ozone depletion can induce death and deformities in frog embryos and may weaken the immune system, making mature amphibians susceptible to parasitic diseases.[8]

Health Effects in Humans

Humans, like other higher organisms, have evolved a range of adaptations in response to the presence of the normal levels of UV radiation found in sunlight. Along with other mammals, they even use UV radiation to their advantage for the production of vitamin D, an essential vitamin associated with calcium metabolism, as previtamin D_3 is formed in epidermal cells of the skin in response to UVB irradiation. To avoid the harmful effects of excessive exposure to UV radiation, human skin has several protective features. These include a thick, keratinized outer layer of epidermis with a high cellular turnover rate, a high capacity to repair damaged cells, an active skin-based immune system to remove dead or nonrepairable cells, and the presence of melanocytes, the melanin pigment-containing cells that are mobilized in response to increased exposure to UV radiation. Dermatologists classify six skin types largely on the basis of the number of melanocytes present. The higher the proportion of melanocytes, the darker the skin and the less likely the risk of sunburn and other adverse effects of UV radiation. Caucasians, with skin scores of 1 and 2 have a relatively high risk of developing skin cancer from prolonged exposure to sunlight. That risk is increased by ozone depletion.

The scope of human health effects of solar UV radiation have been thoroughly reviewed and are not discussed in detail here.[16] The eyes, skin, and immune system are mainly affected. Ocular conditions include severe, noninfectious keratoconjunctivitis or "snow blindness," pterygium formation, droplet keratopathy, and possibly cortical cataracts of the lens. Skin problems associated with UV radiation include sunburn, precancerous lesions such as actinic keratosis, and several forms of skin cancer, including squamous cell carcinoma, basal cell carcinoma, and malignant melanoma. UV radiation can also suppress immune responses, largely in the cellular arm of the immune system in the skin, increasing the risk of skin cancer and also contributing to the expression of certain infections, for example, cold sores, associated with latent herpes simplex infection. In leprosy patients, the lesions of leprosy are more common on areas of the body more consistently exposed to the sun, such as the face and arms. There are also indications that immune responses to vaccinations may be less pronounced following excessive exposure to sunlight.

Health Effects in Domestic Animals

Skin cancers are much less prevalent in domestic mammals than in humans. In large part, this is because the fur or hair coat offers additional protection against the penetration of UV radiation to the skin. Also, the skin of animals tends to be darkly pigmented, especially when the hair color is dark. Nevertheless, several diseases of animals are known to be associated with exposure to UVB radiation. The damaging effect of increased UV radiation exposure in animals is most likely to be expressed on nonpigmented, relatively uncovered portions of the body. These include the eyes, eyelids, ear tips, teats, and mucocutaneous junctions. Epidemiological data on the incidence of UVB-related diseases of animals are sparse, but it is reasonable to assume that as with human skin cancer, increases in effective UVB radiation reaching the Earth because of ozone depletion can result in increased cases.

The animal diseases in which UVB radiation is known to be a causal factor are squamous cell carcinoma in cattle, cats, horses, and sheep; infectious bovine keratoconjunctivitis, or "pinkeye," in cattle; pannus in dogs; and skin lesions in fish. Photosensitization in cattle is certainly associated with exposure to certain wavelengths in sunlight, though UVB has not been specifically implicated. The differential impact of sunlight on pigmented and nonpigmented skin of animals is dramatically represented in clinical cases of photosensitization in Holstein cattle. In these cases, photodynamic agents in the skin react with solar radiation to produce a solar dermatitis that is severe enough to cause skin sloughing on the white-haired and light-skinned portions of the animal but not on the dark-haired, heavily pigmented portions (Fig. 6-7). Sunburn, or solar dermatitis can also be a problem for light-skinned animals, particularly where hair cover is sparse, such as on the teats. Saanen goats and Holstein cows, for example, are prone to getting sunburned teats, which can interfere with milking and predispose to mastitis.

Squamous cell carcinoma is the most widely recognized disease of animals in which occurrence is linked to the intensity and duration of exposure to UV radiation. The disease is of

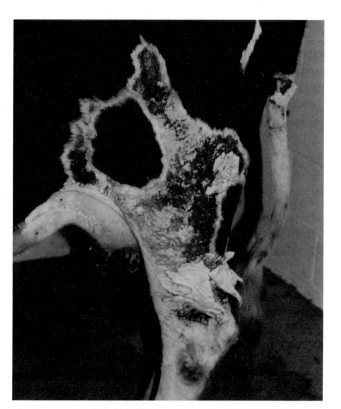

Figure 6-7.   Left flank and hindquarter of a Holstein cow with skin lesions due to photosensitization. Note the characteristic pattern of lesions, with the surface areas of lesser pigmentation and white hair cover far more severely affected than the black areas of hair and skin. The occurrence of photosensitization in domestic animals could increase as a result of ozone depletion and an attendant increase in ultraviolet radiation. (Photo by Dr. David M. Sherman)

considerable economic importance in the beef cattle industry, as it occurs commonly in white-faced Hereford cattle as a neoplastic condition of the eyes and eyelids, often referred to as "cancer eye." Simmental and Holstein cattle, other breeds with relatively little pigmentation around the eyes, also develop ocular squamous cell carcinoma, but not as commonly as Herefords. Economic losses from cancer eye are associated with treatment costs and/or premature culling. The lack of pigmentation on the eyeball and the eyelids of white-faced Herefords predisposes them to the condition, compared with other beef breeds. It is rarely seen in animals less than 4 years of age and has a peak incidence at 8 years of age, suggesting a cumulative radiation dose effect similar to that recognized in humans for skin cancer. In parts of Australia, 6% of all Hereford cattle may be affected with ocular squamous cell carcinoma, and the closer Herefords are kept to the equator, the higher the incidence of the disease. The role of UV radiation in the pathogenesis of bovine ocular squamous cell carcinoma is generally accepted. However, since the linkage was established over 40 years ago, there have been no specific epidemiological studies to identify or correlate changes in rates of ocular bovine squamous cell carcinoma with increased effective UVB radiation due to ozone depletion. Such studies would be of considerable interest.

Other species of domestic animals also develop forms of squamous cell carcinoma associated with exposure to UVB radiation. In cats, squamous cell carcinomas of the eyelids, conjunctiva, and nictitating membranes are most common in white-haired cats over 5 years of age with nonpigmented eyelid margins. White cats are also more likely to develop squamous cell carcinoma of the lips, nose, and ear tips, areas lacking pigmentation and poorly protected by fur. Squamous cell carcinoma of the ear tips is also seen in older white sheep, where cumulative exposure to solar radiation is associated with summer grazing. In horses, squamous cell carcinomas of the eyes and periorbital tissues occur more common in individuals over 8 years of age with lightly pigmented or nonpigmented eyelids. In the United States, Appaloosa and draft breeds of horses are most commonly affected, and the pattern of disease occurrence illustrates the role of UVB radiation in the occurrence of the disease. The incidence is higher at higher altitudes and at latitudes closer to the equator, where mean solar radiation is greater. Cutaneous melanomas are rare in dark-skinned horses, but surprisingly common in older gray or white horses, with up to 80% of gray and white Lipizzaner, Arabian, and Percheron horses affected. The tumors usually develop at the base of the tail or perineum but may be found elsewhere and may metastasize to lymph nodes. While the profile of disease occurrence suggests UV radiation as a potential contributing factor in the pathogenesis, there has been little or no research to establish such a link.

Infectious bovine keratoconjunctivitis (IBK), or pinkeye, is a common disease of cattle worldwide. It is caused by a specific bacterial pathogen, *Moraxella bovis*. However, experimental studies have clearly demonstrated that exposure to UVB radiation increases the clinical severity of infection. It also promotes transmission of the infection between cattle, because UVB exposure itself produces irritation to the eye that prompts cattle to rub their eyes on inanimate surfaces that may be contaminated with the infective lacrimal secretions of other clinically infected cattle. The prospect of increased occurrence of IBK associated with increased effective UVB radiation due to ozone depletion should be of concern to veterinarians. Already, IBK is commonly cited as a predominant disease of cattle in disease surveys carried out around the world. Losses associated with the disease are significant. Acute inflammation of the eyes creates discomfort and impaired vision that is associated with decreased feed intake, especially in grazing animals, which actually may die of starvation. Less dramatic, but still costly effects include weight loss, slower growth of calves, decreased milk production in cows, and associated treatment expenses. Increased occurrence of IBK worldwide would be costly in terms of both animal suffering and economic loss.

Pannus is an ophthalmological condition of dogs, also known as Uberreiter's syndrome, or chronic superficial keratitis. The disease is more common in larger breeds, most notably German Shepherds, and manifests as a progressive, proliferative, superficial keratitis that begins at the lateral limbus and gradually extends to cover the cornea. Epidemiological studies carried out in the 1970s suggested that the disease in the United States was more common in population centers at higher altitudes where incident radiation in the UV wavelength was considerably higher than at sea level. It is hypothesized that chronic, high-intensity exposure to UV radiation in certain breeds produces alterations in corneal tissues that make them appear foreign to the host. An autoimmune response to these antigens manifests as corneal inflammation.

Investigations into the effects of UV radiation on fish health date back to 1930, when mortality in brook trout, *Salvelinus fontinalis*, was observed in response to exposure to certain wavelengths of UV light. As the aquaculture industry continues to expand, the practice of confining fish in cages in relatively shallow water may result in increased manifestations of UVB-related fish diseases of veterinary concern. Fish are susceptible to solar dermatitis, or sunburn. In 1985 it was reported that farmed rainbow trout, *Salmo gairdneri*, kept in shallow, unshaded, clear-water ponds at high altitude in Bolivia developed severe necrosis of the dorsal fin. The fish would actively seek what little shade was available adjacent to the pond walls. Similarly, in 1987, Atlantic salmon, *Salmo salar*, raised in sea cages off the west coast of Ireland developed severe dorsal skin lesions during the summer months and experienced a high mortality rate. While several factors contributed to this disease outbreak, exposure to prolonged summer sunlight was considered an important predisposing factor.[28] The UV effect was intensified by the clarity of the coastal water, which was unusually clear because there had been little rain or coastal water runoff to create turbid conditions.

Veterinarians everywhere and in all types of practice should be alert to the occurrence of animal diseases related to UV radiation and their potential to increase in the future. Animal management practices will need to be changed in response to increased UV radiation, for example, shading of fish ponds, or sun block applications to goat teats or cat's ears. As the role of solar effects in disease pathogenesis varies with latitude and altitude, there is a need for networks of veterinarians in different locales to share data on the incidence patterns of various diseases over time. Well-constructed epidemiological studies can help clarify the role of UV radiation in the pathogenesis of suspect diseases in veterinary medicine and provide further support to policymakers committed to addressing the problems of ozone depletion and its implications for global health.

Issues of Global Environmental Contamination

The power of modern human society to transform Earth is visible everywhere. The impact of the axe, the plow, and the bulldozer on the natural landscape and its inhabitants is readily apparent to even the casual observer. Yet the industrial and technological revolution has spawned other less-visible, but no less powerful instruments of environmental transformation in the form of manufactured chemicals and nuclear radiation, which can serve as environmental pollutants and compromise the health of living organisms on a global scale.

Some damaging chemicals, such as sulfur dioxide, nitrous oxide, and carbon monoxide, which contribute to air pollution and acid rain, are unintended byproducts of the burning of fossil fuels, the principal energy source powering contemporary society. Others, such as organophosphate insecticides or plastic polymers were intentionally developed for benevolent purposes to improve the health, quality, and convenience of life for human beings. Some of the adverse consequences of these products were immediately apparent, and efforts were made to minimize their negative impact. In other cases, adverse consequences were unanticipated, initially undetectable, or simply overlooked because of the net benefits that could be accrued by their use. Yet over time, the cumulative adverse effects of some such chemicals became painfully apparent. The modern environmental movement in the United States can pretty much be traced back to the publication in 1962 of Rachel Carson's *Silent Spring*, in which the unintended effects of herbicides and pesticides on the environment were simply and eloquently revealed to the reading public.

Since the 1960s it has become increasingly clear that chemical pollution is a problem of global proportion and that it is necessary to address chemical pollution from a global perspective. Next to nuclear radiation, nothing underscores the interconnectedness of life on Earth and its collective vulnerability more than chemical pollution. Improved methods of detection and expanded efforts of surveillance have revealed how widespread the distribution of potentially harmful, man-made chemicals is on the planet. There is virtually not a place on Earth where some form of synthetic chemical or chemical breakdown product cannot be found in soil, water, or tissue of plants and animals. Investigators are continuing to locate and identify the diverse and harmful effects of these widely dispersed and cumulative toxins on living organisms.

It is beyond the scope of this book to provide a comprehensive presentation of the science of environmental toxicology, a complex subject for which numerous textbooks exist. However, the relevance of environmental toxicology to the future of veterinary medicine cannot be overemphasized. The subject will offer many professional challenges and opportunities to veterinarians in the coming years. The intention of the following sections is to present information on two contamination issues of global proportion that are of current concern and that pose serious potential environmental and health threats relevant to veterinarians. The first topic is endocrine disruptors, a group of chemicals that act as estrogen mimics with the potential to disrupt reproductive and developmental processes in a wide range of organisms, including the domestic animals that make up the traditional purview of veterinary medicine. The second topic is nuclear radiation.

Finally, if veterinarians are going to play an active role in promoting environmental health, they need to recognize the polluting potential of livestock-production systems and work with livestock producers to correct some of the practices that contribute to environmental contamination, while protecting the livelihood of producers. Contemporary issues of environmental contamination in animal agriculture, including animal waste management and the use of toxic chemicals are discussed at the end of this chapter.

Endocrine Disruptors

The occurrence of substances in the environment with the capacity to mimic the behavior of estrogens is not unfamiliar to veterinarians. Most veterinary students learn about the capacity of phytoestrogens to alter the reproductive performance of livestock. Phytoestrogens are chemical compounds naturally produced by certain plants and fungi that exert estrogenic effects in animals following consumption of the plants. The condition most commonly occurs in sheep grazing legume pastures containing phytoestrogens. The plants most often involved are subterranean, ladino, and red clover. The estrogenic substances they contain are coumestans and isoflavones, which are also found in soybeans. Some pine trees also produce estrogenic substances, and in the case of consumption of pine needles, tips, or branches, cattle rather than sheep are most affected. Molds in the genus *Fusarium* also produce a phytoestrogen, zearalenone, which mainly affects pigs. Zearalenone may be present in high concentration in moldy feeds, especially maize, barley, and oats.

Though the manifestations differ somewhat between species, phytoestrogens consumed by sheep, cattle, and pigs generally disrupt normal reproductive function via their estrogenic activity. Affected animals may show reduced serum progesterone levels; hyperplasia of uterine, vaginal, and cervical epithelium; increased teat size and milk secretion, enlarged external genitalia, with possible prolapse of the vagina and uterus; dystocia;

possible abortion; and feminization of castrated males, who may also show mammary enlargement and even produce milk. Pigs with zearalenone toxicity also exhibit increased incidence of fetal malformation and reduced fetal size. If the phytoestrogen exposure is recognized early and animals are removed from the offending feed, the reproductive changes observed in adult animals are readily reversible. For example, ewes showing abnormalities on spring clover pasture will breed normally in the fall if quickly removed after recognition of the cause. However, if the role of pasture is not recognized or if grazing options are limited and animals are forced to remain on clover pastures for even two grazing seasons, an irreversible process of "defeminization" will occur, and high numbers of ewes may be rendered infertile, unable to conceive.

In general, estrogen mimicry has been a relatively minor aspect of veterinary practice, as its causes are known, and its occurrence is limited. However, in recent years, a more ubiquitous and insidious occurrence of estrogen mimicry has been emerging that may have profound and far-reaching effects on the reproductive future not only of domestic animals, but of a wide range of wildlife species, and human beings as well.

Sources of Endocrine Disruptors

The new estrogen mimicry is associated with a wide variety of manufactured chemicals and their breakdown products. These chemicals are associated with a larger group of synthetic chemicals that have come to be known as POPs, or persistent organic pollutants. The POPs and their breakdown products are widely distributed in the environment, persist for long periods, and accumulate in living tissue. Some of these chemicals are no longer being produced or their use has been banned. However, their effects as endocrine disruptors were not recognized until well after their manufacture and dissemination was widely established. As a result, their potential danger to reproductive health may persist long after their original intended uses have been abandoned. A list of chemicals that have been associated with endocrine disruption is given in Table 6-9. These endocrine disruptors are referred to in the scientific literature and popular press by a number of different names including endocrine disrupters, estrogen mimics, xenoestrogens, pseudoestrogens, pseudoandrogens, and xenobiotic chemicals.

Many different classes and categories of manufactured chemicals are thought to be involved, and new chemicals with estrogenic activity are continually being identified. These chemicals are used in a wide range of applications and are produced in enormous amounts. Colborn, Dumanoski and Myers presented the first comprehensive overview of the endocrine disruptor phenomenon and its implications, in their book *Our Stolen Future*.[14] The book offers some statistics on chemical production and distribution that underscore the scope of the problem:

- U.S. production of carbon-based synthetic chemicals exceeded 435 billion pounds in 1992, while global production is estimated to be four times this amount.

- Globally, 100,000 synthetic chemicals are on the market, with 1000 new ones added annually. Only a few hundred of these compounds have been studied in detail for their health and reproductive effects.

- The world pesticide market is over 5 billion pounds annually, with 1600 specific chemicals being used as pesticides. The United States alone uses 2.2 billion pounds.

- The United States currently uses 30 times more pesticides than it did in 1945. Some of the newer pesticides have 10 times the killing power on a weight basis.

- 35% of the food consumed in the United States has detectable pesticide residues. The percentage is higher in developing countries.

- In Egypt, most milk samples tested showed residues of 15 different pesticides.

- In 1991, the United States exported 4.1 million pounds of pesticides that had been banned, cancelled, or voluntarily suspended in the United States. This included 96 tons of DDT and 40 million pounds of compounds known to have endocrine-disrupting effects.

Routes of Exposure

The POPs, which include the endocrine disruptors, share several important characteristics that facilitate their widespread distribution in the environment and in living tissues:

- They are marketed worldwide through commercial channels for their intended use as pesticides, packaging, insulators, etc.

- These chemicals are structurally quite stable and slow to degrade, so once applied or discarded, they accumulate in the environment.

- Even when they do degrade, some of the degradation products possess endocrine-disruptive potential similar to that of the parent compound.

- Following intentional distribution and use, POPs are unintentionally redistributed around the globe and into various ecosystems on the basis of their physicochemical properties.

- POPs tend to have low vapor pressure, which means that they are readily volatilized and easily enter the atmosphere where they are widely distributed by air currents. Subsequently, they will precipitate out of the atmosphere, particularly in response to colder temperatures, meaning that they will tend to concentrate in the higher latitudes.

Table 6-9 Chemicals Reported to Function as Endocrine Disrupters, Grouped by General Category of Use

Pesticides
  Herbicides
    2,4-D (CPA)[a]
    2,4,5-T (CPA)
    Alachlor (A)
    Atrazine (T)
    Metribuzin (T)
    Nitrofen (NE)
    Trifluralin (D)
  Fungicides
    Benomyl (B)
    Hexachlorobenzene (OC)
    Mancozeb (DTC)
    Maneb (DTC)
    Metiram-complex (DTC)
    Tributyltin (OT)
    Zineb (DTC)
    Ziram (DTC)
  Insecticides
    Isomer of hexachlorocyclohexane (OC)
    Carbaryl (C)
    Chlordane (OC)
    DDT and metabolites (OC)
    Dicofol (OC)
    Dieldrin (OC)
    Endosulfan (OC)

    Heptachlor (OC)
    Heptachlor epoxide (OC)
    Lindane (OC)
    Methomyl (C)
    Methoxychlor (OC)
    Mirex (OC)
    Oxychlordane (OC)
    Parathion (OP)
    Synthetic pyrethroids [b]
    Toxaphene (OC)
    Transnonachlor (OC)
  Nematocides
    Aldicarb (C)
    1,2-Dibromo-3-chloropropane
Industrial chemicals
  Cadmium (HM)
  Dioxins[b]
  Lead (HM)
  Mercury (HM)
  Polybrominated biphenyls[b] (PBB)
  Polychlorinated biphenyls[b] (PCB)
  Pentachlorophenol (PCP)
  Penta- to nonylphenols[b] (AP)
  Phthalates[b]
Styrenes[b] (P)

[a] The class of compound of each chemical is listed in parentheses: A, amide; AP, alkylphenol; B, benzimidazole; C, carbamate; CPA, chlorophenoxy acid; D, dinitroaniline; DTC, dithiocarbamate; HM, heavy metal; NE, nitrophenyl ester; OC, organochlorine; OP, organophosphate; OT, organotin; PBB, polybrominated biphenyl; P, plastic; PCB, polychlorinated biphenyl; PCP, pentachlorophenol; T, triazine.

[b] The family of compounds is identified in the table. Numerous individual compounds within the family have been identified as endocrine disruptors. For example, there are approximately 210 PCB compounds and 75 dioxin compounds.

From Colborn T, vom Saal FS, Soto AM. Developmental effects of endocrine-disrupting chemicals in wildlife and humans. Environ Health Perspect 1993;101(5):378–384.

- POPs also tend to be lipophilic, which means that when they are consumed by living organisms they localize and accumulate in fatty tissues rather than being excreted. When fatty tissues are mobilized, as in lactation, the POPs are mobilized as well, concentrated in the milk, and passed on to the offspring.

Because these chemicals tend to persist in the fatty tissues of living organisms, bioaccumulation or biomagnification occurs progressively through the food chain. A large organism eats numerous small organisms, each containing miniscule amounts of endocrine-disrupting chemical and thereby accumulates the chemical load of its prey. That large organism and many of its kin may in turn be eaten by a larger organism higher on the food chain, who then absorbs and retains the collective load of endocrine-disrupting chemicals in its prey. In this manner, animals high on the food chain, including hu-

mans, amass large loads of endocrine-disrupting chemicals. Concentrations of chemical toxins in fatty tissues can become magnified up to 70,000 times background levels.

So it is that PCBs manufactured in the United States and used to insulate electrical transformers in Brazil could potentially end up in the perirenal fat of otters eating fish in the North Sea off the coast of England. However, endocrine disruptors can be as close as the home pantry. Nonylphenol, for example, is an estrogen mimic added to polystyrene and PVC plastics as an antioxidant to make them less brittle. These plastics have numerous household uses and are common in homes. Other alkylphenols used widely in detergents, pesticides, and personal care products are broken down by bacteria to produce estrogenic substances. Bisphenol is found in polycarbonate laboratory flasks and jugs for drinking water and has been identified in the plastic lining of metal cans used for packaging canned foods. A concentration of 2 to 5 ppb can cause effects in cells.

Mode of Action

One of the first synthetic chemicals to be identified as possessing estrogenic activity was diethylstilbestrol, or DES. Its recognized capacity to mimic estrogen led to its widespread and principal use as a pharmaceutical in human medicine and as a growth promotant in livestock agriculture. Ultimately, significant adverse effects on human reproductive health were recognized with the use of DES in human medicine, and its use was discontinued. However, the drug has become a model for understanding the effects of other endocrine-disrupting chemicals whose endocrine activity was a secondary and unforeseen consequence, unrelated to its primary use.

DES was used widely in human obstetrics during the 1950s to manage problem pregnancies, particularly in women with a history of miscarriages. Then, in 1971, the drug was linked to the increased occurrence of a usually rare, vaginal cancer, clear cell carcinoma, in young women. It became clear that the common thread in these cases was that the mothers of these young women had taken DES in the early stages of the pregnancies that bore these female children. This of course prompted wider epidemiological investigations into other possible associations between genital or reproductive abnormalities in children whose mothers had taken DES. A number of further associations were found. In female children, there were anatomical abnormalities of the female genital tract and, following sexual maturity, abnormal pregnancies. In male children, in utero DES exposure was linked to increased incidence of cryptorchidism and hypospadias at birth and decreased semen and sperm counts at sexual maturity. The DES experience helped to establish a number of biomedical facts that were previously not widely recognized or accepted:

- Living organisms, including humans, can mistake synthetic chemicals for hormones.

- Exogenous drugs and other chemicals can cross the placenta and influence the developing fetus.

- Timing of drug exposure in relation to the stage of fetal development is a critical determinant of whether or not different types of fetal abnormalities occur.

- The effects of developmental abnormalities may not be immediately obvious in the newborn, but may become manifest years later.

- At the cellular level, human beings will respond to chemical or hormonal stimuli in a similar manner as other animals, and experimental data from animal models can be instructive regarding potential dangers to human health.

Studies of DES also helped scientists better understand more about the specific mechanisms by which estrogen mimics exert their influence:

- Estrogen mimics bind effectively to hormone receptor sites on cells.

- The specificity of hormone/receptor binding is not rigidly "lock and key." Many different molecular structures can effectively bind to a given receptor.

- The structure of receptor molecules is retained evolutionarily across species. Hormones that bind to fish or mouse cell receptors are likely to bind to human receptors.

- Adverse effects of estrogen mimics depend not only on the size of the dose, but also the timing of the dose.

- DES, like other estrogen mimics, does not bind to transfer globulins in serum as endogenous estrogen normally does. Therefore estrogen mimics escape normal dose titration controls and are fully available to exert hormonal effects.

As knowledge about estrogen mimics expanded, it became clearer that a number of different mechanisms exist for synthetic, or anthropogenic, chemicals to produce varying effects of endocrine disruption. DES was a "true" estrogen mimic in that it bound to estrogen receptor sites and induced estrogenic responses. However, other endocrine disruptors act differently. The fungicide vinclozolin, for instance, is an androgen-receptor blocker, while DDE, a breakdown product of DDT, accelerates hormonal degradation. As a result, some endocrine disruptors mimic estrogen activity, some are antiestrogenic, and others are androgenic.

Effects of Endocrine Disruptors

Details of the structure, function, and modes of action of steroid hormones, including estrogen, can be found in basic endocrinology texts and are not extensively reviewed here. Normally, estrogen is involved in regulation of the estrus cycle, including ovulation and preparation of the uterus for pregnancy. Estrogen influences sexual behavior including the expression of sexual receptivity, or heat. It modulates the development of secondary sex characteristics in females, including mammary development. Estrogen also exerts influence outside reproductive function. It is involved in calcium metabolism and can stimulate the secretion of angiotensinogen and thyroid-binding globulin. Generally speaking, estrogen exerts its effects at the cellular level in target tissues by binding to receptor proteins in the cytoplasm of target cells. The estrogen-receptor complex then moves to the nucleus of the cell where it induces derepression of part of the genetic information of nuclear DNA. New messenger RNA (mRNA) is formed, and protein synthesis is increased. Finely tuned internal feedback mechanisms prevent the overexpression of estrogen effects in normally functioning individuals.

Estrogen mimics, which escape the regulatory feedback mechanism that normally modulates estrogen activity, can exert powerful effects on mature animals as well as developing fetuses. The recognized, deleterious effects of estrogen mimics in various species of animals from reptiles to humans include:

- Increased susceptibility to cancers in hormone responsive tissues. Two of the four most common cancers in the United States, breast and prostate cancer, are hormone sensitive.

- Abnormal expression of sexual characteristics, including feminization of males, masculinization of females, hermaphroditism, genital malformations such as hypospadias, and decreased sperm counts in males.

- Aberrant expression of normal mating and nesting behaviors.

- Impaired thyroid function and brain development.

- Learning disabilities and attention deficits.

- Immunosuppression, particularly impairment of cell-mediated immunity.

Scope of the Problem

The revelations of the 1970s linking DES administration during pregnancy to genital cancers and reproductive dysfunction in the resulting female offspring raised public awareness about the inherent power and dangers of hormonal therapies. This invoked important policy responses from government and the medical community. The use of DES was severely curtailed, so that current and future generations of citizens could feel secure that they would not experience the same tragedies that DES inflicted on the generation born in the 1950s.

Addressing the problem of today's endocrine-disrupting chemicals will not be as simple or straightforward, and much more may be at stake. DES essentially represented a point-source toxicology problem in human beings. DES was directly and intentionally administered to selected patients with their consent, albeit a poorly informed consent. Even when DES was being used as a growth promotant in the livestock industry, the point of contact was clear for human exposure, and the option to avoid exposure to DES was still retained by the consumer, who could choose not to eat meat.

Today's endocrine disruptors present a very different predicament. These anthropogenic chemicals represent a complex, nonpoint source pollution problem that exposes a wide range of animal species, including humans, to potentially grave risks. The ubiquitous distribution of POPs in the environment and their progressive accumulation in animals throughout the food chain makes avoidance by choice an impossibility. Birds and mammals that have evolved as fish eaters, for example, are impelled, by their natural behavior to consume endocrine-disrupting chemicals every time they capture and consume their natural prey.

There is growing evidence that no place on Earth is wholly safe from environmental contamination with POPs. This was shown by studies of albatross populations at the Midway atoll in the north central Pacific Ocean, a remote, undeveloped site presumed to be relatively free of toxic contamination. Despite the remoteness of the locale, studies revealed that black-footed albatross adults, chicks, and eggs at Midway atoll contain high levels of DDT, PCBs, and dioxins.[23] This population is showing deformed embryos, eggshell thinning, and a drop in nest productivity. The levels of some endocrine-disrupting chemicals in the Pacific albatross are as high as those recorded in bald eagles from the Great Lakes region of North America, an area of intense industrial activity.

Another indication of the pervasiveness and impact of endocrine disruptors is a clear pattern over the last 50 years of a worldwide increase in abnormalities of the human male genital system, including reduced sperm counts and sperm quality, increased occurrence of testicular cancers, and increased occurrence of congenital abnormalities such as cryptorchidism and hypospadias.[40] That such abnormalities may be modulated by estrogens and can be initiated in utero was well established by the DES experience. However, the pattern continues long after the DES ban has been in place, strongly suggesting a role for anthropogenic estrogen mimics accumulated by pregnant women.

Table 6-10 offers examples of some of the situations in wildlife and humans that have been associated with endocrine-disrupting chemicals through direct environmental exposure or by bioaccumulation through consumption of contaminated prey. This list is by no means complete. Even if additional known examples were added, such as those involving polar bears, lake trout, red-eared turtles, and others, the list would still not be complete because so much is still unknown about endocrine disruptors, their impact, and the establishment of direct causality. Information that is partially or fully lacking includes facts about the range of chemicals with endocrine-disrupting effects, their distribution, their breakdown characteristics, the effects of their breakdown products, the susceptibility of different animal species and their tolerance to different doses, synergistic effects that may exist between different combinations of endocrine disruptors, and how different species vary in their clinical expression of endocrine disruption. The scientific challenges in establishing the role of endocrine disruptors on the health of aquatic vertebrates and invertebrates has recently been reviewed.[35]

Challenges for the Future

It seems unlikely that the presence of endocrine-disrupting chemicals in the environment is going to diminish anytime in the near future. There are several reasons for this. First is the growing worldwide demand in chemicals for agricultural, industrial, and consumer use, fueled by global economic expansion and development. Annual worldwide sales in the chemical industry are estimated to exceed $1.5 trillion. Second is the fact that large numbers of new chemicals are continually being developed and introduced to the marketplace. Third is that stockpiles of old chemicals, discarded in the 1960s and 1970s in waste dumps around the world, are beginning to leak out of their old, rusted containers into soil and groundwater. Fourth

Table 6-10 Some Reproductive and Other Abnormalities Observed and Reported over the Last 60 Years Associated with Exposure of Wildlife Species and Humans to Endocrine-Disrupting Chemicals and Other Persistent Organic Pollutants in the Environment

Species Affected	Emergence of Problem	Geographical Location	Source	Abnormalities Observed	Suspected Chemical
Eagles	1940s	Florida	Bioaccumulation: fish consumption	Population declines; abnormal courting, mating, and nesting behavior; sterility	DDT; others, not specifically identified
Mink	1960s	Michigan	Bioaccumulation: consumption of Lake Michigan fish	Reproductive failures	PCBs, DDT
Otters	1950s	England	Bioaccumulation: fish consumption	Population reductions; reproductive failures	PCBs, mercury
Gulls, terns	1970s to present	California, Great Lakes, Washington, Massachusetts	Bioaccumulation: Fish consumption	Feminization and infertility in males; female gull nest pairing	DDT; others, not specifically identified
Alligators	1980s to present	Florida: Lake Apopka, Lake Griffin	Bioaccumulation: agricultural runoff into lakes	Population reductions; reduced egg viability in females; feminization, abnormal genitalia in males	Dicofol; others, not specifically identified
Black-footed albatross	1990s	Midway Atoll: Northern Pacific Ocean	Bioaccumulation: feeding on flying fish and their eggs	Decreased nesting productivity, deformed embryos, eggshell thinning	PCBs, DDT, dioxins
Beluga whales	1970s	USA/Canada: St. Lawrence Estuary	Bioaccumulation: transfer in milk to offspring	Population collapse; decreased fertility and juvenile survival; thyroid abnormalities, adrenal hyperplasia, increased tumor incidence	PCBs and others; up to 24 toxins identifiable in Beluga tissues
Seals and dolphins	1980s	Lake Baikal, Russia; coast of NW Europe; Atlantic coast of USA; Mediterranean Sea	Bioaccumulation: aquatic food sources	Immunosuppression with secondary disease outbreaks of distemper virus (seals) and morbillivirus (dolphins)	Not specifically identified
Dogs, male	1970s	Military dogs serving in Vietnam	Environmental exposure	Twice the rate of testicular cancer as military dogs serving elsewhere	Suspect dioxins (Agent Orange), 2,4-D; 2,4,5-T
Panthers, male	1980s	Florida	Contaminated soil and water	Thyroid dysfunction; immunosuppression; abnormal sperm; undescended testicles; feminization	Mercury, DDT, DDE, PCBs
Human children	Current	Michigan	Bioaccumulation: consumption of Lake Michigan fish	Intellectual impairment; memory loss; attention deficits	PCBs
Human males	1950s to present	Worldwide	Bioaccumulation; environmental exposure	Decreasing sperm counts	PCBs and others

is that regulatory controls, either voluntary or mandatory, are not widely established or practiced with regard to the endocrine-disrupting potential of synthetic chemicals.

In poor countries, the financial resources or technical capacity for regulatory oversight may be lacking. But even in wealthy nations, the regulatory mechanisms that are in place are often inadequate or inappropriate. In developed countries, the mandate of regulatory agencies with regard to chemical toxins has traditionally been to develop testing methods and regulatory policies that identify and limit the risks of acute toxicity or carcinogenicity, whereas key expressions of endocrine-disrupting toxins are developmental defects or diminished reproductive capacities whose clinical manifestations may be delayed for years. The screening and evaluation methods used for assessment of acute toxicity and carcinogenicity are strongly linked to assessments of dose responsiveness, whereas many of the effects of endocrine disruptors may be related more to the timing of exposure to a toxin than to its dose.

A prerequisite to effecting meaningful change in the way society perceives, uses, monitors, and regulates persistent organic pollutants in the future is to develop and present strong scientific documentation of direct links between specific chemicals in the environment and their endocrine-disruptive effects. While firm linkages have already been established in some instances, for many wildlife and some human situations the evidence of a link remains circumstantial. Some efforts are already under way to clarify some of these uncertain areas. In the United States, the Centers for Disease Control and Prevention (CDC), through the National Center for Environmental Health, has undertaken a number of initiatives including critical reviews of existing data on endocrine disruptors and human health, the initiation of case-control studies in the field on the relationship of DDE exposure and accumulation to human breast cancer risk, and surveillance studies using biomarkers to define exposure levels to various endocrine-disrupting chemicals. Conservation and environmental groups, such as the World Wildlife Fund, are supporting research efforts on wildlife models for endocrine disruption.

Some policy initiatives are already under way as well. At the international level, efforts are proceeding to minimize the release of persistent organic pollutants into the environment. In 1998, under the auspices of UNEP and the FAO, a treaty was drafted, referred to as the PIC Convention, for Prior Informed Consent. It sets standards and guidelines to ensure that developing countries do not become the unsuspecting dumping ground for hazardous chemicals. The convention requires full disclosure of the contents of chemical shipments by the shipper and the right of refusal by the importer. UNEP and FAO are also sponsoring efforts for another treaty to focus on agreements to limit the release and emissions of POPs. The initial focus is on managing the so-called dirty dozen: aldrin, chlordane, DDT, dieldrin, dioxins, endrin, furans, heptachlor, hexachlorobenzene, mirex, PCBs, and toxaphene.

Clearly there are challenges and opportunities for veterinarians to participate in solving the endocrine disruptor puzzle.

This is an area of inquiry that will benefit from the broad comparative medical training and perspectives of veterinarians. The differentiation of abnormal structure, function, and behavior across a wide spectrum of species is a fundamental aspect of veterinary medicine and a key requirement in interpreting the effects of endocrine disrupters. Veterinarians can make useful contributions to an interdisciplinary research approach that requires expertise in chemistry, toxicology, ecology, biology, epidemiology, and many facets of clinical medicine. Identifiable research priorities include

- New investigative and diagnostic approaches that can confirm the role of endocrine-disrupting chemicals in the various suspect expressions of clinical abnormality observed in different species in the field.

- Identification of additional, yet-unrecognized situations in which wildlife species are being affected.

- Identification of appropriate biomarker animal sentinels that can signal potentially dangerous accumulations of toxic chemicals in specific environments.

- Additional epidemiological investigations to identify and monitor population declines and their possible linkage to endocrine-disrupting chemicals. Such declines include worldwide decreases in amphibian populations with related developmental abnormalities, regional marine mammal die-offs, and declines in waterfowl populations.

Finally, there is the question of whether or not domestic animals, including pets and livestock, are experiencing problems associated with endocrine-disrupting chemicals. Virtually all the reports of endocrine disruption associated with environmental contamination or bioaccumulation have been situations involving humans or wildlife species. Essentially, there have been no reports of the problem in domestic animals. Is it possible that domestic animals are avoiding problems associated with exposure to endocrine disruptors, or are veterinarians just not recognizing such problems? It is up to the veterinary community to answer that question.

Nuclear Radiation and Global Health

Since 1945, when the awesome destructive power of nuclear weapons was revealed to the world by the atomic bombs dropped on Hiroshima and Nagasaki, all living things on Earth have shared an uncertain future and a common vulnerability. In the nuclear arms buildup of the Cold War, which followed World War II, a nuclear arsenal was created that consisted of thousands of nuclear weapons with the combined explosive power to destroy a million Hiroshimas. A single, small, 2-megaton warhead has destructive power equivalent to that of all the conventional bombs used in World War II combined. Suddenly, human ingenuity had created the capacity for global annihilation. If the existing inventory of nuclear warheads were exchanged, there would essentially be no place to hide. When physicians emerged as outspoken advocates of nuclear disarmament in the 1970s, they made a significant contribution to public awareness by framing the risk of nuclear holocaust as a public health problem. Full-scale nuclear war, they declared, would be "the final epidemic."

Human beings would not be the only victims of nuclear catastrophe. The potential for nuclear war to radically alter the biosphere, to deplete all forms of life on Earth, and to change the course of natural evolution was recognized by physicians, biologists, ecologists, and other scientists. In a landmark paper published 1983, Dr. Paul R. Ehrlich and 19 distinguished colleagues laid out in broad terms the long-term biological consequences of nuclear war.[20] The paper presented a clear message that nuclear warfare would have dramatic ecological consequences, well beyond the more apparent political and social consequences. Humans beings who survived the immediate destruction of nuclear explosions would encounter a very grim and unfamiliar world in which climate was radically altered, the landscape transformed, the natural world diminished, and the capacity to produce, or even find food, severely curtailed.

The explosions, heat, and destruction of a large-scale nuclear war would, in addition to killing hundreds of millions of people, release massive amounts of dust and soot into the atmosphere, blocking most incident solar radiation. For months to years afterward, there would be subfreezing temperatures, low light levels, high doses of ionizing radiation, and increased UV radiation. Plants unable to withstand freezing temperatures would perish, crop production would be severely constrained, fresh water bodies might be frozen, and wild plant foods would be heavily contaminated with radiation. There would be intense competition among surviving organisms for scarce, remaining food supplies, and surviving humans might be disadvantaged in the competition. Intense UV radiation would cause mutations in plants, cause blindness in humans and animals, and could kill off aquatic phytoplankton, causing a collapse of the food chain with large-scale population losses in marine ecosystems. Overall there would be an enormous loss of genetic and species diversity, including the possibility of widespread extinctions.

Current Risks of Global Radiation Exposure

Thankfully, the potential for large-scale nuclear war and its horrific consequences has diminished significantly in recent years following the breakup of the Soviet Union, the end of the Cold War, and the implementation of international nuclear-arms limitation agreements. However, a number of situations and circumstances still exist today that could result in the release of large amounts of ionizing radiation, with or without the attendant impacts of nuclear explosions. These situations potentially involve nuclear power plants, nuclear waste storage sites, nuclear weapons manufacturing sites, aging nuclear weapons arsenals, the emergence of new nuclear nations with

the capacity to engage in an exchange of nuclear weapons, and the growing specter of nuclear terrorism.

In 1997, it was reported that despite significant progress on arms limitations and reduction agreements between the United States and Russia, nuclear weapons in both countries remain on hair-trigger alert, ready to fire at literally a moment's notice.[7] Under these circumstances, mistaken launches of nuclear warheads remain a possibility. Destruction of targeted cities could occur within 43 minutes of the first event that puts the retaliatory launch process into play, say, for example, misinterpreting the launch of a communications satellite seen on radar as the start of a preemptive missile strike.

The risk of such mistakes is aggravated by the ongoing political instability and economic deterioration in Russia, which has resulted in a diminished capacity to oversee and maintain the remaining nuclear arsenal properly. Nuclear submarines sit rusting in Murmansk harbor. Power companies have repeatedly shut off the electricity at nuclear weapons installations for nonpayment of bills. Thieves have disrupted communications at nuclear weapons control centers by stealing the copper telecommunications cables leading into the buildings. Military technicians working in command and control have gone months without pay, and routine maintenance of radar equipment, computers, and other vital tracking and warning systems has become erratic. All of these conditions contribute to the potential risk for accidental launches of nuclear missiles. The failure to regularly pay staff and the associated lack of morale also have led to concerns that some disgruntled workers or military personnel may sell kilogram quantities of plutonium or highly enriched uranium to third parties, thus increasing the risk of nuclear terrorism as well.

While the Comprehensive Test Ban Treaty has been signed by 152 countries, including the 5 major nuclear powers, it has not prevented the emergence of new nuclear nations. In 1998, both India and Pakistan tested nuclear bombs produced for military purposes. The two nations essentially have been adversaries since Pakistan was first created out of former Indian territory in 1947. They have fought three conventional wars since that time and continue to be engaged in an ongoing, low-level conflict over the territorial status of Kashmir, currently a part of India. Repeated efforts toward conflict resolution through negotiations between these two traditional adversaries have yielded no substantial results. Now, the potential for an exchange of nuclear weapons between these two antagonists in south Asia exists as a real possibility. As this is one of the most densely populated regions on the planet, the loss of life would be tremendous. As it is also one of the poorest, with poorly developed infrastructure, efforts to provide relief and rehabilitation following a nuclear exchange would be enormously complex and difficult. The impact would be felt well beyond the region, with fallout and ionizing radiation causing potential health concerns great distances from the local theater of war.

Release of uncontrolled ionizing radiation in the future may arise from sources other than the accidental or intentional use of nuclear weapons. According to U.S. Department of Energy data reported in 1996, there are 432 operating nuclear reactors in the world, used for the generation of electrical power. While nuclear reactors do not explode like nuclear bombs, accidents at nuclear power-generating plants can release substantial amounts of ionizing radiation into the atmosphere, onto the land, and into water supplies. Such releases can have acute and chronic effects on human and animal health and contaminate food supplies for extended periods. Accidents at nuclear power stations require professional responses from veterinarians, as was confirmed in the aftermath of the Three Mile Island nuclear plant accident in Middletown, Pennsylvania, in 1979 and following the explosion and fire at the nuclear power station in Chernobyl, Ukraine, USSR, in 1986. The aging of nuclear power plants, particularly in the republics of the former Soviet Union, raises the level of concern about increased risk of nuclear accidents in the future, as the capacity and budgets for proper monitoring and maintenance are reduced.

Nuclear munitions factories and former test sites may also be sources of radiation release. In the mid-1980s, residents of southwestern Ohio were shocked to learn that the Fernald Feed Materials Processing Plant, a processing plant owned by the U.S. Department of Energy for production of uranium for nuclear weapons, had been releasing radioactive uranium dust into the atmosphere through its smokestacks for about three decades. Perhaps even more disturbing was the fact that such releases from the plant, about 20 miles northwest of Cincinnati, were repeatedly brought to the attention of government authorities by plant managers and workers, but little or no effort was made by government to reduce their occurrence. As the story unfolded, it became clearer that exposure to uranium and other radioactive materials was even more extensive. When the plant was first built in 1951, no provisions were made for solid waste disposal. Later, pits were dug, but rainwater runoff from the pits contaminated nearby land and groundwater. Thousands of pounds of radium and other radioactive wastes were stored in concrete tanks at Fernald. When one of the tanks developed cracks, leaking was allowed to persist until the level of waste fell below the crack. In 1989, at a congressional subcommittee hearing, testimony was given estimating that since the opening of the plant, 6350 tons of uranium waste had been disposed in pits, 83.5 tons had been discharged into the Great Miami River, and 149 tons had been discharged into the air. Citizens in the area filed a suit against the federal government, and in 1989, the Department of Energy agreed to pay $73 million to settle claims of up to 24,000 neighbors of the Fernald plant. The settlement did not acknowledge the occurrence of health problems associated with the uranium releases. Rather, the money was awarded to compensate claims of emotional distress and reduction in property values. Part of the funds were designated to carry out prospective epidemiological studies to assess more accurately whether or not the radioactive releases did in fact produce adverse health effects in the region.

More than 10 years later, such epidemiological studies are still in progress around Fernald, as well as around other U.S. nu-

clear weapons facilities where earlier accidents or problems with nuclear waste management have been identified, such as the Hanford site in Washington, Rocky Flats in Denver, and Savannah River in South Carolina. The CDC, through the Radiation Studies Branch of the National Center for Environmental Health, is working with affected communities to improve data collection and epidemiological monitoring to establish the effects of radiation exposure. Inhalation of radioactive uranium, for instance, is known to be associated with an increased incidence of lung cancer, while ingestion of radioactive uranium in contaminated water may contribute to cancers in other body tissues. However, in situations like that at Fernald, it can be difficult to establish strong cause-and-effect relationships for small increases in certain types of cancer in large populations, as numerous other potentially confounding causes such as cigarette smoking or toxic chemical exposures can exist.

Veterinary medicine could likely play a more active and useful role in data collection and interpretation in such studies. Domestic animals, especially dogs and cats, with shorter life spans, more rapid aging processes, shorter gestations, and greater number of offspring than humans can serve as useful sentinels of increased cancer occurrence. Networks of veterinary practitioners participating in prospective epidemiological studies at incremental distances from nuclear contamination sites might contribute much to the understanding of links between radiation and neoplastic disease.

These examples point out that risks of uncontrolled radiation release of sizable proportions still exist around the world. Because radiation is "invisible" and its effects not widely understood, there is a tendency for people to react very emotionally to real and imagined exposure. As highly educated members of their communities, veterinarians can play an important role in public education and awareness about the real and imagined dangers of nuclear radiation in all its forms, both peaceful and destructive. Furthermore, health professionals, including veterinarians, need to have a basic understanding of the risks associated with different types of radiation exposure and be familiar with the principles and procedures involved in responding rationally and effectively to incidents of uncontrolled release of nuclear radiation. Veterinarians in particular will have front-line responsibilities in minimizing the exposure of domestic animals to ionizing radiation and in ensuring that food from livestock does not pose a health risk to humans consuming it.

Radiation, Animals, and Foods of Animal Origin

A nuclear bomb explosion produces over 200 different radionuclides, with decay rates ranging from a fraction of a second to millions of years. The fissioning of uranium in a nuclear power plant reactor produces 27 different radionuclides. The radionuclides of most concern with regard to safety of the food supply are iodine-131, strontium-90, and cesium-137. Iodine-131 has a half-life of approximately 8 days; strontium-90, a half-life of 28 years; and cesium-137, a half-life of 30.2 years. The differences in their half-lives as well as differences in their essential elemental properties mean that each of these radionuclides will behave characteristically after release into the atmosphere. In the period immediately following the uncontrolled release of ionizing radiation, reduction of exposure for all radionuclides is essentially the same. Animals and people should be sheltered in buildings that prevent direct contact with fallout and that are constructed to reduce exposure to ionizing radiation. Similarly, in that early phase of potential exposure, animals and people should consume stored feeds whenever possible and drink stored water or fresh water only from deep or covered sources. After the acute phase, the strategies and tools available for minimizing the effects of different radionuclides will differ according to their distinct chemical properties and their behavior in living systems.

Iodine-131 once deposited on vegetation may be ingested by animals. It is readily absorbed from the gastrointestinal tract and tends to localize in the thyroid gland, the milk, and, in poultry, the eggs. Cows secrete approximately 8% of the daily intake of iodine-131 into their milk, and cow's milk is the major potential source of iodine-131 exposure for people following nuclear accidents. Iodine-131 ingested by humans also localizes in the thyroid gland and can produce thyroid cancers. Children are more sensitive to radioiodine than adults. Up to 50% of ingested radioiodine ends up in the thyroid glands of children, compared with 20% for adults. Also, thyroid glands in children are considerably smaller than those in adults. These factors result in a higher proportionate dose and greater potential for damage in children. Since the half-life of iodine-131 is 8 days, reducing the risk of iodine exposure both to animals and in turn to humans is less problematic than with other radionuclides. Housing dairy cattle indoors and feeding only stored feeds for up to 2 months would minimize intake by cattle and allow for decay of iodine-131 on crops and in fields to tolerable levels. If milk does become contaminated, it may not be necessary to discard it. If proper facilities are available, the milk can be frozen, dried, or otherwise processed into storable dairy products and those products retained until radioactivity of iodine-131 is reduced to acceptable limits. This could occur within 2 months of initial contamination, depending on initial concentrations. The uptake of iodine-131 by the human thyroid can also be blocked by saturating the thyroid gland with potassium iodide, which must be taken orally for a period of 2 to 3 months. If this is done in cattle, however, iodine-131 diverted from the cow's thyroid gland, may instead end up in the milk.

While radioactive iodine poses a threat to milk drinkers for about 2 months following a nuclear accident, contamination of milk with strontium poses a more persistent problem. Strontium-89 and strontium-90 are produced in fission reactions, but only the latter poses potential long-term problems for food supplies, as strontium-89 has a half-life of 50 days, and virtually all has degraded by the end of 1 year. Strontium-90, with a half-life of 28 years, is more problematic. Strontium-90 behaves like calcium in living systems and is competitive with that mineral. As with calcium, bone is a target organ for strontium-90 deposition. Under experimental conditions, strontium-90 administration is associated with osteosarcoma and other bone

tumors in beagle dogs, laboratory mice, and miniature swine and also produces immunosuppressive effects in some experimental models. Animals, including humans, preferentially absorb calcium over strontium, and this inherent metabolic preference helps to reduce the intensity of strontium exposure. Only about 10% of the strontium present in a cow's diet will be absorbed and end up in milk. In turn, only about 25% of the strontium ingested in the human diet reaches the bone in adults, and about 50% in children.

Strontium-90 falling to earth can contaminate soil for long periods. It can be taken up by plants from the soil via the root system and can also enter plants through the flowers, where it can localize in seed grains. Therefore, crops harvested for the feeding of livestock or directly for human consumption may remain contaminated with strontium-90 for years, depending on the initial level of contamination. In calcium-rich soils, calcium is taken up in preference to strontium, and this can be used to advantage. Application of lime or gypsum to contaminated soil will increase the concentration of available calcium and thus proportionately reduce strontium uptake by plants. If the soil is heavily contaminated, liming alone will not render the soil safe for cultivation. Alternatives are the cultivation of nonfood crops or of food crops such as oil seeds or sugar beets that do not readily accumulate strontium in their edible portions. Deep plowing of contaminated surface soil might also be considered.

Cesium-137 acts biologically like potassium. Upon ingestion by animals, it is absorbed and passed into the milk and to muscle tissues, as potassium would be. Therefore, cesium represents a contamination problem for both meat and milk. Cesium contaminates pastures and croplands by direct contact with plants and by uptake through plant roots. It becomes bound in the matrix of clay soils and is therefore less available for uptake by plants in such soils. More than 10 years after the Chernobyl nuclear power plant accident, the major contributor to low-dose chronic radiation problems is the cesium radionuclides. Cesium has been identified in the new growth rings of trees, raising concerns about increased cesium-137 concentrations in wood harvested from such trees. Wild foods, such as game animals, berries, and mushrooms have persistently high radiocesium levels.

In the case of domestic animals, interventions are available that can effectively reduce cesium levels in the meat and milk. While cesium-137 has a radioactive decay half-life of 30.2 years, its biological half-life in tissues, before it is turned over and excreted, is only 2 to 4 weeks, depending on animal species. Therefore, it is possible to reduce cesium levels significantly in muscle tissue of meat-producing animals by feeding stored, noncontaminated feeds for the appropriate period immediately preceding slaughter. In the case of dairy animals, in which production is continuous, or of meat animals that are managed by direct grazing on pastures and meadows, this is not practical. In these cases, other techniques are available. A group of compounds, the hexacyanoferrates, known collectively as Prussian Blue, will bind radiocesium so that it passes

The Chernobyl Legacy: Human Health, Food Safety, and International Trade

On April 25, 1986, managers at Unit 4 of the Nuclear Power Station in Chernobyl, Ukraine, USSR (see photo, left) initiated a test to determine how long the turbine generator in the plant would provide electricity to run the emergency pumps that provided water to cool the reactor core in the event of a reactor shutdown. At 1:23 am on April 26, a combination of human error, poor reactor design, and disregard of safety systems by the personnel carrying out the test led to a sudden surge of power and heat in the fuel core. This resulted in the instantaneous conversion of the reactor's cooling water to pressurized steam that blew the concrete cover off the reactor. A second explosion of hydrogen generated by water reacting with the cladding of the fuel rods occurred seconds later. As a result, the graphite moderator rods in the reactor caught fire, and radioactive fission products were carried out of the reactor into the atmosphere with the fire's smoke. It was a week before the continued release of radioactivity from the damaged reactor was fully contained. During that time, virtually all of the reactor's gaseous fission products and about 3% of the solid products were released into the outside environment.

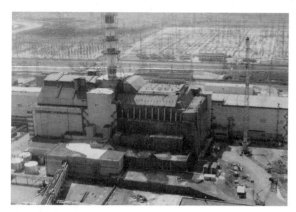

Chernobyl nuclear plant. (Photo courtesy of the IAEAgency; photographer, Petr Pavlicek)

Leaked radioactivity was first detected outside the Soviet Union at a nuclear power station in Sweden. When it was realized that Chernobyl was the source, monitoring stations worldwide began to monitor the dispersion. The radioactive plume was tracked over the European part of the Soviet Union, notably Ukraine, Belarus, and Russia, and into Europe. Northwesterly winds early on accounted for much of the deposition in Scandinavia, the Netherlands, Belgium, and Great Britain. Later the plume shifted to the south and much of central Europe, the northern Mediterranean, and the Balkans received some deposit. Radionuclides associated with heavier particulate debris settled out closer to the accident site. The most radiologically important radionuclides detected outside the Soviet Union were iodine-131, tellurium/iodine-132, cesium-137, and cesium-134. Where the passage of the plume coincided with heavy rainfall, radionuclide deposition was greatest. These places included Austria, southeastern Switzerland, southern Germany, Scandinavia, and the northern U.K. For example, the estimated average deposition of cesium-137 in the province of Salzburg in Austria was 46 kBq/m2. By comparison, the average cesium-137 deposition in drier Portugal was 0.02 kBq/m2. While no deposition was detected in the southern hemisphere, radioactivity from Chernobyl was detectable in the northern hemisphere as far away as Japan and North America.

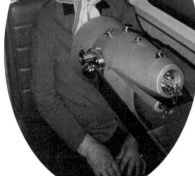

Whole-body radiation count of citizen. (Photo courtesy of the IAEAgency; photographer, Petr Pavlicek)

Map of region affected by Chernobyl accident.

Nine days after the accident, radiation was detected by monitoring stations in Washington state, 9000 miles from Chernobyl. By May 16, detectable increases in radioactive iodine in cow's milk were noted by EPA monitoring stations across the entire United States, though the levels were not considered unsafe. Chernobyl made it painfully clear that a major nuclear accident was a global phenomenon. It produced inevitable transboundary implications, with consequences that would affect many countries, even at great distances from the accident site. Like a malevolent genie released from a bottle, the radiation release from Chernobyl unleashed a myriad of political, social, economic, and health problems, which, along with the radioactivity itself, would linger for a long time.

The effects of Chernobyl on human health were immediately a paramount concern around the world. In the acute phase of the disaster, there were 134 cases of acute radiation sickness in individuals directly involved in the accident and its containment, with 28 deaths resulting from radiation injuries. Assessment of the chronic effects of the Chernobyl accident provoked an intensive, international effort. In the photo at the left, for example, a woman in Novozybkov, Russia, about 110 miles northeast of Chernobyl is being screened for whole-body radiation in a mobile van unit as part of the IAEA International Chernobyl Assessment Project in 1990. To date, the overall impact of Chernobyl appears to be less than originally feared. There has been a significant increase in thyroid carcinomas in children living in contaminated regions of the Soviet Union. In districts of Belarus, for instance, the occurrence of thyroid cancers per million children had increased 100-fold by 1994, compared with the rate in 1984 before the Chernobyl accident. However, 10 years after the accident, monitoring agencies had not yet found increases in other types of cancers, including leukemia, or in the occurrence of congenital abnormalities, adverse pregnancy outcomes, or any other radiation-induced diseases. Long-range epidemiological studies by WHO and other national and international agencies are still ongoing.

A very real effect, cited by all investigators, was the psychological distress that followed Chernobyl. Enormous numbers of people were affected, particularly those exposed to high doses of radiation, including the 800,000 soldiers and workers who participated in the large-scale cleanup, the 135,000 people who were evacuated from around the accident site in the first week, and the 270,000 or so residents of highly contaminated areas of the Soviet Union, such as Belarus where cesium-137 deposition levels exceeded 555 kBq/m2. The fear and anxiety about yet-to-be manifested disease lingers as a disruptive force in the everyday lives of these people.

One transboundary consequence of Chernobyl that raised tensions and tested the capacity for international cooperation was the issue of international trade in food products considered contaminated by radiation. Many countries did not have preexisting standards or legislation to address these issues. As a result, some abrupt decisions were made that were not scientifically grounded or that were politically unpopular. For example, some uncontaminated countries felt justified in refusing importation from contaminated countries and unilaterally established zero tolerance for radionuclides of any kind in imported food. In 1986, the European Commission imposed a ban on importation of milk products with radiocesium levels above 370 Bq/kg and levels above 600 Bq/kg for all other food types, with no attention paid to the amount of food consumed or total dose of exposure. Spices would be banned at the same dose as vegetables, even though the former are consumed in minute amounts relative to the latter. The need for harmonization and standardization of regulations grew increasingly apparent. In 1989, at a meeting in Geneva, some guideline values for radioactivity in food moving in international trade were agreed upon and incorporated into the WHO/FAO Codex Alimentarius (CA). The CA is internationally agreed upon as the accepted standard for food safety with regard to issues of international trade and is recognized as such by the World Trade Organization (WTO). While it was a positive development to have the radionuclide guidelines in the CA established, they did create problems for food producers in some regions, and effective countermeasures needed to be developed and applied to reduce contamination levels in foodstuffs, including foods of animal origin.

For instance, the northern U.K. received high doses of radionuclides as a result of heavy rains as the Chernobyl plume passed overhead. Cesium contamination of soil was high in parts of Wales, Scotland, Ireland, and England. This resulted in restrictions on the movement and slaughter of 4.25 million sheep because of high levels of cesium in muscle associated with the grazing of vegetation on cesium-contaminated peaty soils which, unlike clay soils, permit considerable uptake of cesium by plants. By January 1994, though the situation had improved, some 438,000 sheep were still restricted. As many affected farmers had few options for managing sheep other than grazing on available natural pastures, methods were needed to either reduce the ingestion of cesium or the intestinal absorption of that which was ingested. Building on the experiences of colleagues in Norway and the former Soviet Union who developed techniques for administration of cesium-binding compounds to cattle to reduce meat and milk contamination, researchers at the Institute of Terrestrial Ecology in Cumbria, U.K., have developed wax-coated ammonium ferric hexacyanoferrate boluses that can be administered orally

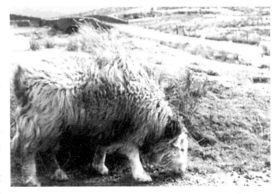

Grazing sheep in Cumbria, UK. (Photo courtesy of N. A. Beresford, Institute of Terrestrial Ecology, Cumbria, UK)

to sheep grazing hill and upland areas. These boluses degrade slowly in the rumen over a period of 7 or more weeks, and reduce cesium-137 concentrations in muscle by about 50% between 3 and 8 weeks after administration.[6] The use of such boluses may provide farmers with a way to reduce muscle cesium levels below the trade limit of 1000 Bq/kg established by the Codex Alimentarius Commission.

unabsorbed through the digestive tract and is eliminated in the feces, from which it is only slowly available to plants. Following the Chernobyl disaster, researchers in Norway, Russia, Ukraine, Belarus, and the U.K. have evaluated different protocols for supplying hexacyanoferrates orally to cattle to reduce radiocesium levels in milk and meat. Two- to eightfold reductions in cesium absorption can be achieved in cattle grazing contaminated fodder, depending on the dose, delivery, and type of hexacyanoferrate administered.[10] Such reductions can bring cesium levels below tolerated limits. Fourteen years after Chernobyl, however, sheep grazing in the U.K. are still acquiring levels of radiocesium in muscle that exclude them from international trade (see sidebar "Chernobyl Legacy: Human Health, Food Safety, and International Trade").

The challenges to the veterinary profession following an accidental release of ionizing radiation can be complex and daunting, as was made clear by the Chernobyl accident in 1986. Norway was a good case in point. Outside the Soviet Union, Norway was the country most widely and severely affected by radioactive fallout, notably cesium-137 and cesium-134. Norway's Official Meat Inspection Acts give responsibility to the veterinary authorities to ensure that radioactivity levels in meat do not exceed official intervention levels and thereby protect the public from hazards posed by contaminants in meat. The fallout created considerable problems related to meat from sheep, goats, and cattle grazing mountain pastures and also from reindeer, which are an important source of livelihood and nutrition in the region. As discussed in Chapter 2, the diet of grazing reindeer is composed largely of lichens, and lichens accumulate radioactivity more than many other plants because of their large surface area and long lifespan.

In an article describing the response of Norwegian veterinarians to Chernobyl, Brynildsen and colleagues acknowledged that the veterinary services were, like other authorities involved, poorly prepared to respond to this type of extensive nuclear emergency.[10] However, veterinarians were able to draw on previous experience and training in contingency planning and emergency management of infectious disease outbreaks to mount a useful and practical response. Effective countermeasures to control cesium levels in meat, such as preslaughter feeding of livestock with uncontaminated fodder and the oral administration of cesium binders were introduced, and new methods to measure levels of radioactive cesium in live animals were developed. While the efforts to reduce the detrimental impact of the Chernobyl radioactive fallout on animal agriculture and reindeer herding in Norway were prolonged and complex, the veterinary services dealt capably with their professional responsibilities to protect human health and the economic well-being of farmers.

Veterinary Response to Nuclear Accidents

More detailed discussion of the fundamentals of radiation biology, health physics, and emergency management is beyond the scope of this book. A primer of sorts for veterinarians appeared in the *Journal of the American Veterinary Medical Association* in 1987 as part of a special issue on veterinary services in disas-

ters and emergencies. Articles by Morrison,[31] Schulte,[39] and Nussbaum[34] specifically address the veterinary implications of nuclear emergencies and provide basic information on the types of nuclear radiation and radioactivity, sources and intensities of radiation exposure, the effects of radiation on biological systems, the potential effects on food-producing livestock, and actions to minimize these effects. They also review the general structure of governmental emergency response plans in the event of nuclear accidents and the role of veterinarians in such radiation emergency response plans. Though published in 1987, these articles still contain useful and relevant information.

Today, most industrialized nations and states and provinces within those nations have developed emergency response plans to deal with nuclear incidents. The design of emergency response plans will vary among jurisdictions, depending on a number of factors including, for instance, the presence or absence of nuclear power plants in the area, the size and location of large population centers, and the extent of agricultural activity. At the state level, emergency response plans are usually developed and coordinated through a state emergency management agency with the cooperation of state environmental protection, pubic health, and public safety agencies. The state departments of agriculture are usually responsible, at least in part, for establishing guidelines and protocols to monitor radiation effects on livestock following accidental exposure to ionizing radiation. State veterinarians may be involved in sampling animals, farm premises, and foodstuffs for detection of radiation levels as well as in providing advice to animal owners in managing their animals to limit contamination.

Veterinary practitioners who want to play a more active role in their communities can do so through community education, training, and participation in emergency responses. The Federal Emergency Management Agency (FEMA), through its Emergency Management Institute, offers independent study courses covering various aspects of emergency management that are available on the internet. A number of these courses are relevant to veterinarians, particularly in the context of radiation emergencies. Courses of interest include IS-10, Animals in Disaster-Awareness and Preparedness; IS-11, Animals in Disaster-Community Planning; IS-3, Radiological Emergency Management; and IS-301, Radiologic Emergency Response. Course descriptions and details for enrollment are available through the Emergency Management Institute home page at http://www.fema.gov/emi/.

The International Situation

While the Three Mile Island accident acutely heightened public awareness of nuclear safety issues in the United States, it was Chernobyl that solidified international recognition that major nuclear accidents in peacetime were global concerns with serious transboundary implications, even for countries far away from the accident site. This recognition resulted in considerable efforts to enlarge and strengthen international cooperation in areas such as communication, harmonization of emergency management criteria, and coordination of protective actions. Major initiatives that evolved in the period following Chernobyl include

- International conventions on early notification and assistance in case of a radiological accident, facilitated by the International Atomic Energy Agency (IAEA) and the European Commission (EC)
- Improved preparedness through development of the international nuclear emergency exercises (INEX) program, by the Nuclear Energy Agency (NEA) of the Organization for Economic Cooperation and Development (OECD)
- A classification scheme for nuclear accidents in the international accident severity scale (INES), facilitated by the IAEA and NEA
- Establishment of radionuclide contamination standards for foods in international trade through the Codex Alimentarius Commission facilitated by the FAO and the World Health Organization (WHO).

The IAEA (www.iaea.org/worldatom) is a specialized agency of the United Nations with headquarters in Vienna, Austria. The agency serves as the world's central intergovernmental forum for scientific and technical cooperation in the nuclear field and as the international inspectorate for the application of nuclear safeguards and verification measures covering civilian nuclear programs. Individual countries join IAEA as member states and are then able to use the services of the agency. There are currently 132 member states. IAEA activities include nuclear safeguards and verification; physical protection of nuclear material; nuclear radiation and waste safety management; and, nuclear power, fuel cycle and waste technology development. There is a technical cooperation unit that conducts training courses and participates in on-site projects in over 90 countries. IAEA also supports a program called the Contact Experts Group, specifically created in 1995 to coordinate international efforts to assist the Russian Federation in dealing with the complicated ecological problems associated with the management of radioactive waste accumulated from past activities in nuclear weapons production, use of nuclear energy for peaceful purposes, and the reductions in nuclear arms. IAEA coordinated much of the monitoring and investigative work that went on in the aftermath of Chernobyl.

While the risks and dangers of nuclear power are real, they should not completely overshadow the fact that nuclear technologies can provide beneficial contributions to society. As such, IAEA also supports the development and application of nuclear technologies for peaceful purposes, including applications directly relevant to veterinarians. The IAEA and FAO together support a program known as the Joint Division of Nuclear Techniques in Food and Agriculture (see http://www.iaea.org/programmes/nafa/). This joint program supports research, training, and analytical support to develop and disseminate nuclear technology in diverse ap-

plications including the improvement of soil and water management, production of better crop varieties, control of insect pests, improvement of food quality and safety, and diagnosis of animal diseases. Some examples of animal health-related projects include the application of progesterone radioimmunoassays to improve artificial insemination programs and improved diagnostic immunoassays for a number of important livestock diseases including rinderpest, foot and mouth disease, trypanosomiasis, and contagious bovine pleuropneumonia, among others.

IAEA maintains laboratories at Seibersdorf, Austria. The facility includes the Training and Reference Centre for Food and Pesticide Control, another joint activity of IAEA and FAO. It was established in recognition of the growing need for countries to implement national legislation and trade agreements ensuring the quality and safety of food in international trade. The centre is intended to address concerns about the presence of pesticide residues, veterinary drugs, microbial contamination, natural toxins, heavy metals, and radioactive contaminants in international food trade through research and training in appropriate analytic techniques.

Environmental Pollution from Livestock Production

The effect of environmental toxins and pollutants on the health and productivity of domestic animals has long been an area of professional concern in veterinary medicine. Veterinary toxicology is an established part of the standard veterinary curriculum, and several good textbooks are available on the subject. The emphasis has been on clinical toxicology, aimed at training veterinarians to recognize the various types of toxic agents that can cause clinical disease in animals, their sources and mechanisms of action, and proper methods for treating and preventing intoxication. In this age of increased environmental awareness, however, there is a need for greater scientific and professional recognition that livestock production itself may add to the pollution of soil, air, and water. Potential causes of environmental pollution associated with livestock production are animal wastes and various chemicals used in animal agriculture, including antiparasitic agents commonly used by veterinarians.

Manure and Animal Waste Management

In our time, manure has been transformed from a valuable agricultural resource to a potentially troublesome environmental contaminant, largely because of the intensification of animal production practices. The confinement of large numbers of animals in controlled environments is a growing trend, and the numbers of animals per livestock operation are increasing. Fewer farms are managing greater numbers of animals. This trend began in the poultry industry about 60 years ago and is now far advanced in the swine industry as well. While the size of cattle makes them less conducive to intensified management, consolidation of beef feedlot production and intensification of dairy production are also occurring. Intensified production offers some advantages to producers and consumers. It improves efficiency of livestock production by creating economies of scale. It allows greater degree of standardization of production and facilitates the production of livestock products of more consistent quality and character. Intensification also creates some problems in animal production: it raises issues about the comfort and welfare of production animals raised in strict confinement; it may increase the risk of disease transmission by congregating large populations of animals; and it concentrates animal wastes, creating problems in waste management. Critics of confinement animal production often refer to it disparagingly as factory farming. In the context of waste management, the factory comparison is valid. Large volumes of animal effluent are accumulated during the production process and must be properly managed, just as a factory must properly manage the waste stream generated during production.

The United States is a leader in intensified animal production. In by 1996, in the poultry industry, 97% of all sales of broiler chickens came from operations producing 100,000 or more birds per year. In the beef industry, with 45,000 beef feedlots nationwide, one third of all marketed cattle came from just 70 of the largest feedlots. In the dairy industry, the number of dairy herds decreased from 250,000 to 150,000 between 1986 and 1996, while average herd size increased by more than 50%. The most dramatic changes have occurred in the swine industry. During the decade up to 1996, the number of hog operations in the nation decreased by 72% while the national hog inventory increased by 18% in the same period. In 1997, 63% of all hogs sold in the United States came from farms marketing over 5000 head annually. In North Carolina, between 1982 and 1992, the average number of swine per farm increased by almost 600% while the number of farms in the state declined by 62%.

Intensification of livestock operations is not limited to the United States. Europe also has embraced large-scale confinement production. For example, two relatively small countries, the Netherlands and Belgium, contain 7.5% of western Europe's human population, but 20% of its swine population. In other parts of the world, where relatively affluent urban populations have increased the demand for meat, the response has been to introduce intensified animal production facilities near cities. However, waste management challenges and associated environmental problems have thwarted these initiatives. Swine operations have been scaled back in Taiwan because of such constraints and virtually eliminated in Singapore.

Animals produce considerable amounts of manure as shown in Table 6-11. It is estimated that U.S. farm animals currently produce almost 1.4 billion tons of manure annually. While manure is often referred to as waste, it has significant potential value as an agricultural resource. Like commercial fertilizers, manure can provide nitrogen, phosphorus, and potassium, which can contribute to the enrichment of agricultural soils. In addition, manure provides a variety of trace minerals to support crop production and organic matter that helps to build the soil humus and retain soil moisture. However, the relative proportions of nitrogen and phosphorus in manure and their bioavailability over time is more variable than that of commercial formulated fertilizers. Therefore, the rational application of manure to soils requires preparatory calculations that take into account the nutrient inventory of the manure, the nutrient requirements of the type of crop to be grown, the existing nutrient status of the soil, and the degree of expected supplementation, if any, with commercial fertilizers. The timing and technique of application of manure also affects its usefulness. Ideally, manure should be integrated into soil, not simply applied to the surface. This means injecting liquid manure or turning over soil after manure application to incorporate solid manure. Manure applied on frozen ground or left on the surface will do less to enrich the soil and is more likely to be washed from fields by melting snow or rain.

Storage of manure has become more challenging and costly with increased concentration of animals in commercial production systems. This is especially true in regions where winters are cold enough to eliminate the possibility of spreading manure on fields for a good part of the year. Various types of storage facilities have been developed, including in-ground and above-ground systems. In-ground systems include underfloor pits directly below animals in housing units or adjacent earthen basins and lagoons, often associated with earthen dams or embankments. Above-ground systems include simple stacking of manure, concrete tanks, or coated steel tanks. Problems have emerged with some of these systems.

Table 6-11 Manure Production and Composition in Various Types of Livestock (in kg per day/454 Kg (1000 lb) of animal unit)

Livestock Type	Total Daily Manure Output (Kg)	Nitrogen Content (Kg)	Phosphorus Content (Kg)
Beef cattle	26.8	0.14	0.05
Dairy cattle	36.3	0.20	0.03
Swine	28.6	0.19	0.07
Broiler chickens	36.3	0.50	0.15

There is nothing intrinsically wrong with earthen basins and lagoons as methods of manure storage. However, if not properly constructed, there can be serious consequences. The most dramatic of these consequences are failures of earthen embankments or retaining walls, leading to the sudden release of vast volumes of liquid manure. Such events have received considerable publicity in the United States in recent years and have focused attention on intensified animal agriculture as a source of pollution. For example, the accidental spill of 25 million gallons of hog waste from an 8-acre waste lagoon into two tributaries of the New River in North Carolina in June 1995, was widely linked in the media to the death of an estimated 10 million fish and the closing of 364,000 acres of coastal wetlands to shell fishing. A less dramatic, but significant, issue with in-ground systems is leaching. The proper placement, construction, and lining of lagoons and basins must take the permeability of local soils into account as well as the depth and proximity of aquifers. Where permeable soils exist, linings of clay or other suitable materials are indicated to prevent leaching of waste constituents into groundwater.

Even when manure is properly stored, it ultimately requires disposition of some sort. Application to fields is the traditional method. Liquid manure can be disseminated by tractor-drawn tank sprayers or irrigation systems, solid manure by tractor-drawn spreaders. However, as animals are concentrated for production, and feeds are trucked in from distant sites rather than grown locally, there is often insufficient cropland adjacent to intensive animal production systems to absorb all the manure safely. Since manure has value as fertilizer, the prospect of transporting manure to distant croplands for application seems reasonable, but the nutrient value of manure on a per volume basis is relatively low, and when transport costs or drying costs to reduce volume are figured in, its value as a saleable commodity is tenuous. This can be a problem of international dimension. It is estimated that all of Dutch farmland can safely accommodate 50 million tonnes of manure per year, but that livestock farms in the Netherlands are producing approximately twice that amount. About 40% of the excess comes from calf fattening and dairy units, 40% from swine production facilities, and 20% from poultry units. Neighboring Belgium, with large animal populations of its own, banned importation of liquid manure from the Netherlands. The Dutch authorities have had to institute a number of strict laws and regulations to control the volume of manure spread on fields and the time of year it can be spread. In 1987, a law was passed requiring farmers to keep a record of farm manure production and to pay a levy if their fixed quota was exceeded.

Pollution Potential of Animal Waste Animal manure has considerable potential as an environmental pollutant of air, soil, and water. Two types of atmospheric pollution are recognized. One is ammonia, which is produced from nitrogen in manure during the microbially mediated anaerobic digestion that occurs while manure is stored in basins or lagoons. The ammonia bubbles into the atmosphere, where it contributes to production of acid rain. Acid rain continues to be a problem in the northeastern region of North America and through much of northern Europe. While the bulk of atmospheric pollutants contributing to acid rain come from industrial sources, agricultural sources contribute. Approximately 20% of the acid depositions that fall in the Netherlands comes from agricultural sources, including animal manure.

The second atmospheric problem associated with manure is odor. This has become a surprisingly contentious issue in the United States in relation to large-scale, intensive, swine operations, and neighbors, including some farmers, have become quite active in pushing for restrictive ordinances on the siting of commercial swine farms and controls on manure handling. Persistent, strong odors that permeate clothes and buildings can clearly be a nuisance for those downwind, but some affected individuals have claimed psychological and physical reactions as well. Uncovered manure reservoirs emit hydrogen sulfide gas, which can contribute to odor and also produce physical effects including nausea and eye irritation. More research is needed to better understand the generation of odors from stored animal waste, to develop new methods to control them. Presently, appropriate technology is more or less limited to covering stored manure with straw or other materials and paying attention to siting of storage facilities relative to prevailing winds and population centers. Above-ground storage in tall tanks is also preferred because the tank produces a chimney effect that may carry odors higher into the air where they are less noticeable to neighbors.

With regard to soil contamination, excessive application of manure to fields can contribute to the occurrence of nitrate poisoning in livestock. Some crops (e.g., oats, ryegrass, and sorghum) under certain conditions will accumulate high concentrations of nitrates from heavily fertilized soil. Livestock that graze or are fed these nitrate-accumulating plants may die acutely from anemic anoxia associated with nitrite-induced methemoglobinemia.

Contamination of ground water occurs either by leaching of manure constituents from manure storage facilities or by runoff from fields into water courses after rains or melting snow. Among the leachates of concern are nitrates, phosphorus, and potential pathogenic organisms such as *Escherichia coli*, especially when these contaminants reach wells or aquifers providing drinking water for humans. Infants are particularly susceptible to nitrate-induced methemoglobinemia, and people of all ages can potentially become ill from ingestion of enteric bacteria.

Under conditions in which excessive runoff from fields into waterways occurs, serious disruptions of aquatic ecosystems can occur through the process of eutrophication. High concentrations of nitrates and phosphates stimulate growth of algae. Dying algae produce extensive organic waste material that is then degraded by bacteria. The metabolic activity of the bacteria in turn depletes dissolved oxygen in the water. The loss of oxygen can kill fish and other aquatic life forms. In recent years, an even more dramatic manifestation of eutrophication has been linked to agricultural runoff into waterways, namely, the proliferation of *Pfiesteria piscicida*, a toxin-producing organism that not only kills fish, but also causes illness in humans.

P. piscicida is a dinoflagellate. The single-celled, motile, aquatic organism was first discovered and described in 1991. It has a complex life cycle, assuming as many as 24 distinct forms, some of which are toxin producing. At least two specific toxins have been identified. One is a fat-soluble toxin that causes skin lesions and the other is a water-soluble neurotoxin. The organism can be found under a variety of aquatic conditions, though it favors an estuarine environment of brackish, slow-moving water with temperatures about 21.1°C (70°F). Increased *P. piscicida* populations are associated with nitrate and phosphorus nutrient enrichment of waters from animal manure, human sewage, and agricultural runoff. Proliferation of the organism has been linked to major fish kills in North Carolina and Maryland.[12] Affected fish may show characteristic circular, ulcerative skin lesions associated with the fat-soluble toxin effect of the organism. People exposed to *Pfiesteria* toxins also have manifested signs of illness including memory loss, confusion, a burning sensation of the skin, and, possibly, headaches, rash, eye irritation, upper respiratory irritation, muscle cramps, and digestive upsets.

The CDC has acknowledged the association of *P. piscicida* with human illness and has established an epidemiological effort in conjunction with state health departments in affected states to better establish a causal relationship. In the Maryland *Pfiesteria* outbreak of 1996, tens of thousands of fish were killed over a 7.2 km length of the Pocomoke River, which flows into the Chesapeake Bay. Human health effects were also reported. As the state has a large intensive poultry industry, the outbreak led to increased scrutiny of waste management practices in the industry. Similarly, in North Carolina, calls for increased oversight of waste management in the swine industry have followed large fish kills in that state, in which *P. piscicida* was also implicated.

The Regulatory Response Not surprisingly, animal agricultural interests have bristled at being identified as the main culprits in *Pfiesteria* outbreaks. While the high concentration of swine in affected areas of North Carolina and of poultry in affected areas of Maryland cannot be denied, the livestock sector argues that there are numerous other sources of nitrogen and phosphorus that can be reaching local waterways and predisposing to algal blooms, including *Pfiesteria* proliferation. Such sources include commercial fertilizer runoff from crop agriculture, effluents from human sewage-treatment plants, and industrial sources. However, there is a historical reason why intensive livestock operations in the United States are currently receiving what sometimes seems like excessive scrutiny and that has to do with the particulars of the Clean Water Act.

When the Clean Water Act was first passed in 1972, the focus of regulation was on so-called point-source polluters. A factory, for example, might have a single large discharge pipe running from the plant out to a nearby river through which it regularly dumped the wastes and residues of its manufacturing process. In 1972, large-scale, confinement livestock operations were still relatively uncommon compared with family farm operations keeping livestock. While the Clean Water Act

recognized the existence of concentrated animal-feeding operations (CAFOs) and gave authority to the Environmental Protection Agency (EPA) to regulate them, most regulatory oversight and enforcement was directed toward industrial polluters and municipal sewage plants. Family farms where manure was spread on farm fields were basically left unregulated by the Clean Water Act, because runoff from fields into local waters was considered a "non-point source" of pollution. The act has succeeded in significantly reducing industrial pollution of the nation's waterways over the last 25 years.

Now, greater attention is being paid to water pollution originating from non-point sources, including crop-based agriculture and intensive livestock production. In 1998, the EPA, in conjunction with the USDA, announced their intention to aggressively enforce those aspects of the Clean Water Act that dealt with CAFOs, proposing that permits be required for any operation with over 1,000 livestock units, defined as 1,000 cattle, 2,500 swine, or 100,000 hens. Granting of permits will require approval of an overall plan for waste management at each facility. As of 2001, the proposed EPA rules on CAFOs are still under consideration by Congress, and the final criteria for defining CAFOs may turn out to be even more stringent than originally suggested. The rules are scheduled to become final in December 2002.

Water pollution and disruption of aquatic environments associated with agricultural practices have emerged as global problems. The widespread use of chemicals directly in support of improved crop production is probably the major source of agricultural pollutants. These chemicals include commercial fertilizers, pesticides, and herbicides as well as animal manure. In addition, loss of soil itself through erosion can disrupt aquatic environments through siltation. Globally, a number of situations have been identified in which agricultural runoff is believed, at least in part, to result in aquatic environmental disruption:

- A 13,000 to 18,200 km² area of lifeless water in the Gulf of Mexico, referred to as the "dead zone," has been linked to algal blooms associated with nutrient enrichment of the Gulf's waters, largely from agricultural runoff throughout the entire Mississippi River Basin that empties into the Gulf.

- In East Africa's Lake Victoria, agricultural pollution from farms in the watershed is contributing to fish kills in the lake that are adversely affecting the livelihood of local fishermen.

- In Ecuador, commercial shrimp farmers practicing aquaculture in coastal estuaries are experiencing increased disease problems in shrimp associated with agricultural pollutants being delivered to coastal waters from inland farms up river.

- In Australia, conservationists are concerned that clearing coastal lands for cattle pastures is producing large amounts of silt that are contributing to the death of corals in the Great Barrier Reef.

Some creative and innovative approaches are being adopted for animal waste management. Diversification of farm activities can allow manure to be redirected to other productive applications such as generation of biogas for use as fuel and use of the solid residue as a nutrient base for fish ponds or hydroponic gardening. Agricultural engineers and environmental scientists have been working on the design of grass and forest buffers between croplands and water sources to serve as artificial wetlands that help to remove excessive nutrients and harmful substances from manure runoff before it reaches streams or rivers.

Whether a veterinarian is interested in environmental health, public health, food safety, or production medicine, there is some aspect of waste management that can offer professional challenges. Veterinarians should work with farmers on the development and implementation of voluntary waste management plans. Many state agriculture departments or environmental protection agencies now have workbooks or software programs available to assist in this process, often referred to as "nutrient management planning." Waste management has also become a contentious issue in many communities, and veterinarians should be visible in these debates, using their scientific training and community standing to help clarify some of the technical, environmental, and health concerns, both real and imagined, that surround these debates. This holds true in the international arena as well. In many countries, regulatory statutes governing oversight of agricultural practices with potential for environmental damage may not exist or, if they do exist, are not strongly enforced. Therefore, veterinarians consulting on livestock development projects abroad can use their opportunities as "foreign experts" to encourage consideration of waste management issues in new livestock production schemes and help to develop reasonable management plans.

Chemicals Used in Animal Agriculture

Since World War II, there has been a steady and dramatic increase in the use of chemicals for farming in industrialized nations. While the vast majority of chemical use is directed toward crop agriculture in the form of synthetic fertilizers, herbicides, and pesticides, there has also been an increase in the use of synthetic chemicals in livestock agriculture. Pesticides are used in livestock production primarily to control external parasites by direct application to animals or farm premises and also to control some internal parasites. Among the most highly effective compounds in use for much of the 1950s through the 1980s were the organophosphates and the organochlorines, which were used widely by veterinarians for the control of flies, lice, mange, ticks, fleas, and some gastrointestinal nematodes. However, the use of chemicals in agriculture and veterinary medicine has come under increasing regulatory control as the potential environmental and public health consequences of their use have become clearer.

In the United States, for instance, the EPA (www.epa.gov) was created in 1970 as a federal agency to protect and enhance environmental quality in the nation. Included in the EPA mandate were the regulation of solid waste disposal, radiation, and toxic substances, including pesticides used in agriculture and veterinary medicine. The EPA considers numerous criteria in evaluating and approving pesticides, demonstrating a broad concern for consumer safety, public health, and environmental health. Tests and data are evaluated to assess human health effects and ecological toxicity as well as the chemical fate and environmental distribution of the pesticides. Applications that are approved specifically designate the conditions under which the pesticide may be used, including targeted species, dose rates, routes of administration, and tolerance levels for residues in food or feed. Pesticides may be denied approval for risks to human health or for environmental reasons. Chemicals that were previously approved for use can be subjected to new reviews as additional scientific information about their potential harm becomes available, and they may be reregistered with more restrictive guidelines for use or have their approval withdrawn altogether. This process has affected veterinary practice with regard to the drugs available for treating ectoparasites in livestock, as many organochlorine and organo-phosphate compounds previously available are no longer licensed for use.

The Emphasis on Environmental Safety Newer compounds in different classes such as the synthetic pyrethroids and the avermectins, including ivermectin, have since emerged to replace the banned chemicals of previous decades for use in ectoparasite control in livestock. In general, these compounds may be safer for humans and for the environment than the organochlorines, organophosphates, and carbamates, though they are still not without some risks. Newer approaches to the formulation and administration of pesticides to animals such as impregnation of ear tags, parenteral injection, oral administration, or localized application over the back (e.g., pour-ons and spot-ons) to effect total body coverage also makes dissemination of pesticides into the environment or high-level exposure to humans less likely. Nevertheless, the level of tolerance for adverse environmental effects has become so narrow that it is the rare compound that does not provoke intensive public and regulatory scrutiny. Ivermectin is a good example.

Ivermectin is a broad-spectrum parasiticide in the avermectin class, a group of compounds derived from soil organisms. These macrocyclic lactones act on chloride channels in nematode and arthropod nerve cells and induce flaccid paralysis of the parasites. Ivermectin was essentially the first drug available to veterinarians that could be given to animals parenterally by injection or oral administration and had efficacy against both internal nematodes and external arthropod parasites. The drug is approved for use in most domestic animal species though not for use in lactating animals and only in lower doses for dogs, as idiosyncratic reactions have been observed in dogs given large-animal doses, particularly collies. In addition, ivermectin has found use in human medicine for the successful treatment of onchocerciasis, or river blindness. Though its occurrence is limited to sub-Saharan Africa, onchocerciasis, caused by a filarial worm, *Onchocerca volvulus,* is the leading cause of human blindness in the world. Ivermectin offered the first safe, inexpensive, and effective means for controlling the disease in humans.

Its numerous beneficial attributes aside, there are still environmental health concerns raised over the use of ivermectin. The drug is mostly excreted in the feces and is slow to degrade in feces and soil, with a half-life of 91 to 217 days in winter and 7-14 days in summer. Ecologists and environmentalists have drawn attention to the fact that the persistence of ivermectin in fecal pats can have adverse effects on a variety of insects, including dung beetles, which play an important role in breaking down ruminant fecal pats to return nutrients to the soil and which also prey on developing stages of insect pests that develop in dung, such as the horn fly. These are not trivial matters. In Australia, for instance, where ruminant animals were not part of the indigenous flora, dung beetles were imported after the introduction of cattle to the continent in recognition of their important role in maintaining pasture quality.

However, the impact of ivermectin on dung beetle development is not uniform and must be studied on a case-by- case basis. A number of research studies have been done that indicate that different dung beetle species show variable susceptibility to the effects of ivermectin. Furthermore, local climate and the timing of ivermectin treatments relative to the local cattle management system also influence whether or not dung beetles are exposed to ivermectin at critical periods in their developmental cycle. In many cases, adverse impacts are minimal. In other situations, the impact on dung beetles can be significant and may be associated with broader ecological impacts. For example, southwest England is home to the largest known roost of a rare bat known as the greater horseshoe bat, (*Rhinolophus ferrum-equinum*) which feed heavily on *Aphodius* sp. dung beetles. Local conservationists claim that administration of ivermectin to cattle in the area may make the dung sterile for 35 to 120 days and kill *Aphodius* larvae that may normally be present at concentrations of up to 100 larvae per pat. When ivermectin use is widespread in the spring, pregnant bats may face a food crisis between April and June, and their young may risk starvation if fecal pats within a kilometer of their roost are still sterile in early August. These claims are disputed by the manufacturer as not scientifically substantiated. The conflict, which was reported in the British press in 1998, is still ongoing.

Ivermectin has also become the focus of a hot debate relating to its safety for use in marine environments. Sea lice have emerged as a serious constraint to production of cultivated salmon off the shores of Scotland, and fish farmers, already under pressure to reduce the use of dichlorvos for sea lice control (see sidebar "Salmon Fishing vs. Salmon Farming in Scotland") increasingly turned to ivermectin to control these ectoparasites of fish, even though the use of ivermectin in fish was not officially approved. When the Scottish Environmental Protection Agency (SEPA) considered approving ivermectin for that specific use in 1996 at the request of salmon-farming as-

sociations, it was met with a storm of protest by environmentalists and consumer advocates who were concerned about tissue residues in marketed fish, the persistence of ivermectin in marine environments, and its toxic effects on a wide variety of marine organisms, including shrimp, mussels, starfish, and sea worms. Scientific studies supported some of the claims but not others. Ultimately, SEPA approved the use of ivermectin to control sea lice, but with restrictions that included a ban on its use within 2 nautical miles of any shellfish farmer.

The environmental challenges to ivermectin on land and at sea underscore the scrutiny to which veterinary drugs are now subjected in relation to their environmental impact. They also underscore the extent to which complex and well-designed scientific research is necessary to substantiate the environmental impact of synthetic chemicals and provide a rational basis for decision making in complex situations that have too often become politically charged issues played out in the media without sufficient scientific input. There are considerable opportunities for veterinarians to be involved in such objective research.

Pesticide Use in the Developing World   In general, compliance with regulatory controls on the use of pesticides for veterinary applications in the United States and other highly industrialized nations is good. There are a number of reasons for this, including a high level of public awareness and concern about pesticides, detailed and enforceable regulations, and routine monitoring by regulatory authorities. For example, in the United States in 1988, the monitoring program of the USDA Food Safety and Inspection Service, the National Residue Program, analyzed 2750 randomly selected samples from 17 animal species or production classes for residues of chlorinated hydrocarbon pesticides and found only 3 violations (0.1%).

Another key reason for compliance is international trade. As described earlier in this chapter with respect to control of radionuclide activity in foods, the Codex Alimentarius Commission, cosponsored by FAO and WHO, serves as a scientific advisory body to establish tolerance limits for pesticide residues in food products entering international trade. The World Trade Organization (WTO) recognizes the Codex Alimentarius as the scientific authority on such matters, and WTO member nations agree to respect the tolerance limits suggested by the Codex Alimentarius for food products offered in international trade.

In many developing countries, the use of pesticides in general and in veterinary medicine in particular remains largely unregulated and continues to pose threats to health and the environment. There are a number of reasons for this. In some cases, politicians and policymakers perceive the value of pesticides for improving agricultural productivity or controlling vector-borne disease to far outweigh the adverse consequences of their use, and the view is not challenged by a citizenry that may be largely uneducated and uninformed about the environmental and human health effects of pesticides. Even if informed, they may be disenfranchised, with little opportunity to influence legislative policy. Even where the potential hazards of unregulated pesticide use are recognized, government may lack the capital, infrastructure, and personnel to carry out the necessary licensing, surveillance, and enforcement activities successfully.

In addition, most poor countries are not active food exporters and therefore lack the incentive to meet Codex Alimentarius standards on chemical residues in food products. Finally, in tropical regions especially, damage by pests to crops and livestock can be considerable, particularly when exotic breeds of plants and animals with high production potential but little local disease resistance are introduced from outside the region. Endogenous breeds, though often less productive, frequently possess natural or selected resistance to local pests while introduced breeds do not. Control of ticks and tick-borne diseases, for example, is essential to maintain health and production when exotic Holstein cattle are introduced from Europe or North America into tropical countries as an element of dairy improvement projects.

Global pesticide use exceeds 5.5 billion pounds per year. While the industrialized world accounts for 80% of the pesticide market, the fastest growing segment of the world market is in the developing countries. This includes the use of pesticides no longer approved for use in developed countries. In fact, some of these pesticides are still manufactured and exported from developed countries in which their use is banned. The situation in poorer countries with regard to pesticide use for livestock is exemplified by the case of Ghana, a small, West African nation of about 18 million people with more than half the population involved in agriculture and fishing. Life expectancy in Ghana is 57 years, the adult literacy rate is 64.5%, and currently only 44% of eligible school-aged children attend grades 1 through 3. The mean annual per capita income is US$ 2032.

Scientists at the University of Ghana carried out surveys to gather information on the use of pesticides in the country, specifically for control of ectoparasites in livestock.[4,6] Twenty-four different products were available within the country from traders, mostly in the city centers. The products included 12 organophosphates, 7 synthetic pyrethroids, 3 carbamates and 2 organochlorines. Both of the organochlorine products were formulations of lindane, one a louse powder for dusting and the other for aqueous applications. The latter lindane product, formulated for dipping, spraying, and hand dressing, was the pesticide product most widely used by Ghanaian farmers and herders for control of ectoparasites in livestock, especially ticks, which carry 10 different hemoparasitic diseases of livestock in Ghana. There are several reasons for the popularity of lindane among livestock owners and managers in the country. Lindane was one of the earliest products available. As such, it has brand name recognition, has a known history of efficacy, and remains cheaper than the newer products such as synthetic pyrethroids. Also, farmers recognize and value the staying power of lindane, with residual protection lasting for extended periods after application. This is important in the Ghanaian context, where pesticide vendors may be located in cities or smaller commercial centers far from the rural locations of animals. With limited access to cash and transportation, farmers prefer products that do not need frequent application.

While state farms and experimental stations use dipping tanks or commercial sprayers for application of pesticides to livestock, the small herd size and low income level of the average Ghanaian farmer does not permit investment in such equipment. The most common form of pesticide application in the country for large animals is hand application or hand dressing. The vast majority of farmers prepared lindane solutions from unmeasured amounts of stock formulations without use of protective gloves, masks, or clothing. Then, a rag or sponge is hand-dipped into the bucket of pesticide solution and dabbed onto those areas of cattle commonly favored by ticks for attachment, such as the ears, perineum, and, notably, the udder. Some farmers use a squirt bottle to apply the pesticide solution to the udder and may do so in conjunction with milking, when animals are already restrained and ticks on the udder are easily noted. No withdrawal times were observed relative to pesticide use before slaughter or for sale of milk, and empty acaricide containers are sometimes sold for reuse and refilled with food products such as vegetable oil.

Lack of farmer education, low levels of consumer awareness, and the absence of a clear-cut government policy regarding use of pesticides in food-producing animals creates a human health risk in Ghana and other developing countries that is now totally unacceptable in developed countries. On a more encouraging note, Ghana's Parliament passed the Pesticides Control and Management Act in 1996, capping 5 years of legislative debate and preparation. The law empowers the Ghana Environmental Protection Agency (EPA) to regulate production, importation, distribution, handling, and use of pesticides and to enforce pesticide laws and promote safe pesticide use through public education. Government officials, however, acknowledged from the outset that its EPA would have a difficult time controlling hazardous pesticide imports because smugglers have the advantage in eluding enforcement of the new regulations.

Statistics on adverse human health effects resulting specifically from pesticide use in livestock are not generally available. However, the situation relative to the overall use of pesticides in agriculture is more widely reported. The WHO estimates that from 2 to 5 million agricultural workers in the developing world may experience an episode of acute insecticide poisoning each year because of inadequate training in pesticide use and the failure to use protective clothing or respirators. This alarming statistic is relevant to veterinarians intending to work in developing countries. Over the last decade there has been a strong trend in international development programs to train farmers and herders as community-based animal health workers, providing them with training to recognize, treat, and prevent the most common diseases of livestock in their areas, using a limited repertoire of veterinary drugs. Often the drug kit contains a broad-spectrum pesticide for ectoparasite control, as ectoparasites are often important constraints on livestock production. Such pesticides must be chosen wisely, with consideration given to environmental and human health effects in addition to more practical concerns such as cost and efficacy. Community-based animal health workers, who are sometimes illiterate, must be properly trained to understand both the risks and the safe use of pesticides in livestock (Fig. 6-8). Community-based animal health programs are discussed further in Chapter 8.

Integrated Pest Management (IPM)

Public concerns about, and greater understanding of, the adverse environmental impacts of pesticide use have led to greater management and oversight of pesticide use. Agricultural states now have regular training programs for farmers and

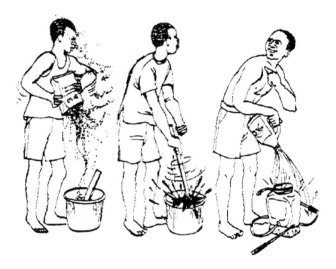

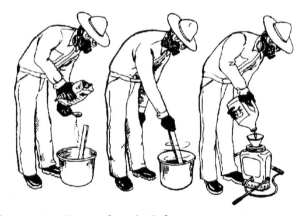

Figure 6-8. The use of visual aids for training is an important aspect of extension activities in developing countries, especially in rural areas, where illiteracy rates are often high. These drawings, developed for use in Africa, demonstrate improper and proper techniques for handling and mixing stock pesticide formulations before application. The drawings emphasize the use of protective clothing and the need to take care. These visual aids, along with others, are available at the website of the International Centre of Insect Physiology and Ecology (ICIPE) in Nairobi, Kenya (http://www.icipe.org/clipart/) for use in preparing posters, flip charts, and other training and extension aids related to pest control. (Drawings by Barbara Shear, from Crop Protection Clip Art Book, vol 1, The Sahel. 1990. USAID. Reproducible without copyright restriction, courtesy of ICIPE, Nairobi, Kenya.)

require certification for application of restricted pesticides. Yet, even with stricter regulation and control of agricultural chemical use, it is estimated that more than 67 million birds are killed by legal application of pesticides to croplands in the United States each year. Up to 25% of U.S. lakes and streams are contaminated with agricultural pollutants, and an estimated 6 to 14 million fish are killed annually. In addition, some approved agricultural chemicals or their breakdown products are now being recognized as having estrogenic activity and may be contributing to the endocrine-disruptor phenomenon discussed earlier.

At the same time, insects and other targeted pests continue to develop resistance to existing chemicals. For instance, in the veterinary arena, the development of ear tags impregnated with pyrethroid insecticide for use in cattle in the 1970s was heralded as a major breakthrough in hornfly control in cattle in the United States. However, by the mid-1980s in the United States and by 1991 in Canada, hornfly resistance to pyrethroids was widespread, causing the need to develop new products and strategies for hornfly control. Currently, there are more than 535 insects, 210 weeds, and 210 plant diseases known to be resistant to at least one pesticide. Despite the heavy reliance on pesticide compounds, with American farmers applying over 1 billion pounds of pesticides to the land annually, approximately $20 billion in pest damage to food crops still occurs each year in the United States. Manufacturers, meanwhile, are increasingly reluctant to invest in the development of new pesticides and to underwrite the ever-widening and costly array of safety tests required for regulatory approval, when the new products they market may be rendered obsolete by the development of resistance in targeted pests within a matter of years.

This situation of heavy reliance on pesticide use in the face of continued losses due to pests, coupled with the persistent demand for new pesticides to control the evolving resistance of agricultural pests, represents a cyclical dilemma for farmers that some critics call the "pesticide treadmill." In response to the pesticide treadmill, there is a growing interest among agricultural scientists, environmentalists, farmers, and consumers in reducing the dependence of agricultural enterprises on pesticide use through the development and application of integrated pest management (IPM) practices.

IPM resists precise definition. In fact, there is a web site that maintains an inventory of evolving definitions of IPM since the 1950s (see http://www.ippc.orst.edu/IPMdefinitions/define.html). The basic concept of IPM is to develop multifaceted approaches to pest control that reduce pest losses to economically acceptable limits, that are cost-effective, that pose minimal risk to human health and environmental quality, and that offer long-term sustainability. Selection of an IPM strategy for any given situation must be based on a thorough understanding of the natural history of the pest and its host, the ecological setting in which the pest and host exist, and the agricultural system and management practices under which the pest problem occurs. Based on such detailed knowledge of a particular pest problem, a set of appropriate and complementary pest control interventions can be applied.

The control interventions used in IPM are drawn from a number of categories. Different authorities on IPM take different approaches to classifying these categories. In the case of parasitic diseases of livestock, Uilenburg suggests that the appropriate categories are ecological control, biological control, genetic control, mechanical control, immunological control, and sanitary control.[43] It is also appropriate to include a category of chemical control, since in some cases IPM can significantly reduce the use of pesticides but may not always be able to eliminate their use altogether.

Control Ecological control involves manipulation of the relationship between the animal host, pest, and environment, based on intimate knowledge of their interactions in space and time. A simple and well-known example of such an intervention, familiar to all veterinarians and livestock owners, is pasture rotation of grazing animals to help control gastrointestinal parasitism. By periodically moving livestock, exposure to infective larvae in pastures is reduced. IPM requires understanding local livestock management practices, to select appropriate interventions. Pasture rotation, for example, while suitable for private farms and ranches, would be much more difficult to implement where communal grazing is routinely practiced. One must also understand the pest life cycle. Pasture rotation, for example, is a much more effective tool for managing one-host ticks than two- or three-host ticks. Other examples of ecological control include setting brush fires to reduce tick populations in grazing lands, a common practice among African herders, or the use of zero-grazing (i.e., total confinement of animals to reduce exposure to ticks), which is increasingly being advocated when high- producing, exotic breeds of livestock are introduced into tropical regions.

Careful study of an animal-management system may be necessary to identify variables that can be manipulated to effect simple, low-cost ecological controls. For example, in South Africa, Karoo tick paralysis, caused by feeding *Ixodes rubicundus* female ticks is a major constraint on small-ruminant production in moister, more hilly portions of the Karooveld between March and August. Researchers there studied tick behavior in relation to the length of veld grasses between 10 and 45 cm and to the crown cover associated with the presence of wild olive trees. They determined that ticks survive longer on tall grasses and are twice as likely to infest sheep grazing tall grasses They also learned that when crown height was raised by cutting lower branches to mimic the effect of browsing goats, tick densities in the vicinity of trees dropped significantly. On the basis of these observations, it was possible to recommend ecological controls for reduction of Karoo tick paralysis, including introducing horses or cattle to graze down long grasses before introducing small ruminants and increasing the proportion of goats in mixed sheep and goat flocks to keep wild olive trees pruned by browsing.

Biological Control Even pests have their own pests. Biological control involves the use of natural predators, parasites, and pathogens that ordinarily attack agricultural pests. Some examples for control of crop pests include the introduction of ladybugs to consume aphids or the release of parasitic wasps or other hymenoptera (parasitoids) that lay eggs in the adult or immature forms of certain insect pests and, in the process of development, destroy them. To date, biological control has found far greater application against crop pests than against livestock pests, but livestock examples do exist, and it is a challenge to future researchers to develop others. Brazilian researchers, for example, are experimenting with a naturally occurring pasture fungus with the capacity to kill trichostrongylid nematode larvae in cattle dung, including *Haemonchus contortus*, a costly gastric parasite of cattle, sheep, and goats worldwide. Researchers at the International Centre of Insect Physiology and Ecology (ICIPE) in Nairobi, Kenya, are looking at a number of different approaches to biological control of ticks such as *Rhipicephalus appendiculatus* and *Amblyomma varieagatum*, which are vectors of important hemoparasitic diseases in ruminant livestock in tropical regions. Approaches under investigation include the use of parasitoids (e.g., the parasitic wasp *Ixodiphagus hookeri*), fungi (e.g., *Beauveria bassiana*), the planting of certain pasture grasses (e.g., *Melinis minutflora*, or molasses grass) that contain tick-repellant substances, and the identification of natural acaricides extractable from local plants that could serve as biopesticides (e.g., the euphorbia, *Margaritaria discoidea*). More information about ICIPE activities in biocontrol of livestock pests can be accessed at their website (www.icipe.org).

Genetic Control The category of genetic control methods takes advantage of the role that genetics plays in reproduction and the development of natural resistance to pests. Techniques for the genetic control of reproduction focus on disruption of normal breeding in insect pests. The most successfully applied techniques to date have involved the sterilization of male insects by irradiation and then releasing them to breed with fertile females in the wild. The elimination of the New World screwworm, *Cochliomyia hominivorax*, from North America has been accomplished using this method. Screwworms can cause serious losses in livestock. Female flies lay eggs on wound edges, and the developing larvae (screwworms) feed in the wounds, causing severe, necrotizing lesions. Taking advantage of the biological fact that female flies mate only once, the USDA in 1958 initiated the sterile male-release eradication program. Females mated with sterile males laid eggs that did not hatch. Within a year of the program's inception, the screwworm flies had been eliminated from Florida, at a cost of approximately US$ 11 million, compared with a preprogram cost of over US$ 200 million annually due to animal losses and treatment and control costs.

In recent years, there has been increased interest in using the sterile, irradiated male technique for the control of tsetse flies (*Glossina* spp.), the vectors of human and animal trypanosomiasis in Africa. The reproductive patterns of tsetse flies favor the sterile male control method. The IAEA, discussed earlier in this chapter with regard to issues of nuclear radiation, has active research programs using irradiation to produce sterile insects to combat tsetse, screwworms, and other animal and crop pests and to develop improved techniques for mass rearing, genetic sexing, quality control, aerial release, and field monitoring for more cost-effective implementation of genetic control. IAEA scientists are also exploring the application of molecular biology for the development of modified strains of insects for future pest control applications.

The selection of pest-resistant livestock for animal-production systems has been a traditional method of pest control, but the potential for wider application of this technique has exploded with the advent of modern biotechnology. Some breeds of animals are known for specific disease resistance. For example Ndama and West African Shorthorn breeds of cattle are recognized as trypanotolerant. This means that they can limit proliferation of trypanosomes after infection and manifest milder clinical disease than other breeds, independent of their pre-existing immune status. In another example, tropical *Bos indicus* breeds of cattle generally show greater resistance to tick infestation than temperate *Bos taurus* breeds. Using computer models, Barnard et al. looked at economically feasible approaches to controlling the tick *Amblyomma americanum* in beef cattle in the southern United States using IPM techniques over a 5-year period.[5] Among the techniques considered were host resistance through breed selection (*B. indicus* vs. *B. taurus*), pasture rotation, habitat conversion, topical acaricide use in animals, systemic acaricide use in animals, and application of acaricides to pastures. Manipulation of the model revealed that the single most effective control strategy for controlling *A. americanum* in beef forage areas was the selection of tick-resistant *Bos indicus* cattle over *Bos taurus* cattle. However, economically feasible control strategies that took into account other production and market factors required a combination of breed selection, acaricide use, and pasture rotations.

The development of transgenic science in the past few years will no doubt lead to remarkable advances in the exploitation of genetic resistance to pests as a tool of IPM and reduce dependence on insecticides. Already there is considerable interest in identifying different breeds of livestock that show putative resistance. Once such breeds are identified, it must determined whether their resistance is genetically based or acquired through endemic exposure and subsequent immunity. If genetic, the gene(s) for resistance must be located. This can then potentially be followed by transgenic manipulation to transfer resistant genes into other breeds of animals. In such a manner, high-producing breeds can be made resistant to pests such as ticks that currently inhibit their introduction into areas where their production potential is needed but their traditional susceptibility to disease has made their introduction impractical.

Mechanical Control Mechanical control involves the use of traps and barriers to keep insects away from hosts. The best-known use of traps relevant to veterinary and human medicine is for tsetse fly control, where a variety of low-cost capture traps have been developed that attract and passively capture tsetse flies. These traps use shapes and colors known to attract flies, based on research into tsetse fly behavior. Traps are shaped to cast a horizontal shadow to attract the flies, which then approach from the underside and move upward

into the trap. Swatches of blue or black cloth also will draw tsetse flies to land on the traps (Fig. 6-9). In addition, traps can be baited with odor attractants such as cow urine that lure the flies.

In recent years, there have been numerous efforts by governments, NGOs, and international agencies to encourage community participation in the construction, siting, maintenance, and monitoring of tsetse fly traps in endemic countries in which the local people can most benefit from reduction of human and animal trypanosomiasis. Community-maintained trapping programs are a far cry from the tsetse-control approaches of the 1960s and 1970s, which depended primarily on the widespread destruction of tsetse habitat, aerial spraying of insecticides, and the wholesale slaughter of wild ungulates to reduce food sources for the blood-feeding flies.

Immunological Control Parasitologists have long envisioned the use of vaccines for the control of internal and external parasites, though the challenges of producing vaccines against complex organisms like nematodes and arthropods have been considerable. The identification of critical antigens and their production as effective recombinant proteins remains a significant obstacle. Nevertheless, there is some progress in the development of vaccines against arthropod pests of livestock. In Australia, work has progressed on vaccines against the "buffalo" fly of cattle, *Haematobia exigua*, and the sheep blowfly, *Lucilia cuprina*, but the most significant advance has been made in the development of an effective vaccine against *Boophilus microplus*, a one-host tick of cattle with a wide geographical distribution in tropical and subtropical regions of the world. It is of great economic importance as a vector of babesiosis. Recently, vaccines containing the recombinant *Boophilus microplus* gut antigen Bm86 have been developed and are now available commercially. One, Gavac, was developed in Cuba and tested in Cuba and Brazil.[9] The other, TickGARD, was created and tested in Australia.[24] Antibodies stimulated against the recom-

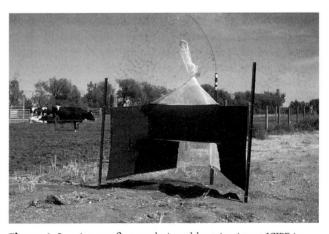

Figure 6-9. A tsetse fly trap designed by scientists at ICIPE in Nairobi, Kenya. Traps such as these can be built and maintained by villagers who have a stake in tsetse fly control to reduce the occurrence of trypanosomiasis in humans and livestock. (Photo courtesy of Dr. Steve Mihok)

binant antigen damage tick gut cells and either kill ticks outright or diminish their reproductive potential. The use of such a vaccine can drastically reduce dependence on synthetic chemicals for tick control. In Cuban field studies, use of the vaccine permitted a 60% reduction in the number of required acaricide treatments and reduced livestock losses due to tick burdens and babesiosis. Australian trials reduced fertility up to 70% in ticks feeding on vaccinated cattle and reduced the number of required acaricide applications by two or three per season.

Sanitary Control In some cases, as with infectious diseases, control of movement of livestock infested with arthropod pests can limit their spread and economic impact. Mange mites, for example, are readily spread between animals by contact and can cause considerable fleece and skin damage. Severe infestations can be fatal. In poor countries, with limited veterinary infrastructure, mange in small ruminants can be a pervasive national problem causing great economic loss. Effective regulatory programs that permit quarantine of infested animals with mandatory treatments or destruction of animals with compensation to owners can effectively control the spread of infestations and limit the need for widespread pesticide use. Sheep scab, for example, a form of mange caused by *Psoroptes ovis*, has been eliminated in the United States through a federally regulated quarantine program. In 1905, a quarantine was established, restricting movement of sheep from all territory west of the eastern border of N. Dakota, S. Dakota, Nebraska, Kansas, Oklahoma, and Texas. The last case of sheep scab in the United States was confirmed in a small flock of sheep in New Jersey in 1970.

Chemical Control Avid proponents of IM envision that it will someday offer enough tools and strategies to control all major crop and livestock pests cost-effectively without the use of synthetic chemicals. Practically speaking, however, chemical pesticides will continue to play a role in pest control, particularly with regard to livestock for the foreseeable future. The immediate challenge, therefore, in attempting to balance animal productivity with environmental safety is to use strategic applications of synthetic chemicals timed to minimize the amount of pesticide necessary, while maximizing their effectiveness in the overall pest-control effort. This requires a thorough understanding of the life cycle and ecology of targeted pests and the environment and management system in which the host animal is maintained.

New technological developments in the formulation of pesticides are also helping to reduce the environmental impact of synthetic chemical use in livestock. Traditionally, in tropical and semitropical regions where ticks and tick-borne diseases are a major constraint on livestock production, the regular whole-body immersion of cattle and small ruminants in dipping races has been routine (Fig. 6-10). A dipping race or tank may contain thousands of gallons of water-based acaricide solutions. These dipping solutions become dirty and periodically need replacement. The careless discard of old dip solutions or con-

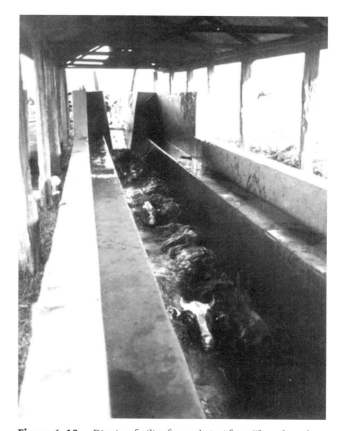

Figure 6-10. Dipping facility for cattle in Africa. Though such dipping facilities are extremely useful for controlling tick-borne diseases in cattle, the handling and disposal of acaricides used in such dips is fraught with environmental and public health hazards, if not properly managed. (Photo courtesy of International Livestock Research Institute (ILRI); photographer, Dave Ellsworth)

tainers of undiluted stock solutions can cause acute poisoning, particularly when dumped into streams, ponds, or rivers used by humans and animals for drinking, or can cause chronic problems of groundwater and soil contamination around old dip sites, as has occurred with arsenic and chlorinated hydrocarbons at some locations in the United States and Australia. However, newer formulations of acaricides allow the use of very small volumes of acaricide applied directly to animals in the form of pour-ons or spot-ons. These preparations diffuse from the site of application to give general protection to the treated animal. Pesticide-impregnated ear tags also limit environmental dispersal of acaricides. The efficacy of impregnated ear tags or tail bands can be further enhanced by combining attractant pheromones in addition to pesticides. Attractant pheromones against *Amblyomma* ticks have been identified and have been put to such use in Africa. There are even new technologies for improving the environmental safety of dipping sites. Researchers in Texas have reported on the development of a field-scale biofilter able to treat 11,000-L batches of dip solution containing the organophosphate insecticide coumaphos and to reduce concentrations of coumaphos in the solution from 2000 to 10 mg/L over a 14-day period.

Another new development in the area of chemical control is the search for new classes of pesticides that are derived from natural sources and have minimal environmental impact. Many plants and other organisms have evolved natural resistance to pests and predators, including chemical defenses. Pyrethrin, from chrysanthemum, and rotenone, from derris, are examples of pesticides derived from plants that have found large-scale commercial application in pest control. However, these compounds still possess some environmental toxicity, since their mode of action is not specific to insects. Pyrethrin and rotenone, for example, both can be toxic in aquatic environments and kill fish. There are, however, natural insecticides with a mode of action more specifically limited to insects. One important source for such a natural pesticide was identified in the early 1980s. This was the bacterium *Bacillus thuringiensis*, referred to widely as Bt. Different strains of Bt produce different toxins, and scientists have identified the genetic coding for more than 50 of these toxins, which are activated in the alkaline environment of the midgut of mosquitos and various leaf-eating insects, including important crop pests such as gypsy moth caterpillars, Colorado potato beetles, cotton bollworms, and the European corn borer. Once activated, these toxins work specifically on gut cell membranes to lethally disrupt osmotic regulation and water balance.

Bt has been available commercially for a number of years for topical application to crops and, more recently, through genetic engineering technology, the capacity for Bt biopesticide production has been incorporated into corn, potato, cotton, and other plants, so that farmers can plant seeds to produce crops that are naturally resistant to common insect pests. Yet even this technological wizardry may not eliminate the potential for harmful environmental effects. Early in 1999, experimental findings suggested that Monarch butterfly caterpillars that consumed milkweed leaves dusted with pollen from genetically engineered Bt corn plants ate less, grew more slowly, and died more quickly than control caterpillars consuming milkweed free of the corn pollen. Other researchers have since challenged the notion that Bt corn presents a risk to monarch butterflies (see http://www.ars.usda.gov/is/br/btcorn).

There are tremendous opportunities for veterinary scientists to participate in the research and development of new IPM tools and strategies for animal pest control. There is also an important extension and outreach role for veterinary practitioners to work with clients and industry to promote wider adoption and application of IPM approaches that are cost-effective and offer relief to a global environment heavily burdened by the stresses of widespread, and sometimes inappropriate, pesticide use.

Addressing the Challenge of Environmental Health

As human beings, we live in an unprecedented time of rapidly expanding human populations, increasingly powerful technology, growing global affluence, and rising expectations for material wealth and comfort. Yet Earth itself cannot and does not expand to meet our expectations. Many of Earth's resources are either finite or renewable at a pace that is often exceeded by our collective demands. Furthermore, we share the planet with a diverse array of other living organisms and natural ecosystems whose benefits to us go unrecognized and are ultimately lost as we continue to transform the planet primarily to serve our own short-term material needs.

Scientists are increasingly able to recognize and document the deleterious effects of human activity on the environment and draw attention to the fact that our actions bear harmful consequences, not only to the natural world and its denizens, but to ourselves, to our own children, and to their children in turn. There is growing recognition that environmental health is an essential prerequisite for long-term human happiness and prosperity. The maintenance of ecological function and resiliency on Earth is necessary to generate biological resources such as trees, fish, wildlife, and crops and to support ecological services such as watershed protection, air purification, climate stabilization, and erosion control that ultimately support and sustain the growth of human society on our planet. We can not ignore the biological and geophysical foundations of human existence. We must acknowledge, through our collective actions, that we are not only on this Earth, but of this Earth.

The tension between meeting human needs and preserving environmental health is well represented in the sphere of agriculture. As the discussions in this chapter have illustrated, efforts to produce food on the planet often have adverse environmental consequences on soil, water, and air quality; on ecosystem health; and on biodiversity. This is true of animal agriculture as well as crop agriculture. Yet the demand for food steadily increases, not only in quantity but in variety, as populations and affluence grow, and consumer demand for animal products in the diet expands worldwide. At the same time, concerns about environmental health have emerged as important social priorities to the point where many modern agricultural practices are coming under increasing regulation with regard to their environmental impact. These parallel developments-an increasing demand for food and an expectation that it will be produced with minimum adverse impact on the environment-have created significant tension between environmentalists and agriculturists, particularly with regard to modern animal agriculture. Veterinarians need to see the integration of environmental health with animal production not as a threat but as an opportunity, and they need to lead the way.

Discussion Points

1. What issues of land degradation exist in Australia? How are they similar to historic problems in the United States? What role does livestock grazing play in land degradation there?

2. Identify a pastoralist society somewhere in the world of interest to you and identify the pressures that have come to bear on their traditional herding practices. If you were a veterinarian serving as an international consultant on a project to reinvigorate their traditional livelihood, what recommendations would you make to the host government?

What interventions and services would you offer to the pastoralists themselves?

3. What are the important diseases of farmed salmon and farmed shrimp? Identify a specific disease of interest to you and evaluate the usefulness of available diagnostic tools, therapeutic interventions, vaccines, and management practices that might predispose to the disease.

4. Potential implications of global warming on the health and management of grazing animals in the U.K. are presented in this chapter. What specific changes might occur in animal agriculture as a result of global warming where you live? What new vectors and animal diseases might you be confronted with? What zoonotic diseases?

5. How would you design and carry out a study to determine if the incidence of bovine ocular squamous cell carcinoma has changed in relation to ozone depletion and increased effective UVB radiation?

6. How would you design and carry out a study to determine the role of animal waste in creating conditions that lead to *Pfiesteria* blooms in estuarine waters in the mid-Atlantic region of the United States?

7. While DES was banned as a growth promotant for use in the livestock industry years ago, livestock producers still rely on implants to improve rates of gain. One such product is zeranol, a synthetic estrogen. Gather information on zeranol and review it. Can zeranol be considered an endocrine disruptor? Do you believe there is any risk of endocrine-disrupting effects to people who consume beef produced with the use of zeranol? Do you feel this aspect of zeranol has been adequately evaluated? What agency is responsible for such reviews? How would you advise cattle-owning clients on the use of zeranol?

8. Where is your nearest potential source for uncontrolled release of sizable quantities of ionizing radiation? Identify the agencies responsible for emergency response. Review emergency response plans and evaluate their effectiveness and appropriateness for dealing with animal-health and food-safety issues.

9. Does your state or province have waste-management plan requirements for livestock producers? If so, obtain the materials available in support of this program. Contact a willing livestock producer in the area and work through a waste management plan for that facility. Consider recommendations you could make to reduce environmental hazards associated with manure management.

References

1. Aitken ID. Environmental change and animal disease. In: The Advancement of Veterinary Science: The Bicentenary Symposium Series. Veterinary Medicine Beyond 2000. Wallingford, UK: C.A.B. International, 1993:179–193.

2. Altieri MA, Farrell J. Traditional farming systems of south-central Chile, with special emphasis on agroforestry. Agroforestry Syst 1984;2:3–18.

3. Awumbila B. Acaricides in tick control in Ghana and methods of application. Trop Anim Health Prod 1996;28:50S–52S.

4. Awumbila B, Bokuma E. Survey of pesticides used in the control of ectoparasites of farm animals in Ghana. Trop Anim Health Prod 1994;26:7–12.

5. Barnard DR, Mount DR, Haile GA, et al. Integrated management strategies for *Amblyomma americanum* (Acari: Ixodidae) on pastured beef cattle. J Med Entomol 1994;31(4):571–585.

6. Beresford NA, Hove K, Barnett CL, et al. The development and testing of an intraruminal slow-release bolus designed to limit radiocaesium absorption by small lambs grazing contaminated pastures. Small Ruminant Res 1999;33:109–115.

7. Blair BG, Feiveson HA, von Hippel FN. Taking nuclear weapons off hair-trigger alert. Sci Am November, 1997:74–81.

8. Blaustein AR, Kiesecker JM, Chivers DP, et al. Ambient UV-B radiation causes deformities in amphibian embryos. Proc Natl Acad Sci USA 1997;94:13735–13737.

9. Boue O, Redondo M, Montevo C, et al. Reproductive and safety assessment of vaccination with Gavac against the cattle tick (Boophilus microplus). Theriogenology 1999;51(8):1547–1554.

10. Brynildsen LI, Sandvik O, Ormstad I. The role of the veterinary services in efforts to introduce measures to reduce harmful effects of the Chernobyl fallout. Norsk Veterinaertidsskr 1995;107(10):929–942.

11. Brynildsen LI, Selnaes TD, Strand P, et al. Countermeasures for radiocaesium in animal products in Norway after the Chernobyl accident-techniques, effectiveness, and costs. Health Phys 1996;70:665–672.

12. Buck EH, Copeland C, Zinn JA, Vogt DU. Pfiesteria and related harmful blooms: Natural resource and human health concerns. Report for Congress. Washington, DC: Congressional Research Service, 1997. (Also at http://www.cnie.org/nle/mar-23.html#Summary)

13. Colborn T, vom Saal FS, Soto AM. Developmental effects of endocrine-disrupting chemicals in wildlife and humans. Environ Health Perspect 1993;101(5):378–384.

14. Colborn T, Dumanoski D, Myers JP. Our Stolen Future. New York: Dutton, 1996.

15. Colwell RR. Global climate and infectious disease: the cholera paradigm. Science 1996;274(5295):2025–2031.

16. De Gruijl FR. Health effects from solar UV radiation. Radiat Protect Dosimetry 1997;72(3–4):177–196.

17. de Haan C, Steinfeld H, Blackburn H. Livestock and the Environment: Finding a Balance. Report of a study coordinated by the Food and Agriculture Organization of the United Nations, The United States Agency for International Development, and the World Bank, 1997.

18. Dodd JL. Desertification and degradation in sub-Saharan Africa: the role of livestock BioScience 1994;44(1):28–34.

19. Dunbar R. Scapegoat for a thousand deserts. New Scientist 1984;104:30–33.

20. Erlich PR, Harte J, Harwell MA, et al. Long-term biological consequences of nuclear war. Science 1983;222:1283–1292.

21. Gardner G. Shrinking Fields: Cropland Loss in a World of Eight Billion. Worldwatch Paper no. 131. Washington, DC: Worldwatch Institute, 1996.

22. Heath SE. Animal Management in Disasters. St. Louis: Mosby, 1999.

23. Jones PD, Hannah DJ, Buckland SJ, et al. Persistent synthetic chlorinated hydrocarbons in albatross tissue samples from Midway Atoll. Environ Toxicol Chem 1996;15(10):1793–1800.

24. Jonsson NN, Matschoss AL, Pepper P, et al. Evaluation of TickGARD(PLUS), a novel vaccine against Boophilus microplus, in lactating Holstein-Friesian cows. Vet Parasitol 2000;88 (3/4):275–283.

25. Kurlansky M. Cod: A Biography of the Fish That Changed the World. New York: Walker & Co, 1997.

26. Lewis CE, Burton GW, Monson WG, et al. Integration of pines, pastures, and cattle in south Georgia, USA. Agroforestry Syst 1983;1:277–297.

27. Lobitz B, Beck L, Huq A, et al. Climate and infectious disease: use of remote sensing for detection of *Vibrio cholerae* by indirect measurement. Proc Natl Acad Sci USA 2000;97(4):1438–1443.

28. McArdle J, Bullock AM. Solar ultraviolet radiation as a causal factor of "summer syndrome" in cage-reared Atlantic salmon, *Salmo salar* L.: a clinical and histopathological study. J Fish Dis 1987;10:255–264.

29. McNaughton SJ, Banyikwa FF, McNaughton MM. Promotion of the cycling of diet-enhancing nutrients by African grazers. Science 1997;278:1798–1800.

30. Mitchell JH. Ceremonial Time: Fifteen Thousand Years on One Square Mile. Boston, Houghton Mifflin, 1984.

31. Morrison JE. Radiologic hazards and defense. J Am Vet Med Assoc 1987;190:746–761.

32. Murphy D. The rise of robber barons speeds forest decline. Christian Science Monitor, August 24, 2001:8–9.

33. Naylor RL, Goldburg RJ, Mooney H, et al. Nature's subsidies to shrimp and salmon farming. Science 1998;282:883–884.

34. Nussbaum SR. The New Jersey Plan for response to nuclear plant accidents. J Am Vet Med Assoc 1987;190:790–792.

35. Oberdorster E, Cheek AO. Gender benders at the beach: endocrine disruption in marine and estuarine organisms. Environ Toxicol Chem 2001;20(1):23–36.

36. Ponting C. A Green History of the World. The Environment and the Collapse of Great Civilizations. New York: Penguin Books, 1991.

37. Repetto R. Deforestation in the tropics. Sci Am 1990; 262(4):36–42.

38. Savory A. Holistic Resource Management. Washington, DC: Island Press, 1988.

39. Schulte SJ. Nuclear disaster. J Am Vet Med Assoc 1987;190:762–789.

40. Sharpe RM, Skakkebaek NE. Are oestrogens involved in falling sperm counts and disorders of the male reproductive tract? Lancet 1993;341:1392–1395.

41. Tucker CJ, Dregne HE, Newcomb WW. Expansion and contraction of the Sahara desert from 1980 to 1990. Science 1991;253:299–301.

42. Tustin JR, Knowles RL, Klomp BK. Forest farming: a multiple land-use production system in New Zealand. Forest Ecol Manage 1979;2:169–189.

43. Uilenberg G. Integrated control of tropical animal parasitoses. Trop Anim Health Prod 1996;28:257–265.

44. United Nations Environment Programme. Global Environment Outlook, 1997. New York: Oxford University Press, 1997.

45. World Resources Institute. Chap 9, Forests and land cover. World Resources 1996–97, A Guide to the Global Environment. London: Oxford University Press, 1997.

Suggested Readings

Durning AB, Brough HB. Taking Stock: Animal Farming and the Environment. Worldwatch Paper no. 103. Washington, DC, Worldwatch Institute, 1991.

McMichael AJ. Planetary Overload. Global Environmental Change and the Health of the Human Species. Cambridge, England: Cambridge University Press, 1993.

Nell AJ, ed. Livestock and the Environment. Proceedings of the International Conference on Livestock and the Environment, Ede/Wageningen, the Netherlands, 16–20 June 1997. Wageningen, the Netherlands: International Agricultural Centre, 1998.

Pimentel D. Global warming, population growth, and natural resources for food production. Soc Nat Resource 1991;4(4):347–363.

Safina C. Song for the Blue Ocean. New York: Henry Holt, 1997.

Strauch D, ed. Animal Production and Environmental Health. World Animal Science Series, B6. Amsterdam: Elsevier Science, 1987.

Tyler CR, Jobling S, Sumpter JP. Endocrine disruption in wildlife: a critical review of the evidence. Crit Rev Toxicol 1998;28(4):319–361.

United Nations Environment Programme: The Impact of Climate Change. UNEP/GEMS Environment Library no. 10. Nairobi: UNEP, 1993.

Wolfson R. Nuclear Choices. A Citizens Guide to Nuclear Technology. Cambridge, MA: MIT Press, 1991.

Chapter 7
Preservation of Biodiversity, Wildlife, and Conservation Medicine

OBJECTIVES FOR THIS CHAPTER

After completing this chapter, the reader should be able to

- Recognize the factors contributing to loss of biodiversity and accelerating rates of animal and plant extinctions
- Identify the tools available to protect habitat and endangered species
- Appreciate the potential for veterinarians to apply their skills to wildlife conservation and management in cooperation with other scientists and conservationists in the emerging field of conservation medicine

Introduction

The late president of the Nature Conservancy, John C. Sawhill, observed that "In the end, our society will be defined not only by what we create, but by what we refuse to destroy." We live in a period when human beings are creating enormous material wealth. Too often, however, the cost of this material gain is the loss of enormous natural wealth manifested as the widespread degradation of habitat, the extensive loss of biodiversity, and accelerating rates of species extinction. In many places on Earth, unknown species are being obliterated before they can even be identified, catalogued, or studied, and alarm bells are being sounded. There is growing concern about what we are destroying and the impact that such destruction will have on our own prospects for survival. There is also a growing movement to refuse to destroy more and to conserve what still exists. Veterinarians can contribute significantly to global efforts in wildlife conservation and the preservation of biodiversity, though the full potential for veterinary medicine to participate in such efforts remains largely unrealized. In this chapter, biodiversity is defined and the threats to biodiversity discussed, along with the factors contributing to accelerating rates of extinction, including disease. Efforts to preserve biodiversity are presented and the tools available for use in wildlife conservation described. Finally, the emerging field of conservation medicine is introduced. Throughout all these discussions, the implications for veterinary medicine and the current and potential involvement of veterinarians are highlighted.

Defining Biodiversity

The term *biodiversity,* a contraction of *biological diversity,* refers to the full range of organisms that together constitute the sum of life on Earth. Biological diversity is expressed at three levels. First, there is the genetic diversity that exists within any given species of microorganism, plant or animal. Second, there is the diversity of the myriad species themselves. Third, there is the ecological diversity of distinct ecosystems composed of different assemblages of organisms adapted to a certain physical environment, be it desert, grassland, coral reef, or rainforest.

Biodiversity at the Gene Level

Genetic diversity at the organism level occurs as allelic variation in gene pairs within individuals of the same species. Alleles in oth-

erwise similar genes occur spontaneously as a result of genetic mutations. Mating results in potentially different allelic combinations of genetic expression in offspring and can lead to the development of new and different phenotypic traits. Some of these traits may continue to be transmitted to subsequent generations of offspring. Such new traits can represent useful anatomical, physiological, or behavioral adaptations that allow individuals of the phenotype to exploit a new ecological niche or compete more effectively in their existing ecological niche. This process of adaptation can lead to the emergence of distinct new species from common ancestors. Perhaps the best-known example of this process are Darwin's finches of the Galapagos Islands, a group of isolated and relatively inhospitable islands off the coast of Ecuador. Charles Darwin, during his travels on the HMS Beagle in the 1830s, observed 14 distinct species of finches on these islands and postulated that they all derived from a single common ancestral flock of seed-eating, ground-feeding finches probably blown onto the island from the mainland by a storm millennia earlier. The evolution of these distinct species from a single source in a geographically isolated area is termed *adaptive radiation.* As a result of adaptive radiation, Darwin's finches have become distinct species with varied beak shapes and feeding behaviors that allow them to exploit a wide variety of ecological niches and associated feed sources on the Galapagos Islands while largely avoiding direct competition with each other (Fig. 7-1). Other examples of adaptive radiation include the avian honeycreepers of Hawaii, with 54 distinct species derived from one ancestral species; the lemurs of Madagascar; the moa bird species of New Zealand; and the cichlid fishes of Lake Victoria in eastern Africa. Notably, the moa of New Zealand are now extinct, and virtually all these other examples of adaptive radiation are threatened.

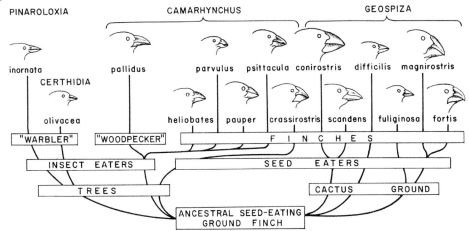

Figure 7-1. Beak characteristics of the 14 distinct finch species of the Galapagos Island finches postulated by Charles Darwin to be derived from a single species of ancestral seed-eating, ground-feeding finch and to have evolved into separate species through the process of adaptive radiation. Geographical isolation facilitates the process of adaptive radiation and helps to explain why island environments often host a rich variety of endemic species and are "hotspots" of genetic diversity. (Reproduced with permission from Welty JC. The Life of Birds. 2nd Ed. Philadelphia: WB Saunders, 1975.)

Domestic animal breeders exploit allelic variation in a very controlled manner to promote traits in domestic animals that best serve the breeders' cultural or economic purposes. The extent to which allelic variation can be expressed phenotypically in domestic animals is clear in the diversity of dog breeds that have been developed, ranging in size from the Chihuahua to the Saint Bernard, but all representing the species *Canis familiaris*. The diversity within livestock species is also evident, for example, with phenotypically distinct breeds of goats selected for cashmere fiber production (Chinese Liaoning goat), mohair fiber production (Angora goat), high milk production (Toggenburg goat), meat production (Boer goat), or adaptation to arid climates (Black Bedouin goat), while all representing the species *Capra hircus*.

Biodiversity at the Species Level

There is tremendous expression of genetic diversity at the species level. At present, approximately 1.5 million living species, from viruses to mammals, have been identified and described. Two thirds of these known species are insects and plants, with about 751,000 and 248,500 species, respectively. The remaining third of known species are divided among all the other taxonomic categories as presented in Table 7-1. Scientists feel confident that most vertebrate animals and a considerable portion of the world's plant species have been identified, but this is far from true in other taxonomic groups.

Current estimates of the number of unidentified insects range from 5 million to over 30 million species. A great deal is known about a relatively small number of bacteria, about 4000 species, and any veterinary student who has struggled to remember the cultural and biochemical characteristics that distinguish the various pathogenic bacteria from each other may feel that this is a sufficient number to know about. Yet estimates of the number of bacteria as-yet undiscovered or unclassified range from the tens of thousands to the millions. A single gram of soil alone may contain up to 4000 distinct species of bacteria. The known fungi presently number about 47,000, but the number of unknown fungi may exceed a million. Tropical soils likely harbor a myriad of unknown fungal species, any one of which may, like the blue-green mold, *Penicillium*, produce a potent antiinfective agent of incredible value to humanity. In fact, an endophytic fungus has recently been isolated from inside a twig in a national park in Costa Rica that produces a potent antiinfective agent, apicidin, with strong activity against pathogenic protozoa of the Apicomplexa group, including *Plasmodium falciparum* and *Cryptosporidium* and *Toxoplasma* spp.[11] Currently there are no safe drugs with reliable efficacy against *Cryptosporidium* spp, and most of the existing antimalarials are becoming ineffective because of development of drug resistance by *Plasmodium* spp.

Biodiversity at the Ecosystem Level

The collection of organisms that live together in a particular locality is referred to as a *biological community*. The biological community, in conjunction with the physical environment and climatic conditions of that locality, is referred to as an *ecosystem*. Distinctly defined ecosystems may vary considerably in size, depending on the criteria used for definition. The broadest terrestrial ecosystem categories are *biomes*, defined primarily by climatic factors. While different classification systems exist, there are essentially six main biomes on Earth: tropical rain forest, tropical savanna, midlatitude deciduous forest, desert, sub-Arctic taiga, and polar tundra. In addition, aquatic environments can be classified into several broadly defined biomes. Marine, or salt water biomes include tidal zones, shallow waters (including coral reefs), and the deep ocean. Fresh water biomes include lakes, rivers and streams, wetlands, and estuaries.

Interactions between living organisms and the physical environment help to define and shape a given ecosystem. Soil types, altitude, terrain, temperature variations, and patterns of rainfall influence the types of organisms that reside and survive within the physical environment. In turn, the biological community in a given locale may help shape the character of the local environment by modulating temperature, retaining moisture, regulating sunlight, and enriching soil. Plants may provide food for herbivorous animals, and various animals and insects may assist in the fertilization and dissemination of seeds to ensure future plant growth. A keystone species in the ecosystem, such as a mammalian predator, may keep other herbivorous animal populations in check so that the vegetative carrying capacity of the ecosystem is not exceeded. Each distinct ecosystem has its own characteristic interdependency, be it coral reef, mangrove swamp, alpine meadow, or montane forest. This functional interdependency is closely linked to, and depends upon, the maintenance of biological diversity.

Ecosystems vary considerably in the variety and quantity of life they can support and therefore differ in the extent of their biological diversity, or species richness. Environments with the most biodiversity are tropical rain forests, coral reefs, and large tropical lakes. Tropical rain forests, while they represent only 7% of the earth's land area, are believed to contain over half of the world's species. Other species-rich environments include tropical dry habitats, such as the East African savanna, and temperate shrub lands with Mediterranean climates (i.e., predominantly winter rainfall) such as, for example, southwestern Australia. The southwest botanical province of Australia, an area of about 310,000 km² south and east of Perth, contains a total of 5649 known native plant species, of which 79.2% are endemic, meaning that they occur naturally only within this particular ecosystem. Endemic species are of particular interest and concern in discussions of biodiversity and its preservation, as endemic species may exist in very narrow ranges of distribution, such as a single small island or a particular mountaintop. Disruption of such a small ecosystem can easily lead to the extinction of an endemic species.

Earth As a Unified Ecosystem

The concept of biodiversity extends beyond a library of genes, an enumeration of species, or a catalog of ecosystems. There is

Table 7-1 Number of Described Species of Living Organisms[a]

Kingdom and Major Subdivision	Common Name	No. of Known Species	Totals
Virus	Viruses	1,000	1,000
Monera			
Bacteria	Bacteria	3,000	
Myxoplasma	Bacteria	60	
Cyanophycota	Blue-green algae	1,700	4,760
Fungi			
Zygomycota	Zygomycete fungi	665	
Ascomycota	Cup (lichen) fungi	28,650	
Basidiomycota	Basidiomycete fungi	16,000	
Oomycota	Water molds	580	
Chytridiomycota	Chytrids	575	
Acrasiomycota	Cellular slime molds	13	
Myxomycota	Plasmodial slime molds	500	46,983
Algae			
Chlorophyta	Green algae	7,000	
Phaeophyta	Brown algae	1,500	
Rhodophyta	Red algae	4,000	
Chrysophyta	Chrysophyte algae	12,500	
Pyrrophyta	Dinoflagellates	1,100	
Euglenophyta	Euglenoids	800	26,900
Plantae			
Bryophyta	Mosses, liverworts, hornworts	16,600	
Psilophyta	Psilopids	9	
Lycopodiophyta	Lycophytes	1,275	
Equisetophyta	Horsetails	15	
Filicophyta	Ferns	10,000	
Bymonsperms	Gymnosperms (e.g., evergreen trees)	529	
Dicotolydonae	Dicots (e.g., deciduous trees)	170,000	
Moncotolydonae	Monocots (e.g., grasses)	50,000	248,428
Protozoa	Protozoans	30,800	30,800
Animalia			
Porifera	Sponges	5,000	
Cnidaria, Ctenophora	Jellyfish, corals, comb jellies	9,000	
Platyhelminthes	Flatworms	12,200	
Nematoda	Roundworms	12,000	
Annelida	Annelids (earthworms and relatives)	12,000	
Mollusca	Mollusks	50,000	
Echinodermata	Echinoderms (starfish and relatives)	6,100	
Arthropoda	Arthropods (insects and others)		
Insecta	Insects	751,000	
Other arthropods	Other arthropods	123,161	
Minor invertebrate phyla		9,500	989,761
Chordata			
Tunicata	Tunicates	1,250	
Cephalochordata	Acorn worms	23	
Vertebrata	Vertebrates		
Agnatha	Lampreys and other jawless fish	63	

(continued)

Table 7-1 Number of Described Species of Living Organisms[a] (Continued)

Kingdom and Major Subdivision	Common Name	No. of Known Species	Totals
Chrondrichthyes	Sharks and other cartilaginous fish	843	
Osteichthyes	Bony fish	18,150	
Amphibia	Amphibians	4,184	
Reptilia	Reptiles	6,300	
Aves	Birds	9,040	
Mammalia	Mammals	4,000	43,853
Total, all organisms			1,392,485

[a]In 1986, noted biologist E. O. Wilson compiled this tabulation of approximately 1.4 million known species. By 2000, the number of known species has increased to 1.5 million, and estimates of the number of species that remain undiscovered and/or unidentified range from 5 to 150 million. Wilson suggests that there are may be as many as 5 million additional, unknown insect species alone.

From Wilson EO. The current state of biological diversity. In: Wilson EO, ed. Biodiversity. Washington, DC: National Academy Press, 1988.

dynamic interplay among living things that makes the whole of the world's living organisms greater than the sum of its parts. Through their complex interactions, living organisms not only support themselves, but work in concert to ensure that the conditions that make life possible for each species on Earth are properly met and maintained. Regulation of atmospheric gases, for example, is in large part a collective function of the earth's diverse biomass involved in exchanges of oxygen, carbon dioxide, and other atmospheric gases that regulates an atmospheric composition conducive to life.

The notion of Earth itself as a large, living, and self-regulating organism is expressed in the Gaia hypothesis, proposed by Dr. James Lovelock and named after the Earth goddess of Greek mythology, Gaia. The Gaia hypothesis postulates that living things and the physical Earth itself make up a unified, physiological system that functions as a living organism. While this theory is considered highly controversial in the scientific community, it does serve to draw attention to the interconnectedness of life on this planet. Viewing photographs of Earth taken from space, one can, emotionally at least, embrace the premise of Gaia theory. As seen floating in the blackness of space, Earth's blue oceanic "cytoplasm"; its green, brown, and white terrestrial "organelles"; and its hazy atmospheric "cell membrane" do indeed suggest a self-contained, living organism that depends on the integrated function of all of its component parts for survival. Such a view underscores the importance of maintaining biodiversity on Earth.

The Economic Value of Biodiversity

Whether the Gaia hypothesis proves to be scientifically valid or not, it is clear from ongoing scientific research that biological diversity is associated with a variety of ecosystem services that support life on the planet and offer distinct benefits to human society. At least 17 such biodiversity-dependent

ecosystem services have been identified and are presented in Table 7-2, with examples.

Many of these ecosystem services, though now recognized, remain only partially understood. The Biosphere 2 Project in Oracle, Arizona, for example, attempted to create a 3.15-acre self-sufficient, self-contained, enclosed ecosystem based on current principles of earth science and biology. Despite tremendous technical input, design expertise, and a considerable budget, this "human terrarium" was unable to support its 8 human inhabitants with adequate food, water, and air for 2 years. As Cohen and Tilman conclude in their assessment of the lessons learned from Biosphere 2,[8] "There is no demonstrable alternative to maintaining the viability of Earth. No one yet knows how to engineer systems that provide humans with the life-supporting services that natural ecosystems produce for free."

One of the greatest challenges of the coming decades, a time when biodiversity will be under enormous threat, is for scientists, government leaders, and policymakers to help people understand the vital role that biodiversity plays in their everyday lives through provision of essential ecosystem services, and thereby encourage efforts to preserve that biodiversity. The natural world is too often viewed as a backdrop for human activity rather than an integral part of it. Even when the value of nature is appreciated, the ecosystem services that maintain global equilibrium, such as atmospheric regulation, seem too abstract or remote to focus citizen attention or to encourage a sense of personal responsibility. So collectively, we continue our assault on Earth's living resources without any clear knowledge of how or when we may reach a point of irreparable damage that destabilizes key environmental functions and alters the viability of the planet for human habitation (see sidebar "A Simple Metaphor of Biodiversity").

We live in an age and a culture in which virtually all things, material or aesthetic, are now measured and valued in economic terms. One approach to raising awareness about the importance of biodiversity is to quantify, in economic terms,

Table 7-2 Ecosystem Services and the Functions They Perform, with Examples

Ecosystem Service	Ecosystem Functions	Examples
Gas regulation	Regulation of atmospheric chemical composition	CO_2/O_2 balance; O_3 for UVB protection; SO_x levels
Climate regulation	Regulation of global temperature; precipitation and other biologically mediated climate processes at global or local levels	Greenhouse gas regulation; dimethylsulfide production affecting cloud formation
Disturbance regulation	Capacitance, dampening, and integrity of ecosystem response to environmental fluctuations	Storm protection, flood control, drought recovery, and other aspects of habitat response to environmental variability mainly controlled by vegetation structure
Water regulation	Regulation of hydrological flow	Provisioning of water for agricultural (e.g., irrigation) or industrial (e.g., milling) processes or transportation
Water supply	Storage and retention of water	Provisioning of water by watersheds, reservoirs, and aquifers
Erosion control and sediment retention	Retention of soil within an ecosystem	Prevention of loss of soil by wind, runoff, or other removal processes; storage of silt in lakes and wetlands
Soil formation	Soil formation processes	Weathering of rock and the accumulation of organic material
Nutrient recycling	Storage, internal cycling, processing and acquisition of nutrients	Nitrogen fixation; N, P, and other elements or nutrient cycles
Waste treatment	Recovery of mobile nutrients and removal or breakdown of excess or xenic nutrients and compounds	Waste treatment, pollution control, detoxification
Pollination	Movement of floral gametes	Provisioning of pollinators for reproduction of plant populations
Biological control	Trophic-dynamic regulation of populations	Keystone predator control of prey species; reduction of herbivores by top predators
Refugia	Habitat for resident and transient populations	Nurseries, habitat for migratory species, regional habitat for locally harvested species, or overwintering grounds
Food production	Portion of gross primary production extractable as food	Production of fish, game, crops, nuts, fruits by hunting, gathering, subsistence farming, or fishing
Raw materials	Portion of gross primary production extractable as raw materials	Production of lumber, fuel, or fodder
Genetic resources	Sources of unique biological materials and products	Medicine; products for materials science; genes for resistance to plant pathogens and crop pests; ornamental species (pets and horticultural varieties of plants)
Recreation	Providing opportunities for recreational activities	Ecotourism, sport fishing, and other outdoor recreational activities
Culture	Providing opportunities for noncommercial uses	Aesthetic, artistic, educational, spiritual, and/or scientific values of ecosystems

Reproduced with permission from Costanza R, et al. The value of the world's ecosystem services and natural capital. Nature 1997;387(6630):253–260.

A Simple Metaphor for Biodiversity

The U.S. Fish and Wildlife Service offers an interesting metaphor on their website concerning the unforeseen and potentially dangerous consequences of ongoing biodiversity loss as a result of human activity.

Imagine this nightmare. You're sitting on a plane that's ready to take off, looking out the window. Suddenly a mechanic walks up to the wing and removes several of the rivets that hold the wing on. You wonder what he's up to, but the plane takes off before you 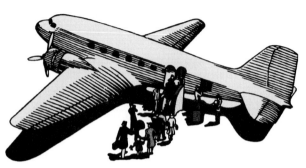 can find out, and you figure that a few less rivets won't make much difference anyway. At the next airport, two mechanics start removing rivets from the wing, and you start to worry. But the plane takes off again before you can find out what's going on. When you land again, five mechanics start removing rivets like crazy! Now you're really worried! How many rivets can be removed before the wing falls off and causes the plane to crash? Which rivet will be "the last one"? Before the plane takes off again, you wake up. This wouldn't be such a ridiculous scene, if it weren't for the fact that it's a good metaphor for what humans are doing to the complex web of life on this planet. If you compare species with the rivets on that plane's wing, it makes you wonder how many more species might disappear forever before our ecosystem or life on our planet is irreversibly damaged. (From the website of the United States Fish and Wildlife Service, http://endangered.fws.gov/kids/biodivrs.htm)

the value of goods and services traditionally considered to be provided "free" by natural processes. A new intellectual discipline has evolved that focuses on this issue, referred to as *ecological economics*. Ecological economists recognize that short-term economic gain is often an underlying motivation for activities that lead to environmental damage and the depletion of natural resources. However, such gains may be not only short-term but also short-sighted, leading to unforeseen environmental and social costs. By calculating the economic value of ecosystem services and goods that are lost due to environmental degradation and biodiversity loss and by factoring those costs into human activities, ecological economists can begin to demonstrate the real impact to society of biodiversity loss and environmental degradation in economic terms. Such information can be extremely valuable in raising public awareness and influencing development planning and policy making.

For example, in recent years, the city of New York has worked with the state of New York to ensure protection of its safe drinking water supply by restricting development and controlling pollution in the city watershed. The city's water comes from a network of reservoirs in the Catskill Mountains north of the city, and it represents the largest unfiltered urban water supply in the nation. Much of the Catskill Mountain watershed region is heavily forested, and the forests themselves serve to catch and retain water and allow it to be naturally filtered as it seeps through the forest floor and heads ultimately into the reservoirs. It would cost the city of New York an estimated 4 billion dollars to construct and operate water treatment facilities that could accomplish what the forested Catskill watershed accomplishes naturally in terms of water purification.

Ecological economics would say that the water purification value of the Catskill watershed is $4 billion and should be recognized for its monetary value. In addition, the Catskill Mountain forests function as a biologically diverse ecosystem that provides numerous aesthetic and recreational services to visitors and residents that also add to the forests' economic value. Cutting down the trees of the Catskills would cost society far in excess of their value as timber.

Ecosystem services and natural capital can be assigned values in a number of different categories. *Direct economic value* refers to those natural products that are directly collected and used by people. Direct economic value is further subdivided into *consumptive use value* and *production use value*. The former refers to products that are harvested and consumed locally and do not enter marketing channels. Such products might include fuel wood, forest animals that are trapped or hunted, or plants harvested as traditional medicines. Such consumptive use is common among poorer rural peoples in developing countries. *Production use value* refers to natural harvested products that are destined for commercial market channels and may be involved in national or international trade, such as timber, fish, natural fibers, and plant extracts such as gums and resins with commercial application.

Indirect economic value is a measure of the economic benefit of ecosystem services that accrue without the harvesting or destruction of natural resources. *Nonconsumptive use value* refers to the value of ecosystem services that are not consumed through use, such as atmospheric and climatic regulation, water purification, disturbance regulation such as flood control, and soil retention. *Option value* refers to the potential for a species to provide some presently unknown future economic benefit to human society, for example, a yet undiscovered medicine such as an anticancer drug, which might have commercial value in the hundreds of millions or billions of dollars. Finally, *existence value* is the intangible emotional, aesthetic, or spiritual value that human beings place on a living species, biological community, landscape, or ecosystem. Existence value assumes economic importance as people seek to visit natural places that they hold in high regard. Ecotourism, for example, is a burgeoning industry that depends primarily on the existence value of certain charismatic species or unique environments.

Factoring Nature into Productivity Indices

Ecological economist Robert Costanza and colleagues made an ambitious and important effort to promote a new way of thinking about the importance of biodiversity by undertaking a global valuation of the world's ecosystem services and natural capital.[9]

Sixteen distinct biomes and 17 ecosystem services were identified, and monetary value was calculated for each of the ecosystem services provided by a particular biome, as presented in Table 7-3. In total, it was estimated that the cumulative monetary value of the world's ecosystem services fell in the range of US$16 to 54 trillion, with an average of US$33 trillion per year, even though such services are usually outside the market system, neither valued or paid for. By comparison, the annual global gross national product (GNP) is approximately US$18 trillion. Thus, the cash value of ecosystem services exceeds the value of all the world's traditionally measured economic activity by a factor of 1.8.

This work emphasizes that ecosystem services provide a vital underpinning to virtually all human commerce. Yet these services remain overlooked or undervalued in traditional measurements of economic activity. If these services were actually paid for, the price of commodities that depend directly or indirectly on ecosystem services would be much higher. Costanza et al. propose that the value of ecosystem services be incorporated into project appraisals so that the potential loss of ecosystem services can be weighed against the anticipated benefits of the project.[9] For example, shrimp farming is often carried out in coastal areas that are first cleared of mangrove forests. While the shrimp farmers may benefit from the sale of shrimp, the costs of clearing mangrove forests include a loss of protection against coastal flooding and hurricane wind damage, increased loss of coastal land to erosion, and the loss of nursery habitat for a wide range of marine organisms including species of fish vital to traditional commercial fisheries. Shrimp farming looks less lucrative when these lost services are accounted for in monetary terms equal to the cost of having to replace them.

The Cost of Biodiversity Loss to Medicine

As the discussion above indicates, all segments of society are diminished by the loss of biodiversity. However, veterinarians, as health professionals, have a particular stake in seeing that plant and animals species are preserved, because of the potential contribution that plants and animals can make to the development of new medicines and as medical models. The contributions of biodiversity to medicine and human health have been recently reviewed by Grifo and Rosenthal.[22] Some examples of this important association are given below in the sections on naturally derived medicines and wild species as medical models.

Naturally Derived Medicines

Animals, plants, and microorganisms have historically been a major source of new medicines. Of the 10 most frequently prescribed drugs in the United States, only 2 are synthetic; the remaining 8 originate from natural sources. Four are derived from animal sources, 2 from fungi, 1 from a bacterium, 1 combination drug from a fungus and bacteria, and 1 from a plant. Three quarters of the drugs used to control infectious disease are derived from natural sources. The best-selling drug of all time, aspirin, is derived from willow trees of the genus *Salix*.

Some of the most exciting drug discoveries of recent years have been medicines derived from natural sources, often involving groups of plants and animals that are under heightened risk of extinction because they reside in habitats under siege, such as, rainforest amphibians and reptiles, or marine species associated with coral reefs. For example, Capoten, which is used to treat hypertension, was discovered as a result of research on the venom of a New World rainforest viper. Soft corals produce a variety of valuable compounds. For instance, pseudopterosins are natural products isolated from the Caribbean soft coral *Pseudopterogorgia elisabethae* which possess novel antiinflammatory properties, while Pacific soft corals of the genus *Eleutherobia* produce eleutherobins, potent anticancer drugs similar in function to Taxol, which itself is a revolutionary anticancer drug derived from a plant, the Pacific yew (*Taxus brevifolia*). It is disheartening to think that other such corals are actually in danger of disappearing before scientists have a chance to evaluate them for their pharmaceutical treasures.

Wild Species As Medical Models

Wild animals can serve as valuable medical models for studying physiological responses that could illuminate our understanding of disease pathogenesis and provide new insights into disease management and prevention. Bears, for example, hibernate but do not lose bone mass despite being immobile for 4 to 5 months. No other vertebrate is known to do this. Understanding how the bear can maintain bone density in the face of total inactivity could provide major insights into the prevention or treatment of osteoporosis, a largely untreatable condition that affects about 25 million Americans, results in approximately 1.5 million bone fractures annually, and carries a societal cost of over US$10 billion in medical costs and lost productivity. Bears also do not urinate for months during hibernation, whereas humans would become uremic and die

Table 7-3   Estimated Monetary Value of 17 Ecosystem Services Distributed over 16 Separate Biomes

Ecosystem Services (1994 US$ ha^{-1}yr^{-1})[a]

Biome	Area (ha × 10^6)	1 Gas Regulation	2 Climate Regulation	3 Disturbance Regulation	4 Water Regulation	5 Water Supply	6 Erosion Control	7 Soil formation	8 Nutrient Cycling
Marine	36,302								
Open Ocean	33,200	38							118
Coastal	3,102			88					3,677
Estuaries	180			567					21,100
Sea grass/algae beds	200								19,002
Coral reefs	62			2,750					
Shelf	2,660								1,431
Terrestrial	15,323								
Forest	4,855		141	2	2	3	96	10	361
Tropical	1,900		223	5	6	8	245	10	922
Temperate/Boreal	2,955		88		0			10	
Grass/Rangelands	3,898	7	0		3		29	1	
Wetlands	330	133		4,539	15	3,800			
Tidal marsh/Mangroves	165			1,839					
Swamps/Floodplains	165	265		7,240	30	7,600			
Lakes/Rivers	200				5,445	2,117			
Desert	1,925								
Tundra	743								
Ice/rock	1,640								
Cropland	1,400								
Urban	332								
Total (US$ 3 10^9)	**51,625**	**1,341**	**684**	**1,779**	**1,115**	**1,692**	**576**	**53**	**17,075**

[a]The total estimated value of all the services combined is US$33.2 trillion. Numbers in the body of the table are in $ ha^{-1} yr^{-1}. Row and column totals are in $yr^{-1} × 10^9. Column totals are the sum of the products of the per hectare services in the table and the area of each biome, not the sum of the per hectare services themselves. Shaded cells indicate services that do not occur or are known to be negligible. Open cells indicate lack of available information.

9 Waste Treatment	10 Pollination	11 Biological Control	12 Habitat/Rerfugia	13 Food Production	14 Raw Materials	15 Genetic Resources	16 Recreation	17 Cultural	Total Value per ha	Total Global Flow Value
									577	20,949
		5		15	0			76	252	8,381
		38	8	93	4		82	62	4,052	12,568
		78	131	521	25		381	29	22,832	4,110
					2					3,801
58		5	7	220	27		3,008	1	19,004	375
		39		68	2			70		4,283
									6,075	
									1,610	
									804	12,319
87		2		43	138	16	66	2	969	4,706
87				32	315	41	112	2	2,007	3,813
87		4		50	25		36	2	302	894
87	25	23		67		0	2		232	906
4,177			304	256	106		574	881	14,785	4,879
6,696			169	466	162		658		9,990	1,648
1,659			439	47	49		491	1,761	19,580	3,231
665				41			230		8,498	1,700
	14	24		54					92	128
2,277	**117**	**417**	**124**	**1,386**	**721**	**79**	**815**	**3,015**		**33,268**

Reproduced with permission from Costanza R, et al. The value of the world's ecosystem services and natural capital. Nature 1997;387(6630):253–260.

after a few days of being unable to urinate. Understanding the mechanisms by which bears avoid uremia while retaining excretory products could lead to new approaches to managing chronic renal failure in human or veterinary patients. Yet, all eight of the world's bear species are threatened with localized or generalized extinction.

Poison dart frogs produce a variety of paralytic alkaloids that act by binding selectively to sodium and potassium channels, calcium pumps, and acetylcholine receptors in nerve and muscle membranes. Tremendous insights into cellular function have been derived by scientists studying this diverse group of alkaloids. However, the 100 or so species of poison dart frogs that live in the rainforests of Central and South America are in grave danger of disappearing as a result of habitat loss and the ongoing phenomenon of worldwide amphibian decline, the causes of which remain unclear.

Threats to Biodiversity

Earth has a dynamic history. The fossil record tells us that deep oceans once existed where grassy plains now prevail. These oceans teemed with diverse living forms that are now extinct. Dinosaurs once dominated Earth but are now known to us only by the excavated bones displayed in museums. Clearly, there has been dramatic change and upheaval on the planet. Yet life has persisted, with some forms disappearing, and new forms emerging over a span of millions of years.

Given this record of resiliency, why do we need to be concerned about current threats to biodiversity? The key variable that distinguishes our present time from the distant past is the power of humanity to transform the environment and the alarming rate at which this transformation is being accomplished. We are eliminating in hundreds of years what took millions of years to make, with seemingly little regard for, or understanding of, the possible adverse consequences to all living forms on the planet, including ourselves. If we deplete natural capital and disable ecosystem services through the unmindful destruction of biodiversity, our own future as a species may be at risk. Yes, new species may evolve to replace us in the course of millions of years, but this will be of little consolation to our children and our children's children, within whose lifetimes a major, humanity-driven loss of biodiversity will occur if we continue on our present course.

There are four major threats to biological diversity. These are habitat loss; overexploitation of resources; the introduction of invasive species; and the spread of disease. Other notable threats include pollution and climate change, which are important in their own right but also can be considered subcategories of the four major threats. In the category of habitat loss, for instance, habitat may retain its physical character but be made inhospitable to certain species as a result of contamination with pollutants or by alterations in ambient temperature or rainfall patterns due to climate change. In the follow-

ing sections, the impact of the major threats to biodiversity are discussed in more detail.

Habitat Loss

Habitat loss can occur either as the absolute destruction of an ecosystem or as the diminished capacity of a given ecosystem to support the species associated with it. In addition to outright habitat destruction, three causes of diminished capacity are discussed below, including habitat fragmentation, pollution, and climate change.

Habitat Destruction

The outright obliteration of habitat by human activity is commonplace in the world today. The most notable and widely publicized example is the rapid rate of rainforest destruction. The patterns and causes of global deforestation are discussed in more detail in Chapter 6.

In general, life on Earth follows a latitudinal biodiversity gradient, with more abundant biodiversity at the equator than at the North and South poles. Among tropical ecosystems, tropical rainforests are considered the most biologically diverse terrestrial ecosystems on the planet. For instance, 300 different tree species have been identified in a single hectare of Peruvian forest, compared with only about 700 tree species total for all of North America. Based on extrapolations from transect surveys of rainforest insect populations, the total number of living species in tropical rainforests has been estimated to be as high as 30 million. Tropical rainforest originally covered about 16 million square kilometers of Earth. By 1991, this area had been reduced by more than half to 6.7 million square kilometers. Currently, rainforest is being cleared at a rate in excess of 130,000 square kilometers annually. The annual rate of rainforest loss as a proportion of total rainforest varies among countries, with annual rates as high as 3.5% in the Philippines and Haiti. Many rainforests have unique flora and fauna found nowhere else. For example, Madagascar is home to 28 species of endemic lemurs that are increasingly endangered as the island's forests are cleared at a rate of 1100 sq km per year. At that rate, all remaining forest and the lemurs in them will be gone by the year 2020, except for a small area under protection.

It is not only tropical rainforest habitat that is being lost at alarming rates. Other habitats under pressure include dry tropical forests and grasslands; wetlands, including mangrove forests; coral reefs; and lakes and rivers. Like the soils of temperate forests, the soils of dry tropical forests are better able to support crop agriculture and animal grazing than those of tropical rainforests. The dry forests on the Pacific coast of Central America have been cleared systematically, and only 2% of the original dry forest area remains intact. Grasslands are being lost to urbanization and conversion to agricultural use. When not managed properly, they are also subject to degradation through overgrazing by livestock as discussed in Chapter 6.

Growing urbanization associated with the filling of wetlands for housing and commercial development, and results in the loss of critical habitat for a wide variety of birds, fish, and invertebrates. In addition to the loss of species, important ecosystem services are compromised when wetlands are destroyed, including water purification and flood control. Mangrove forests are being cut for coastal resort development, to clear land for rice cultivation, and to develop shrimp hatcheries for aquaculture enterprises. India has already lost 85% of its coastal mangrove habitat, often in association with aquaculture activities.

Coral reefs are the tropical rainforests of the marine environment, supporting enormous biodiversity. Though they take up only about 0.2% of the oceans' total area, they are estimated to contain up to one third of all marine fish species. Up to 10% of the world's coral reefs have already been destroyed. Reefs around Madagascar, the Philippines, Indonesia, the Malay Peninsula, and much of the Caribbean are projected to be lost within the next 10 to 20 years, based on current levels of destruction. Coral reefs are subject to a number of ruinous processes including chemical pollution, silting and sedimentation, algal blooms, and reckless fishing practices, including the use of dynamite and cyanide as discussed in more detail in Chapter 6.

Lakes and rivers are also under assault, being damned for electrical power, drained for irrigation purposes, or diverted for other uses including flood control and transportation.[55] There are more than 36,000 operational dams on rivers around the world. In the United States, only 2% of rivers run unimpeded. The adverse effect on salmon breeding and the fate of salmon species is well publicized and is currently the focus of conservation efforts involving heated policy debates over the wise use of rivers. Little of the outflow of major world rivers such as the Ganges, Nile, and Colorado reach the sea because so much water is diverted for agricultural irrigation along their routes. The Aral Sea in Uzbekistan is literally disappearing along with its native fish species as a result of ill-planned irrigation diversions to support cotton and rice cultivation. Lake Chad in Africa is also undergoing volume depletion as a result of irrigation schemes.

Habitat Fragmentation

Even when a given habitat is perceived to be intact, its functionality may be impaired by fragmentation. Fragmentation occurs when an expansive habitat is broken up into circumscribed islands by human activity. Roads can seriously fragment habitat. They can deter animal movement either physically or behaviorally and may result in the deaths of animals by traffic accidents or separate animals from breeding grounds, food supplies, or mates. Equally important, roads or developed parcels of land adjacent to undisturbed habitat create "edge" effects. Edges on forest habitat, for example, allow easier access of predators such as raccoons, snakes, and cats into areas that were formerly inaccessible and thereby decrease the breeding success of birds that nest on the ground, for instance the ovenbird (*Seiurus aurocapillus*) and the black and white warbler (*Mniotilta varia*) in North America. The protection provided by deep woods disappears when habitat is fragmented by edge

effects. The fauna of a single unfragmented 10-ha plot of forest will differ substantially from the fauna of 10 1-ha plots on the same site if the large plot is transected by a grid of roads. Furthermore, the protection offered to hunted species by deep woods is diminished when a road is cut into a forest. The increase in logging roads in western and central Africa in recent years is having a devastating effect on primate populations as poachers with trucks and automatic weapons gain easier access to forest primate communities and slaughter monkeys and apes for the bushmeat trade (i.e., wild animals killed specifically for human consumption of their meat).

Fragmentation of large habitats into habitat islands is particularly important for large species and migrating species. Large mammals often require a large land area to support their food gathering or hunting efforts or they need to migrate seasonally with changing weather to find adequate food supplies year round. Large highways, pipelines, irrigation channels, housing developments, or other physical disruptions of continuous habitat may effectively exclude large mammals from portions of their habitat necessary for survival or block effective migration. Conservation efforts have increased to protect or create corridors that allow large blocks of habitat to be joined, thus maintaining the carrying capacity of the overall ecosystem. The issue of corridors is discussed later in this chapter.

Pollution

Various forms of chemical pollution can degrade a habitat and diminish its capacity to support biodiversity even when superficially the habitat appears intact. The phenomenon of acid rain illustrates such a process. Nitrogen and sulfur oxides are released into the air by human industrial activities such as smelting and generation of electrical power with coal and other fossil fuels. These compounds combine with atmospheric moisture to produce nitric and sulfuric acids that are returned to the earth in rainwater. Accumulation of this acidic precipitation in lakes and ponds can lower the water pH to levels incompatible with life processes. When the pH reaches 5.0, fish may fail to spawn. When it reaches 4.0, fish may die outright. Over a third of the lakes in Sweden and Norway, far from industrial sources of pollution, are acidified. Acid rain also acidifies soil and can produce more readily apparent destructive effects on forests. Large diebacks of forest in Europe and eastern North America have been linked to acid rain and air pollution. In addition, acid rain weakens trees and makes them more susceptible to disease and parasitism.

Heavy metal contamination can contribute to biodiversity loss without seemingly altering the environment. For example, Scheumhammer and Norris report on the ecotoxicology of lead shot and lead fishing weights.[50] Environmental contamination with these byproducts of recreational hunting and fishing presents a risk to a variety of susceptible species including waterfowl, upland game birds, shorebirds, and raptors. Common loons (*Gavia immer*) ingest small lead sinkers during their feeding efforts in freshwater lakes and ponds. Lead poisoning accounts for 10 to 50% of recorded adult loon mortality. Raptors can bioaccumulate lead by eating prey that contains lead shot. An estimated 10 to 15% of bald eagle and golden eagle postfledgling mortality in Canada and the United States is associated with lead poisoning.

The widespread use of DDT as a pesticide in the 1950s and 1960s is a well-known example of chemical pollution affecting biodiversity without visibly altering the landscape. The devastating impact of DDT on raptors, songbirds, beneficial insects, and other life forms was brought to the public's attention by Rachel Carson in her book *Silent Spring* and led eventually to the banning of the use of DDT, at least in developed countries. A rebound of eagles, ospreys, and other bird populations followed the cessation of its use. Today, the entire world is faced with new environmental pollutants that can undermine the reproductive capacity of living species around the globe while not visibly altering habitat. These chemicals, which function as endocrine disruptors, are discussed in Chapter 6. The endocrine disruptors include a wide range of herbicides, fungicides, insecticides, and industrial chemicals that are widely distributed throughout terrestrial and aquatic environments.

Climate Change

Global warming has the potential to cause profound habitat loss. The genesis of global warming is discussed in Chapter 6. One effect of global warming is the melting of glaciers and polar ice. The loss of polar ice has been associated with declines in Adelaide penguin populations as their habitat melts away. A more widespread impact of melting is a resultant rise in sea levels. Some estimates suggest that sea level may rise as much as 1.5 m in the next 100 years, resulting in the outright disappearance of some islands and island nations such as Kiribati, Tuvalu, and the Marshall Islands in the south Pacific, along with their unique endemic biodiversity. In addition, there may be widespread submersion of low-lying coastal areas on all of the continents, including, for example, parts of Florida and Bangladesh, leading to tremendous disruptions of human society as well as the loss of coastal wetland habitat. Rising sea levels may also promote the local extinction of certain species of coral with specific depth-dependent adaptations, along with multiple other marine species that depend on these specific coral. Rising ocean temperatures have also been associated with diebacks of coral reefs through "coral bleaching" due to the death of temperature-sensitive symbiotic algae that live inside the corals.

Rising temperatures associated with global warming can also affect terrestrial biodiversity. Atmospheric warming is already resulting in shifts in species ranges toward the poles. Two thirds of European butterfly species are now found as much as 35 to 250 km more northward than several decades ago.[41] Species already present in more-northern climes may not be able to adapt to the increasing temperature or may succumb to increased competition with the more-recent, warmth-adapted arrivals. Climatic records in Iceland indicate that average winter temperatures there increased 2°C between 1870 and 1970. During that same time, local populations of two birds, the dovekie (*Alle alle*) and the long-tailed duck (*Clangula hyemalis*), fell dramatically, while several more southern species of birds,

including lapwings (*Vanellus vanellus*) and tufted ducks (*Aythya fuligula*), began to regularly frequent the island and established successful breeding colonies. Warming temperatures can also be associated with the spread of disease by favoring an increased range for arthropod vectors of infectious agents, as discussed in Chapter 6 and later in this chapter.

Overexploitation

Since at least Neolithic times, the killing of wildlife by humans for food and other cultural purposes has been a major cause of species extinction. In his book *The Diversity of Life*, E. O. Wilson describes strong circumstantial evidence that the movement of Paleo Indian hunters into North America from Asia about 12,000 years ago was in large part responsible for the rapid extinction of three species of mastodons on the North American continent, which until that time had flourished for 2 million years. More recent effects of human overexploitation of wildlife are better documented. Archeological evidence on Hawaii indicates that between 35 and 55 species of birds were extirpated from the Hawaiian Islands following the settlement by Polynesians about AD 300. Following the arrival of European colonists in the late 18th century, an additional third of the remaining 50 or so species were eliminated by a combination of overexploitation and habitat loss. In New Zealand, the impact of hunting on birds following the arrival of humans about AD 1000 was dramatic. The New Zealand islands contained 13 species of moas, large flightless birds ranging in size from turkeys to larger than ostriches. Hunting by Maoris had virtually eliminated all the moas from New Zealand by the time European settlers arrived there in the 19th century. Overexploitation is not a vestige of the distant past. In North America, European settlers almost eliminated the bison (*Bison bison*) in the 19th century and succeeded in eliminating the passenger pigeon (*Ectopistes migratorius*) in the early 20th century through unrestricted and unmanaged hunting.

The overexploitation of wild species continues today. The wanton destruction of large mammals to obtain specific body parts for frequently questionable medicinal uses, arcane cultural uses, or as status symbols is well publicized. The slaughter of elephants for ivory, rhinoceros for horn, bear for gall bladders, tigers for humeral bones, the Siberian musk deer (*Moschus moschiferus*) for its scent gland, and the Tibetan antelope (*Pantholops hodgsonii*) for cashmere fiber are reasonably well known examples of this form of overexploitation. However, there are many other lesser known examples of overexploitation involving the harvest of plant and animal species for use as traditional medicines. TRAFFIC, the wildlife trade monitoring program of the World Wildlife Fund (WWF) and the World Conservation Union (IUCN) identifies 102 medicinal plant species and 29 animal species in southern and East Africa alone that currently require conservation management efforts.

An increased trade in bushmeat has emerged as a major concern in recent years. Traditionally, indigenous peoples dwelling near forest communities or grasslands supplemented their food supplies with animal protein obtained by hunting or trapping wild birds and mammals. When traditional hunting and trapping methods were used and human populations were relatively low, the taking of wild animals was, in many cases, sustainable. The situation has changed drastically, however. Increased populations, the availability of firearms and vehicles, and an increase in logging roads have given a new, deadly boost to the bushmeat trade. Reports in the year 2000 indicate that already threatened primates such as the chimpanzee, bonobo, and gorilla in central Africa are now under further pressure as they are increasingly targeted as a source of meat, not only for local consumption but, incredibly, for export. Chimpanzee meat has even showed up in Congolese restaurants and African food shops in Europe. In 1999, eight headless gorilla carcasses were found in cases at Heathrow airport. It is estimated that in the northern Congo, chimpanzee and gorilla populations are being destroyed at the rate of 5 to 7% per year.

The international wildlife trade extends well beyond the disturbing use of endangered primates as bushmeat. In our era of relative affluence, high-speed transportation, and expanded global trade, a wide variety of living organisms have become marketable commodities in high demand. Table 7-4 lists some major wildlife groups, both plant and animal, which are targeted in international trade, the approximate numbers traded each year, and their general use. Smuggling of animals into the United States has become an enormous industry, comparable to drug smuggling. In the first 7 months of 2001, Mexican authorities seized over 50,000 smuggled animals bound for the United States, including rare species such as Siberian tigers (*Panthera tigris altaica*) and Tibetan antelopes (*Pantholops hodgsonii*).[43] Veterinarians should particularly note that a great many birds, reptiles, and fish are taken for the exotic pet trade. Veterinari-

ans concerned about wildlife conservation can educate clients about the connections between exotic pets, the illegal animal trade, and the loss of biodiversity and can become involved in developing new techniques and strategies for successful captive breeding and management of exotic pet species to relieve pressures on wild populations.

The biodiversity of marine ecosystems is also threatened by overexploitation. Commercial whaling has had a major impact on the populations of some whale species, bringing at least two species to the brink of extinction. While commercial whaling is subject to much greater control and constraint today, whales still are threatened by problems of aquatic pollution and critical injuries from collisions with boats and fishing gear. Many species of fish with commercial value for human consumption have been overfished to the point that local populations of some species have been severely diminished. As many commercial fish are predators at the top of their respective food chains, their disappearance can result in significant alterations in the population dynamics of other species, often with unknown consequences. The impact of modern commercial fishing practices on the environment and biodiversity are discussed further in Chapter 6.

Invasive Species

Either intentionally or unintentionally, humans have been moving other living organisms around the world with them in their travels or in relation to their various vocations and avocations. Often, these nonindigenous or exotic organisms find favorable ecological niches in their new surroundings and become well established in their new location, frequently to

Table 7-4	Major Groups Targeted by the Worldwide Trade in Wildlife[46]	
Group	**Number Traded Each Year**	**Comments**
Primates	25–30 thousand	Mostly used for biomedical research, also for pets, zoos, circuses, and private collections
Birds	2–5 million	Zoos and pets; mostly perching birds, but also legal and illegal trade in parrots
Reptiles	2–3 million	Zoos and pets; also 10–15 million raw skins; reptiles are used in some 50 million manufactured products (mainly coming from the wild but, increasingly from farms)
Ornamental fish	500–600 million	Most saltwater tropical fish come from the wild and may be caught using illegal methods that damage other wildlife and the surrounding coral reef
Reef corals	1000–2000 tons	Reefs are being destructively mined to provide aquarium decor and coral jewelry
Orchids	9–10 million	Approximately 10% of the international trade comes from the wild, sometimes deliberately mislabeled to avoid regulations
Cacti	7–8 million	Approximately 15% of the traded cacti come from the wild, with smuggling a major problem

the detriment of local species. When exotic species become established, they are considered invasive species. Historically, the impact of invasive species on biodiversity has been profound, and the process continues today in relation to the steady expansion of global trade and economic development. The ongoing introduction of invasive species has come to be known as biological pollution. Invasive plant species now account for more than half the vegetation species present on some islands and 20% or more on continental mainlands.

Exploration, colonization, and trade have historically been important factors in the dissemination of invasive species. During the age of sail, roughly from the 15th to the 19th century, domestic animals were purposely left on ocean islands along trade routes to provide an easy source of food during long voyages by sailing ships with limited storage capacity. Animals such as pigs and goats, prolific species with no natural enemies, destroyed vegetation and contributed to the elimination of native animal species by predation, competition, or outright habitat destruction. Rats, left inadvertently by visiting ships, also did their share of damage to nesting birds and other species.

In contemporary times, ships still play a role in disseminating invasive species, though no longer intentionally. Ballast water and soil released from ships at ports of entry has been found to contain a variety of living forms carried from distant sources, including weed seeds, arthropods, algae, bacteria, small fish, and shellfish. Approximately 79 million tons of foreign ballast water are released in the United States each year. Zebra mussels (*Dreissena polymorpha*), which are native to the Black Sea, have fouled the North American Great Lakes and driven out native mussel species. They were likely introduced in ballast from a European tanker in 1988, and the invasion is expected to cause $5 billion in damage by 2002, mostly by clogging infrastructure. In the 1990s, pathogenic strains of the cholera organism, *Vibrio cholerae*, were found in ballast water on ships arriving in the United States and Australia from Latin American ports.

The brown tree snake, *Boiga irregularis*, an invasive reptile originating in the South Pacific and Australia has been introduced onto many Pacific islands. On the island of Guam alone, the snake has extirpated 10 of 13 native bird species, 6 of 12 native lizard species, and 2 of 3 bat species. The snakes most likely arrived on Guam in ship cargo from the New Guinea area. In the early 1950s the snakes were seen primarily around the main port area, but they became conspicuous throughout central Guam by the 1960s, and by 1968, with no natural predators present, they had spread throughout the island.

Agriculture, horticulture, and homesickness have been major driving forces in the intentional introduction of invasive species. During the period of European colonization, many European species were brought to the colonies to provide familiar foods, garden flowers, or birdsong to remind people of the homeland, often displacing local species. Unusual cultural motivations can also spur the introduction of invasive species. In the late 19th century, the American Acclimatization Society fos-

tered the idea of introducing every bird species mentioned in the works of William Shakespeare into the United States, including the European starling. In 1890, 60 European starlings were introduced into Central Park in New York. Within a century, the number of starlings in North America increased to well over 200 million. This remarkably successful adaptation to a new environment came at a cost to indigenous species of birds. The European starling is a cavity-nesting bird. Its pursuit of desirable nesting sites has caused serious dislocation of native cavity-nesting birds such as the Eastern bluebird (*Sialia sialis*). Local populations of Eastern bluebirds became alarmingly low in the mid-20th century and required a concerted response by conservationists and concerned citizens to build and set out nesting boxes for use by bluebirds, with entry holes that would not allow access by starlings.

One of the world's most dramatic ecological disruptions associated with misguided introductions of invasive species is occurring in Lake Victoria in East Africa, the world's largest tropical lake. This freshwater ecosystem is suffering a dual assault of invasive species, one fish and one plant. Lake Victoria was a freshwater ecosystem of great biodiversity. Of particular interest there are the cichlid fishes, of which there were over 300 species in the lake. In 1954 the Nile perch, *Lates niloticus*, was introduced into Lake Victoria by the British colonial administration with the benign intention of improving fish catches for local fishermen. This, however, turned out to be an ecological disaster. The Nile perch is a fast-growing, predatory fish that can reach a weight of 200 kg and a length of 2 m. The voracious perch have consumed many of the algae-eating cichlid fishes in the lake. With the cichlids depleted, the biomass of algae in the lake has increased. Large mats of algae fall to the lake bottom and decompose in a process that has depleted oxygen in the lower portions of the lake and rendered the waters uninhabitable. The endemic cichlids of the lake have been all but eliminated, and the Nile perch itself, having consumed its food supply, may itself be in jeopardy.

More recently, an invasive plant, the water hyacinth, *Eichhornia crassipes*, has wreaked further havoc in Lake Victoria. This water plant, with a showy purple-blue flower, is originally from South America. It was introduced into East Africa as an ornamental plant and found its way into the region's lakes and rivers. The plant multiplies rapidly and floats on the surface, preventing sunlight and oxygen from getting into the water. Decaying plant matter also reduces oxygen in the water. Thus, water hyacinth infestations reduce fisheries, shade out submersed plants, crowd out surface plants, and reduce biological diversity. The plant has become so abundant in East African waterways that it has clogged rivers and blocked dams, interfering with hydroelectric power generation. Furthermore, the freshwater snails that harbor the causative agent of schistosomiasis attach to the suspended roots of the hyacinth and are carried to new locations, thus spreading the risk of disease for people entering the water. Together, the Nile perch and the water hyacinth have turned one of the world's richest sources of aquatic biodiversity into an empty vessel.

Invasive species, a threat to biodiversity in their own right, may also carry dangerous pathogens and transmit them to local naive populations of wildlife. The red-fin perch (*Perca fluviatilis*), for instance, was introduced into Australia from Europe in the 1860s and rapidly spread through the country's lakes and rivers. It is a predatory species that through consumption and displacement has depressed populations of local indigenous fish, crayfish, and amphibians. More recently, it has been recognized that the red-fin perch carries a viral pathogen, epizootic hematopoietic necrosis virus (ENHV), which can be transmitted to indigenous fish species as well. The virus is being spread by birds through regurgitation of infected fish or mechanical transfer on feathers, feet, or bills. Movement of fish by anglers as well as mechanical transfer on boats, nets, and other equipment is exacerbating the problem. Tasmania has introduced a conservation plan to keep red-fin perch out of its waterways to protect a number of species of endemic fishes in the family *Galaxiidae*. EHNV is a ranavirus in the family Iridoviridae, members of which are affecting fish and amphibians worldwide. The iridoviruses have been implicated in the global amphibian die-off that has been occurring over the past several years.

In addition to carrying disease agents, invasive species may harbor disease vectors or serve as disease vectors themselves. The Asian tiger mosquito (*Aedes albopictus*) reached the United States in 1985 in a shipment of water-laden, used tires entering Texas from Japan. Within 2 years, the mosquito had spread to 17 states, and by 1995 had reached as far north as New Jersey. This mosquito can carry the viruses responsible for dengue fever, yellow fever, and La Crosse encephalitis in humans and can also transmit dog heartworms.

In 2000, the United States Department of Agriculture (USDA) issued a ban on the importation of several species of African tortoises that are popular as pets. It was recognized that some tortoises were entering the United States with infestations of ticks of the species *Amblyomma*, including the tropical bont tick, *A. variegatum*, and the African tortoise tick, *A. marmoreum*. These ticks are competent vectors of the organism *Cowdria ruminantium*, which causes the fatal ruminant livestock disease cowdriosis, or heartwater. The ban was spurred by the fact that breeding colonies of the ticks had been identified in Florida on premises where imported tortoises had been housed, suggesting that the ticks could become locally established. Heartwater poses a serious threat to the cattle industry and potentially to wild ruminants, including whitetail deer (*Odocoileus virginianus*) and pronghorn antelope (*Antilocapra americana*), if competent, infected vectors become established in the United States.

Climate change can further facilitate the invasion of disease vectors. The occurrence and persistence of African horse sickness in equids in Spain from the late 1980s following the importation of infected zebras from Namibia is considered to be associated with increasing seasonal temperatures that have allowed persistence of the insect vector, *Cullicoides imicola*.[34] Prior to this time, African horse sickness was restricted to sub-Saharan Africa. When it did occur outside the region, the infection was usually self-limiting because competent vectors did not survive colder periods of the year to maintain the infection.

Disease

Ecologists, conservation biologists, and veterinarians are increasingly recognizing the spread of infectious agents as a major threat to biodiversity, referring to the dissemination of parasites and microorganisms as *pathogen pollution*. It is difficult to know with certainty to what extent the occurrence of disease is increasing in wild animals and plant populations as historically, there has been little scientific documentation or investigation of disease outbreaks in the natural world. Even after the germ theory of disease was well established, disease investigation focused on humans and domestic animals. The first major infectious disease outbreak in wild animals that was described in some detail was the rinderpest panzootic that occurred in wild African ungulates following the introduction of infected cattle into sub-Saharan Africa at the end of the 19th century. This disease outbreak and others that have affected mammals and birds and attracted investigative attention are summarized in Table 7-5.

In the last 20 years, in conjunction with growing awareness of the biodiversity threat, there has been a surge of interest in the role of disease in wildlife conservation. While mammals and birds continue to get a good deal of attention, disease issues affect a wide range of plant and animal species, including terrestrial and aquatic invertebrates and many coniferous and deciduous plants. Daszak et al. present a good overview of the issue of emerging diseases in terrestrial ecosystems,[12] while Harvell et al. have published a similar overview on the emergence and impact of disease on marine ecosystems.[24] These authors and others identify a variety of factors that contribute to the emergence of disease as an important threat to biodiversity. These include increased trade and movement of animals and plants, shrinking habitats and restricted ranges, stressors associated with degraded habitat, incursions of people and livestock, and climate change. Each is discussed briefly below.

Disease and Increased Trade

The increased trade and movement of animals and plants around the world augments the risk of disease spread. Global trade in wildlife is a multibillion dollar business, with an estimated 350 million plants and animals traded each year. This includes species considered to be at risk under the international agreement of the Convention on International Trade in Endangered Species of Wild Flora and Fauna (CITES), which calls for the 145 participating nations to require trade permits for species movements. The scale of wildlife trade is reflected by the number of these CITES permits. Between 1990 and 1994, for example, the following approximate numbers of plants and animals were traded worldwide under CITES: primates, 146,000; wild cats, 3,400; parrots, 1.82 million; tortoises, 215,000; live monitor lizards, 228,000; chameleons, 278,000; boas and pythons, 652,000; poison arrow frogs, 21,000; and live plants in the Appendix I endangered species category alone, 563,000. This of course, reflects only the legal, documented trade. A great deal of illegal smuggling of living wildlife also occurs. In the United Kingdom alone, in a single year, customs

Table 7-5 Notable Disease Episodes Affecting Wild Mammal and Bird Populations

Species Affected	Disease	Years	Causative Agent	Source	Comments and Reference
Ungulates, especially African buffalo (Syncerus caffer) and wildebeest (Connochaetes taurinus)	Rinderpest	1890–1899	Morbillivirus	Introduced domestic cattle	Up to 90% of some populations killed off; predators secondarily affected; lasting effects on the distribution of African ungulate wildlife[44]
Chimpanzees (Pan troglodytes)	Polio	1966	Poliovirus	Humans	Presumptive diagnosis in outbreak of paralysis and death[19]
Harbor seals (Phoca vitulina)	Distemper	1988	Phocine distemper virus	Probably migrating harp seals (Phoca groenlandica)	Epizootic killed about 18,000 seals[25]
Lions (Panthera leo)	Distemper	Early 1990s	Canine distemper virus	Most likely sympatric domestic dogs	Unusual crossover of canine virus to feline species causing clinical disease[49]
Black-footed ferrets (Mustela nigripes)	Distemper	1985	Canine distemper virus	Sympatric domestic dogs	Plague contracted from prairie dog prey important cause of population decline, but last free-living colonies eliminated by canine distemper[53]
African elephant (Loxodonta africana)	Flaccid trunk paralysis	1989	Unknown	Unknown	Peripheral neuropathy; possibly infectious, but not fully elucidated[29]
Ethiopian wolf (Canis simensis)	Rabies	Early 1990s	Rabies virus	Sympatric domestic dogs	Only about 400 Ethiopian wolves remain in the wild[31]
Arctic foxes (Alopex lagopus semenovi)	Mange	1983–1995	Otodectes cynotis	Seafaring trappers	Only 90 endangered individuals remained; treatment attempted to save the species[18]
African wild dogs (Lycaon pictus)	Rabies	1990s	Rabies virus	Sympatric domestic dogs	Vaccination has been attempted in some packs to reduce losses[32]
Caspian seals (Phoca caspica)	Distemper	Spring 2000	Canine distemper virus	Unidentified	Over 10,000 seals died.; this species limited to the Caspian Sea; vulnerable to extinction[28]
House finch (Carpodacus mexicanus), and goldfinch (Carduelis tristis)	Mycoplasmal conjunctivitis	Beginning in 1994 and ongoing	Mycoplasma gallisepticum	Possibly domestic poultry	Backyard bird feeders have served as focal points for dissemination of the disease[15]
Hawaiian endemic bird species	Avian malaria and avian pox	Beginning in 1826 and ongoing	Plasmodium relictum and avian pox virus	Competent mosquito vector (Culex quinquefasciatus) introduced by ship in 1826	40% of the birds on the US Endangered Species list are Hawaiian endemics[54]

officials made over 30,000 seizures of CITES listed plants and animals illegally entering the UK. Of course the number of successfully smuggled plants and animals cannot be known precisely.

For many species of plants and animals, the range of pathogens and parasites they may harbor has not been fully ascertained. For legally traded imports, the practice of testing for known diseases and enforcement of extended quarantine periods reduce the likelihood that diseases, known and unknown, will be introduced into native populations of related plants and animals. However, it is not foolproof. Commercial transport of packaged bees and queens, along with accidental transport of bees on ships or aircraft has led to global spread of the parasitic bee mite, *Varroa jacobsoni*. Originally identified in Asia, the parasite now infests honey bees (*Apis mellifera*) on every continent except Australia. Varroasis causes high mortality in honey bees, leading not only to commercial losses in reduced honey production, but also to reduced pollination services for wild and agricultural plants.

Rational controls such as testing and quarantine are impossible to implement in the case of smuggled or illegally transported species, and the risks for introduction or spread of disease in these situations are significant. The introduction of rabies into the northeastern United States in the late 1970s represents a costly, serious, and ongoing public health hazard and a threat to indigenous wildlife and livestock populations. It most likely resulted from the illegal capture and translocation of infected raccoons from an endemic rabies area in the American southeast to more northern locations for hunting purposes. Subsequently, the disease spread throughout the northeast.

Disease and Habitat Alteration

Alteration of habitat can occur in many ways, often as the result of human transformations such as reduction in habitat area, fragmentation of habitat area, isolation by fencing or ring development, contamination by chemical pollutants, climate change, or introduction of exotic species. These degradations can, alone or in concert, predispose animal and plant species to disease. Reduction or fragmentation of habitat can reduce carrying capacity and increase competition for limited food resources, resulting in undernutrition. Lowered nutritional status can compromise immune defenses and make animals more susceptible to the effects of parasitism, expression of latent infections, or the spread of new infections. Crowding around limited water sources or within lekking sites and birthing areas can increase the buildup of pathogens in localized environments where animals are likely to concentrate, leading to eruptions of disease. Such diseases may spread rapidly through animal species that exhibit close herding behavior, such as range ungulates, or that live in close knit family groups, such as primates.

Even when direct efforts are made to protect biodiversity, through the creation of parks and protected areas, the results are not always as intended. The boundaries of parks and preserves do not always accommodate the needs of all species contained within, and constraints on behavior or resource availability can be linked to disease problems. Delineated habitats or restricted range can lead to increased concentrations of wildlife populations per unit area. This can lead to increased environmental contamination with pathogens and parasites, which in turn can increase the risk for disease outbreaks and their rapid spread through susceptible populations. This process threatens biodiversity. An example is provided by the situation at Etosha National Park in Namibia in southwest Africa. This park is home to a variety of plains ungulates including blue wildebeest (*Connochaetes taurinus*), plains zebra (*Equus burchelli*), springbok (*Antidorcas marsupialis*), and gemsbok (*Oryx gazella*).

In the 1970s, an 850-km game-proof fence was completed on the park perimeter that prevented the normal migrations of wildebeest. On the southern edge of the park boundary, artificial waterholes were built. The animals, no longer able to migrate, congregate around the waterholes, which leads to overgrazing, habitat degradation, and contamination of the water supply and surrounding grazing areas with pathogens, notably the spores of *Bacillus anthracis*, the cause of anthrax. Anthrax has emerged as a major endemic disease problem at Etosha. Researchers have shown that these ungulate populations are well below the carrying capacity of the park, based on calculations of the food resource ceiling, and have concluded that anthrax is the major constraint working to limit herd expansion.[4] Linked to this is the fact that the carnivores and scavengers at Etosha, including lions (*Panthera leo*) and spotted hyenas (*Crocuta crocuta*), are resistant to anthrax, so their numbers do not decline proportionately as a result of consuming infected herbivore prey. This distortion of the predator-prey balance adds further pressure to the dwindling herds in the park. Census figures on wildebeest in the 1950s before the game-proof fence was built were approximately 25,000. Currently they range from 2,200 to 2,600, about one tenth of their former strength.

Disease and Human Incursions

One of the main driving factors of habitat destruction is the conversion of wild areas to human use. This process is most dramatically evident in the steady clearing of rainforest for agricultural and other commercial purposes, but virtually all the world's biomes are being altered by human activity, including aquatic and marine ecosystems. One of the effects of ongoing human incursion into wild areas is the increased risk of the transfer of pathogens to indigenous animals through increased contact with humans, their domestic animals, and the detritus of their economic and social activity. While the potential transfer of pathogens between humans, domestic animals, and wildlife is multidirectional, the present discussion focuses on the impact of disease spread to wildlife as a threat to biodiversity. Nevertheless, human incursion into formerly wild areas is increasingly recognized as a key factor in the appearance of several important emerging diseases in humans, notably acquired immunodeficiency syndrome (AIDS) and Ebola virus infection.

Table 7-5 offers several examples of situations in which increased contact with humans and domestic animals is leading to outbreaks of wildlife disease. The spread of rabies and distemper to wild canids, including African wild dogs (*Lycaon pictus*), bat-eared fox (*Otocyon megalotisis*), jackal (*Canis aureus*), and hyena (*Crocuta crocuta*) as well as lions (*Panthera leo*) and possibly other felids in Africa, is linked to closer contacts between wildlife and domestic dogs. This results from increased human settlement on the peripheries of game parks and reserves and the increased presence of pastoralist herders with domestic dogs on rangelands exploited by canid and felid carnivores. Such transference of disease from domestic animals to sympatric wildlife is referred to as *spillover*.

In addition to spillover of disease from domestic canids to wild carnivores, there are also well-known cases of spillover from domestic ruminant livestock into wild ruminants. Rinderpest has been mentioned in a historic context, but rinderpest continues to threaten wildlife, albeit more locally and sporadically. In 1994 and 1995 an outbreak of rinderpest in Tsavo National Park in Kenya eliminated 60% of the Cape buffalo (*Syncerus caffer*) and 60% of the lesser kudu (*Tragelaphus imberbis*). The outbreak was associated with illegal movement of domestic cattle.

Tuberculosis is a notable and important example of spillover. In eastern and southern Africa, the disease has long been present in domestic cattle. Wild ruminants vary in their susceptibility to bovine tuberculosis, but some species, notably the Cape buffalo, are particularly vulnerable. Several major disease outbreaks in buffalo have occurred over the last 30 years, with high morbidity and mortality in buffalo in Queen Elizabeth Park in Uganda and Kruger National Park in South Africa. Veterinary services in many African countries have diminished in recent years for various reasons, as discussed in Chapter 8. When livestock diseases such as tuberculosis are left unregulated and unchecked, the risk for spread to wildlife populations increases.

The tuberculosis connection between wildlife and livestock is not limited to Africa. Badgers (*Meles meles*), a native wildlife species in southwestern England are now recognized as a reservoir of bovine tuberculosis in that country. In New Zealand, at least two wildlife reservoirs of bovine tuberculosis are recognized, and both, the brushtail possum (*Trichosurus vulpecula*) from Australia and the ferret (*Mustela furo*) from Europe, are invasive species introduced in the 19th century. The possum, in addition to being a potential source of infection for livestock, is also recognized as destructive to endemic beech forest vegetation. Ferrets were introduced from Europe in the 1880s to control rapidly expanding rabbit populations. By 1900, ferrets were well established in the wild and contributed to the decline of native birds including the kiwi (*Apteryx australis*), weka (*Gallirallus australis*), and blue duck (*Hymenolaimus malacorhynchos*) and to the extinction of kakapo (*Strigops habroptilus*) on the mainland.

Currently, in Michigan, state officials are dealing with an endemic focus of bovine tuberculosis in whitetail deer (*Odocoileus virginianus*) in the northeastern lower peninsula of the state. Eighteen of 354 hunter-killed deer examined from this endemic region in 1995 showed evidence of tuberculosis. In addition, *Mycobacterium bovis* has been isolated from small numbers of coyotes (*Canis latrans*), raccoons (*Procyon lotor*), black bear (*Ursus americanus*), bobcats (*Lynx rufus*), red fox (*Vulpes fulva*), and opossums (*Didelphis marsupialis*) in the endemic area, with the most likely source of infection for these animals considered to be the consumption of tuberculous white-tailed deer. The occurrence of a reservoir of tuberculosis in whitetail deer is causing serious concern among cattle owners and regulatory authorities because of the growing risk of infection of cattle by deer through contact in pasture or woodland. In 1979, Michigan was declared a bovine tuberculosis-free state, with no infected cattle herds. In 2000, the state once again had 8 of 5142 cattle herds confirmed as infected with bovine TB. The USDA downgraded Michigan's tuberculosis accreditation status, and several neighboring states are restricting importation of Michigan cattle. This return of a domestic animal disease from a wildlife reservoir back into the domestic animal population is referred to as *spillback*. Another current instance of potential spillback in the United States attracting great public attention involves the bison of Yellowstone National Park and the possibility that they might infect cattle adjacent to the park with brucellosis.

Primate species are especially vulnerable to close contact with human beings as they are susceptible to many of the same infectious organisms as humans. This is particularly true of the great apes, who share over 97% of our genome and are our closest living relatives. In Africa, there have been several instances of disease outbreaks in gorillas and chimpanzees associated with human pathogens. In 1988, a disease outbreak in mountain gorillas (*Gorilla gorilla beringei*) in the Virunga region of Zaire (now the Democratic Republic of Congo) was most likely due to human measles, based on histological examination of lesions. Polio was strongly suspected as the cause of paralytic disease in chimpanzees (*Pan troglodytes*) in Gombe Stream National Park, Tanzania, as the outbreak in chimps occurred in association with a confirmed polio outbreak in humans in a nearby village. The Gombe chimps also periodically experience flulike respiratory disease outbreaks that are sometimes fatal and are believed to be derived from human contact. In Indonesia, captive orangutans (*Pongo pygmaeus*) that had contracted tuberculosis in captivity were released into the wild, leading to the spread of tuberculosis in wild orangutan populations, with some documented fatalities. Not all of the health problems occurring in primates because of increased contact with humans are infectious. Many poor villagers living around protected areas set snares to trap wild game to supplement their diets and income. Even though snaring primates may not be the primary objective, these animals sometimes do become ensnared and may lose limbs or succumb to secondary infections associated with their wounds.

The full impact of disease on biodiversity remains unknown. Clearly, however, the risk of disease is widespread. It appears that few environments visited by humans have escaped exposure to new, potentially dangerous pathogens. There is even evidence of alien disease exposure in Antarctica, where a serosurvey of Antarctic penguins revealed antibodies to infectious bursal disease virus, a pathogen of domestic chickens.[17] The presence of the virus in Antarctica is presumed to be associated with human activity such as improperly disposed kitchen wastes from ecotourism expeditions or research stations. Similarly, crab-eating seals (*Lobodon carcinophagus*) in Antarctica in 1955 were infected with canine distemper virus, presumably from sled dogs used in an Antarctic expedition.

Disease and Climate Change

Global warming associated with greenhouse gases and the occurrence of El Niño/southern oscillation (ENSO) events are described in Chapter 6. These climate perturbations are increasingly being considered underlying factors in the occurrence of wildlife disease. Harvell et al. report on emerging marine diseases in which climate change has very likely played a role in disease occurrence.[24] For example, death of coral due to bleaching has been associated with persistently warmer ocean waters from extended ENSO events. Prolonged warm water temperatures may promote opportunistic bacterial infections and trigger the expulsion of the coral's symbiotic algae, which leads to the fatal bleaching. ENSO events are also linked to outbreaks of Dermo disease in Eastern oyster populations in the Gulf of Mexico. The disease is caused by the protozoan parasite *Perkinsus marinus*. The intensity of infection in Gulf oyster populations fluctuates with ocean temperatures during alternating El Niño and La Niña events.

In the spring of 1996, there was an alarming epizootic of fatal disease in Florida's endangered manatee population. The total population of Florida manatees (*Trichechus manatus latirostris*) at the time was only about 2600. Suddenly, seemingly healthy manatees began dying, and in a matter of weeks, 155 had perished. Ultimately, veterinarian Greg Bossart and colleagues identified the cause of death as brevetoxicosis, caused by the potent neurotoxin elaborated by the marine dinoflagellate, *Gymnodinium breve*.[6] This dinoflagellate was associated with algal blooms occurring in Florida waters at the time. The occurrence of harmful algal blooms, known commonly as red tides, has been increasing steadily over the last 20 years. While the occurrence of harmful algal blooms is caused by multiple factors, some researchers consider that warmer ocean temperatures associated with global warming and ENSO events contribute to this phenomenon.

Terrestrial disease events are also being associated with climate change. Baylis et al. have demonstrated a link between periodic epizootics of African horse sickness (AHS) in South Africa and warm-phase ENSO events in which pronounced drought early in the ENSO year is followed by heavy rains.[2] It is postulated that during drought, zebras, which are a reservoir for the AHS virus, congregate heavily around limited water sources and increase the infection rate of midge vectors (*Culicoides imicola*) that feed on the zebra. During subsequent wet periods, when the midge vector populations expand, a large proportion of the susceptible horse population is infected and becomes ill. In the largest recorded AHS outbreak in South Africa, over 40% of the nation's horse population died.

Daszak et al., in their paper on emerging infectious diseases of wildlife, cite a newly discovered fungal disease, cutaneous chytridiomycosis, which has been identified as a cause of amphibian mortality linked to population declines in Central American and Australian rain forests.[12] The disease is unusual in that it has occurred seemingly spontaneously in distant locations at sites that are relatively undisturbed ecologically. One postulated cause of the disease is an alteration of preexisting host-parasite relationships resulting from climate change. Spread of the disease agent is believed to be associated with the active and extensive international trade in amphibians as pets, for outdoor pond stocking, for laboratory specimens, and for zoological collections.

The distribution of arthropod disease vectors can be strongly influenced by changing climate. Warming temperatures allow dispersion of mosquitoes and other cold-intolerant insect vectors into new regions, where naive populations of wildlife may succumb to pathogens carried by these vectors. Warming temperatures can extend vector range both horizontally across a landscape and vertically up mountainsides. The full impact of such climate-related vector dissemination as a threat to biodiversity is not known, as the full inventory of vector-transmitted wildlife diseases has not been completely elucidated. However, some specific examples are emerging. The situation with avian malaria in Hawaii is one such example. The endangered i'iwi (*Vestiaria coccinea*), one of nine endemic Hawaiian honeycreepers found in the cloud forests of East Maui, has survived in the higher forest elevations because mosquitoes that transmit deadly avian malaria apparently cannot breed successfully at the cooler temperatures found at these higher elevations. A warmer climate might allow the mosquito to move farther up the mountain and transmit avian malaria to the i'iwi just as it has been doing to susceptible honeycreeper species living at lower elevations.

Disease and Conservation Efforts

As habitat is lost, fragmented, and invaded by exotic species, wildlife populations diminish. For some species, population sizes become so small that the threat of extinction looms large. The impact of disease in such small, remnant populations can be devastating, be it rabies or canine distemper in African wild dogs (*Lycaon pictus*), brevetoxicosis in manatees (*Trichechus manatus latirostris*), or the spread of contagious human pathogens into great ape species, as mentioned. To protect these dwindling populations, veterinarians have to be actively involved in conservation efforts to help identify disease risks, monitor health status, intervene therapeutically when necessary, and develop appropriate strategies for disease prophylaxis consistent with the behavior and ecology of the beleaguered species.

Furthermore, as populations of endangered species in the wild diminish, efforts to maintain these species in captivity have increased, along with efforts to return captive-bred individuals to their original wild habitats. These captive breeding and reintroduction efforts are also fraught with the risk of disease, as discussed later in the section on reintroductions and translocations. With so many wildlife species at risk and relatively little known about the diseases of wildlife and their natural histories, there are tremendous opportunities and challenges for veterinarians to become professionally involved in the preservation of biodiversity. The emerging field of conservation medicine represents an avenue for veterinarians to become more actively involved. Conservation medicine is discussed in more detail at the end of this chapter.

Accelerating Rates of Extinction

The ultimate expression of biodiversity loss is species extinction, the utter and total obliteration of a unique form of life. That each living species expresses a set of unique structural, functional, and behavioral characteristics that allow it to thrive in a particular ecological niche is certainly a source of wonderment. Biologist E. O. Wilson has referred to each and every species as a masterpiece of evolution. That so many masterpieces currently face the prospect of being erased from Earth is a cause for great sadness and concern. Two important facts are emerging with regard to extinction. First, the rate at which species are being extinguished is rapidly accelerating relative to the paleobiological record, and second, this accelerated extinction rate is essentially the result of human activity.

Interpretation of the fossil record by paleobiologists indicates that extinctions are a normal part of the evolutionary process. Over time, the adaptive characteristics of individual species may no longer provide a competitive edge, and the species will die off. Studies of fossilized marine invertebrates indicate that the life span of ancient species was in the range of 1 to 10 million years and that the rate of extinction, calculated as the number of species extinctions (E) per million species-years (MSY), was between 0.1 and 1 E/MSY. This was the pattern before the arrival of human beings. Archeological studies indicate that the Polynesian peoples who first colonized the Pacific islands and who possessed only Stone Age technology were responsible for the extinction of approximately 2000 bird species, about 15% of the world total of bird species. In just the last few hundred years, human society, equipped with modern technology, has accelerated the pace of extinctions even further.

The study of extinction events in circumscribed environments such as the Pacific islands provides a good framework for studying how habitat loss from human activity is linked to species extinctions. Island biogeography models suggest that generally, a 50% loss of habitat leads to a 10% loss of the species within a defined ecosystem. E. O. Wilson estimates that the current extinction rate is 1,000 to 10,000 times greater than the rate of 0.1 to 1.0 E/MSY determined from the fossil record, which suggested that for every million species on Earth, one species per year on average became extinct.[59] Today, for every million species on Earth, 1,000 to 10,000 can be projected to become extinct annually, based on certain reasonable assumptions. Species diversity is richest in tropical rainforests, and in contemporary times, rainforests are being cleared at the rate of 1% per year. Island biogeography models indicate that a 1% habitat loss leads to a 0.2 to 0.3% species loss. Wilson makes a conservative estimate that there are at least 2 million distinct rainforest species, which translates into a loss of at least 4000 to 6000 species per year, or an average of about 14 species extinguished daily. At this rate, one fourth of all existing biological species may become extinct in the next 30 to 40 years.

Such a rate of species loss can be categorized as mass extinction. Paleontologists identify five earlier mass extinctions in the Earth's biological history, when large numbers of species disappeared over a relatively short period, perhaps in relation to some catastrophic astronomical, geological, atmospheric, or climatic event. The first mass extinction occurred over 438 million years ago, the most recent, and best known, because it brought the demise of dinosaurs, occurred some 65 million years ago. What distinguishes our own current mass extinction, however, is that it is occurring primarily as a result of human agency. Never before has one species been directly responsible for the extermination of countless other species in what could reasonably be considered a biological holocaust.

In his textbook *A Primer of Conservation Biology*, Richard B. Primack summarizes the characteristics that make a species vulnerable to extinction.[46] Recognition of all these characteristics can help identify relative risks for individual species extinctions and aid in the development of conservation strategies. The list of species vulnerability characteristics includes the following:

- Species with narrow geographical ranges
- Species with only one or a few populations
- Species in which population size is small or declining
- Species with low population densities
- Species that need large home ranges
- Animal species with large body sizes
- Species with limited behavioral or physiological adaptability
- Species that are seasonal migrants
- Species with little genetic variability
- Species with specialized niche requirements
- Species that are characteristically found in stable environments
- Species that form permanent or temporary aggregations
- Species that are hunted or harvested by people

Human impact can be especially destructive in locations where numerous endemic species with small population sizes exist within a narrow geographic range. When this restricted habitat is disrupted or obliterated by human intrusion, large numbers of species can be lost in what has been termed the "cookie cutter" pattern of extinction. One new approach to slowing the rate of extinction is based on the recognition of factors that increase species vulnerability as well as the devastating impact of cookie cutter habitat loss. Myers et al. have put forward the concept of identifying and protecting biological "hotspots."[37] Hotspots are specific environmental regions rich in biodiversity in which the number of unique species present is proportionately high relative to the area of habitat that must be protected and managed to save them from extinction. Not surprisingly, a good many, though by no means all, of the biodiversity hotspots they identify are associated with tropical rainforests.

Myers and colleagues reason pragmatically that while it would be desirable to be able to ensure the protection of all endangered and threatened species, the scope of global habitat destruction is so rapid and extensive and the financial resources for conservation efforts are so relatively limited, that it is rational and prudent to focus conservation efforts as much as possible on the "hotspots," so that the greatest number and diversity of species can be saved in the shortest period with the limited resources available. The 25 biodiversity hotspots proposed for conservation priority are presented in Table 7-6. These hotspots are estimated to compose only 1.4% of the earth's land area, but they contain 44% of all vascular plant species and 35% of all the species contained in four major vertebrate groups, namely, mammals, birds, reptiles, and amphibians.

Conservation initiatives such as the protection of biological hotspots offer some hope for success in preserving biodiversity. In the meantime, however, the acceleration of extinction rates continues. The IUCN issued its most recent global survey on extinctions in 2000, the IUCN Red List of Threatened Species. The Red List categorizes threatened species living in the wild as critically endangered, endangered, or vulnerable (Table 7-7). Since the last survey in 1996, many worsening trends were noted. In total, 11,046 species of the world's known plants and animals are considered to be threatened with extinction. The total number of threatened animal species has increased in just 4 years from 5205 to 5435. The number of primates in the critically endangered category increased from 13 to 19 in that 4-year period. The number of mammals overall in that category increased from 169 to 180, and the number of birds from 168 to 182. This represents approximately one in four mammalian and one in eight of the world's bird species currently at risk of extinction. More information on the findings reported in the 2000 Red List are available on the internet at www.redlist.org.

Efforts to Preserve Biodiversity

That the major threats to biodiversity result from human activity is a cause for both dismay and hope. Dismay because, as human beings, we are heedlessly prosecuting a biological holocaust that ultimately may threaten our very own survival. Hope, because, as human beings, we are capable of learning and modifying our own behavior in the service of enlightened self-interest. Human activity can be changed through a process of increased awareness, education, shifts in cultural values, and the establishment of new priorities and practices expressed through personal choice, political consensus, and the rule of law.

Ecologist and author David Ehrenfeld, writing in the volume *The Last Extinction* suggests that the ultimate success of all conservation efforts will depend on a revision of the way we use the world in our everyday living when we are not specifically thinking about the issue of conservation.[14] He sees our current approach to environmental resources and natural capital as essentially exploitative, emphasizing quantity, production, consumption, waste, and perpetual growth. Instead, Ehrenfeld suggests, we must learn and embrace a position of stewardship toward environment resources and natural capital that celebrates quality, equilibrium, durability, stability, and, ultimately, sustainability.

In the United States, the journey toward stewardship began, at least symbolically, on Earth Day, April 22, 1970. Earth Day was conceived and promoted by U.S. Senator Gaylord Nelson as a national "teach-in" to promote citizen awareness of environmental problems, to bring environmental issues into the arena of public debate, and to encourage the political establishment to consider laws and policies that addressed important environmental issues. By the end of that same year, the U.S. Environmental Protection Agency (EPA) was established, the Clean Air Act was signed into law, and nearly 81,000 ha of land in the United States was designated protected wilderness. In 1972, the Clean Water Act was signed into law, and DDT was banned from use in the United States. In 1973, the Endangered Species Act was signed into law.

Earth Day and its influence in the United States notwithstanding, grave environmental challenges persist worldwide, particularly with regard to the preservation of biodiversity. The next few decades are a critical period in which the fate of many species will be decided forever. Intensified efforts for problem solving are required. A growing number of concerned citizens, scientists, politicians, and policymakers are working to expand knowledge and to develop strategies, partnerships, and policies in a concerted effort to slow the rate of habitat loss and species extinctions and to preserve global biodiversity. Specific areas of focus include:

- Scientific inquiry to understand and document loss of biodiversity and its causes

- Increased data collection and monitoring of environmental quality and natural capital

- Expanded public awareness and educational programs focused on biodiversity issues

- Creation of new partnerships for global governance of the earth's resources

- Increased citizen activism through nongovernmental organizations (NGOs) and internet communication

- Development and enforcement of international conventions, laws, and treaties

Table 7-6 Biodiversity Hotspots

Hotspot[a]	Principal Biome Types[b]	% of Earth's Land Area	Vascular Plant Species Present (Total/Endemic)	Bird Species Present (Total/Endemic)	Mammalian Species Present (Total/Endemic)
Tropical Andes	TRF/TDF/HAG	0.21	45,000/20,000	1,666/677	414/68
Mesoamerica (Central America)	TRF/TDF	0.16	24,000/5,000	1,193/251	521/210
Caribbean	TRF/TDF/XV	0.02	12,000/7,000	668/148	164/49
Choco-Darien-Western Ecuador	TRF/TDF	0.04	9,000/2,250	830/85	235/60
Atlantic forest region (Brazil)	TRF/STRF	0.06	20,000/6,000	620/73	261/160
Brazilian Cerado	TDF/WS/OS	0.24	10,000/4,400	837/29	161/19
Central Chile	M	0.06	3,429/1,605	198/4	56/9
California Floristic Province	M	0.05	4,426/2,125	341/8	145/30
Madagascar and Indian Ocean Islands	TRF/TDF/XV	0.04	12,000/9,704	359/199	112/84
Eastern Arc Mountains (Eastern Africa)	TRF	0.001	4,000/1,400	585/22	183/16
Cape Floristic Province (South Africa)	M	0.01	8,200/5,682	288/6	127/9
Succulent Karoo (South Africa)	XV	0.02	4,849/1,940	269/1	78/4
Guinean forests of West Africa	TRF	0.09	9,000/2,250	514/90	551/45
Mediterranean basin	M	0.07	25,000/13,000	345/47	184/46
Caucasus	TPF/G	0.03	6,300/1,600	389/3	152/32
Sundaland (Malay peninsula and nearby islands)	TRF/TDF	0.08	25,000/15,000	815/139	328/115
Wallacea (central Indonesian islands)	TRF/TDF/XV	0.04	10,000/1,500	697/249	201/123
Philippines	TRF	0.02	7,620/5,832	556/183	201/111
Indo-Burma (southeast Asia)	TRF/TDF	0.07	13,500/7,000	1,170/140	329/73
Mountains of south central China	TPF/G	0.04	12,000/3,500	686/36	300/75
Western Ghats (India) and Sri Lanka	TRF	0.001	4,780/2,180	528/40	140/36
New Caledonia	TRF/TDF/MS	<0.001	3,332/2,551	116/22	9/6
New Zealand	TPF/G	0.04	2,300/1,865	149/68	3/3
Polynesia/Micronesia	TRF/TDF	0.001	6,557/3,334	254/174	16/9
Southwestern Australia	M	0.02	5,469/4,331	181/19	54/7
TOTALS		1.41	287,762/131,049	14,254/2,713	4,925/1,401

[a]These 25 ecoregions are high priorities for global conservation efforts. While composing only 1.4% of Earth's land area, they contain approximately 44% of the world's known vascular plant species, 28% of bird species, 29% of mammalian species, 38% of reptile species, and 54% of amphibian species.[35]

[b]Biome types: G, grassland; HAG, high altitude grassland; M, Mediterranean type; MS, Maquis shrubland; OS, open savanna; STRF, subtropical rainforest; TDF, tropical dry forest; TPF, temperate forest; TRF, tropical rain forest; WS, woodland savanna; XV, xerophytic vegetation.

Table 7-7   Categories of Endangered and Threatened Species As Defined by the IUCN

EXTINCT (EX)—A taxon is Extinct when there is no reasonable doubt that the last individual has died.

EXTINCT IN THE WILD (EW)—A taxon is Extinct in the Wild when it is known only to survive in cultivation, in captivity or as a naturalized population (or populations) well outside the past range. A taxon is presumed Extinct in the Wild when exhaustive surveys in known and/or expected habitat, at appropriate times (diurnal, seasonal, annual), throughout its historic range have failed to record an individual. Surveys should be over a time frame appropriate to the taxon's life cycle and life form.

CRITICALLY ENDANGERED (CR)—A taxon is Critically Endangered when it is facing an extremely high risk of Extinction in the Wild in the immediate future.

ENDANGERED (EN)—A taxon is Endangered when it is not Critically Endangered but is facing a very high risk of Extinction in the Wild in the near future.

VULNERABLE (VU)—A taxon is Vulnerable when it is not Critically Endangered or Endangered but is facing a high risk of Extinction in the Wild in the medium-term future.

LOWER RISK (LR)—A taxon is Lower Risk when it has been evaluated, does not satisfy the criteria for any of the categories Critically Endangered, Endangered or Vulnerable. Taxa included in the Lower Risk category can be separated into three subcategories:

1. *Conservation Dependent (cd)*. Taxa which are the focus of a continuing taxon-specific or habitat-specific conservation programme targeted towards the taxon in question, the cessation of which would result in the taxon qualifying for one of the threatened categories above within a period of five years.

2. *Near Threatened (nt)*. Taxa which do not qualify for Conservation Dependent, but which are close to qualifying for Vulnerable.

3. *Least Concern (lc)*. Taxa which do not qualify for Conservation Dependent or Near Threatened.

DATA DEFICIENT (DD)—A taxon is Data Deficient when there is inadequate information to make a direct, or indirect, assessment of its risk of extinction based on its distribution and/or population status. A taxon in this category may be well studied, and its biology well known, but appropriate data on abundance and/or distribution is lacking. Data Deficient is therefore not a category of threat or Lower Risk. Listing of taxa in this category indicates that more information is required and acknowledges the possibility that future research will show that threatened classification is appropriate. It is important to make positive use of whatever data are available. In many cases great care should be exercised in choosing between DD and threatened status. If the range of a taxon is suspected to be relatively circumscribed, if a considerable period of time has elapsed since the last record of the taxon, threatened status may well be justified.

NOT EVALUATED (NE)—A taxon is Not Evaluated when it is has not yet been assessed against the criteria.

More information on these categories and the criteria used to place species into the appropriate category are available from the IUCN on the internet at www.redlist.org/info/categories_criteria.html.

- Strengthening of local capacity in nations around the world to successfully implement programs and policies that protect biodiversity

Each of these efforts is discussed briefly below.

Scientific Inquiry

Experience with environmental issues such as air pollution, water pollution, the biological effects of DDT, ozone depletion, and global warming have made it abundantly clear that good science must inform policy debates about environmental matters. This is especially true when proposed remedies for environmental problems are perceived to diminish economic activity or to increase costs and reduce profits for commercial interests. Emotions will run high under such circumstances,

and the objectivity of well-established scientific fact can help all parties to see beyond their own special interests in developing solutions to complex problems. For example, accurate scientific information about the extent of lead contamination in the environment, its health effects on humans and animals, and the role of leaded gasoline in motor vehicles as a major source of lead contamination resulted in a successful phase-out of leaded gasoline in the United States despite initial objections by automobile manufacturers and oil-refining interests. Almost 30 years later, with the phase-out of leaded gasoline in the United States virtually completed and lead levels dropping in the nation's soil and water, there is little evidence that the transition had any lasting adverse impact on the fortunes of these two industries.

The same situation holds in the matter of preserving biodiversity, in which efforts to protect habitat and save species can mean restrictions on the extraction of natural resources, the building of roads, the expansion of agriculture, the use of synthetic chemicals, or the release of pollutants and greenhouse gases. Scientific inquiry and analysis are necessary to better understand and define the character, function, and value of threatened ecosystems so that the impact of change can be more adequately measured. Scientific assessment also allows rational management plans to be developed so that meaningful protection of biodiversity can be achieved while the reasonable imperatives of human enterprise are accommodated.

Advances in the discipline of ecological economics as discussed earlier in this chapter offer an example of how analytical studies can inform decision making on matters of biological resource use. Ecological economics allows comprehensive cost/benefit analysis to be carried out so that the advantage of short-term gains from resource exploitation, such as clearcutting a forest, can be accurately compared with the long-term gains possible from sustainable management of a natural resource base, such as harvesting forest products and promoting ecotourism. Such analyses can promote "wise use" of environmental resources that retain biodiversity while supporting economic activity.

Perhaps the most significant development in the application of science to the preservation of biodiversity has been the emergence of the field of conservation biology. *Conservation biology* is a multidisciplinary science that integrates various aspects of biogeography, ecology, economics, evolution, genetics, population biology, and taxonomy to assist in solving critical problems in the preservation of biodiversity. It draws on the knowledge and methods of more traditional biological disciplines of resource management such as agriculture, forestry, wildlife management, and fisheries biology, but unlike these disciplines, it focuses on the long-term preservation of entire biological communities rather than on specific biological resources that are being managed primarily for commercial extraction or recreational activities. Conservation biology also integrates the perspectives and practices of nonbiological fields such as environmental law, environmental ethics, sociology, anthropology, and climatology.

In his excellent introduction to the subject, *A Primer of Conservation Biology*, Primack identifies three specific goals for the science[46]:

- To investigate and describe the diversity of the living world

- To understand the effects of human activities on species, communities, and ecosystems

- To develop practical interdisciplinary approaches to protecting and restoring biological diversity

Primack stresses the multidisciplinary nature of conservation biology and the importance of scientists with different training and expertise working together on the complex problems of ecosystem management, which often have economic, sociological, and political causes as well as biological ones. Interestingly, veterinary medicine receives scant mention in Primack's text. This is not a slight on the part of the author. Rather, it represents a failing of the veterinary profession so far to fully recognize its potential contribution to conservation biology and to reach beyond the confines of its own professional sphere to collaborate with scientists in other disciplines. Part of this failure relates to limitations within the traditional veterinary curriculum, as discussed later in the section on conservation medicine.

Any veterinary student or graduate interested in issues of biodiversity in general and wildlife conservation in particular should become familiar with the science of conservation biology and become more actively involved in the conservation biology community. The Society of Conservation Biology (SCB) was established in 1985 to help develop the scientific and technical means for the protection, maintenance, and restoration of life on this planet through research, publication, and educational activities. The SCB began publishing a peer-reviewed journal, *Conservation Biology*, in 1987. Information on the SCB and its goals and activities can be found on the internet at http://conbio.net/scb/. By becoming familiar with the perspectives, priorities, and practices of conservation biology, veterinarians will be better able to define the effective contributions that veterinary science can make to the preservation of biodiversity.

Data Collection and Monitoring

Much work has been done in recent years by conservation biologists, climatologists, oceanographers, and other scientists to develop baseline data on the state of the world's biological resources and other, related environmental parameters, such as atmospheric and climatic changes, which influence the state of the world's biodiversity. The technical capacity now exists to track and document a variety of indicators of environmental health, including patterns and rates of rainforest destruction, species extinctions, atmospheric warming trends, changes in greenhouse gas composition, increases in sea level, and the size and location of ozone holes in the stratosphere. In our information-based society, information is a powerful tool. It becomes difficult for politicians and policymakers to ignore trends that are carefully documented through a steady accumulation of credible data, particularly when informed and concerned citizens have access to the same information.

Data collection and dissemination is carried out by a variety of organization under numerous auspices. The Red List of Threatened Species, for example, is produced by the IUCN (http://www.iucn.org). This organization, founded in 1948, is a unique worldwide partnership of over 10,000 scientists and experts from 181 countries linked through the participation of 78 states, 112 government agencies, 735 NGOs, and 35 affiliates. Through its Species Survival Commission (SSC), the IUCN has been assessing the conservation status of species, subspecies, varieties, and selected subpopulations of animals and plants on a worldwide basis for almost 40 years. Starting in 2001, the Red List will be updated annually, with an updated analysis published in hard copy at least once every 4 to 5 years.

Similarly, the Intergovernmental Panel on Climate Change (IPCC) (http://www.ipcc.ch/) is a network of scientists assembled under the auspices of the United Nations Environmental Programme (UNEP) and the World Meteorological Organization to periodically assess the scientific, technical, and socioeconomic information relevant for understanding the risk of human-induced climate change. The IPCC does not carry out new research or monitor climate-related data, but does carry out detailed, periodic assessments based mainly on published and peer-reviewed scientific literature. IPCC assessment reports were published in 1990, 1995, and 2001, and these assessments have steadily moved toward a clearer implication of human activity as a principal cause of increased atmospheric greenhouse gases and global warming. As such, these reports have played a pivotal role in informing international efforts to control greenhouse gas emissions, such as the Kyoto Protocol of 1997, and the subsequent efforts to implement it, as discussed in more detail in Chapter 6.

Other sources of data relevant to environmental health in general and biodiversity in particular are readily available. The World Resources Institute (WRI) has a large collection of tabulated data available at its website that can be downloaded in PDF format (www.wri.org). WRI resources include specific databases on agriculture, biodiversity, climate change, economics, forestry, oceans, and water resources as well as country profiles, global trends, and global statistics. There are also numerous links to other valuable sources of information such as the National Library for the Environment. The Worldwatch Institute (www.worldwatch.org) annually produces a paperback volume called *Vital Signs* that reports statistical data and narrative summaries on environmental trends, with an emphasis on social and economic parameters that influence environmental health and natural capital.

In 1995, UNEP initiated the Global Environment Outlook (GEO) Project to address the environmental reporting requirements contained in Agenda 21, the international environmental agreement that resulted from the UN Conference on Environment and Development, more commonly known as the Earth Summit, held in Rio de Janeiro in 1992. The GEO Project coordinates a global environmental assessment and periodically produces comprehensive GEO reports that detail the state of the world's environment and provide guidance for the formulation of environmental policies and resource allocation. The latest GEO report, *Global Environment Outlook-2000*, can be accessed on the internet at http://www.unep.org/Geo2000/.

The World Conservation Monitoring Centre (WCMC), was founded in 1988 as a joint effort of the IUCN, the WWF, and the United Nations Development Program. In 2000, the WCMC became an office of the UNEP. The WCMC (www.unep-wcmc.org/) provides informational services on conservation and sustainable use of the world's living resources and helps others develop information systems of their own. WCMC informational programs concentrate on species, forests, protected areas, marine and fresh waters as well as habitats affected by climate change, such as polar regions. The WCMC also focuses on the relationship between trade and the environment and the wider aspects of biodiversity assessment.

Public Awareness and Education

During the period that this chapter was in preparation, I attended a social gathering where a cousin introduced me to a thoughtful 12-year-old boy named Alex from suburban New Jersey. Knowing I am a veterinarian who had some interest in wildlife, the cousin wanted Alex, a family friend, to meet me. It turned out that Alex was a fervent and knowledgeable conservationist, deeply concerned about the future of snow leopards and tigers on this planet. When I asked him what he knew about these animals, he provided a wealth of information about their habitat, the various tiger species that were endangered, the size of their remaining populations, the major threats to their survival, and efforts that were under way to protect these species in the wild. He further indicated that he intended to build his life's work around the survival of these species. He had already formulated a plan to become a mammalogist and had already picked out the university where he would receive his training. He even described the fieldwork he intended to do in support of snow leopard conservation. When I asked him how he developed his interest and obtained all his valuable information, Alex indicated it was a mixture of schoolwork, class projects, nature shows on television, web searches, and visits to the library. Following our conversation, I was left with the feeling that I had benefited much more from meeting Alex than he had from meeting me.

Alex represents hope for the future of biodiversity on Earth and reflects the growing importance of public awareness and environmental education in shaping attitudes and behavior toward the natural world. In recent years the United States has experienced a virtual explosion of information available to the general public concerning matters of wildlife conservation, preservation of biodiversity, and other aspects of environmental health through the various media, as well as through the activities of museums, zoos, and aquariums.

In addition, there has been a significant effort to formalize environmental education through incorporation of environmental issues into primary and secondary school curricula and the training of teachers to deliver those curricula. In 1971, the North American Association for Environmental Education (NAAEE) was established to serve the education community. The NAAEE is a network of professionals, students, and volunteers working in over 55 countries around the world to develop science-based environmental curricula and train teachers to effectively integrate environmental education into their teaching efforts. EE-Link, a resource for environmental education on the internet is a project of the NAAEE and offers extensive information about available resources and programs in environmental education (http://www.nceet.snre.umich.edu/). The nonprofit educational organization, Second Nature, provides similar support and resources for environmental education at the university level (http://www.secondnature.org/).

Despite such progress, there is still a long way to go, both in the United States and around the world. Williams, writing in *Audubon Magazine* about environmental education, indicated that the latest available figures from 1994 showed only 13% of secondary education majors and 14% of elementary education majors were required to take a course in environmental education and that only three states required it as part of teacher training.[57] Furthermore, Williams indicates that a backlash to environmental education is occurring in the United States, with some opponents suggesting that environmental education is hostile to free enterprise and private property. At least some of the these opponents are on record as claiming that the EPA provides financial support to educational programs that distort scientific evidence on important environmental issues such as global warming, acid rain, air pollution, and water quality and then manipulate children to become political activists who support misguided environmental policies.

Veterinarians can play a valuable role in their communities as credible sources of information and learning about conservation issues. A Gallup poll released in November 2000 indicated that veterinarians are considered the third most trusted trade or profession in America by their fellow citizens, following only nurses and pharmacists. In addition to this high level of respect, the public has a general inclination to consider veterinarians reliable sources of information and advice on all matters related to animals. As such, there is a remarkable opportunity for veterinarians interested in wildlife conservation and the preservation of biodiversity to encourage public awareness about conservation issues and to participate in conservation education. Veterinarians can participate through dissemination of conservation information at their veterinary practices; as volunteers in the public schools, nearby parks, conservancies, and nature centers; or as instructors at community colleges and adult education programs.

Unlike young Alex in New Jersey, a great many school children in developing countries have little or no access to information about threatened species in particular or conservation issues in general. Often rural children know indigenous wild animals only as potential sources of bushmeat, as pests who damage crops, or as predators who prey on livestock or even, sometimes, humans. The fear of being eaten by a tiger may be a more immediate and realistic concern than trying to protect that tiger. Urban children in many developing countries may have no knowledge or experience with wildlife at all. It is becoming clear to the conservation community that local people must be involved in local conservation efforts if such efforts are going to succeed. The good intentions and financial contributions of foreigners will not suffice to save the day if local people are not knowledgeable about environmental issues. Education is an essential prerequisite for local people to become committed stakeholders for conservation efforts.

In recognition of this need for environmental education in developing countries, a number of international conservation organizations and multinational agencies have made a commitment to conservation education in primary and secondary schools of developing countries around the world. For example, Wildlife Trust, formerly Wildlife Preservation Trust International, supports the Wild Ones program, which was initiated in 1995. By 2000, The Wild Ones made up a network of more than 30,000 children, teachers, and conservation pro-

fessionals in 30 countries around the globe. The program provides students ages 7 to 14 with an international perspective, opportunities for cooperative science activities, and a sense that each individual has the capacity to improve the prospects for endangered species (www.thewildones.org/).

In Uganda, the Uganda Wildlife Education Centre (UWEC), formerly the Entebbe Zoo, has become an important force in conservation education in the country, with active programs for Uganda's schoolchildren, who are now visiting the Centre by the thousands. This effort exemplifies the kind of international partnerships that are evolving to support local conservation education. UWEC receives financial support and technical input from the government of Uganda, the Wildlife Conservation Society in New York, The Jane Goodall Institute, and the Zoological Park Board of New South Wales, Australia, among others.

Grassroots Activism

Citizen groups can play an important role in the promotion of environmental health, the wise use of natural capital, and the preservation of biodiversity. For instance, the Chipko Movement, which gained prominence in India in the 1970s, exemplifies the growing trend of citizen environmental activism. *Chipko* is the Hindi word for "tree-hugger." In northern India, where deforestation was a severe problem, local villagers banded together to prevent commercial timber harvesting through acts of civil disobedience including climbing into trees that were about to be cut by commercial contractors. Now, 30 years later, participatory forestry in India has become institutionalized, with the Indian Forest Service working directly with local villagers in forest management and use. More recently, the name Chico Mendes became a household word when the Brazilian rubber tapper led a movement of local forest workers to promote sustainable use of Amazon forests as "extractive reserves" of renewable forest products rather than clear-cutting forest for timber and cattle ranching. In 1988, Chico Mendes paid for his ideas and actions with his life, but not before demonstrating how grassroots activism could bring international attention to important biodiversity issues such as rainforest destruction and the wise use of natural resources.

In Chapter 5, the expanding role of NGOs in rural development and sustainable agriculture is discussed. NGOs have also been playing an expanded role in the area of environmental health, including the preservation of biodiversity and wildlife conservation. The number of environmental NGOs is growing. One estimate indicates that the number of environmental NGOs, as a percentage of all NGOs involved in social change, increased from 2% in 1953 to 14% in 1993. Citizen support for environmental NGOs has also increased. Membership in the WWF, for example, grew from about 570,000 in 1985 to 5.2 million in 1995. In the United States, the number of land trusts (i.e., NGOs involved in protecting biodiversity through the purchase and management of open space) has increased from 743 in 1988 to 1213 in 1998, and the amount of land set aside by these groups has more than doubled.

NGOs work at the local level through the organization and support of citizen education and action focused on local environmental issues and by incorporating an environmental dimension into social and economic development projects. Community conservation, a process by which local communities play a direct and active role in the management of natural resources such as forests and wildlife has become a major focus of NGOs interested in wildlife conservation

NGOs are also increasingly influencing public policy at the national and international levels. For example, the IUCN and the WWF played important roles in the successful efforts to ban the international trade in ivory in 1990 under the auspices of the CITES agreement by providing sound evidence of elephant population declines and by mobilizing public concern. While individual NGOs can be influential, NGO partnerships can be even more powerful. A number of powerful global NGO networks have been established to address specific environmental issues. Examples of such international environmental networks include BirdLife International, Pesticide Action Network, Climate Action Network, and the Biodiversity Action Network. Such networks strengthen the credibility of local member organizations and improve their capacity to influence national policy within their own countries. They have also given NGOs and the citizens they represent a stronger voice in multinational deliberations on global environmental matters, as welcomed participants at United Nations conferences on environmental policy or as unwelcomed protesters at international meetings such as the World Trade Organization meeting in Seattle in 1999.

The outreach and influence of environmental NGO networks has been further enhanced by access to the world wide web. The advent of the internet with its powerful capacity for dissemination and exchange of information has become an important catalyst for bringing people together around common causes. The internet engenders global awareness and support for local issues and has been an important tool for empowering local groups to address environmental concerns through grassroots activism.

Global Governance and Agreements

The scope of many environmental problems extends beyond national borders and must be addressed through international cooperation. There are two key elements to such cooperation. One is the establishment of durable institutions that can take on the responsibility of global governance pertaining to issues of the environment. The second is the promulgation, observance, and enforcement of international agreements on specific environmental issues that create a framework for defining problems and solutions, establishing rules of conduct, creating mechanisms for ensuring compliance, and providing avenues for conflict resolution.

The United Nations was created in 1945 as an institution of global governance to help maintain international peace and security, to promote human rights, and to foster international cooperation in solving international problems of economic, social, cultural, and humanitarian nature. Not surprisingly, as the global nature of environmental problems began to be re-

alized and documented over the last 50 years or so, the United Nations also expanded its role in addressing environmental issues. Initially, environmental mandates were integrated into existing UN agencies. The Food and Agriculture Organization (FAO), for example, began to consider environmental implications of agricultural development schemes in their work and, over time, became a strong advocate for sustainable agricultural practices that incorporate responsible management of natural resources. In 1972, a separate UN program was established, the UNEP (http://www.unep.org/), with headquarters in Nairobi, Kenya, to coordinate international efforts on environmental matters. UNEP has logged some significant achievements since its inception. In the area of biodiversity, UNEP coordinated efforts leading to the international Convention on Biodiversity in 1992. UNEP also administers CITES, the major international agreement protecting threatened species from extinction.

A number of important international environmental agreements have gone into effect in recent years to control hazardous wastes, ensure atmospheric quality, promote wise use of natural resources, conserve wildlife, and protect biodiversity. Major treaties and agreements, their objectives, and examples of their accomplishments are provided in Table 7-8. While the creation of treaties and agreements has been beneficial, more needs to be done. In examining the relationship between globalization and environmental health, French emphasizes the importance of strengthening global governance both through the strengthening of institutions such as UNEP and by improving compliance with existing multinational treaties.[16] To achieve greater compliance, French suggests that the following actions are required:

- Updating treaties in response to new scientific information or changing political circumstance

- Reliable and transparent reporting by signatories on progress with treaty implementation

- Provision of adequate funding and authority for administrative secretariats to oversee agreements properly

- Centralization, coordination, and streamlining of various administrative offices established to oversee different, but often related, environmental treaties and agreements

- More powerful enforcement tools, such as trade restrictions, to encourage treaty compliance

- Greater available financing to help signatories, especially in developing nations, to develop the human resources, technical capacity, infrastructure, and rule of law to comply with the terms of treaties

In addition to global treaties, there are also national laws and institutions that are extremely important in promoting environmental health and conservation of natural resources. In the

Table 7-8 Important Multinational Environmental Treaties Including Treaties Directly Related to Preservation of Biodiversity

Treaty or Agreement[a]	Inception	Parties	Objectives	Sample Accomplishments
International Whaling Convention *http://www.unep.ch/seas/main/legal/iwc.html*	1946	40	To protect whales from excessive harvesting; amended in 1992 to ban all commercial whaling of large whales	Significant reduction in the taking of whales from more than 66,000 in 1961 to about 1,500 annually at present
Antarctic Treaty *http://sedac.ciesin.org/pidb/texts/antarctic.treaty.protocol.1991.html*	1959	44	To promote scientific research and to protect Antarctica from dumping, development, and military activities	Mining exploration forbidden in Antarctica for 50 years
Convention on International Trade in Endangered Species of Wild Fauna and Flora (CITES) *http://www.cites.org*	1973	146	To protect endangered species by restricting trade in plants and animals threatened with extinction	Successful ban on ivory trade in 1990 to protect the African elephant
UN Convention on the Law of the Sea *http://www.un.org/Depts/los/index.htm*	1982	132	Establishes a framework for ocean development including 200-mile exclusive economic zones and provisions for reducing pollution, conservation of marine resources, and restoration of diminished species	Established a system for settling disputes on fishing and other matters of ocean use; in 1993, a global moratorium was imposed on all large-scale pelagic driftnet fishing on the high seas, including enclosed and semienclosed seas
Montreal Protocol on Substances that Deplete the Ozone Layer *http://www.unep.org/ozone/*	1987	172	End the use of chlorofluorocarbons (CFCs) and restrict the use of other ozone-depleting substances	Successful phaseout of manufacture and use of (CFCs) in industrial countries by 1996
Basel Convention *http://www.basel.int/*	1989	133	To control the international movement of hazardous wastes and to ban export of such wastes to developing countries	International agreement on definitions of which wastes are hazardous and nonhazardous; established rules on liability and compensation for damages caused by accidental spills of hazardous waste during export, import, or disposal
UN Framework Convention on Climate Change *http://www.unfccc.de/resource/conv/index.html*	1992	176	To slow the pace of global warming by stabilizing CO_2 emissions at 1990 levels and for countries to produce emissions inventories	Led to Kyoto Protocol in 1997 plus follow-up meetings to establish specific targets and timetables for control of carbon emissions
Convention on Biological Diversity *http://www.biodiv.org/convention/articles.asp*	1992	176	Creates an international framework for conservation and sustainable use of biological diversity; recognizes national sovereignty over biological resources and supports fair and equitable sharing of the benefits derived from use of genetic resources	Signatory nations developing national biodiversity inventories, biodiversity management plans, and the technical capacity to implement them
Convention on Desertification *http://www.unccd.int/main.php*	1994	159	To combat desertification through sustainable management of land and water resources with an emphasis on community participation	Developed national action programs for affected countries to combat desertification

[a]Internet addresses identify sources of the complete texts of treaties and subsequent amendments plus relevant links.

United States, for example, the Endangered Species Act (ESA), enacted in 1973, has been a valuable tool for conservationists involved in efforts to save a number of plant and animals species from imminent extinction in the United States. These animals include the bald eagle (*Haliaeetus leucocephalus*), the California condor (*Gymnogyps californianus*), the peregrine falcon (*Falco peregrinus*), the red wolf (*Canis rufus*), the California gray whale (*Eschrictius robustus*), the Virginia big-eared bat (*Plecotus townsendii virginianus*), the least Bell's vireo (*Vireo bellii pusillus*), and the black-footed ferret (*Mustela nigripes*) (Fig. 7-2). The ESA also has been instrumental in efforts to save many foreign species from extinction, because its terms include prohibition of importation of live specimens or products from endangered species into the United States. As of 1995, the ESA listed 535 nonindigenous species, including 252 endangered and 22 threatened mammalian species, which are banned from importation.

Not all countries however, have sufficient resources to enforce international treaties or national conservation laws. In many cases, countries that are the richest in biodiversity are the poorest in terms of economic development. Furthermore, in many nations, preservation of biodiversity and conservation of natural resources remain low governmental priorities because of indifference, corruption, cultural attitudes, or political expediency. The result is that international treaties and national laws written to protect wildlife are ignored or even flaunted (see sidebar "Houbara Brouhaha in Pakistan"). In

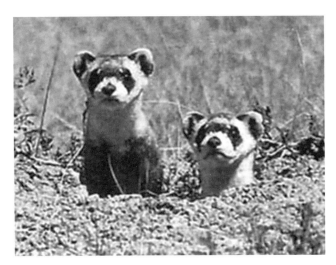

Figure 7-2. Black-footed ferrets looking out from a prairie dog hole. The story of the near extinction and subsequent recovery of the black-footed ferret is an important example of the role of disease in extinction. Disease has affected the conservation efforts of the black-footed ferret on two counts. First, outbreaks of the plague in prairie dogs threatened the ferret, as prairie dogs are its primary food supply. Then, outbreaks of canine distemper in the ferrets themselves almost completely eliminated the remaining population. Protection through the Endangered Species Act, captive breeding efforts, and comprehensive wildlife management plans have given the black-footed ferret a second chance. (Photo by Luther C. Goldman/ U.S. Fish and Wildlife Service)

such cases, grassroots efforts, often with the support of NGOs and other external agencies, assume greater importance in conservation efforts.

Local Capacity Building

Since much of the economic resources, technical expertise, and enthusiasm for wildlife conservation resides in developed countries, partnerships and outreach are important mechanisms for building local enthusiasm and capacity for efforts to preserve biodiversity within less-developed countries and to achieve actual progress in wildlife conservation. NGOs that focus on environmental issues are assuming an important and growing role in such efforts. International NGOs are increasingly forming partnerships with local NGOs, communities, schools, government officials, zoos, research institutions, and other interested parties to promote wildlife conservation through research, education, training, and action. The Wildlife Preservation Trusts (WPT) offers a good example to illustrate the scope and impact of such NGO action.

The WPT initially evolved out of the efforts of famed writer, naturalist, and zookeeper, Gerald Durrell, who founded the Jersey Zoological Park on the isle of Jersey in the English Channel Islands in 1959 and the Durrell Wildlife Conservation Trust in 1963. In 1971, Durrell established a sister organization in the United States, Wildlife Preservation Trust International, and in 1985, Wildlife Preservation Trust of Canada. Together these organizations have accomplished a great deal in protecting critically endangered species through a combination of efforts in the areas of species management, research, professional training, public education, and cultivation of international partnerships. Local capacity building has been a critical element in all of these efforts.

Species management efforts by WPT have included development of successful captive breeding techniques through careful studies of nutrition and behavior both in captivity and in the wild, restoration and protection of habitats, reintroduction of captive-bred individuals into natural habitats, and the ongoing management and protection of those habitats, all with direct involvement of local communities, indigenous scientists, in-country NGOs, and government officials. Through its species-management programs, WPT has brought some species back from the verge of extinction. For instance, there were only four known individuals of the Mauritius kestrel (*Falco punctatus*) when WPT became involved in their recovery. Now, through captive breeding and reintroduction, there are currently over 650 individuals in the wild, including over 100 breeding pairs.

The Jersey Zoological Park serves as an important site for research on reproductive techniques and other aspects of the captive breeding and rearing of endangered species, including identification and control of wildlife diseases. It is also, however, an important center for professional training of conservation workers from around the world. Over 800 trainees from 80 countries have received training at the International Training Centre for Breeding and Conservation of Endangered

Houbara Brouhaha in Pakistan

Enacting legislation to protect threatened wildlife is an important element in the conservation toolbox. However, if the spirit of the law is ignored and the letter of the law remains unenforced, little tangible benefit results. If the spirit and letter of the law are flagrantly violated, particularly by the very government responsible for enacting the laws, real harm can be done. Such appears to be the case in Pakistan relative to the Houbara bustard.

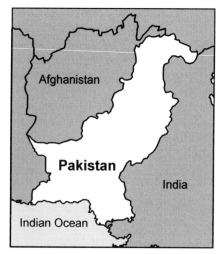

Map of Pakistan.

The Houbara bustard, *Chlamydotis undulata macqueenii,* is a large, striking bird of the deserts and semiarid grasslands of Asia, ranging from the Middle East to Mongolia. It is a migratory bird that nests in summer mainly in Central Asia and winters in South Asia, including Pakistan and the Middle East, though some populations are known to reside year round in these southern areas of the range. Houbara are capable of strong flight but have large powerful legs and, in daily activities, prefer to run or crouch and hide in the face of danger. The bird is mainly mottled brown, blending easily with its dryland habitat. During breeding season, males exhibit an elaborate courtship display. The bird is omnivorous, feeding on grains, berries, insects, lizards, and snakes. The nest is a shallow scrape on the ground, lined with feathers and leaves. The IUCN-World Conservation Union lists the Houbara bustard as a vulnerable species, with certain local populations threatened with extinction, particularly in the Gulf states of the Middle East. One significant pressure on this bird is habitat destruction from overgrazing of grasslands by livestock and conversion of grasslands to agricultural use with irrigation. The other important pressure is hunting, which brings the story back to Pakistan and the Arab hunting princes.

The Houbara bustard plays an important role in the cultural history of the nomadic peoples of the Arabian peninsula. The Arabs, over centuries, became great falconers, as falconry was a useful tool for ancient desert people to hunt game as a supplemental source of animal protein in an otherwise limited diet. The Houbara bustard, a large and meaty bird, became a prime target for Arab falconers. Today, hunting for the Houbara bustard persists in Arabian culture, but primarily as a recreational pastime for the wealthy elite. While falcons are still used, the arsenal of today's sheiks and princes has expanded to include fleets of four-wheel-drive vehicles, radar tracking equipment, and even infrared spotlights to find birds at night, which has made the Houbara hunt deadly efficient. As a result, most indigenous populations of Houbara bustard in the Gulf states have been brought to the verge of extinction, and the sheiks have looked elsewhere for their recreation, primarily Pakistan, which has become the principal venue for Houbara hunting by the Gulf states' elite.

Pakistan has been a party to the CITES since 1976. Three provinces in Pakistan, Punjab, Sindh, and Balochistan, where most of the Houbara occur, have provincial laws banning hunting of the Houbara bustard. Pakistani citizens themselves have been prohibited

Species. These trainees learn the fundamentals of conservation biology, get hands-on experience with a variety of animals and animal-management techniques, and conduct research, when possible, with the species they will be responsible for managing in their home countries. Much additional professional training occurs on-site and in-country through direct participation in WPT field projects. In Brazil, for instance, over 50 Brazilians have been trained in primate behavior, reintroduction and translocation methods, and census techniques in support of conservation efforts focused on lion tamarins.

Public education also plays an important role in promoting the success of local conservation efforts in developing countries where access to schools and electronic media may be limited. WPT began an education program in Brazil in communities close to the range of the endangered golden lion tamarin (*Leontopithecus rosalia rosalia*). Interviews revealed that many local peo-

ple simply did not know that the animal was endangered and occurred nowhere in the world but in their own backyard! An education campaign was then built on the foundation of establishing a strong sense of local pride of ownership for this beautiful and threatened animal. Through local efforts such as poster campaigns, school talks, art festivals, and the building of a local nature center, a strong sense of community conservation was created, and hunting of the golden lion tamarin for the illegal pet trade has been curtailed.

Linking conservation efforts directly to the needs of local people is another technique that the WPT have used in implementing their conservation programs. The Angonoka, or ploughshare tortoise (*Geochelone yniphora*), of Madagascar offers an example. Surveys of local villagers determined a number of factors that threatened their livelihood, including both uncontrolled bushpigs that trampled crops and brush fires that

from hunting the Houbara bustard since 1972. Yet each year, the federal government issues special permits to sheiks from Saudi Arabia and the emirates to come and hunt the Houbara bustard in Pakistan. While limits are ostensibly set on the number of birds that can be taken, no game wardens are permitted to accompany the hunting parties, and it is generally accepted that the limits are routinely exceeded. One conservative estimate is that the Arab hunters are taking at least 6,000 birds each year, even though an expert committee convened in 1983 set the country's total Houbara population (including migrants) at somewhere between 20,000 and 25,000.

Pakistan, as an Islamic republic, maintains strong cultural ties to the Gulf states. More to the point, it also maintains strong economic ties. Many Pakistanis emigrate to Saudi Arabia and the United Arab Emirates to find employment and income as service workers. The Arab nations also provide a considerable amount of direct economic aid to Pakistan. In 1992, it was estimated that the Gulf states supplied over US$3.5 billion annually to Pakistan in military aid, economic aid, and remittances to Pakistani workers. This is a substantial amount for a poor country like Pakistan, with an annual per capita income of US$350. Not surprisingly, critics of the Pakistan government argue that permission to hunt Houbara in Pakistan is a quid pro quo for the largesse of the wealthy Gulf state leaders.

The Houbara hunt gained international attention in 1992 in large part because of an article in the *New Yorker* magazine that detailed the extravagances and seeming illegality of the annual appearance in Pakistan of the Arab sheiks and princes.[56] Subsequently, conservationists in Pakistan, with support from international wildlife NGOs such as the WWF created much public awareness of the situation within Pakistan, including demonstrations to protest the apparent flaunting of provincial conservation law by the federal government. In 1993, in the face of this public outcry, the federal government vowed to discontinue granting special permits to foreigners to hunt the Houbara bustard. However, as recently as August 2000, internet postings on the subject still indicate that the federal government continues to grant special permits to wealthy Houbara hunters from the Gulf nations, and Houbara numbers continue to decline.

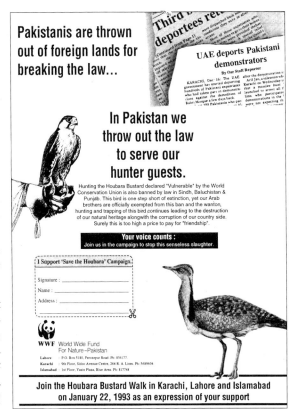

Pakistani newspaper advertisement for conservation rally.

spread to forests and destroyed trees needed for cooking and building homes, boats, and fences. Conservationists recognized that brush fires and rooting pigs also disrupted tortoise nesting in forest areas. Subsequently, efforts were made to set up village environmental committees to control fires, set up bush-pig traps, and establish tree nurseries for replanting. As a result of these efforts to protect the forest for the benefit of local people, the nesting habitats of the Angonoka tortoise also would be protected.

Tools for Wildlife Conservation

Conducting scientific inquiries, collecting accurate data, monitoring environmental trends, creating public awareness, establishing institutions of global governance, abiding by environmental treaties, and building local capacity for implementation of conservation programs are all important elements of the framework necessary to achieve progress in preserving biodiversity. Once the framework is in place, there are a number of tools that conservationists can draw upon to accomplish specific goals in the protection of wildlife species. These tools can be applied in two broad areas of effort: *in situ* conservation activities, which focus on the protection and management of wild species where they naturally occur, and *ex situ* conservation activities, which focus on the propagation and safe keeping of particular species in places apart from their natural habitats, which often are under siege. *In situ* and *ex situ* conservation efforts are linked through the hope that threatened species can be maintained in captivity until such time that degraded habitats are restored and protected sufficiently to allow the reintroduction of captive populations into the wild.

In Situ Efforts in Wildlife Conservation

Tools available in the conservation toolbox for *in situ* protection of wildlife include the creation and management of protected areas and the wild species they contain, community participation in conservation efforts, and the development of sustainable opportunities for the nonconsumptive and consumptive use of wildlife resources.

Establishing Protected Areas

As habitat degradation is a principal cause of species loss, the creation of protected areas where human activity is restricted represents a major tool for conservationists in the fight to protect wildlife. As part of its overall conservation mission, the IUCN maintains the Program on Protected Areas to promote the establishment and successful management of a global network of terrestrial and marine preservation sites. In 1994, IUCN published a classification system for protected areas based on the amount of human activity permitted. These areas can be grouped into strictly protected areas and partially protected areas. Strictly protected areas include strict nature reserves, wilderness areas, national parks, and national monuments. Partially protected areas include habitat/species-management areas, protected landscapes and seascapes, and managed resource-protected areas. More-detailed descriptions and definitions of these categories is available at the IUCN website, http://wcpa.iucn.org/

In 1998, according to data from the World Resources Institute, there were 4502 strictly protected areas around the world, encompassing approximately 500 million hectares. In addition, there were 5899 partially protected areas, covering an additional 348 million hectares. This represents about 6% of Earth's total land surface, with only 4% in the strictly protected categories, although some biodiversity advocates suggest that at least 10% of Earth's land area needs strict protection to forestall a global extinction crisis. With regard to marine ecosystems, only about 1% of Earth's marine environment is currently included in protected areas. Among the largest and best known are the Great Barrier Reef Marine Park in Australia, Greenland National Park, Galapagos Marine Park in Ecuador, and the Netherlands's North Sea Reserve. While there has been a general positive trend over the last 50 years in the increased acquisition and designation of protected areas, there is still a good deal to be accomplished.

In an analysis of the state of the world's protected areas at the end of the 20th century, Green and Pierce identified several major gaps in the protected areas network at global, regional, and national levels.[20] These include

- A very limited marine component, in comparison to the terrestrial component

- A preponderance of small, rather than large, protected areas, jeopardizing their integrity and long-term ecological viability

- A lack of application of the full range of IUCN management categories in some regions, limiting benefits from the full spectrum of services for which protected areas are intended

- Unmet targets in the representation of major biomes within the global network, particularly with respect to temperate grasslands and lake systems

- A majority (66%) of countries and dependent territories with less than 10% of their total land area represented in protected areas, and 20% with less than 1% represented

Historically, protected areas have been acquired and managed by governments, but increasingly, land is being acquired for conservation purposes by NGOs, including private land trusts and wildlife conservation groups. Partnerships between national and local governments, local NGOs and international NGOs, commercial interests, and local communities for the acquisition and management of protected areas are a growing phenomenon. The Nature Conservancy, for example, is the largest land trust in the United States, with over 4.8 million ha protected within the United States. However, Nature Conservancy also protects 25.0 million ha outside the United States, focusing on the acquisition of land to protect biodiversity in over 27 nations around the world, with a strong emphasis in Latin America, the Caribbean, and the Asian Pacific region. In 1990, the organization launched the Parks in Peril Program specifically to strengthen the management of 37 parks encompassing over 11.3 million ha in 15 countries of Latin America and the Caribbean. Many of these parks existed "on paper" only, with few resources available and little enforcement authority exercised to actually protect the biodiversity contained within. With funding from the US Agency for International Development, Nature Conservancy worked with governments in Mexico, Belize, Jamaica, Dominican Republic, Dominica, Guatemala, Honduras, Costa Rica, Panama, Colombia, Ecuador, Peru, Bolivia, Paraguay, and Brazil to strengthen local capacity for park management through training, research, policing, infrastructure development, and greater involvement of local communities (http://nature.org/aboutus/projects/parks/).

Acquiring Land for Targeted Species

Selection of lands for protection may be driven by a number of purposes including recreational use, the existence of unique land forms, or traditional cultural uses. While these are worthwhile reasons for protection in their own right, they may not necessarily optimize efforts to conserve wildlife. A 1998 study in Massachusetts by the Nature Conservancy and the Massachusetts Division of Fisheries and Wildlife underscores this point.[3] Fully one fourth of the land area of Massachusetts is protected from development, with 0.5 million ha of open space having been acquired over the last century for a variety of purposes including protection of water supplies, farmland, and recreational areas. While the preservation of biodiversity was accomplished in some cases, it was not always the overriding priority in selecting land for protection. Therefore, while Massachusetts has an admirable record in the preservation of open space, a large number of plant and animals species remain threatened. This is because the historic pattern of land acquisition did not reflect the ecological distribution of threatened species in certain areas of the state. For example, all the mountaintops in the Berkshires are protected, while only 15% of the lower elevations of the mountains are protected. The mountaintops are home to only 12 rare species, while the lower, unprotected portions harbor 112 rare species. Overall, Massachusetts has 424 plant and animal species on its threatened and endangered list. Over half the reptile species in the state, such as the bog turtle (*Clemmys muhlenbergii*) and the redbelly turtle (*Pseudemys rubriventris*) remain threatened through habitat loss, as well as 16% of all plant and vertebrate animal species, despite the 0.5 million ha already protected. The report concludes, however, that it would require acquisition of only 36,500 additional ha of land specifically targeted as important habitat in key locations to protect an additional 70% of the imperiled plant and animal species in the state.

Linking protected areas to biodiversity preservation of course requires considerable scientific knowledge about the distribution and behavior of, and threats to, endangered species and underscores how important valid scientific information is in helping to shape public policy. On a global scale, the same process is taking place with regard to the Biodiversity Hotspots Initiative discussed earlier in this chapter. Accumulated knowledge about biodiversity obtained by conservation biologists and other scientists working in the field has led to the understanding that advantageous "rates of return" can be calculated for investments in habitat protection with regard to the number of species protected when the appropriate areas are targeted for protection.

Corridor Development

Even when land is set aside for the purpose of protecting biodiversity, the results may be less than intended. In some cases, the size of the area of land protected does not suffice to fully support the populations of animals residing within. This is particularly true for large mammals, who may require extensive acreage to provide sufficient food resources. For instance, it is estimated that a population of 390 grizzly bears requires an area of over 80,600 km² to thrive in the Rocky Mountain environment. This is over 9 times the size of Yellowstone National Park and almost 12 times the size of Banff National Park in Canada. Migratory behavior also may not be accommodated by the existing layout of protected areas, with roads, canals, fences, and large-scale development disrupting access to seasonal food supplies or breeding grounds. Unfortunately, such fragmentation of habitat by human artifact is widespread and often poses a threat to the viability of isolated populations and, in some cases, entire species populations.

One important development in conservation science to overcome the obstacles of fragmentation in protected areas is the development of corridors that link habitat islands and reconnect isolated populations to necessary breeding sites, food supplies, or other population groups for mating. The corridor concept may be applied locally on a small scale or regionally on a grand scale. Localized efforts to overcome the constraints of fragmentation include placing culverts under country roads in rural England to help frogs and salamanders reach aquatic breeding sites in the spring, constructing overpasses on the Trans-Canada highway to allow wolves to cross safely in search of prey, and suspending ropes between trees over roads to create aerial bridges for howler monkeys or black lion tamarin in Latin America. On a larger scale, some major initiatives are under way to establish corridors to link protected areas. Two in particular are the Yellowstone to Yukon Initiative in North America, and the Meso-American Biological Corridor that is planned to run through all of Central America.

The Yellowstone to Yukon (Y2Y) Initiative (http://www.rockies.ca/y2y/) is a carefully planned, long-range effort to restore the Rocky Mountain range of North America, fragmented by two centuries of development, to a fully functional mountain ecosystem able to support secure and viable populations of a wide range of species, including grizzly bear (*Ursus horribilis*), black bear (*Ursus americanus*), gray wolf (*Canis lupus*), cougar (*Puma concolor*), lynx (*Lynx canadensis*), wolverine (*Gulo luscus*), fisher (*Martes pennanti*), marten (*Martes americana*), moose (*Alces alces*), elk (*Cervus canadensis*), woodland caribou (*Rangifer caribou*), bighorn sheep (*Ovis canadensis*), mountain goat (*Oreamnos americanus*), bull trout (*Salvelinus confluentus*) and Arctic grayling (*Thymallus arcticus*). The intended corridor will be approximately 3200 km long and 480 km wide. Coordination of the Y2Y Initiative began in earnest in 1991 and involves the active participation of over 80 organizations including the governments of Canada and the United States, various provincial and state agencies, Native American groups, environmental NGOs, commercial interests, and communities within or bordering the corridor area. It involves acquisition of new protected lands as well as agreements with private land owners to secure a network of strategic core wildlife reserves linked by wildlife movement corridors and protected by surrounding transitional or buffer zones that allow human activity but keep major industrial transformations at a distance.

Central America accounts for only 1% of Earth's land mass but contains at least 8% of the world's known plant and animal species. Habitat fragmentation has been severe in Central America, due to high rates of human population growth, deforestation, agricultural expansion, and urbanization. The 2400-km Meso-American Biological Corridor (MABC) was launched in 1996, building on earlier efforts aimed at reestablishing a natural corridor throughout the original range of the Florida panther (*Puma concolor coryi*), which included North, Central, and South America. The MABC is intended to create a continuous ribbon of forest from northern Belize, on the border with Mexico, through southern Panama, to the border with Colombia. Prior to the MABC initiative, Central American countries collectively had established 461 protected areas in the region. However, over half of these areas are considered too small to play a significant role in protecting biodiversity, hence the need for, and value of, the corridor concept.

While the creation of corridors is a valuable tool for conservationists, it is not a panacea. One potential problem with corridor development and the attendant facilitation of extensive animal movement is the spread of disease. Some man-made obstacles to animal movement were created purposely to prevent the spread of disease. For example, in South Africa and Botswana, hundreds of kilometers of cordon fences have been erected to keep migrating wildlife separate from cattle to prevent the transmission of foot and mouth disease, which would interfere with the cattle export business. In general, various diseases of wild animals may spread from infected to naive populations of the same species, may spill over into domestic animal species, or may have zoonotic potential as well. There is a real and necessary role for veterinarians to play in the planning, design, management, and long-term monitoring of proposed wildlife corridors. For example, veterinarians with the Center for Conservation Medicine at Tufts University (http://www.tufts.edu/vet/ccm/Y2Y.htm) are involved in assessing the risks of disease, particularly zoonotic disease, associated with the Y2Y initiative. Among the diseases of concern already identified for study are brucellosis, tuberculosis, plague, hantavirus infections, and chronic wasting disease of elk, which appears to be a transmissible spongiform encephalopathy similar to bovine spongiform encephalopathy and scrapie, though its potential as a zoonotic infection remains unknown.

Protection of Keystone Species

The dictionary defines a *keystone* as the stone at the top of an arch that supports the other stones and keeps the whole arch from falling. Conservation biologists define a *keystone species* as a plant or animal in a given ecosystem that plays a critical or central role in maintaining the overall balance of biodiversity within that ecosystem by providing key services that if lost can produce a domino, or cascade, effect leading to the gradual degradation or collapse of the ecosystem. There are numerous well-known examples. Fig trees are critical to rainforest ecosystems because their fruit are a major source of food for a wide variety of birds, mammals, insects, and reptiles. Elephants are considered keystone species in grassland savanna systems as they are critical to maintaining grass growth by controlling brush incursion, which is vital to the large populations of grass-grazing ungulates in the ecosystem. Many predatory species such as wolves are keystone species because they keep prey populations in check, prohibiting them from expanding beyond the carrying capacity of the ecosystem's forage supply. Pollinating species such as bees and bats can be keystone species because the major plant species in the ecosystem depend on them for propagation.

The sea otter (*Enhydra lutris*) is a keystone species in the marine kelp forest ecosystem. Kelp forests provide food and shelter for large numbers of species of fish and shellfish. Sea otters prey on sea urchins, which in turn consume kelp. If sea otters are not present to keep sea urchins in check, the urchins cause severe declines in the kelp forests and their associated species. Wherever otters been eliminated, kelp forest communities decline. Where otters are reintroduced, kelp communities have returned.

The black-tailed prairie dog (*Cynomys ludovicianus*) is a keystone species of the American prairie. This animal is believed to provide critical services to as many as 170 different vertebrate species, including the endangered black-footed ferret. The near extinction of the black-footed ferret (*Mustela nigripes*) is linked to the persecution of the prairie dog as a rangeland pest. When farmers and ranchers poisoned prairie dogs, ferrets, which consume prairie dogs as a principal food source, suffered relay toxicity. A solid understanding the natural history of a keystone species and its role in the ecosystem are important prerequisites for developing meaningful conservation efforts and habitat-management plans.

Certain species may also serve as "flagship," or "umbrella," species. If a species is charismatic enough to capture the attention, concern, or affection of the public, it may serve as a catalyst for conservation efforts in its particular habitat, even if it does not necessarily provide key services in the ecosystem. Generating public support for protecting the charismatic species can be good for the species itself and also can have a distinct umbrella effect of protecting all the other species that share its habitat. Wildlife Trust, in its work with the black lion tamarin (*Leontopithecus chrysopygus*) in Brazil, promotes the animal as a flagship species to mobilize efforts to help preserve the severely threatened Atlantic forest and all its denizens. Listed as one of the 25 global biodiversity hotspots, the Atlantic forest today is highly fragmented and has been reduced to only 7% of its original land area. The black lion tamarin is now the logo of Wildlife Trust, just as the panda (*Ailuropoda melanoleuca*), another flagship species, is the logo of the WWF.

Reintroductions and Translocations

Reintroduction of wild species into natural habitats has emerged as an important tool for wildlife conservation. Scientific advances in captive breeding of animals and plants in zoos, aquaria, and plant conservatories have not only protected an increasing number of species from extinction, but also have created opportunities for placing species back into the wild in sufficient numbers to allow them, at least potentially, to become reestablished in their natural environment. Similarly, successful wildlife-management efforts in some locales have protected certain species to the point that "excess" animals are available for translocation to other sites where populations of the same species have been dramatically reduced or eliminated.

The successful reintroduction of native species, of course, is not simply a matter of having enough individuals to return to the wild. Every imperiled species is threatened for varied and complex reasons related to issues of habitat degradation, overexploitation, disease, competition from invasive species, or cultural prejudice. Underlying problems must be identified, addressed, and corrected before reintroductions are made, so that the reintroduced plants or animals have a reasonable chance for a new start. For example, in Uganda, during the civil unrest of the 1970s and 1980s, wildlife populations in the country's national parks were decimated by roving bands of soldiers and bandits with automatic weapons. Now that the rule of law has returned to the country, efforts to restore wildlife resources can be addressed. Some residual populations of indigenous animals are rebounding on their own, while in other cases, reintroductions are required. In remote Kidepo Park in Uganda's northeast corner, for instance, three Rothschild giraffes were reintroduced from Lake Nakuru National Park in Kenya in 1997. In the Luwero region of the country, elephant numbers have so rebounded that the animals are causing problems for farmers by raiding crops. Translocation of these elephants to Murchison Falls National Park, where elephant numbers are still low, was initiated in 1999.

Translocation is the general term for the movement of living organisms from one area, with free release in another. While translocations for conservation purposes are increasing, most translocations are done for sport and recreational purposes and involve the introduction or restocking of game animals, game birds, and sport fish. Other translocation activities include release of rescued or rehabilitated wildlife or the release of pets into the wild, as well as the movement of captive wild species for commercial purposes, such as deer farming or private game parks. These alternative livestock and captive wildlife industries are expanding rapidly, especially in the United States. In Texas alone, between 1966 and 1996, the number of non-indigenous ungulates, increased from 37,500 to 198,000. The American bison industry is reported to be growing by 30% per year, with over 250,000 bison present in 1997, compared with 30,000 in 1972. In reviewing recorded translocations in the United States, Canada, Australia, and New Zealand between the years 1973 and 1986, Griffith et al. found that translocations occurred at an average rate of 515 per year. Only 7% involved threatened or endangered species, while 92% involved game species and 1% involved other species.[21]

In many cases, species introduced in translocation efforts may not be indigenous to the area of release and therefore must be considered as invasive species with the potential to transmit disease or displace local species. The widespread practice of translocation is a major concern to conservation organizations, agricultural agencies, and animal and public health officials. One example of a translocation which had the potential to adversely affect wildlife, domestic livestock, and humans involved an outbreak of bovine tuberculosis in captive bison in South Dakota in 1985. Epidemiological investigations found that the bison herd had been exposed in 1982 to tuberculous ranched elk that were later depopulated. In the interim, over 370 potentially infected bison had been shipped to 87 herds in 20 states, exposing over 2450 additional bison and approximately 4190 cattle to possible tuberculosis. Subsequently, 18 bison herds were identified as infected, requiring implementation of control measures, and payment of indemnity.

Disease transmission has clearly emerged as a major concern associated with translocations. The specter of disease is especially worrisome in wildlife reintroductions involving endangered species with small extant populations, as the introduction of disease into such populations can have devastating consequences. The situation with the golden lion tamarin (*Leontopithecus rosalia*) illustrates this potential danger. The golden lion tamarin, a primate native to the Atlantic coastal rain forest in Brazil, is classified as critically endangered by the IUCN. Efforts to raise golden lion tamarin in captivity have been reasonably successful. However, efforts to reintroduce captive-bred tamarin into the wild were derailed by disease. As reported by Montali et al., captive tamarin at a zoo in the United States contracted viral hepatitis as a result of being fed mice infected with lymphocytic choriomeningitis virus (LCMV).[36] This arenavirus is not a naturally occurring infection in free-living tamarin, so wild populations would have to be considered naive for LCMV. The reintroduction of infected individuals to the wild, therefore, could be catastrophic for indigenous populations of the primate. The presence of this disease now means that all captive tamarin have to be screened for LCMV before reintroduction can be considered.

Not only may introduced animals spread disease to existing wild populations, but the reverse may occur as well. Captive-bred animals born and raised far from their native habitat often have no experience with indigenous parasites and pathogens that are enzootic in the area where they are to be released and, therefore, may succumb to these infectious agents or parasites following reintroduction. Even wild-caught animals that are reintroduced into new regions may fall prey to local diseases if those diseases were not present in their home range, but exist at the reintroduction site. Additional examples of reintroduced animals bringing disease to local populations and local populations transmitting disease to introduced animals are given in Tables 7-9a and 7-9b, respectively. Woodford strongly recommends that captive breeding facilities be established near release areas, to increase the likelihood that captive and wild animals will experience the same pathogens and parasites prior to release and at the same time be less likely to be exposed to exotic parasites present in foreign environments such as zoos on other continents.[60]

To minimize the effects of disease in reintroductions, a number of things are required. First is for more-complete information about the infectious, parasitic, and hereditary diseases of wild animal species and their susceptibility to diseases for which they may not be known natural hosts, but to which they may be exposed in captivity. Health-monitoring programs should be in place wherever source populations of animals are maintained for reintroduction. Second, all animals should be examined and appropriately tested by knowledgeable veterinarians prior to release. Griffith et al., in their translocation survey, discovered that in 24% of the translocations recorded, no professional examination of animals for parasites, disease, or injury was carried out.[21] Third, more information is needed about disease and parasite occurrence in wild populations present in release areas and their potential impact on reintroduced animals. Fourth, all reintroductions need to include some follow-up effort to track disease occurrence in reintroduced individuals and native populations, including, whenever

Table 7-9 Examples of Disease Problems Associated with Translocations

Part a. Situations in Which the Translocated Animals Introduced Disease into the Area of Release and Caused Disease in Local Animals of the Same and Other Species

Species Translocated	Source of Animals	Disease(s) Introduced	Release Area	Species Affected
Reindeer (*Rangifer tarandus*)	Captive bred in Norway	Warble flies, nostril flies	Greenland	Woodland caribou (*Rangifer tarandus*)
Mojave desert tortoise (*Gopherus agassizii*)	Pet shops in California	Mycoplasmal respiratory infections	Mojave Desert	Wild tortoises
Plains bison (*Bison bison*)	Captive bred in Montana	Tuberculosis and brucellosis	Canada	Wood bison (*Bison bison athabascae*)
Rainbow Trout (*Oncorhynchus mykiss*)	Captive bred in the US	"whirling disease"	United Kingdom	Trout
Raccoons (*Procyon lotor*)	Wild caught in southeastern US	Rabies	Northeastern US	Raccoons and other wild and domestic mammals
Bighorn sheep (*Ovis canadensis*)	Wild caught in Arizona	Viral pneumonia	New Mexico	Bighorn sheep

Part b. Situations in Which Introduced Animals Contracted Disease from Animals or Animal Disease Vectors Already Present in the Release Area

Species Translocated	Source of Animals	Disease Encountered	Release Area	Source of Pathogen
Koala (*Phascolarctos cinereus*)	Wild caught in Victoria, Australia	Tick paralysis	Victoria, Australia	Toxic agent in saliva of *Ixodes* spp. ticks
Lechwe (*Kobus leche*)	Wild caught in Zambia	Heartwater (*Cowdria ruminantium*) in *Amblyomma* spp. ticks	South Africa	Enzootic in local wild ruminants
Caribou (*Rangifer tarandus*)	Wild caught in Eastern US	Cerebrospinal nematodiasis (*Parelaphostrongylus tenuis*)	Ontario, Canada	White tail deer (*Odocoileus virginianus*)
Hawaiian goose (*Branta sandivicensis*)	Captive bred in the UK	Avian tuberculosis (*Mycobacterium avium*)	Hawaii	Local birds
Black rhinoceros (*Diceros bicornis*)	Wild caught in the Kenya highlands	Trypanosomiasis	Lowland Kenya	Via tsetse flies from local wildlife and domestic livestock.

Adapted from Woodford MH. International disease implications for wildlife translocation. J Zoo Wildl Med 1993;24(3):265–270.

References for each example are provided in this paper.

possible, necropsies on dead animals and, if feasible, periodic sampling of relevant indices such as serological titers, fecal examinations for parasites, or microbial isolations from available excretions or discharges. Radio tracking and other identification methods can help facilitate this process. Again, Griffith et al. found that in less than 25% of the translocations they surveyed were there sufficient data collected to determine the proportion of translocated animals that were lost to disease.[21]

Cooperative international efforts are also needed to ensure that timely information is available about disease problems occurring in different countries. The Office International des Epizooties (OIE), based in Paris, has been involved in monitoring and reporting disease statistics in livestock to assist in matters of trade and disease control since 1924 and also sets the standards for accepted diagnostic testing for livestock disease. The OIE now has a working group on wildlife diseases that compiles and reports wildlife disease occurrence around the world as well. The Federation of American Scientists (FAS) has also organized an email network of animal disease reporting known as AHEAD, an acronym for animal health and emerging animal diseases, which is part of the FAS ProMED disease-reporting system. AHEAD is available on the internet at http://www.fas.org/ahead/index.html.

The Veterinary Specialist Group (VSG) of the IUCN is also involved in trying to improve information and standards associated with disease risks in wildlife translocation. The VSG is working with the OIE to improve wildlife disease surveillance, to develop risk-analysis methods and procedures for proposed international wildlife translocations, to harmonize regulations for international translocations, to standardize diagnostic procedures for wildlife diseases, and to standardize vaccination procedures and immunization schedules for wildlife. In 2000, the VSG announced the publication of a relevant and important booklet entitled *Quarantine and Health Screening Protocols for Wild Animals prior to Translocation and Release into the Wild* in support of their effort to limit disease spread associated with animal movement.

Clearly, there is a tremendous need for veterinarians to become involved in addressing disease issues related to reintroduction efforts. While veterinarians have already contributed much in this area, their contributions may not be adequately recognized beyond the confines of the veterinary profession. Cunningham, writing on the disease risks of wildlife translocations in the journal *Conservation Biology*, made the following observation[10]: "Threats posed to conservation programs by translocation of pathogens along with the translocation of host species are being increasingly recognized. However, publications on this subject have appeared primarily in veterinary literature which often is not read widely by those who fund, plan, or carry out the majority of wildlife translocations." The message is clear. Veterinarians need to become better integrated with the conservation community at large, make their knowledge and skills more widely known, help to establish conservation priorities, and then work as part of the conservation team to ensure successful outcomes.

Species Management Plans

Many threatened and endangered species, especially those with small populations, require special, focused conservation efforts if they are going to survival in the wild. The IUCN, the leading independent, science-based, multinational agency involved directly in wildlife conservation, plays a major role in these efforts through its Species Survival Commission and the Species Specialist Groups (SSGs) contained within it. The headquarters of the Species Survival Commission (SSC) is in Gland, Switzerland. However, the SSC is described by the IUCN itself as a "knowledge network" of approximately 7000 volunteers working in almost every country in the world. This widely dispersed knowledge network includes wildlife researchers, wildlife veterinarians, zoo specialists, marine biologists, park managers, government officials, and recognized experts with special expertise in various biological groupings including birds, mammals, amphibians, reptiles, plants, and invertebrates. The SSC serves as the main source of advice to the IUCN and its members on the technical aspects of species conservation.

One important role the SSC plays in species conservation is in the preparation and distribution of the IUCN Red List of Threatened Species discussed earlier in this chapter. Other activities of the SSC include: providing technical and scientific advice to governments, secretariats of international environmental treaties, and conservation organizations; publication of conservation-related information; organization of training, technical, and policy workshops; implementation of field-based conservation projects; and raising funds for conservation research. The current strategic plan of the SSC is available on the internet at http://www.iucn.org/themes/ssc/news/stratplanintro.htm.

The SSC network of members is organized into approximately 110 (SSGs), which are primarily taxon-based and focus on the challenges of conserving individual species, for instance, the African elephant (*Loxodonta africana*), or groups of related species, for instance, wild canids. A full list of the IUCN SSGs is available on the internet at http://www.iucn.org/themes/ssc/sgs/sgs.htm. Each SSG, with its volunteer group of specialists, maintains current information about the species on which it focuses, including their biology, habitat, distribution, population status, protection status, principal threats, and conservation action plans. These data have multiple uses such as updating the Red List, identifying research priorities for species protection, advising governments on policy formulation, and providing technical information to other conservation agencies and organizations.

In addition to the taxon-based SSGs, there are a number of discipline-based SSGs, including the Veterinary Specialist Group, the Re-introduction Specialist Group, the Invasive Species Specialist Group, the Sustainable Use Specialist Group, and the Conservation Breeding Specialist Group. The VSG provides technical, advisory, and policy-related services to the conservation community at large and within the SSC. The VSG has also been involved in developing policies and guidelines for the capture, restraint, and care of wildlife during research or conservation efforts.

The Conservation Breeding Specialist Group (CBSG) has developed a very valuable program for the conservation of threatened species with small remaining populations, known as the Population and Habitat Viability Assessment (PHVA). PHVA workshops are conducted as an exercise to assess the extinction risks facing a particular species and to develop and test management strategies that can serve as the basis of policies and actions in the field aimed at protecting that species. PHVA workshops are organized and conducted in coordination with other agencies and organizations that have a stake or interest in the preservation of the particular species to be assessed. The PHVA is held in the country or region where the species is found so that local conservation groups and government officials from relevant agencies can attend and participate.

In December 1997, for instance, a PHVA for the mountain gorilla (*Gorilla gorilla beringei*) was held in Kampala, Uganda. The workshop was held as a collaborative effort of the CBSG in conjunction with the Primate Specialist Group of the IUCN SSC, and representative agencies from the governments of the three countries where gorillas reside, Uganda and its neighbors Rwanda and the Congo. The focus of the workshop was captured in its rather direct title "Can the Mountain Gorilla Survive?" Over a period of 5 days, about 70 participants divided into working groups to characterize and discuss various threats to the mountain gorilla in its natural habitat and to develop recommendations for addressing those threats. The working groups included Health and Disease; Human Population Issues; Population Biology and Simulation Modeling; Management and Research; Governance; and Finance, Revenue, and Economics. These working group designations illustrate the range of expertise represented in the workshop and the diversity of problems and challenges that need to be considered to devise and implement an effective species-survival plan for the mountain gorilla (see sidebar "Gorillas in the Midst . . . of Trouble").

One important feature of the PHVA workshops is the use of a computer-simulation modeling tool known as VORTEX.[30] The program name draws on the concept of the extinction vortex, in which populations diminish to a small enough size that they cannot sustain or rebound and, therefore, spiral to extinction. VORTEX models population dynamics as discrete, sequential events that occur according to defined probabilities. Workshop participants, with their diverse expertise, provide specific data or best estimates on the various parameters to be included in the model: male-female population ratios, age at first breeding, prolificacy, life span, foraging range, etc. Veterinarians provide information about the species susceptibility to different diseases, the risks of such diseases occurring, and expected morbidity and mortality associated with each disease. All the input is analyzed by the VORTEX program to produce statistics that summarize the demographic and genetic stability of the population under study. This information allows conservationists to assess the short-, medium-, and long-range prospects of the species for survival or extinction and identifies the factors that pose the greatest threat to extant populations. Thus, VORTEX helps conservationists and policymakers develop strategies and programs that promote species survival. A list of the PHVAs that have been carried out by the CBSG is available on the CBSG website at http://www.cbsg.org/.

Rescue and Rehabilitation

The rescue and rehabilitation of wild animals has become a well-organized activity over the past 20 years. Wild animal rescue gained wide public attention and considerable public support in association with the strong animal rescue response that

occurred after highly publicized oil spills such as the Exxon Valdez in Alaska in 1989. Veterinarians have played an ever-increasing role in wildlife rescue and rehabilitation. Many veterinary colleges now maintain wildlife clinics, and students rotate through these clinics as part of their clinical training as veterinarians. An extensive network of rehabilitation and rescue centers exists in the United States, and rehabilitation efforts are increasing elsewhere around the world at a rapid rate. Professional associations of rehabilitators exist at the national and international levels. Veterinarians from developed countries are often involved in rehabilitation efforts and the creation of rehabilitation centers in developing countries. Special considerations for working on wildlife rehabilitation in developing countries have been reviewed by Dr. William Karesh of the Field Veterinary Program of the Wildlife Conservation Society in New York.[26]

Considerable debate exists about the role of rescue and rehabilitation in wildlife conservation. Some conservationists are critical of these efforts because they divert important energy and resources away from protecting populations of species and their habitats to save individual animals that may represent species neither endangered nor threatened. For example, costs per oiled bird treated in rehabilitation efforts following the Exxon Valdez spill have been estimated in the range of $600 per bird to as high as $15,000 per bird, while mortality rates in treated and released birds were high. Critics of such efforts argue that the money could be better spent on other conservation efforts, for example, targeted land purchase to protect habitat for endangered species. Ethics and politics notwithstanding, the fact is that efforts to save individuals from non-threatened species have generated a significant and important body of knowledge about the handling, restraint, behavior, nutrition, and clinical management of disease and injury in wild species.

In the case of critically endangered species, where a small, countable number of individuals represents the entire existing population, the distinction between individual animals and populations of animals becomes moot. In such cases, efforts to save individuals become equivalent to saving populations. At such times, the conservation community can be thankful that rescue and rehabilitation efforts have produced a cadre of confident and accomplished practitioners armed with relevant experience and knowledge of procedures and practices that save the lives of animals in trouble.

Take for example, the case of the Kemp's ridley sea turtles (*Lepidochelys kempi*), one of the rarest sea turtles in the world, and categorized as critically endangered in the IUCN Red List. Only 6000 to 7000 breeding adult Kemp's ridley sea turtles are estimated to be alive today. These turtles are migratory, moving each autumn from the North Atlantic, along the eastern coast of the United States, to the Gulf of Mexico. If water temperatures in Cape Cod Bay drop below 50°F before the turtles have cleared the area, then the turtles will become cold shocked and, with mobility impaired, may be driven onto the beaches of Cape Cod where exposure and wind will quickly lead to death from hypothermia. In 1999, up to 300 Kemp's ridley sea turtles washed up on the north-facing beaches of Cape Cod, some already dead on arrival. However, because of organized rescue efforts involving local citizens, the Massachusetts Audubon Society, and the New England Aquarium, as many as 127 of the stranded turtles were quickly located by citizen beach patrols, rewarmed, stabilized, and then transported to the New England Aquarium for veterinary assessment (Fig. 7-3). Fully recovered turtles were then transported by air to Florida for further rehabilitation and, when possible, release. About 80% of the treated turtles survived and were released to the wild. The cold-shock strandings and the rescue efforts are potentially an annual event, and the rescue teams remain vigilant, with successful protocols in place to assist an endangered species that might otherwise perish.

Community Participation in Conservation

The old adage that you can't please all of the people all of the time certainly pertains to the issue of wildlife conservation. Efforts to protect wildlife often come into direct conflict with competing human needs or interests. To be successful and sustainable, conservation programs must take these competing needs and interests into account. Toward this end, in recent years, there has been a growing effort among policymakers to identify and include all potential stakeholders in the planning of new proposed wildlife conservation initiatives and actions.

A case in point is the effort to develop a management plan for the bison (*Bison bison*) of Yellowstone National Park. These bison have been determined to carry brucellosis and are thus perceived as a threat to the cattle industry in the state of Montana and a potential threat to the public health. Development of a long-range management plan and an environmental impact statement for protecting the bison of Yellowstone while satisfying the concerns of the cattle industry, local residents, and health officials required numerous revisions over many years and involved the input of hundreds of state and federal agencies, Native American tribes, interested organizations, and individuals during public comment periods. The Final Environmental Impact Statement was published in August 2000 by the National Park Service of the U.S. Department of Interior. Initial discussions between federal and state agencies began in 1992. Not incidentally, the technical input of veterinary authorities was a critical element in developing the management plan.

While consensus may be hoped for in conflicts surrounding conservation issues, it is inherent in the process that everyone's desired outcomes will not be fully met. In developed countries, resolution of conflict is usually achieved nonetheless. In strong economies, stakeholders hurt financially by conservation agreements can often find alternative livelihoods or can negotiate some compensation for their perceived losses. Even when there are "sore losers," a strong legal system, general respect for the rule of law, and adequate resources for law enforcement and regulatory oversight usually result in compliance with decisions, actions, and programs that favor the protection of wildlife, once they are initiated.

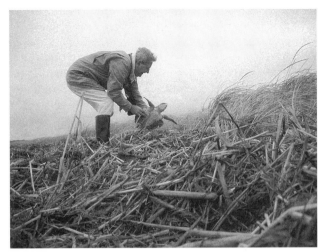

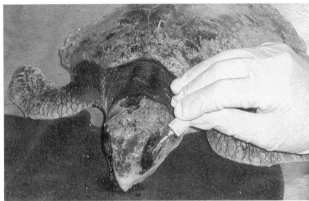

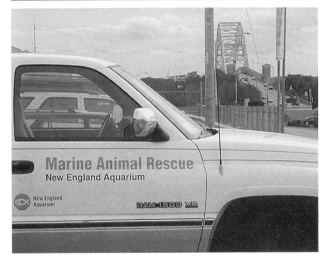

Figure 7-3.   Rescue and rehabilitation effort for Kemp's ridley sea turtles on Cape Cod, Massachusetts. Cold-shocked turtles were picked up from beaches by resident volunteers (top) and brought to a warming and first aid station at the Massachusetts Audubon Sanctuary in Wellfleet (middle). Turtles that required more-aggressive treatment were picked up on Cape Cod and transported to the New England Aquarium in Boston (bottom). Efforts such as these are a vital part of species conservation when populations are low as those of the Kemp's ridley turtle. (Photos courtesy of Mr. Don Lewis, Cape Cod Consultants, So. Wellfleet, MA)

Gorillas in the Midst . . . of Trouble

Wildlife conservation is as much about geopolitics and socioeconomics as it is about biology and ecology. No conservation effort illustrates that more than the turbulent past and troubled future of efforts to protect the mountain gorilla (*Gorilla gorilla beringei*). There are only 650 to 700 mountain gorillas alive in the world today. None are in zoos. All reside within two sites, the small Virunga volcanic mountain range that is trisected by the political borders of Rwanda, the Democratic

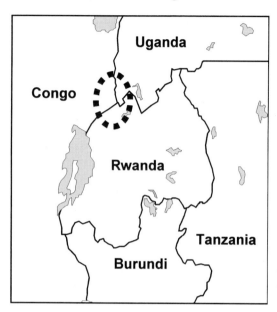

Map of gorilla region of East Africa.

Republic of the Congo (formerly Zaire), and the nearby Bwindi Impenetrable forest of Uganda, about 20 km to the north (All within the *dotted circle* on the map). Approximately half of these gorillas live in Bwindi, and the other half live in Virunga. All live in montane rainforest on volcanic mountain slopes at elevations above 10,000 feet in family troops led by a dominant silverback male. These peaceable animals spend much of their time foraging for plant foods including bamboo, bracket fungi, wild celery, thistles, and other locally abundant plants.

The first outsider to describe the mountain gorilla was a German Army officer, Oscar von Beringe, who was climbing in the Virunga range in 1902. Discovered just at the beginning of the 20th century, the future of the mountain gorilla looks quite precarious at the beginning of the 21st century. Following their discovery, mountain gorillas were captured and hunted extensively by foreign collectors and trophy seekers. Carl Akeley of the American Museum of Natural History himself shot five mountain gorillas in 1921, but recognizing the uniqueness and majesty of the animals, he persuaded the Belgian colonial government in Congo to establish a protected park for them in 1925, which became Parc National de Virunga. The mountain gorillas were then reasonably well protected until the 1960s, when civil war broke out in the Congo, and government policing of the park broke down. Many gorillas were lost in this period to poaching and accidental snaring.

Significant habitat loss occurred during this period as well, when forest was cleared by local villagers for agricultural purposes. Dian Fossey took up residence in the Virungas in 1963 to begin serious study of mountain gorillas. Fossey was instrumental in reducing poaching, raising awareness about the animals, and encouraging conservation efforts.

By the late 1970s a new era in gorilla conservation began when a group of conservation organizations initiated the Mountain Gorilla Project to promote gorilla tourism and to create awareness of the value of mountain gorillas among the people of Rwanda. This effort was highly successful. Rwandans embraced the mountain gorilla as a proud symbol of their national heritage and also recognized the economic returns generated by gorilla tourism. Tourism revenues became the third-largest foreign exchange earner in the country. The Congo and Uganda took note of these developments and also began to promote gorilla tourism. Bwindi Impenetrable Forest was upgraded to the status of a Ugandan national park in 1991, and two groups of gorillas in the forest were gradually habituated for viewing by tourists.

While the 1990s began on a positive note for gorilla conservation, the optimism soon faded. The first major blow was the Rwanda civil war that broke out in 1994. The war basically shut down tourism and made Parc National des Volcans virtually off limits. Re-

In developing countries, however, the situation may be very different. Many developing countries, particularly in the tropics, are rich in biodiversity, but wanting in economic opportunity and lacking in strong government and observance of the rule of law. In the poorest countries, direct conflicts between the interests of wildlife conservation and the needs of poor rural people are a daily occurrence. There is often tremendous human pressure on wildlife habitat and wildlife itself. Grasslands are used for livestock grazing, harvested for fodder, or planted with crops. Forests are cut for fuel wood or building materials or cleared for cropland. Wild animals are

trapped and hunted for food or for cash sale. Rapidly expanding populations and few alternatives for employment intensify pressure on natural-resource use in rural areas where subsistence farming or livestock grazing is the main source of livelihood.

In many countries of Africa, the situation is critical. Large tracts of land were set aside during colonial times as game reserves with an eye toward conservation but also with an eye toward sport hunting for Europeans. These colonial reserves were strictly protected areas, carefully policed to pre-

markably, few gorillas were actually killed during the war, though park infrastructure was significantly degraded. The real impact of the Rwandan conflict on gorillas was in Zaire, where an estimated 1.5 to 2 million Rwandan refugees took up residence, many on the periphery of Parc National de Virunga. These refugees, desperate for shelter and fuel wood, were responsible for extensive deforestation in the park, including almost 5% of the gorillas' forest habitat. In 1996, civil war broke out in Zaire as well, and the region around the park was the site of considerable fighting. Much of the park infrastructure was looted and destroyed. Automatic weapons left behind by fleeing soldiers were seized by poachers and local bandits. As a result of these events, more than 44 park guards and 12 mountain gorillas have been killed since 1995 in Zaire/Congo. By the mid-1990s, gorilla tourism had virtually shut down in Rwanda and Zaire/Congo, park security was not ensured, habitat encroachment and degradation was accelerating, and the gorillas were in peril. In the population and habitat viability assessment carried out for the mountain gorilla by conservationists in 1997, participants were obliged to consider four different war scenarios of varying severity in building population-survival models.

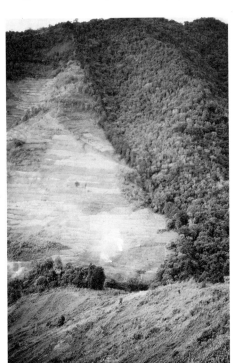

Bwindi National Park edge with farmers' fields adjacent. (Photo courtesy of Dr. Gary M. Tabor)

At least for a time, the situation in Uganda seemed more peaceful and secure. While direct armed conflict was averted at Bwindi, the precariousness of the future for mountain gorillas was still apparent. Uganda is an extremely poor country with a largely agricultural economy and a high population growth rate. The pressure for agricultural land around Bwindi is severe and has turned the forest into an island. The accompanying photograph shows the hard edge of the Bwindi Impenetrable Forest abutting crop land cultivated by local villagers. Incredibly, tourists can easily ascend the mountain slope along the cleared edge of cropland, enter the forest about halfway up, and encounter a habituated troop of mountain gorillas as close as 100 to 200 yards into the forest. There is simply no buffer zone to separate human activity and potential human disease from mountain gorillas. Unfortunately, poachers can gain access as easily as tourists.

In 1995, four adult gorillas were speared and killed by poachers in Bwindi who intended to abduct two gorilla infants, presumably on contract to a private collector. The period following this episode was rather stable at Bwindi, with steady increases in tourism activity and renewed optimism that Uganda's mountain gorillas might be reasonably secure. All that changed again in March of 1999, when a band of Hutu rebels raided Bwindi, overran the tourist encampments, and abducted dozens of tourists, ultimately killing eight of them as well as a park ranger. This appeared to be a calculated move against the government of Uganda, which was supporting ethnic Tutsi in Rwanda against the Hutu during the Rwandan civil war. The Hutu recognized the value of gorilla tourism to the Ugandan economy and set out to destroy the foundation of the nation's tourist industry. At present the future of the mountain gorillas remains uncertain. They exist precariously in poorly protected islands of habitat surrounded by a seething turmoil of poverty, desperation, ethnic hatred, and political instability. The situation would seem all but hopeless were it not for the profound commitment of dedicated conservationists from Rwanda, Uganda, the Congo, and around the world, who persist in the face of adversity to secure a future for this unique and special creature.

vent poaching, encroachment, extraction of natural resources, or use of grasslands by pastoralist communities who depended on livestock grazing. These reserves served as the basis of the national park system in many of the independent African nations that emerged during the 1960s. Gradually, as the economic fortunes of these African nations declined, their capacity to protect wildlife within the borders of protected areas also declined. At the same time, the needs of impoverished rural peoples steadily increased. As the occurrence of poaching and other infractions intensified, it became increasingly clear to conservationists and policymakers that in many cases, it was no longer feasible or conscionable to protect wildlife by fencing out local people. In addition, it was apparent that exclusionary, protectionist wildlife policies actually made local people hostile to wildlife conservation efforts. Since a considerable portion of a country's wildlife actually live outside the borders of protected areas (e.g., an estimated 60% in Kenya), the future of those wildlife populations depended on the goodwill of local people and instillation of a conservation ethic in local communities. Out of these conditions, the community conservation movement arose.

Community-based conservation is a strategy in which the direct participation of local people in the management and sustainable use of natural resources is encouraged and a fair proportion of the economic benefits derived from conservation efforts are returned to the local community. The process is participatory and democratic and encourages local decision-making. Generally, local people are integrated into community-based conservation projects by

- Inviting people living near protected lands to participate actively in land-use policy and management decisions
- Providing local people with proprietary rights or ownership of wildlife resources
- Sharing the economic benefits of wildlife conservation activities (e.g., park gate receipts) with local people

Perhaps the best-known and best-studied community conservation effort is the Communal Area Management Programme for Indigenous Resources, known most commonly by its clever acronym, CAMPFIRE, which began in Zimbabwe in the mid-1980s (see http://www.campfire-zimbabwe.org/). Zimbabwe was formerly the white-ruled nation of Rhodesia. Under white rule, the areas of the country best suited for intensive agriculture were taken over by white farmers, and indigenous Africans were resettled to communal land areas, largely in the northern area of the country. The communal lands tended to be semiarid grasslands unsuitable for cropping and infested with tsetse flies, making them also unsuitable for livestock grazing. What these areas were most suitable for was as wildlife habitat, and indeed, most of the wildlife reserves and parks set up by the white government were in fact adjacent to, or surrounded by, the communal lands. So, hundreds of thousands of black Africans were displaced from their traditional tribal homelands, relegated to dry, seemingly nonproductive communal lands, and then prohibited from using large tracts of adjacent land because they were set aside to protect wild animals. It is not too difficult to see how indigenous Africans in such a situation might become hostile to the notion of exclusionary, protectionist policies of wildlife conservation and even to the animals themselves.

Opportunities to change attitudes and approaches to conservation came with the downfall of Rhodesia and the establishment of the Zimbabwe nation in 1980. The need to address injustices of the past, to encourage economic opportunity for the rural poor, and to facilitate the equitable distribution and use of natural resources all came together in the CAMPFIRE plan. In 1975, the Rhodesian government had given private property holders the right to claim ownership of the wildlife on their land and to benefit from its use. Under CAMPFIRE, which was formally incorporated into Zimbabwe's national conservation strategy in 1985, these same proprietary rights to wildlife resources were given to the people living on the country's impoverished communal lands, which represented 42% of the nation's land area.

Rural communities that wish to participate in CAMPFIRE request legal authority from the government wildlife department to manage their own wildlife resources. The community must demonstrate to the wildlife department its capacity to manage the resources requested. The types of resource use chosen by communities varies, depending on a number of factors, not the least of which is the type of wildlife resources locally available. For communities with considerable big game on their communal lands, selling concessions to tour operators for hunting safaris or photographic safaris is the main revenue generator. Other communities have been involved in hunting and cropping animals themselves: selling crocodile eggs to licensed crocodile farmers, issuing rafting licenses, selling skins and hides and meat, or harvesting and selling Mopane worms. These are actually moth caterpillars (*Gonimbrasia belina* and *Gynanisa maia*) that feed on the Mopane tree. Mopane worms are part of the traditional Zimbabwean diet. They are almost 60% protein and contain significant amounts of phosphorus, iron, and calcium. When dried, they have a long shelf life and can be sold or exchanged for household goods such as sugar, tea, or cooking oil.

Though it varies among communities, the income generated by CAMPFIRE communities can be substantial. Overall, it has been estimated that since its inception, the CAMPFIRE program has increased rural community incomes by 15 to 25%. Some communities, particularly those able to sell hunting concessions, have benefited dramatically. In the first two districts to get approval from the wildlife department, overall gross income increased from Z$650,000 in 1989 to more than Z$10 million in 1993. Income generation has been a strong incentive for conscientious wildlife management and conservation by participating communities. This has been repeatedly demonstrated in the CAMPFIRE program by the establishment of antipoaching units, protection of crocodile nests to reduce egg losses, and other activities that reflect the self-interest of the communities and, at the same time, the well-being of the wildlife resources. Communities have put their increased revenues to a variety of uses. Some income is distributed directly to individual households for discretionary use, but other income is used for community development projects such as wildlife fences to protect crops from trampling.

While community-based conservation may be a useful tool for building support for wildlife conservation in rural communities, it is not a panacea. Some observers, even those friendly to the community conservation concept, have expressed reservations and concerns. Hackel for instance, warns that if desperately poor rural communities accept community-based conservation for its economic benefits, with little or no sense of stewardship, then these same communities may reject community-based conservation at some later time if better economic alternatives arise.[23] In the interim, however, control of wildlife resources will have been ceded to local communities as part of the community-based conservation process. For this reason, future policies relating to conservation of wildlife resources must be considered in a balanced fashion. While the benefits and advantages of successful community-based conservation need to be encouraged, some centralized protectionist authority over wildlife resources may need to be retained until the economic future of the rural poor is more secure. Then, rural communities can embrace conservation not simply out of economic desperation, but also out of a sense of stewardship.

The fundamental concept of community conservation is that human social and economic needs must be actively integrated into conservation plans for conservation efforts to be meaningful and sustainable. This concept has been adopted as the basis of broader regional efforts to protect biodiversity through implementation of the biosphere reserve concept. As described by the United Nations Educational, Scientific and Cultural Organization (UNESCO), biosphere reserves are areas of terrestrial and coastal/marine ecosystems where, through appropriate zoning patterns and management mechanisms, the conservation of ecosystems and their biodiversity is combined with the sustainable use of natural resources for the benefit of local communities, including relevant research, monitoring, education, and training activities. More information about biosphere reserves and the Man and the Biosphere Program is available at the UNESCO website (http://www.unesco.org/mab/).

Exploitation of Wildlife for Conservation Purposes

In the preceding discussion on community-based conservation, the problems associated with an exclusionary, protectionist approach to wildlife conservation are noted. Community-based conservation initiatives try to resolve these conflicts by encouraging participation of local people in the management and protection of wildlife resources in exchange for a share of those resources and the revenues they generate. The incentive for responsible management of the wildlife resource by local people is an ongoing economic return. Inherent in this exchange is the principle that wildlife can be exploited to economic advantage in responsible ways that further conservation objectives.

Several categories of activity link conservation objectives to the use of wildlife resources. Some activities are nonconsumptive, meaning that wildlife resources are neither extracted from their habitat nor killed. The main form of nonconsumptive wildlife use linked to conservation objectives is ecotourism. Other activities are categorized as consumptive, in that they intentionally result in the killing of wildlife under managed circumstances. Consumptive uses include trophy hunting, game ranching, and game farming. Each of these nonconsumptive and consumptive uses and its relationship to conservation is discussed in the sections below.

Ecotourism Tourism is big business. In the year 2000, the world travel and tourism industry accounted for approximately 11% of the world's gross domestic product (GDP), or about US$3.5 trillion, and recorded almost 700 million international

travelers. While all countries produce and receive tourists, overall there is a net flow of tourism revenues from the developed countries to the developing countries. For some developing countries, tourism has become the major revenue earner and source of foreign exchange.

One of the fastest growing segments of the tourism industry is what has come to be known as ecotourism, though exact statistics are hard to obtain, since there is no single, agreed-upon definition of ecotourism. Economic projections related to tourism often lump ecotourism under the larger umbrella of nature tourism, which encompasses all forms and scales of tourism that involve the enjoyment of natural areas and wildlife (Fig. 7-4). Since developing countries in tropical regions are home to much of the world's biodiversity, a number of these countries have had enormous growth in nature tourism in general and ecotourism in particular. Costa Rica, for instance, is now one of the top nature tourism destinations in the world. The tourism boom in Costa Rica began around 1987, and by 1995, tourism had become the largest foreign exchange-earning sector in the nation's economy, surpassing bananas, coffee, and beef and accounting for 7.5% of the nation's GDP. Over 66% of the 781,000 tourists visiting Costa Rica in 1996 visited a natural protected area.

Despite the lack of a precise definition for ecotourism, there is good overall agreement about the general concept. Drawing on a variety of published definitions of the term, several key elements emerge. Characteristics that help define ecotourism include:

- Purposeful travel made specifically to natural areas that are, as much as possible, pristine and undisturbed

- Travel that involves a specific intent to study, appreciate, contemplate, and understand aspects of the natural and/or cultural history of the site being visited

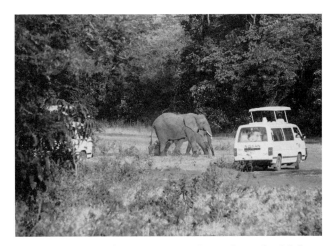

Figure 7-4. East Africa, with its abundant and varied wildlife species, has long been a favored destination for nature tourism. Here, tourists view elephants from a minibus in Serengeti National Park in Tanzania. (Photo by Dr. David M. Sherman)

- Travel that does not contribute to the degradation of the site being visited because the infrastructure supporting the site visits is small scale and low impact

- Travel that may involve failure to see the main attraction at a particular destination (e.g., great apes, jaguars, or tigers) and acceptance of that failure by the tourist

- Travel that respects local traditions and cultures and directly supports the economic well-being of local people

- Tourism activity that directly supports efforts to conserve and protect the natural resources that the tourist came to experience

In terms of the present discussion, the last point is the most important. Many conservationists have embraced ecotourism as a promising conservation strategy. Brandon identifies five potential benefits that can accrue to conservation efforts through ecotourism that are frequently cited by conservationists[7]:

- Providing a source of financing for parks and conservation

- Providing economic justification for natural-resource protection

- Providing local people with economic alternatives to encroachment into conservation areas

- Helping to build a constituency to promote conservation ethics and efforts

- Providing a stimulus for conservation efforts in the private sector

There is no question that well-designed ecotourism enterprises can raise awareness and appreciation of conservation challenges among ecotourists and that such heightened awareness can translate into political and financial support for conservation activities both locally and globally. Well-known conservation organizations, for example, Conservation International and the Nature Conservancy, sponsor their own ecotourism programs. Many ecotourism enterprises successfully meet most or all of the conservation goals envisioned for ecotourism. Some of these enterprises involve complex arrangements between government agencies, NGOs, corporate investors, and local community groups, while others are small, privately owned ventures that combine commercial enterprises with conservation (see sidebar "Ecotourism and Leatherback Turtles in Trinidad").

However, ecotourism has its critics, many of whom suggest that the idealistic rhetoric of ecotourism is often not realized in practice and that many of the problems of mass tourism are also inherent in ecotourism, albeit on a smaller scale. There are ecotourism sites, for example, where carrying capacity must be carefully regulated to avoid environmental degradation or negative impact on the wildlife species that serve as the inducement for visiting the particular site in the first place. Roe et al. reviewed the environmental impact of wildlife tourism/ecotourism and identified a number of direct and indirect negative effects on wildlife.[48] The indirect effects involve various aspects of environmental degradation such as off-road driving, soil erosion, trampling of vegetation, excessive development of infrastructure, and careless solid waste disposal leading to pollution of waterways. Direct impact on wildlife can result from unregulated contacts with, or inappropriate behavior of, tourists and can include disturbance of feeding and breeding patterns, disruption of parent-offspring bonds, increased vulnerability to predators and competitors, death of individual animals, and transmission of diseases.

Clearly, there is an important role for veterinarians in the conceptualization, planning, management, and monitoring of ecotourism enterprises to ensure that the health risks to both wildlife and human visitors are minimized. While ecotourism may present disease risks to a variety of species, the great apes are of particular concern. Gorillas, chimpanzees, and orangutans hold enormous appeal for human beings and have been the focus of intensive ecotourism efforts, while at the same time being subject to serious threats of extinction. Being closely related to human beings, great apes are susceptible to a wide range of human pathogens and may be naive to many of them. They may be exposed to these pathogens from either direct or indirect contact with human beings. As a result, the risk of disease spread and the potential impact on population health is high. The mountain gorilla situation in East Africa is illustrative.

The host countries for mountain gorillas, Rwanda, the Congo, and Uganda, have all recognized the economic potential of mountain gorilla viewing and have attempted to develop their mountain gorilla habitats as ecotourism sites. In recent years, however, prolonged civil unrest in Rwanda and the Congo have dramatically reduced tourism there and increased the interest in Uganda for gorilla ecotourism. Uganda's Bwindi Impenetrable Forest National Park is the home of the nation's mountain gorilla population of under 300 individuals. As a testament to the appeal of gorilla viewing, Bwindi earns more revenue per year in visitor permits and other concessionary fees than the rest of Uganda's National Parks combined, all of which are enthralling in their own right but lack gorillas. The experience of viewing habituated groups of gorillas has become so popular at Bwindi that reservations for a spot on the visitor list often have to be made a full year in advance, since daily visiting groups are limited to six to eight visitors per habituated group. While gorillas are already exposed to disease risk from local people living in the vicinity of the park, the regular arrival of tourists poses a significant, additional risk.

This risk of exposure of mountain gorillas to foreign pathogens is a daily occurrence. Given the nature of modern travel, it is routine for ecotourists to leave their homes in various locations around the world (e.g., the United States, Canada, Germany, Italy, Japan, and Australia), travel to Uganda, and be at Bwindi Impenetrable Forest within 36 to 48 hours of their initial departure from home. These visitors, commingling in Bwindi with each other, local people, and mountain gorillas may be incubating a wide variety of respiratory viral strains or enteric pathogens foreign to great apes in Uganda. There are visiting rules at Bwindi that state that no one who is obviously sick is allowed to actually enter gorilla viewing areas and that visitors are not supposed to get closer than 5 m to gorillas or to use the forest as a toilet. However, in practical terms, these rules may be hard for local rangers and trackers to enforce with zero tolerance of infraction. While ecotourists are supposed to be mindful of minimizing their impact, there are some, unfortunately, who put their own interests first. A wealthy tourist from a developed country with a strong sense of entitlement, who has traveled thousands of miles and spend thousands of dollars to see gorillas and is allowed 1 hour to do so, might become rather aggressive in defending his presumed right to enter the forest, whether he is sneezing or not. Once in the forest, such a tourist may quickly breach the 5-m separation gap when an irresistible photo opportunity presents itself.

Not surprisingly, the gorillas of Bwindi have experienced a number of disease problems in recent years that are most likely transmitted from human beings or contact with human activity. These disease problems have been observed, documented, and addressed by veterinary professionals from the Uganda Wildlife Authority, the Mountain Gorilla Veterinary Project, and other wildlife NGO and research organizations active in gorilla conservation. These conditions include cryptosporidiosis, giardiasis, unspecified respiratory infections, and scabies, from which an infant gorilla died in 1996, though others were successfully treated (Fig. 7-5). Additional disease risks of great concern to veterinarians caring for great apes include influenza, measles, tuberculosis, and polio.

Several veterinary initiatives are under way to improve disease prevention, surveillance, and control among the mountain gorillas. The Morris Animal Foundation's Mountain Gorilla Veterinary Project (MGVP), with a field hospital in Rwanda and links to the Makerere University Faculty of Veterinary Medicine in Uganda, has increased its diagnostic surveillance of mountain gorilla populations by applying molecular techniques for identification of infectious agents in samples that are collected noninvasively, such as feces and urine. They are also screening banked samples and tissues that have been collected from autopsies or during treatment interventions over the years. The newer molecular techniques are allowing identification of agents not previously detectable.

For example, it now may be possible to confirm that the suspected measles outbreak in mountain gorillas in Virunga Park in 1988 was in fact measles. Through such efforts, a better baseline of biomedical data can be established so that the medical history of the gorilla population can be more clearly known, and the appearance of new infections can be more-readily spotted and tracked. In addition, through its field veterinary hospital, the MGVP can respond more quickly and effectively to provide greater support to park officials and government veterinarians to diagnose and control disease outbreaks that could tip the mountain gorilla population into the vortex of extinction.

Trophy Hunting Human society is full of contradictions. While there is a significant population of well-to-do ecotourists who travel the world to view wild animals in their natural habitats and admire them, another significant population of well-to-do tourists travel the world to track wild animals in their natural habitats and kill them. While the animal admirer and the trophy hunter may have more than a bit of difficulty understanding each other's worldview, some in the conservation and rural-development communities recognize both ecotourism and trophy hunting as legitimate and important tools for wildlife conservation when properly managed. While some animal advocates may consider the concept

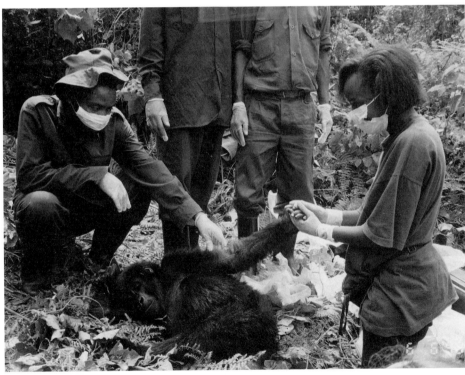

Figure 7-5. Dr. Gladys Kalema, Veterinary Officer of the Uganda Wildlife Authority examines a young mountain gorilla with sarcoptic mange in Bwindi National Park in 1996. This is one of many diseases transmissible from humans to primates that pose a threat to endangered great apes. An outbreak of sarcoptic mange also affected chimpanzees in Gombe National Park in Tanzania in 1997. (Photo courtesy of Dr. Gladys Kalema, Uganda Wildlife Authority)

Ecotourism and Leatherback Turtles in Trinidad

The leatherback turtle (*Dermochelys coriacea*) is one of the world's oldest living creatures, believed to have been present on Earth in the age of the dinosaurs 120 million years ago. Today, it runs the risk of going the way of the dinosaurs — toward extinction. The 2000 IUCN Red List identifies the leatherback as a critically endangered species with Pacific Ocean populations in drastic decline. Atlantic populations are also decreasing overall but not at the same dramatic rate. In 1980, the world population of female nesting leatherback turtles was estimated to be 115,000 individuals. By 1995, that number had dropped to less than a third, an estimated 34,500.

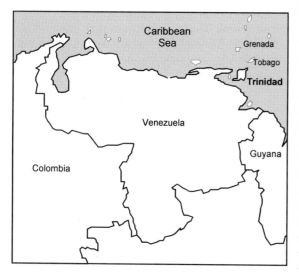

Leatherbacks are remarkable creatures. They have a life span of 80 years. Though males are almost never seen, females return at sexual maturity to the site of their own birth to climb out of the water onto the beach at night, dig a nest in the sand, lay their eggs, cover them, and return to the ocean, usually under cover of darkness. Returning to their birth site annually to nest is all the more amazing when one considers that in the intervening year, the turtles migrate around the oceans for distances up to 12,000 km, following their prime food source, the iridescent jellyfish. The leatherback faces a number of dangers that are contributing to its rapid decline. The turtles are frequently entrapped in fishing nets and drown. It is believed that coastal gill net fishing has virtually eliminated the leatherback populations in Mexico and Central America. Other turtles ingest plastic debris in ocean waters, mistaking it for their preferred food, the jellyfish, and die of intestinal obstructions. Those turtles that make it to the beach for nesting may be taken by poachers for meat, for ornamental shell, or for preparation of traditional medicines. If they are successful in laying eggs before they are discovered and butchered by poachers, the eggs themselves may be taken by scavengers. If they are lucky enough to hatch, considerable losses occur among the hatchlings through predation by birds on their journey from the nest back into the ocean. Clearly, the leatherback turtle could use a helping hand.

One of the largest nesting sites for Atlantic leatherbacks is on the northern coastal beaches of Trinidad, notably Grande Riviere and Matelot. While Trinidad has a reasonably strong economy and a good standard of living due to oil reserves and revenues, the northeastern corner of the island remains relatively undeveloped, with few employment opportunities. The taking of turtles for meat and sale was not uncommon in the area until an expatriate Italian entrepreneur, Piero Guerrini, decided to open a small ecotourism lodge on Grande Riviere beach and dedicate himself to turtle con-

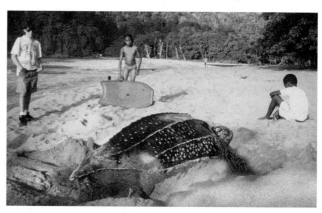

Turtle at nest on beach. (Photo courtesy of Mr. Pierro Guerini, Mt. Plaisir Estate)

of responsibly managed trophy hunting an oxymoron, there is substantial evidence that economic incentives associated with hunting can assist in achieving conservation goals, particularly outside protected areas.

The geographical area where this concept has been most widely implemented and evaluated has been in the savanna regions of Africa, where both wildlife and human populations are high and increasingly compete for the same space. Safari hunting has been used as a conservation tool on communal lands in community-based conservation schemes such as CAMPFIRE and also on privately held lands (Fig. 7-6). While nonconsumptive animal viewing enterprises might be desirable, in reality, not every location has the density of wildlife or mix of species to attract nature tourists in significant enough numbers to make the enterprise financially feasible. Such areas may be more suitable for trophy hunting, which provides both income and an incentive to manage wildlife resources responsibly. If the population dynamics of a game species are well known and properly monitored and limits are properly set and adjusted, there is minimal danger that well-managed trophy hunting will lead to significant population declines. In

servation. Mt. Plaisir Estate is small and unobtrusive but has become an important engine for sustainable economic growth and natural resource conservation. Mr. Guerrini employed local people to build the lodge and all the furniture in it, using local materials. Many local people in Grande Riviere have found employment in the lodge and associated service activities. A farm has been established to grow local produce for meals for the guests, and a goat and cow dairy is under consideration to make fresh cheese for the hotel kitchen.

The hotel owners and staff have assumed stewardship of the beach and the turtles during nesting season, under arrangement with the government and local conservation groups. Hotel employees take turns on night watch to make sure that turtles are not molested and to wake the small number of hotel guests so they can see the marvel of leatherback nesting. They also work with conservation groups to take measurements on turtles and tag them so that they can be tracked and studied over the years. They serve as escorts and bodyguards for the young hatchlings to help maximize the number that safely reach the ocean after hatching. In addition, the hotel serves as a field base during periodic visits from turtle researchers affiliated with Hubbs-San Diego Sea World Research Institute and other institutions. These scientists are conducting a variety of investigations including auditory research to determine if they can develop audible underwater warning signals that can be attached to fishing nets to alert the turtles to the presence of nets and help them avoid entanglement.

Signboard posting protected turtle area. (Photo by Dr. David M. Sherman)

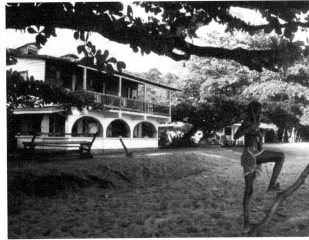

Mt. Plaisir hotel. (Photo courtesy of Mr. Pierro Guerini, Mt. Plaisir Estate)

Though it might be difficult to claim a direct association with the effort at Mt. Plaisir, it is interesting to note that of the 20 or so known leatherback nesting populations in Mexico, the Caribbean, and Central and South America, only 4 are documented to be increasing, and one of these is Trinidad. Thus, Mt. Plaisir Estate appears to represent a successful blend of private business, tourism, conservation, and community development that benefits the people and the turtles of Trinidad and the nature-loving tourists who are lucky enough to find their way to Grande Riviere during the turtle nesting season.

some cases, the number of problem animals killed by animal-control officers and villagers for crop damage exceeds the number permitted for trophy hunting.

The CAMPFIRE example of communal management of wildlife resources in Zimbabwe has demonstrated that communities recognize the income from game hunting permits as a strong conservation incentive. Communities receiving such income, for instance, are much more vigilant about controlling poaching of desirable trophy species on their communal lands, and poachers are far less bold when trophy hunters are roaming the landscape. One CAMPFIRE community even dug waterholes and arranged food deliveries for elephants during a period of drought. In 1997, controlled trophy hunting, consistent with CITES regulations, accounted for 90% of the income received by CAMPFIRE, with 60% of this coming from elephant hunting. In that year, there were an estimated 64,000 elephants in Zimbabwe while the Department of National Parks and Wild Life Management considered the appropriate carrying capacity of the country's elephant habitat to be about 35,000. The department set a nationwide trophy hunting quota of 276, or 0.43% of the population. There

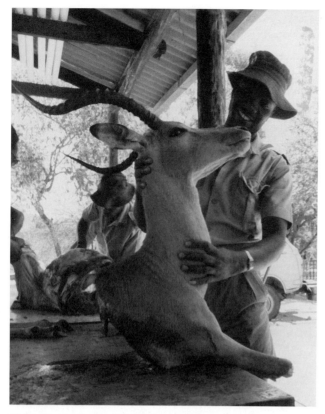

Figure 7-6. Trophy hunting has become an important source of income in southern Africa, both for private landowners and for communal landholders involved in community-based conservation programs. Trophy hunting is proving to be an effective tool for promoting overall wildlife conservation objectives. For instance, where supervised trophy hunting is permitted, poaching of endangered species often drops dramatically. In this picture, an impala is being prepared for taxidermy in Zimbabwe. (Photo courtesy of Mr. Ian B. Leach, Triple Line Consulting, London, U.K.)

are poor districts of Zimbabwe, where elephant harvesting represented the prime source of income, with the full trophy fee of US$12,000 going to the community. In a country where a rural family might subsist on less than US$ 400 per year, this represents a substantial source of income for community-development projects such as wells, schools, and clinics. Surveys estimate that average household income in communal areas participating in CAMPFIRE has increased between 15 and 25%.

Many communal landholders, especially pastoralists who depend on livestock for their primary livelihood, are skeptical about encouraging wildlife populations to expand into areas where livestock are grazed. Increased predation is one concern. Competition for forage with wild ungulates is another. However, the most important concern is the prospect of increased disease transmission. There are many valid considerations, but also some misconceptions, about disease interactions. One valid concern, for instance, is that wildebeest in calving season can readily spread malignant catarrhal fever to livestock. A misconception is that wildlife are responsible for the resurgence of contagious bovine pleuropneumonia (CBPP) that is cur-

rently sweeping East Africa. In fact, despite the presence of disease in areas where livestock and wildlife cohabit, there is no known wild animal reservoir for CBPP and no epidemiological evidence of transmission of the disease from wildlife to cattle.[33] The spread of CBPP in East Africa is due largely to the breakdown of veterinary service delivery associated with inadequate vaccination and the unregulated movement of infected cattle, as discussed in Chapter 8. For other diseases, definitive answers about the risk of disease transmission between wildlife and livestock are currently unavailable and require further research by veterinary microbiologists, parasitologists, and epidemiologists interested in the subject. Some of the animal diseases of current concern in East Africa from the standpoint of wildlife-domestic animal interaction are listed in Table 7-10. A good overview of the issues relating to wildlife and livestock on African rangelands, with a detailed focus on disease interactions, can be found in the recently published work *Can Livestock and Wildlife Co-Exist?*[5]

Many private cattle ranchers in the southern African countries of Namibia, Botswana, South Africa, and Zimbabwe have also seen safari hunting as a profitable alternative or supplement to livestock rearing. For example, in southeast Zimbabwe, in the Chiredzi River Valley, white ranchers began to recognize that they could make more money from wildlife tourism, controlled trophy hunting, and game harvesting for sale of venison than they could from cattle ranching. Even though some of these ranches were tens of thousands of hectares, they were still not large enough to support the range of some of the larger, more desirable game and viewing species such as the white rhinoceros (*Ceratotherium simum*). So gradually, over the years, as many as 15 ranchers agreed to take down their fences and manage their lands cooperatively as a private wildlife reserve. While numerous game species are hunted there, the reserve and nearby Save River Valley Reserve, composed of 23 cooperative properties, are also managed to serve as a protected area for endangered species such as the black rhinoceros (*Diceros bicornis*).

Such efforts can have a considerable positive impact on conservation. In the 1920s, for example, the southern white rhinoceros (*Ceratotherium simum*) was on the brink of extinction, with a population of only 50 to 100 individuals remaining in southern Africa. Today, there are over 8000 southern white rhinoceros. While many factors contributed to the recovery of the white rhino, the development of private game reserves in southern Africa and the potential income from trophy hunting were significant factors in this conservation effort. Today sufficient white rhino exist in Namibia and South Africa to permit controlled trophy hunting. With a 4-day white rhino hunt in South Africa bringing between US$23,000 and $33,000 in revenue to be distributed between wildlife authorities, private game reserve owners, and tour operators, there is considerable incentive for ensuring that the white rhino population remains well managed and that the same success can be achieved with black rhino populations.

Governments too have opted to permit hunting of wild game to help promote conservation efforts. In Tanzania,

Table 7-10.   Some Diseases Affecting Wildlife and Domestic Animals in East Africa

Disease	Causative Agent	Route of Transmission	Animals Affected	Control in Domestic Animals
African malignant catarrhal fever	Alcelaphine herpesvirus I (AHV-I)	Inhalation or ingestion of virus excreted by wildebeest	Cattle, wildebeest	Separation of cattle from calving and young wildebeest
African trypanosomiasis	*Trypanosoma* spp.	Tsetse fly feeding and, less significantly, other biting flies	Domestic livestock and man; wildlife reservoir of infection	Vector control, trypanotolerant livestock, trypanocidal drugs
Anthrax	*Bacillus anthracis*	Intake of spores by ingestion of contaminated soil, food, or water; by inhalation; or through skin	All mammals, especially herbivores	Vaccination, careful disposal of infected carcasses
Bovine cysticercosis	*Taenia saginata*	Ingestion of cysts in meat	Larval form: cattle, rarely wild antelope. Adult form: humans	Meat inspection and thorough cooking of meat
Canine distemper	Morbillivirus	Inhalation of aerosol or through contaminated objects	Domestic dogs, wild canids, some wild felids	Vaccination
Contagious bovine pleuropneumonia	*Mycoplasma mycoides* subsp. *mycoides,* small colony type	Inhalation of infective aerosols from active or carrier cases	Cattle, possibly buffalo	Vaccination, restricted movement and quarantine, removal of infected animals
East coast fever	*Theileria parva*	Feeding by tick vector, *Rhipicephalus appendiculatus*	Cattle and African buffalo	Tick control; vaccination and treatment
Foot and mouth disease	Aphthovirus	Air-borne spread and inhalation, or ingestion of infective material	All cloven-hoofed domestic and wild animals	Vaccination, quarantine and slaughter policy
Rabies	Rhabdovirus	Bite from an infected animal	All warm-blooded animals, including humans	Vaccination, control of domestic dog population
Rift Valley fever	Bunyavirus	Mosquito bite; inhalation of aerosol	Wide range of domestic animals, wild animals, and humans	Vaccination, vector control
Rinderpest	Morbillivirus	Close contact and inhalation of aerosol; ingestion of contaminated feed	Domestic and wild ruminants, pigs	Vaccination of cattle; movement control
Tuberculosis	*Mycobacterium bovis*	Inhalation or ingestion	All domestic livestock, humans, and many wildlife species	Testing and slaughter policy

Adapted from Bourn D, Blench R, eds. Can Livestock and Wildlife Co-exist? An Interdisciplinary Approach. An ODI Research Study. London: Overseas Development Institute, 1999.

wildlife authorities have long recognized safari hunting as an important source of revenue for financing overall conservation efforts in the country. The operating costs of the Selous Game Reserve are covered by the revenue from hunting within that reserve. The indirect conservation value of hunting in the reserve was demonstrated during the period 1973 to 1978, when hunting was temporarily banned. As soon as the licensed tour operators and their staff left the park, illegal poachers, emboldened by the low likelihood of detection, moved in, and elephant numbers in the reserve plummeted.

Game Ranching *Game ranching* is the raising of wild hoofed stock under extensively managed conditions for commercial purposes. As with livestock ranching, game ranching is most often found in semiarid grassland regions where crop cultivation is not feasible. In some cases, game ranching can extend into places where even livestock ranching is not possible because of physiological adaptations of wild game not possessed by cattle. Southern and eastern Africa are the areas of the world where game ranching has become most firmly established as a commercial venture. It is estimated that 10 to 20% of all commercial ranching enterprises in Botswana, Kenya, Malawi, Mozambique, Namibia, South Africa, Tanzania, Zambia, and Zimbabwe are involved in game ranching to some extent. One obvious reason for this is the abundance and variety of wild ungulate species on the African savanna relative to other regions of the world. However, other suitable areas such as the southwestern United States and Australia have fledgling game ranch industries as well, often involving imported hoof stock.

One of the advantages of wild game ranching over cattle ranching is that wild game offers more-varied income streams for ranchers than livestock. While cattle serve primarily for meat production, wild hoof stock on a ranch gives owners the opportunity to develop revenues from nature tourism, trophy hunting, and wildlife translocation activities in addition to slaughter of animals for meat and skins. Game ranching has become so well established in South Africa that there are consulting firms that will help farmers and cattle ranchers develop a customized business plan for game ranching, recommending a specific mix of species and activities suitable for the geography and ecology of the property, and consistent with the marketing goals and financial condition of the client. During the 1990s, the number of game ranches in South Africa grew to over 3500 properties, with the network of private reserves and game ranches in the country expanding from less than 0.8 million ha in 1979 to over 6.5 million ha in 1996.

From a production point of view, many wild ungulates offer advantages over domestic ruminants.[40] For example, weight gains for Thomson's gazelle on rangelands in East Africa average 0.33 kg/day, compared with only 0.14 kg/day for poorly managed cattle maintained under similar conditions. Live-weight production per unit area for the Thomson's gazelle in Kenya was found to be 17% higher than that of cattle. Under range conditions in Africa, many cattle do not breed until 3 to 4 years of age, while many of the antelopes and gazelles begin breeding between 1 and 2 years of age. Similarly, wild ungulates normally bear offspring annually, barring severe drought conditions, while calving intervals for cattle under range conditions may typically extend from 1.6 to 2 years. Meat yields for wild ungulates are also favorable compared with those of domestic livestock. Dressed weights for African game animals are reported in the range of 50 to 63% of live weight, compared with 44 to 50% for domestic stock. Wild-game meat also tends to be much leaner, with fat content in dressed carcasses in the range of 1.9% for impala to 5.6% for the African buffalo, compared with 13.7% for Zebu cattle.

The main drawbacks to wild game ranching as a commercial enterprise is the difficulty of harvesting and processing wild animals. Not being domesticated, they are difficult to handle or transport humanely. Therefore, they often must be killed and dressed on site, requiring hunting teams, vehicles, mobile abattoirs, refrigerated storage, and good transportation infrastructure to get to market. Nevertheless, when the added opportunities of diversifying income from tourism and hunting are added in, properly managed game ranches can be more profitable than livestock ranches and can be more compatible with conservation goals.

The key conservation value of game ranching is in habitat preservation relative to land degradation, particularly in fragile semiarid rangelands. Cattle, as essentially strict grazers, use a very limited range of the forage available in a mixed shrub and grassland habitat such as the South African bushveld. The potential for overgrazing and land degradation exist when cattle are overstocked or otherwise improperly managed as discussed in Chapter 6. Wild ungulates have evolved varied feeding niches in bushveld habitats that allow multiple species to be present and use a diverse array of forage resources without overtaxing the resource base or degrading the habitat for other species such as birds, reptiles, insects, and small mammals. By diversifying forage use with wild ungulates, overall carrying capacity of rangelands may be higher with mixed wild species than with cattle. The addition of goats and sheep to cattle ranches can approximate such diversification of forage use but not as efficiently as a diverse mix of wild ungulates.

The water requirements for many wild ungulates also differ significantly from those of domesticated ruminants. Wild ungulates such as oryx (*Oryx beisa*), impala (*Aepyceros melampus*), wildebeest (*Connochaetes taurinus*), and eland (*Taurotragus oryx*) have excellent physiological adaptations for conservation of water that allow them to disperse more widely through the environment and to tolerate periods of drought more successfully than cattle. The oryx, for instance, has half the drinking water requirement of Dorper sheep, and one quarter that of Boran cattle when the species are standardized on a metabolic weight basis.

Consumer demand for meat is increasing at a rate of 0.6% in developed countries and 2.8% per year in developing countries. In developed countries, increased demand most likely will continue to be met through intensive livestock production based on the ready availability of grain surpluses for livestock feed. In developing countries, particularly in Africa, where per capita grain production in many nations has been static or falling, intensive livestock production is not likely to be the answer to an increasing demand for meat. Therefore, increased production will require increased offtake from rangelands. Game ranching can play a significant role in increasing offtake in sustainable ways.

Game Farming Though the taking of wild animals by the rural poor for food or for sale is a traditional practice, it is also becoming an important factor in the overexploitation of wildlife resources, contributing directly to the loss of biodiversity. There is great variety in what is preferred, hunted, and locally consumed by different cultural groups. Targeted species range from insects and snails to wild birds, rodents, bats, and monkeys. For example, Anadu et al. investigated the wild meat preferences and trade practices in Bendel State of southwestern Nigeria by interviewing hunters and retailers.[1] They found that hunting took place year round but was more intense during the dry season. Some 27 species of mammal were hunted, with 22 species of mammal and 5 species of reptile found on sale. Retailers reported that the grasscutter (*Thryonomys swinderianus*), a rodent also known as the cane rat, was the most popular species among their customers, followed by Maxwell's duiker (*Cephalophus maxwellii*), the brushtailed porcupine (*Atherurus macrourus*), and the bushpig (*Potamochoerus porcus*). The grasscutter was also the most widely sold species, followed by the giant rat (*Cricetomys* spp.), monkeys, and Maxwell's duiker. Interviews revealed that game animals were shot and sold with little regard for existing laws. As a result, the larger mammals had become rare in Bendel, and populations of the smaller ones had come under severe pressure. It was clear that the bushmeat trade is highly commercialized, and substantial profits accrue to middlemen.

As human population continues to increase in many developing countries, pressures on wildlife as a source of protein in the human diet will continue to increase as well. This may imperil species that are directly sought as food, as well as others opportunistically or inadvertently caught. One approach to reducing the pressure on wild species is to identify those that are most popular in a region and develop husbandry practices for rearing them economically in captivity. If market demand can be met by captive raised animals at prices competitive to those for hunted animals, then hunting, snaring, and trapping of those animals and other hapless victims could be reduced. Thus, some conservationists see the development of game farming as an important tool for protecting biodiversity.

Game farming is the rearing of wild animal species in confinement in a semidomesticated state for commercial exploitation. While many game-farming efforts are directed primarily at food production, some enterprises have different primary production goals. However, they may still serve a conservation function. For instance, crocodile farming has become an economically successful business in Africa, with crocodiles being raised primarily for their skins for use in specialty leather products. Prior to the development of crocodile farming as an industry, crocodile hunting (and poaching) in the wild had seriously diminished wild populations of all three crocodile species (*Crocodylus niloticus, Osteolaemus tetraspis,* and *Crocodylus cat-*

aphractus) on the continent to the point that trade controls were initiated under CITES and, in response, crocodile husbandry practices were developed. Under managed-farming systems, crocodile eggs are still harvested in the wild, by permit, and hatched under controlled conditions. By agreement with authorities, however, a certain percentage of the young hatchlings are returned to the wild, while the remainder are raised for slaughter. Crocodile numbers in Zimbabwe have actually increased under this system.

With regard to primary food production through game farming, attempts have been made with quite a variety of species. In Africa, these species include eland (*Taurotragus oryx*), bushpig (*Potamochoerus porcus*), warthog (*Phacochoerus aethiopicus*), various duiker species, guinea fowl (*Numida meleagris*), francolin (*Francolinus* spp.), giant snails (*Achatina* and *Archachatina* spp.), giant rats (*Cricetomys* spp.), and cane rat (*Thryonomys* spp.). In Latin America, species include guinea pigs (*Cavia porcellus*), capybara (*Hydrochoerus hydrochaeris*), agouti (*Dasyprocta* spp.), and paca (*Agouti paca*). Success has varied, depending on a number of factors. Production factors include the biological characteristics of the animal, behavioral constraints, husbandry requirements, growth rates, and disease problems. Marketing factors include startup costs, cultural acceptance of the animal as food, and its production costs and market price relative to meat from similar domestic species or to the same game species when hunted in the wild. The book *Microlivestock* provides useful overviews of a wide range of small-rodent, bird, reptile, and ungulate species from around the world that have the potential to be exploited under managed conditions as food sources in the areas where they occur.[38]

Clearly, there are considerable opportunities for veterinarians to be directly involved in research, development, extension, and training efforts associated with game farming. Fundamental questions about issues of captive management and husbandry, reproduction, disease occurrence and control, nutrition, productivity, and welfare remain unanswered for many of the species that might be adapted to game farming. Wildlife conservationists have been ringing alarm bells about the rampant overexploitation of wild species in Africa for the bushmeat trade in recent years. Game farming potentially serves the dual objectives of improving human nutrition and alleviating the relentless pressure of the hunt on wild populations of game species in rural areas of developing countries.

Ex Situ Efforts

In addition to field efforts to protect endangered species and protect biodiversity, complementary activities are ongoing at zoos, museums, universities, research facilities, and rehabilitation centers around the world. These efforts focus on the study, protection, and propagation of wild animals in captivity. It is in the area of such *ex situ* activity that veterinarians have made their most direct and visible contribution to wildlife conservation to date and that veterinarian knowledge of wild species has made the most advances, although the opportunity for veterinary participation in *in situ* conservation activities is considerable and expanding.

Zoos As Agents of Conservation

While the general public may continue to view zoos primarily as entertainment venues, for conservationists, zoos have become safe houses in the biological holocaust, where endangered species may find refuge. Zoos have also become staging areas for the return of endangered species to their native habitats, whenever and wherever threats to habitat can be resolved and the security of wildlife can be ensured.

Zoos have multiple roles in wildlife conservation. Public education is one extremely important and expanding function. Zoos attract enormous numbers of visitors, especially school-age children. Given the general fascination of children with animals, considerable opportunity exists to focus attention on the plight of specific species, promote awareness of biodiversity issues, and cultivate a conservation ethic in the young, both at zoos and in outreach programs to schools. Closely linked to public education is fund raising. Zoos, by virtue of their high attendance rates, educational activities, and community standing, have the potential to raise considerable funds, not only for the zoo itself, but also in support of field conservation and training programs and other local zoo and NGO conservation initiatives around the world. The World Zoo Organization (http://www.wzo.org/) has developed a World Zoo Conservation Strategy that considers the key function of zoological institutions to be education, linked to in situ and ex situ research and educational programs.

A key function of zoos is to continue to improve their capacity to manage the health and well-being of wild species in captivity. Many zoos in developed countries have undergone remarkable transformations in recent years as captive animals are removed from bare cages and cramped enclosures and transferred to more naturally constructed habitats that better accommodate the animals' unique behaviors and physiological requirements. Regrettably, many zoos in developing countries can not afford the considerable expense associated with such transformations. However, many zoos in developed countries are embracing "sister" zoos in poorer nations and are providing technical and financial assistance to improve the condition of animals in these facilities. The Taronga Zoo, in Sydney, Australia, for instance, has been instrumental, along with the Jane Goodall Institute, in improving the facilities for chimpanzees at the Uganda Wildlife Education Centre, formerly the Entebbe Zoo. New housing and a moated island exhibit have been developed at the zoo site, and a separate 100-acre forested island in Lake Victoria, 45 minutes by boat from Entebbe, was established at the end of 1998 as the Ngamba Island Chimpanzee Sanctuary.

As increasing numbers of species become threatened and endangered in the wild, the role of zoos as safe havens for these species assumes greater importance. As such, zoos are increasingly involved in efforts to fully understand and address the needs of individual animals that may represent the future of a species. This includes research into species' nutritional and physiological requirements, social behaviors, reproductive behaviors, biomedical parameters, and susceptibility and responses to disease. Some animals are being trained through operant conditioning techniques to provide blood samples or receive medications without the need for, and associated trauma of, chemical capture or mechanical restraint. Once a species' requirements for health and well-being are understood and met, the potential exists to expand threatened populations through captive breeding, with the ultimate goal of rebuilding populations in the wild. Propagation of endangered species through captive breeding has become an important conservation activity of zoos. Significant advances in research and technology have been made by reproductive biologists and veterinarians, including the use of artificial insemination and embryo transfer in a wide range of species. At the same time, technologies for controlling breeding in prolific captive species such as the lion have been advanced to reduce the potential for captive populations to exceed the ability of zoos to care for them.

In 2000, the cloning of a wild animal species was announced as the newest advance in reproductive technology with potential application as a conservation tool. Scientists at a Massachusetts-based biotechnology firm successfully produced the first clone of a potentially endangered species, the Asian gaur (*Bos frontalis*). The gaur is a wild ox of south Asia found in the tropical woodlands of India, Indochina, and the Malay Peninsula and is listed as vulnerable to extinction in the IUCN Red List. The cloning procedure involved transferring the skin cell DNA of a recently deceased male gaur into the evacuated egg cell of a domestic bovine and having the pregnancy carried in a domestic dairy cow. Also in 2000, Spanish scientists announced plans to reverse the extinction of a species by cloning cells from a Pyrenean mountain ibex (*Capra pyrenaica pyrenaica*). This ibex was the last known individual of the species and was killed by a falling tree in Ordesa National Park in Spain. There will undoubtedly be considerable debate about the ethics of cloning and its use as a conservation tool. Some critics have already dismissed the procedure as inappropriate because it produces multiple genetic replicates of the same individual, thus contributing further to the narrowing of genetic diversity in already small populations. Others counter by saying that with tissue banking, the procedure offers an opportunity to reintroduce the genes from dead individuals back into living populations to increase genetic diversity.

Species Survival Plans

While the technology of captive breeding is interesting in its own right, the true significance of captive-breeding programs lies in their application to assist the survival of species in danger. Toward this end, the American Zoo and Aquarium Association (AZA), made up of 185 accredited zoos and aquariums in North America, developed a comprehensive program called the Species Survival Plan (SSP) Program, which began in 1981. As described by the AZA, the mission of the SSP Program is to help ensure the survival of carefully selected wildlife species by a combination of implementation strategies that include:

- Organizing scientifically managed captive-breeding programs for selected wildlife species as a hedge against extinction

- Cooperating with other agencies and institutions to ensure integrated conservation strategies
- Increasing public awareness of wildlife conservation issues through development of educational strategies at member institutions and in the field
- Conducting basic and applied research to contribute to the overall knowledge of various species
- Training wildlife and zoo professionals
- Developing and testing various technologies relevant to field conservation
- Reintroducing captive-bred wildlife into restored or secure habitat as appropriate and necessary

The goal of each SSP is to carefully manage the breeding of selected species to maintain a genetically diverse and demographically stable captive population that is healthy and self-sustaining. Species are selected for the SSP Program on the basis of a number of criteria. They are usually endangered or threatened species and frequently are "flagship" species that generate strong interest and support among the general public. They need to be supported by a cadre of qualified specialists with expertise and interest in the particular species, including veterinarians, who are willing and able to invest time and effort into developing and maintaining the SSP activity. At the time of this writing, AZA had 119 individual species in their SSP Program. More information about the SSP Program is available on the internet at http://www.aza.org/ConScience/ConScienceSSPFact/.

When reintroduction becomes part of an SSP, international collaborations are called into play. For example, the CBSG of the IUCN (discussed earlier in the section on species-management plans) operates a program called Global Animal Survival Plans (GASPs). GASPs are part of a collaborative process for managing species at an international level. These global management plans emphasize the linkage of captive programs to the conservation of wild populations. The red-crowned crane, for example, is one of four crane species for which SSPs are managed by the AZA. About 700 red-crowned cranes reside in zoological facilities worldwide, representing one third of the total population alive today. The AZA crane SSP group cohosted a GASP for the red-crowned crane in China in 1993. This was the first attempt at a global captive management program for a bird species. Strong links between SSPs and GASPs have also been forged for conservation of the world's endangered tiger species.

Zoo Medicine

Veterinarians play an extremely important role in conservation by safeguarding the health of endangered animals in captivity. Zoo veterinarians have made significant advances in the ability to diagnose, treat, and prevent disease in the last half-century. Zoo veterinary medicine has become a well-established branch of the veterinary profession with its own specialized texts and journals, professional organizations, clinical and research training programs, and specialty certifications. One need only look at the proceedings of the annual conference of the American Association of Zoo Veterinarians or a current issue of their journal *Zoo and Wildlife Medicine* to get a sense of scope, depth, and sophistication of zoological medicine today.

The vigilance of zoo veterinarians is especially important in recognizing when animals in captivity are exposed to, and succumb to, diseases that they might not otherwise encounter in their native habitats, for instance, the recent occurrence of fatal herpesvirus infections in Indian elephants (*Elephas maximus*) housed in captivity with African elephants (*Loxodonta africana*) at various zoos around the United States. Though the epizootiology is not yet fully elucidated, disease investigations indicate that African elephants are latent carriers of this virus in the wild and manifest clinical disease infrequently, whereas the Indian elephant has no experience with this specific herpesvirus under natural conditions and may become fatally ill when exposed to the virus under conditions of confinement with African elephants.[47] Another recent and dramatic example is the death of 27 captive birds in 1999 at the Bronx Zoo in New York as a result of the sudden and still-unexplained introduction of the exotic West Nile virus into the New York area. The vigilance of the zoo's veterinary pathologist, Dr. Tracey S. McNamara, in working up the cause of death in these captive birds as well as wild dead birds in the surrounding neighborhood led the Centers for Disease Control and Prevention to recognize the problem as exotic West Nile virus.[39]

Another important and emerging responsibility of zoo veterinarians essential to conservation efforts is to ensure that animals that are to be involved in reintroduction programs are not going to introduce diseases into wild populations that would jeopardize the health of those wild populations. The example of arenavirus hepatitis in captive golden lion tamarin is discussed earlier in this chapter. Another chilling example is the discovery of transmissible spongiform encephalopathy (TSE) in a wide range of species of zoo animals in the U.K., including greater kudu (*Tragelaphus strepsiceros*), gemsbok (*Oryx gazella*), nyala (*Tragelaphus angasii*), Arabian oryx (*Oryx leucoryx*), eland (*Taurotragus oryx*), cheetah (*Acinonyx jubatus*), puma (*Puma concolor*), tiger (*Panthera tigris*), and ocelot (*Felis pardalis*). It is believed that these varied species were infected by eating zoo diets that contained bovine tissues contaminated with the agent causing bovine spongiform encephalopathy. Reintroduction of ungulate animals who appear healthy but carry a latent TSE could wreak havoc in wild populations.

The Field of Conservation Medicine

The conservation community has come to recognize the significant role of disease in the loss of biodiversity, and disease has become an important consideration in the design and implementation of wildlife management and conservation efforts such as captive management, corridor development, reintroduction, translocation, and community conservation. Veterinarians can contribute greatly to these design and implementation efforts. However, the conservation community has not fully used the training, interest, and experience of veterinarians. Likewise, the veterinary profession itself has not fully recognized or explored the range of participation possible for veterinarians in wildlife conservation and the preservation of biodiversity. Some veterinarians and conservation biologists have recognized this lack of synergy and are working closely to foster collaboration and integration of their activities. For instance, the wildlife conservation NGO, Wildlife Trust, has an active field veterinary program that is well integrated with its worldwide conservation efforts (http://www.wpti.org/index.shtml).

At the same time, a growing number of disease ecologists, epidemiologists, and physicians are looking more carefully at the role of environmental factors such as habitat transformation, climate change, and the movement of wildlife, humans, and domestic animal populations as critical elements in the emergence of new diseases such as AIDS, Lyme disease, and hantavirus infections, as well as the resurgence of known diseases previously thought to be under control such as malaria, dengue fever, and tuberculosis. These health professionals also see increasing reason and opportunity to collaborate with veterinarians and conservation biologists. This nascent collaboration of the conservation community and the health science community is emerging as the new field of conservation medicine.

As the interdisciplinary field of conservation medicine is quite new, the term still has different meaning to different people, and no one definition has yet been firmly established. The Consortium for Conservation Medicine (CCM), established in 1997, is a collaboration between Wildlife Trust, the Center for Health and the Global Environment at Harvard University Medical School, and the Tufts University School of Veterinary Medicine. CCM defines *conservation medicine* as an emerging discipline that links human and animal health with ecosystem health and global environmental change. By bringing together veterinarians, physicians, ecologists, and other conservation professionals, the CCM attempts to provide an ecological context for health management and the preservation of biodiversity.

Pokras et al. consider the goal of conservation medicine to be integration of the diagnostic and problem-solving tools of medical professionals with the ecological and management knowledge of conservation professionals to preserve biodiversity and maintain the health of interdependent species including humans.[45] This end entails the following tasks:

- Training environmentally literate health professionals
- Breaking down disciplinary barriers to communication and cooperation
- Establishing the scientific underpinnings of the interrelationships among human, animal, and environmental health
- Encouraging broad participation in public education about health and the environment

- Being active in developing conservation and health policies that integrate human and animal concerns
- Encouraging broader definitions for concepts of health
- Developing new technologies to support research and conservation efforts

Australian veterinarians are moving in a similar direction[27] and have formed the Australian Association of Veterinary Conservation Biologists. The aims of the group are

- To provide a forum for veterinarians involved in any aspect of conservation biology, to enhance the contribution of veterinary science in the field of wildlife studies, resource management, and animal welfare
- To encourage research and development of veterinary conservation biology
- To promote cooperation between veterinarians, other biologists, administrators, researchers, and research and teaching institutions
- To provide continuing education programs for veterinarians and others involved in conservation biology

Deem et al. of the Wildlife Conservation Society in New York define *conservation medicine* simply as the application of medicine to augment the conservation of wildlife. They identify a number of key areas in which veterinarians can be directly involved in wildlife conservation efforts[13]:

- Identifying critical health factors in wildlife populations to elucidate the role of disease in population dynamics and to ensure that health and disease issues are properly and fully considered in wildlife management programs
- Monitoring the health of wildlife populations to develop baseline information and detect change in response to environmental perturbations, initiation or modification of wildlife management plans, ecotourism initiatives, livestock incursions, reintroduction programs, or any other activities that might affect wildlife population health
- Participating in wildlife crisis management to providing diagnostic services and to advise on therapeutic or prophylactic interventions when and if appropriate
- Developing new technologies in support of wildlife conservation such as noninvasive diagnostic and

therapeutic techniques, field-based diagnostic test kits, standardization of existing laboratory tests for wildlife species, improved systems of animal identification, safer capture and anesthetic protocols and products, and baited oral vaccines

- Improving animal handling and welfare in association with research activities, translocations, capture of problem animals, or any other project that involves the handling of wildlife
- Training veterinary professionals, biologists, and wildlife managers on matters relating to the health of wildlife, particularly in developing countries in which threats to wildlife are high and opportunities for professional development may be limited

Clearly, a growing number of veterinarians are thinking seriously about issues of biodiversity loss, environmental health, and wildlife conservation and are looking to broaden the participation of the veterinary profession in addressing these global problems. It can be reasonably argued that veterinary expertise has been underused in conservation efforts and that veterinary medicine has much to offer the conservation community. On the other hand, the veterinary perspective is but one of many professional perspectives. Veterinarians interested in participating effectively in wildlife conservation must know and appreciate the contributions and activities of the wide array of scientists and professionals who work in the field. They must be prepared to participate in, and contribute to, interdisciplinary team efforts and understand where and how they can make the most-effective contributions.

Sherman et al. conducted a workshop at the 7th International Theriological Congress on preparing veterinarians for meaningful participation in wildlife conservation.[51] The workshop included nonveterinarians as well as veterinarians, and some interesting points emerged. There was no lack of agreement that veterinarians have a vital role to play in wildlife conservation efforts. However, workshop participants agreed, in general, that the current general veterinary curriculum does not suffice to prepare graduates to work effectively in wildlife medicine and conservation without some additional, wildlife-specific training. Some suggestions offered at the workshop are as follows:

- Provide opportunities for clinical electives during veterinary training in the form of externships at zoos, aquariums, or relevant government agencies
- Develop opportunities for veterinary students to participate in interdisciplinary field research projects while still in veterinary school, for example, during summer breaks
- Provide informal opportunities for students to focus on wildlife issues in veterinary medicine through journal

clubs, discussion groups, symposia, field trips, etc.

- Have veterinarians join appropriate professional groups such as the World Association of Wildlife Veterinarians after graduation and participate in relevant electronic information exchanges
- Although formal zoo residencies may be useful preparation for wildlife medicine, they may encourage "techno-fixes" at the expense of *in situ* solutions to conservation problems; to counter this tendency veterinarians should get formal training in conservation biology before, during, or after veterinary school
- Develop new, non-zoo residency or graduate degree programs in conservation medicine that combine clinical training, course work, and participation in interdisciplinary field research
- In the future, consider competency examination, certification, or special licensing for veterinarians intending to work with wildlife; such requirements are beginning to emerge in certain African countries as a result of the demand for veterinary services associated with the expansion of game ranching and translocation activities

Some progress has been made in addressing these concerns, though veterinary training institutions do vary in their commitment to preparing graduates for work in wildlife conservation. A growing number of veterinary faculties have wildlife clinics through which students rotate for clinical training. Makerere University Faculty of Veterinary Medicine in Uganda has a mandatory field course in wildlife medicine for its fourth-year veterinary students, which takes students into Uganda's National Parks for hands-on training (Fig. 7-7), and has established the Wildlife and Animal Resource Management Unit within the faculty.[52] The Faculty of Veterinary Science at the University of Sydney has added a veterinary conservation biology course to its second-year curriculum. Tufts University School of Veterinary Medicine has been arranging field-based summer research opportunities for those Tufts students interested in wildlife health issues for well over a decade. The University of California at Davis now offers 19 different elective courses for students interested specifically in different aspects of wildlife medicine and encourages graduate students in the Masters of Veterinary Preventive Medicine to focus on wildlife-related issues in their graduate training.

The Envirovet Summer Institute, based at the University of Illinois, College of Veterinary Medicine, offers a field course entitled Terrestrial and Aquatic Wildlife and Ecosystem Health in which veterinary students study ecosystem health concepts and wildlife medicine in a developed country context (United States) and a developing country context (Kenya), to appreciate the role that socioeconomic and ecological factors play in wildlife conservation and ecosystem health

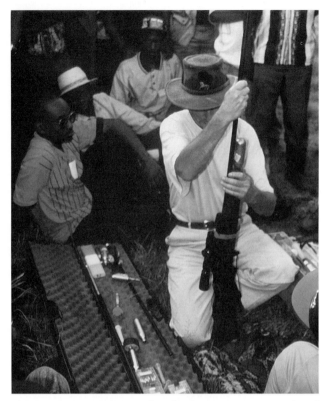

Figure 7-7. Dr. Ludwig Siefert of Makerere University Faculty of Veterinary Medicine reviews darting gun preparation with Ugandan veterinary students during a field course in wildlife medicine at Lake Mburo National Park. In recognition of the important role that wildlife play in the nation's economy, the veterinary faculty has created the Wildlife and Animal Resource Management Unit and expanded the training of Ugandan veterinary students in wildlife medicine and conservation. (Photo by Dr. David M. Sherman)

(http://www.cvm.uiuc.edu/vb/envirovet_2001/index.html. Wildlife veterinarians in South Africa have organized and offer an annual 2-week course in wildlife veterinary medicine held at Parados Game Ranch, in Karino, South Africa that is open to veterinary students and veterinarians from the United States and elsewhere (www.wildlifevets.com). Another short course available in South Africa focuses specifically on wildlife capture techniques (www.parawild.co.za). Additional training, experiential, and employment opportunities for veterinary students and veterinarians interested in wildlife conservation are discussed in Chapter 10.

Discussion Points

1. Are domesticated cats a threat to wild bird populations? Some think so, others do not.[42] Evaluate the evidence yourself. Design a study to determine rates of bird loss from cats, owned and feral. Think about the ethical issues in weighing the value of an unowned domesticated cat versus a potentially threatened or endangered migratory songbird.

2. What is the current status of the role of iridoviridae in the world amphibian crisis? How is the occurrence of this pathogen linked to other factors threatening biodiversity, such as habitat loss, human encroachment, and climate change?

3. What are the main disease risks to different great ape species that must be considered in ecotourism programs? What tools are available for minimizing or eliminating these risks? What practical constraints exist in implementing disease control interventions? Pick a particular site and species and make your recommendations site specific.

4. What role did international NGOs concerned about wildlife conservation play in the demonstrations at the World Trade Organization meeting in Seattle in November of 1999? What linkages between global trade and wildlife conservation were they concerned about?

5. Game farming and game ranching are increasingly recognized as useful tools for promoting the conservation of wildlife species, but animal welfare groups often disagree. For instance, the Canadian Federation of Humane Societies holds the stated position that wild animals should be free to live naturally in the wild and, therefore, is opposed to game farming and game ranching. As a veterinarian interested in conservation of wild animals, defend the exploitation of some individual wild animals to protect the species at large. As a veterinarian interested in animal welfare, defend the prohibition of game farming and game ranching.

6. Pick a species for which there is interest in its potential in game farming. Develop a plan for raising this species commercially. What disease issues and captive management problems might you anticipate, based on the species and the method of husbandry chosen?

References

1. Anadu PA, Elamah PO, Oates JF. The bushmeat trade in southwestern Nigeria: a case study. Hum Ecol 1998;16(2):199–208.

2. Bayliss M, Mellor PS, Meiswinkel R. Horse sickness and ENSO in South Africa. Nature 1999;397(6720):574–579.

3. Barbour H, Simmons T, Swain P, Woolsey H. Our Irreplaceable Heritage. Protecting Biodiversity in Massachusetts. Westborough, MA: Massachusetts Division of Fisheries and Wildlife, Natural Heritage and Endangered Species Program, 1998.

4. Berry HH. Aspects of wildebeest *Connochaetes taurinus* ecology in the Ethosha National Park-a synthesis for future management. Madoqua 1997;20(1):137–148.

5. Bourn D, Blench R, eds. Can Livestock and Wildlife Co-exist? An interdisciplinary Approach. An ODI Research Study. London: Overseas Development Institute, 1999.

6. Bossart GD, Baden DG, Ewing RY, et al. Brevetoxicosis in manatees (*Trichechus manatus latirostris*) from the 1996 epizootic: gross, histologic and immunohistochemical features. Toxicol Pathol 1998;26:276–282.

7. Brandon K. Ecotourism and conservation: a review of key issues. Paper no. 033. Washington, DC: Environment Department, Global Environment Division, World Bank, 1996.

8. Cohen JE, Tilman D. Biosphere 2 and biodiversity: the lessons so far. Science 1996;274:1150–1151.

9. Costanza R, d'Arge R, de Groot R, et al. The value of the world's ecosystem services and natural capital. Nature 1997;387(6630):253–260.

10. Cunningham AA. Disease risks of wildlife translocations. Conserv Biol 1995;10(2):349–353.

11. Darkin-Rattray SJ, Gurnett AM, Myers RW, et al. Apicidin: a novel antiprotozoal agent that inhibits parasite histone deacetylase. Proc Natl Acad Sci USA. 1996;93(23):13143–13147.

12. Daszak P, Cunningham AA, Hyatt AD. Emerging infectious disease of wildlife-threats to biodiversity and human health. Science 2000;287(5452):443–449.

13. Deem SL, Cook RA, Karesh WB. International opportunities in conservation medicine. In: Convention notes, 136th annual convention, American Veterinary Medical Association, July 10–14, 1999, Schaumburg, IL: American Veterinary Medical Association, 1999: 860–862.

14. Ehrenfeld D. Life in the Next Millennium: Who Will Be Left in the Earth's Community? In: Kaufman L, Mallory K, eds. The Last Extinction. Cambridge, MA: MIT Press, 1987:167–186.

15. Fischer JR. Mycoplasmal conjunctivitis in wild songbirds: the spread of a new contagious disease in a mobile host population. Emerg Infect Dis 1997;3(1):69–72.

16. French H. Vanishing Borders: Protecting the Planet in the Age of Globalization. New York: WW Norton, 2000.

17. Gardner H, Kerry K, Riddle M, et al. Poultry virus infection in Antarctic penguins. Nature 1997;387(6630):245.

18. Goltsman M, Kruchenkova EP, MacDonald DW. The Mednyi arctic foxes: treating a population imperiled by disease. Oryx 1996;30(4):251–258.

19. Goodall J. The chimpanzees of Gombe. Boston: Houghton Mifflin, 1986.

20. Green MJB, Paine J. State of the world's protected areas at the end of the twentieth century. In: Protected Areas in the 21st Century: From Islands to Networks. Proceedings of IUCN World Commission on Protected Areas (WCPA) Symposium, Albany, Australia, 24–29 November 1997.

21. Griffith B, Scott JM, Carpenter JW, Reed C. Animal translocations and potential disease transmission. J Zoo Wildl Med 1993;24(3):231–236.

22. Grifo F, Rosenthal J, eds. Biodiversity and Human Health. Washington, DC: Island Press, 1997.

23. Hackel JD. Community Conservation and the Future of Africa's Wildlife. Conserv Biol 1999;13(4):726–734.

24. Harvell CD, Kim K, Burkholder JM, et al. Emerging marine diseases-climate links and anthropogenic factors. Science 1999;285(5433):1505–1510.

25. Heide Jorgensen MP, Harkonen T, Dietz R, et al. Retrospective of the 1988 European seal epizootic. Dis Aquatic Organisms 1992;13(1):37–62.

26. Karesh WB. Wildlife rehabilitation: additional considerations for developing countries. J Zoo Wildl Med 1995;26(1):2–9.

27. Kelly JD, English AW. Conservation biology and the preservation of biodiversity in Australia: a role for zoos and the veterinary profession. Aust Vet J 1997;75(8):568–574.

28. Kennedy S, Kuiken T, Jepson PD, et al. Mass die-off of Caspian seals caused by canine distemper virus. Emerg Infect Dis 2000;6(6):637–639.

29. Kock ND, Goedegebuure SA, Lane EP, et al. Flaccid trunk paralysis in free-ranging elephants (Loxodonta africana) in Zimbabwe. J Wildl Dis 1994;30(3):432–435, 1994.

30. Lacy RC. Vortex: a computer simulation model for population viability analysis. Wildl Res 1993;20:45–65.

31. Laurenson K, Sillero-Zubiri C, Thompson H, et al. Disease as a threat to endangered species: Ethiopian wolves, domestic dogs and canine pathogens. Anim Conserv 1998;1:273–280.

32. MacDonald DW. Rabies and wildlife: a conservation problem? Onderstepoort J Vet Res 1993;60(4):351–355.

33. Masiga WN, Domenech J, Windsor RS, et al. Manifestations and epidemiology of contagious bovine pleuropneumonia in Africa. Rev Sci Tech OIE 1996;15:1283–1308.

34. Mellor PS, Boorman J. The transmission and geographical spread of African horse sickness and bluetongue viruses. Ann Trop Med Parasitol 1995;89(1):1–15.

35. Mittermeier RA, Myers N, Mittermeier CG. Hotspots. Earth's Biologically Richest and Most Endangered Terrestrial Ecoregions. Washington, DC: Conservation International, 2000.

36. Montali RJ, Scanga CA, Pernikoff D, et al. A common-source outbreak of callitrichid hepatitis in captive tamarin and marmosets. J Infect Dis 1993;167(4):946–950.

37. Myers N, Mittermeier RA, Mittermeier CG, et al. Biodiversity hotspots for conservation priorities. Nature 2000;403(6772):853–858.

38. National Research Council. Microlivestock. Little-Known Small Animals with a Promising Economic Future. Washington, DC: National Academy Press, 1991.

39. Nolen RS. Veterinarians key to discovering outbreak of exotic encephalitis. J Am Vet Med Assoc 1999;215(10): 1415,1418–1419.

40. Ntiamoa-Baidu Y. Wildlife and food security in Africa. FAO Conservation Guide no. 33. Rome: Food and Agriculture Organization of the United Nations, 1997.

41. Parmesan C, Ryrholm M, Stefanescu C, et al. Poleward shifts in geographical ranges of butterfly species associated with regional warming. Nature 1999;399:579–583.

42. Patronek GJ. Free-roaming and feral cats-their impact on wildlife and human beings. J Am Vet Med Assoc 1998;212:218–226.

43. Peters G. Mexico's latest illegal migrants: exotic animals. Christian Science Monitor, August 9, 2001:1,8.

44. Plowright W. Effects of rinderpest and rinderpest control on wildlife in Africa. Symp Zool Soc London 1982;50:1–27

45. Pokras M, Tabor G, Pearl M, et al. Conservation medicine: an emerging field. In nature and human society: the quest for a sustainable world. Washington, DC: National Academy Press, 1999:551–556.

46. Primack RB. A Primer of Conservation Biology. 2nd Ed. Sunderland, MA: Sinauer Associates, 2000.

47. Richman LK, Montali RJ, Garber RL, et al. Novel endotheliotropic herpesviruses fatal for Asian and African elephants. Science 1999;283(5405):1171–1176.

48. Roe D, Leader-Williams N, Dalal-Clayton B. Take only photographs, leave only footprints: the environmental impacts of wildlife tourism. IIED Wildlife and Development Series no. 10. London: International Institute for Environment and Development, 1997.

49. Roelke-Parker ME, Munson L, Packer C, et al. A canine distemper virus epidemic in Serengeti lions (*Panthera leo*). Nature 1996;379(6564):441–445.

50. Scheumhammer AM, Norris SL. The ecotoxicology of lead shot and lead fishing weights. Ecotoxicology 1996;5(5):279–295.

51. Sherman DM, Pokras M, English AW. Preparing veterinarians for meaningful participation in wildlife conservation. J Vet Med Educ 1999;26(1):26–29.

52. Siefert L, Opuda-Asibo J, Nakasala-Situma J, et al. Improved training in wildlife utilisation of veterinarians in Uganda. S Afr J Wildl Res 1996;26(4):171–174.

53. Thorne ET, Williams ES. Disease and endangered species: the black-footed ferret as a recent example. Conserv Biol 1988;2:66–74.

54. Van Riper C III, Van Riper SG, Goff ML, et al. The epizootiology and ecological significance of malaria in Hawaiian USA land birds. Ecol Monogr 1986;56(4):327–344.

55. Vitousek PM, Mooney HA, Lubchenco J, Melillo JM. Human domination of Earth's ecosystems. Science 1997;277(5325):494–499.

56. Weaver MA. Hunting with the sheiks. New Yorker 1992;68(43):51.

57. Williams T. Classroom warfare. Audubon 2000;102(5):38–49.

58. Wilson EO. The current state of biological diversity, In: Wilson EO, Ed. Biodiversity. Washington, DC: National Academy Press, 1988.

59. Wilson EO. Threats to biodiversity. Sci Am 1989;261(3):108–116.

60. Woodford MH. International disease implications for wildlife translocation. J Zoo Wildl Med 1993;24(3):265–270.

Suggested Readings

Daily GC, ed. Nature's Services: Societal Dependence on Ecosystem Services. Washington, DC: Island Press, 1997.

Epstein PR. Is global warming harmful to health? Sci Am 2000;283(2):50–57.

Epstein PR. Climate change and emerging infectious diseases. Microb Infect 2001;3(9):747–754.

Fowler ME, Miller RE. Zoo and Wild Animal Medicine. Current Therapy 4. Philadelphia: WB Saunders, 1998.

Heywood VH. Global Biodiversity Assessment. Cambridge, England: Cambridge University Press, 1995.

Kricher J. A Neotropical Companion. An Introduction to the Animals, Plants and Ecosystems of the New World Tropics. 2nd Ed. Princeton, NJ: Princeton University Press, 1997.

McKenzie AA, ed. The Capture and Care Manual. Capture, Care, Accommodation, and Transportation of African Wild Animals, Wildlife Decision Support Services, South Africa, 1993. On the internet, see http://www.wildlifeservices.co.za/captureandcare/

Terborgh J. Diversity and the Tropical Rain Forest. New York, Scientific American Library, 1992.

Terborgh, J. Requiem for Nature. Washington, DC: Island Press, 1999.

Western D. In the Dust of Kilimanjaro. Washington, DC: Island Press, 1997.

Wilson EO. The Diversity of Life. Cambridge, MA: Belknap Press, 1992.

Chapter 8
Delivery of Animal Health Care Services Worldwide

OBJECTIVES FOR THIS CHAPTER

After completing this chapter, the reader should be able to

- Distinguish between veterinary services aimed at the "public good" and at the "private good"

- Identify the main activities and services provided by organized veterinary medicine

- Recognize the different ways that veterinary services are structured in different parts of the world and the reasons for these differences

- Understand the different needs that different societies must address in establishing veterinary service priorities

- Appreciate the various constraints affecting the delivery of veterinary service

- Identify alternative approaches to animal health care delivery that would improve access by the end user, particularly in developing countries

Introduction

Currently, about 2.5% of all the veterinarians in the United States are employed by government, and 86% are in private clinical practice. In Israel, the distribution of veterinarians between government employment and private practice is more equal, with 22% employed by government and 26% in private clinical practice. In India, as in many developing countries in Africa and Asia, the employment distribution of veterinarians is essentially opposite that in the United States, with over 80% of veterinarians working for government and less than 5% in private clinical practice.

What accounts for such variation in the pattern of veterinary employment in different countries of the world? What are the implications of having a nation's veterinarians work for the government or in private practice? Just what services need to be delivered by a nation's veterinarians? Does the pattern of employment in a country have any bearing on the availability, efficiency, and quality of veterinary service delivery? What constraints exist on improving veterinary service delivery in different parts of the world, and what can be done to improve veterinary service delivery in the context of such constraints? Such questions are not simply academic. They reflect the very real issues of whether or not animal owners can reliably gain access to good veterinary care to ensure the health and productivity of their animals, whether or not the public can be protected effectively from zoonotic diseases and whether or not nations can participate competitively in international trade of livestock and livestock products.

To investigate these questions, and provide some answers, this chapter begins with a discussion of the concepts of "public good" and "private good" and the application of these concepts as a foundation for the rational delivery of veterinary services. This is followed by a description of the various activities and services for which organized veterinary medicine is usually responsible in society. The subsequent section of the chapter addresses the organizational differences in veterinary services in different regions of the world and gives some of the historical reasons for these differences. This is followed by a review of the constraints on veterinary service delivery in developing countries and a discussion of some of the approaches being taken to overcome these constraints, including privatization of veterinary services and community-based animal health programs.

We live in an era characterized by the emergence of new infectious diseases and the resurgence of diseases previously thought to be under control, in both animals and humans. As this is also an era of unprecedented international travel and trade, the risk of further disease spread is high, making the need for effective veterinary services greater than ever. Yet, in many areas of the world, veterinary service delivery is not achieving its intended purposes. Improvement in global veterinary service delivery is an important and significant challenge to the profession and a collective obligation. It is also a task that offers a tremendous variety of international career opportunities for veterinarians with a global perspective.

The Concepts of Private Good and Public Good

In recent years, many policymakers, seeking to find ways to improve the quality and efficiency of veterinary services, have found it useful to frame the discussion of veterinary service delivery in the context of three key questions:

- What services need to be provided by a nation's veterinarians and their supporting staff?
- Who benefits from each of the services provided?
- Who pays for these services?

To answer these questions, these policymakers have found it useful to consider the concepts of public good and private good.

Private Good

Any given service can be classified in economic terms according to who receives the benefits of the service. In the context of veterinary service delivery, a purely private good is one that solely and exclusively benefits the owner of the animal receiving the service. This means that no other animal owner or member of the public directly benefits from the veterinary intervention provided. So, when a veterinarian tends to a distal limb laceration on a pleasure horse, manages a case of urethral obstruction in a house cat, vaccinates a dog against Lyme disease, or administers anthelmintic to a flock of sheep grazing on a farmer's own pasture, then the veterinarian is providing services for the private good, as only the owner of the animal and the animal itself benefit. It seems logical that veterinarians delivering such services should be in private clinical practice and that the animal owners receiving such services should pay for such services entirely out of their own pocket. Such is the case in the United States, Canada, and most other developed countries of the world where free market forces prevail and high consumer demand for clinical veterinary services encourages most veterinarians to work in private clinical practice, providing individualized clinical services for the private good.

Public Good

A public good is a service that benefits society at large and to which no one can be denied access. In the context of veterinary service delivery, meat inspection is an example of a pure public good. Anyone who chooses to eat meat benefits from the assurance of a reliable supply of hygienic meat on supermarket shelves. No one can be excluded from receiving the benefit of inspected meat, and since there is no mechanism for exclusion from the benefit, there is also no incentive for individual consumers to pay for meat inspection. In other words, if some consumers were willing to pay, but others were not, there would be no mechanism to require the "free riders" to pay. As a matter of social and economic policy, therefore, it serves society as a whole to recognize, finance, and manage meat inspection as a public good, using tax dollars as the source of revenue to fund the activity.

Another reason that meat inspection needs to be considered a public good is the matter of moral hazard arising from the asymmetry of information. Consumers, in general, are not in a position to reliably assess the wholesomeness of purchased meat. They do not have the technical information, training, or monitoring equipment necessary to validate the safety of the product. The supplier has greater access to such information and, in addition, can potentially misrepresent the wholesomeness of the product, since the buyer cannot easily detect the presence of surface bacteria or residues of drugs or toxins. To avoid such unscrupulous behavior, society again has a vested interest in making meat inspection an independent function carried out by government as a public good. In practice, government could hire independent contractors to carry out the function, but underwriting the activity would still require public funding.

Public Good with Externalities

Not all services to society can be clearly categorized as exclusively private goods or public goods. A number of services fall somewhere in between. For example, the vaccination of a dog for Lyme disease was cited earlier as a purely private good. This is because Lyme disease is transmitted by ticks to other animals and humans. So vaccinating a dog only protects that dog from getting Lyme disease, but does not protect others. On the other hand, consider the vaccination of a dog against rabies. This cannot be considered a purely private good. Rabies can be transmitted directly from an infected dog to other animals and humans. So, when a dog owner has a dog vaccinated, there is a spillover effect. The risk of rabies to others has been reduced at the dog owner's expense, and there is no way that the owner can recoup the costs of vaccination from these secondary beneficiaries. This is an example of a public good with externalities, an externality being a spillover effect that has an impact on others, separate from the direct effect of the service.

Many veterinary services have externalities or spillover effects, and these effects have implications for public policy. When some individuals benefit without directly participating in a service, it is difficult to solicit voluntary participation in, and payment for, that service. In the livestock sector, for instance, it may only be necessary to vaccinate 90% of a susceptible cattle population in a given region to effect general immunity in that population to a specific contagious disease. However, for highly contagious diseases of cattle for which organized vaccination programs are carried out, it would be problematic to allow vaccination to be voluntary. Some livestock owners would quickly deduce that their cattle might be protected if all their neighbors vaccinated their cattle, but they did not. Obviously, it would not require too many like-minded livestock

owners to think along those same lines before vaccination coverage fell below 90%, leading to increased risk of disease occurrence in the region. Therefore, the externality of protection without participation is controlled by legislation that mandates compulsory vaccination for the disease in question.

Table 8-1 provides a summary list of various veterinary functions and services and categorizes them as private goods, public goods, and/or public goods with externalities. Subsequent discussions in this chapter on the structure of veterinary services, the effectiveness of veterinary service delivery, and policy considerations for improving veterinary service delivery depend to a great extent on recognition of the notion of public good and private good.

General Functions of Veterinary Services

Veterinarians and their support staff provide a variety of useful services to society, for both public and private good. In this section, different veterinary functions are identified and briefly explained. In addition, to provide a frame of reference for subsequent discussion of veterinary service delivery around the world, the agencies and organizations responsible for each function in the United States are identified.

There are three major functions generally defined for veterinary service: protection of the national herds and flocks; protection of human health; and clinical service delivery to individual animals. In support of these primary functions, several additional activities need to be provided by society, including education, research, and extension. Each of these primary and ancillary functions is discussed in the following sections.

Protection of the National Herds and Flocks

The *national herd* is a term used to refer collectively to all the hoofed livestock in a given country, and *national flock* refers to its aggregate poultry population. Though the magnitude of the contribution of animal agriculture to the overall economy varies considerably among countries, virtually all nations recognize their own livestock as a valuable economic and social resource. Thus each nation commits some financial and human capital toward an organized effort to protect the national herd and flock from disease and to improve productivity. In countries in which export of livestock or livestock products represents an important sector of the national economy, disease control takes on added importance, as continued export requires compliance with international standards of animal health set forth by individual importing countries and through cooperative agreements among member countries of the Office International des Epizooties (OIE) and the World Trade Organization (WTO), as discussed in more detail in Chapter 9.

The various activities involved in protection of the national herds and flocks are essentially public goods, some with externalities that require legislation and enforcement to protect the common interest. These activities are disease surveillance,

Table 8-1   Various Veterinary Services Categorized As Private Goods or Public Goods

Type of Service	Type of Good	Management Responsibility	Payment Responsibility	Comments
Disease reporting	Public	Government	Treasury	Externalities require regulations identifying lists of mandatory diseases reportable to authorities by private practitioners
Disease investigation	Public	Government	Treasury	Externalities require regulations for mandatory compliance by farmers with disease investigators
Disease control	Public	Government[a]	Treasury and, in some cases of vaccination, animal owners	Externalities require regulations for mandatory compliance with control measures such as vaccination, quarantine, or test and slaughter
Emergency response	Public	Government[a]	Treasury	Externalities require legislation granting special authority and mandating cooperation during times of emergency
Disease surveillance	Public	Government	Treasury	Requires participation and coordination at local, regional, national, and international levels
Control of animal movement	Public	Government[a]	Treasury	Externalities require regulations for mandatory health inspection of animals moving to and from market or across political boundaries
Quality control of veterinary drugs and biologicals	Public	Government	Treasury	Potential moral hazard from misrepresentation of product safety and efficacy
Animal welfare	Public	Government	Treasury	Considered a general concern of society enforceable by law
Zoonotic disease control	Public	Government[a]	Treasury	Externalities require regulations for mandatory compliance by animal owners with vaccination, testing, and other procedures to ensure human health
Meat inspection and food hygiene	Public	Government[a]	Treasury	Potential moral hazard from misrepresentation of quality
Clinical interventions	Private	Private practitioners	Animal owners	Government may continue to provide clinical service where market conditions cannot support private clinical practice
Veterinary education	Public and private	Public and private educational institutions	Student fees and government subsidy	It is in the national interest to have veterinarians, but many graduates go into private practice
Registration and licensure	Public	Government and professional organizations	Veterinarians	Potential moral hazard from lack of regulation of professional credentials and performance

(continued)

Table 8-1	Various Veterinary Services Categorized As Private Goods or Public Goods *(Continued)*			
Type of Service	**Type of Good**	**Management Responsibility**	**Payment Responsibility**	**Comments**
Research	Public and/or private	Government and/or private industry	Treasury and/or producer groups	A specific commodity group may want research resources focused on its own issues, in which case, the group provides its own funding
Extension and outreach	Public and/or private	Government and/or private industry	Treasury and/or producer groups	A specific commodity group may want extension activities focused on their members, in which case, the group provides funding

ᵃGovernment may subcontract private veterinarians or organizations to assist government veterinarians to carry out this work.

disease investigation, disease control, emergency response, disease reporting, control of animal movement, control of veterinary drugs and biologicals, and animal welfare. They are discussed individually in the following paragraphs.

Disease Surveillance and Reporting

Disease surveillance, also referred to as epidemiological intelligence, is the methodical collection and epidemiological assessment of information on diseases of animals in the national herds and flocks. Increasingly, disease data are being correlated with demographic, geographical, production, and market information on animals in the national herd and flock, collected over similar time periods. Collectively, these interrelated data make up an national animal health-monitoring system. Data on diseases transmissible to humans may also be collected and analyzed by agencies responsible for control of zoonotic diseases. Likewise, information on disease in wildlife populations may be collected when wildlife serve as a reservoir for disease potentially transmissible to livestock, companion animals, and humans.

Surveillance is not an end unto itself. Data that are collected must serve some useful purpose. Persons who have willingly contributed information in the past to a disease surveillance effort will not do so in the future if they believe data collection is a nonproductive exercise. Data must be analyzed, interpreted, and reported in a systematic way. When done properly, a number of objectives are well served by an organized surveillance system of data collection and analysis. These objectives are to

- Provide periodic assessments of the productivity and overall health status of livestock populations in a country, and make the information available to the public
- Monitor specific diseases of particular concern within a country so that proper control strategies can be formulated and appropriately reformulated as the situation changes over time

- Identify and track emerging diseases that threaten national herds and flocks or present a risk to humans
- Facilitate export trade through credible certification of a nation's true disease status
- Comply with international treaty obligations, such as the prompt notification of reportable animal disease occurrences to international organizations such as the OIE and to trading partners
- Develop and establish technically justifiable requirements for importation of animals and animal products, to minimize the risk of disease introduction
- Facilitate timely recognition and notification to the public of the occurrence of foreign animal diseases
- Provide adequate and reliable information to the Chief Veterinary Officer, Chief Public Health Officer, and other relevant government policymakers so that they may rationally plan, fund, and implement animal disease-control policies that safeguard animal and human health

Disease surveillance programs depend on a variety of sources for information on animal disease. The main sources are likely to include veterinary practitioners and technicians in private practice or government-run clinics, veterinary diagnostic laboratories, and slaughterhouse inspection data. Additional sources may include veterinary teaching hospitals, census data from agriculture department surveys, import/export records, records of milk marketing boards, or standardized, retrievable data from producer databases, for example, the Dairy Herd Improvement Program.

Surveillance data can be obtained passively or actively. Most routinely collected data are passive data. For passive data collection, protocols are set up for regular, periodic reporting of specific disease observations by veterinarians in the field, regular filing of summary reports of disease findings from diagnostic laboratories, and inspection reports from abattoirs.

Programs of active data collection are initiated when a specific disease problem is of concern to regulatory authorities. In such cases (e.g., the introduction of an exotic disease or the emergence of a disease with public health implications), an organized sampling and testing effort of the target population is developed and undertaken. Such an active sampling program might involve the systematic collection of milk, blood, or other sample materials from a subpopulation of herds in a region. These samples are submitted to a central diagnostic laboratory for bacterial isolation, serological testing, or other such evaluation, as the disease under consideration might dictate. The recent introduction of West Nile virus into the United States prompted such an active disease surveillance program, with federal, state, and local regulatory authorities initiating sampling of mosquito pools, wild birds, and horse populations to track the spread of the disease and to plan appropriate control interventions.

Disease surveillance programs are vertically integrated. Data from the field are progressively transferred to centralized authorities for analysis, interpretation, and reporting. As such, veterinarians in the field, along with district laboratories and local slaughterhouses may report to state, provincial, or regional veterinary authorities who, in turn, transmit their findings to the national level. Most countries have a central veterinary authority, often identified as the Chief Veterinary Officer, who is responsible for the national program of regulatory veterinary medicine. Administratively, regulatory veterinary medicine usually exists as a division or section within a national ministry or department of agriculture. Within the section, there is usually an epidemiology office responsible for analyzing the disease surveillance data and reporting their findings to the government and the public.

In the United States, the hub of disease reporting is at the state level. Each state usually has a State Veterinarian's Office, a Bureau or Division of Animal Health, and a State Veterinary Diagnostic Laboratory, possibly with branch laboratories located around the state, if animal agriculture represents a large sector of the state's economy. Each state develops and maintains a list of reportable diseases that veterinarians practicing within the state are obligated to report when they are diagnosed. In general, diseases reportable to the state fall into a number of expected categories:

- Diseases exotic to the United States, such as foot and mouth disease, rinderpest, or African Swine fever

- Diseases that occur in the United States, but not in that particular state or region, for example, anaplasmosis

- Diseases with important public health implications, such as brucellosis, tuberculosis, and rabies

- Diseases of local economic importance reflecting the major livestock industries of the state or region, for example, paratuberculosis in dairy cattle

- Diseases for which an active management or control plan is in effect, for example, pseudorabies in swine

At the federal level, the Animal and Plant Health Inspection Service (APHIS) of the U.S. Department of Agriculture (USDA) is the principal agency for regulatory veterinary medicine in the United States. An overview of APHIS and other USDA agencies involved in animal disease control is provided in Table 8-2. APHIS, through its Veterinary Services branch, operates the Center for Epidemiology and Animal Health, in Fort Collins, Colorado, which is responsible for analyzing and reporting national animal disease data through the National Animal Health Monitoring System (NAHMS).

Disease Investigation

Formal disease investigations are carried out by veterinarians empowered by government to undertake such investigations. Disease investigation is generally considered a public good with externalities, in that such activity, while protecting livestock owners in general, may lead to quarantine, the destruction of animals, or other disease-control measures that may adversely affect individual livestock owners. Therefore, the cooperation of livestock owners with official disease investigations is usually mandated by law.

Two types of situation may lead to a formal disease investigation. One is to confirm a suspected case of a reportable disease after the regulatory authorities are notified by a veterinarian that such a disease has been tentatively diagnosed in the field. The second is to establish, when possible, the cause of an unfamiliar, unrecognized, or poorly characterized animal health problem being reported by producers or their veterinarians in a particular locale or in a particular species. The purposes of a disease investigation are to

- Confirm the cause of a disease outbreak

- Evaluate the extent of the outbreak

- Assess the risk of spread to susceptible populations of animals and/or humans

- Initiate preliminary measures to prevent such spread

To accomplish these objectives, investigators must carry out a thorough clinical examination, select and submit appropriate samples for evaluation at diagnostic laboratories, and conduct an epidemiological assessment. The clinical examination includes a detailed history, physical examination, and necropsy evaluations. Laboratory testing requires adequate and proper selection of samples, a clear description of the outbreak with suspected causes identified, careful handling and packaging of samples along with appropriate paperwork, and safe and timely transport of samples to the appropriate laboratories.

The epidemiological assessment requires contact and interviews with livestock owners whose herds are either affected or in contact with affected herds; description of the herds in terms of location, numbers, and animal characteristics (age,

Table 8-2   Organizational Chart of Agencies within the USDA Actively Involved in Veterinary Service Delivery in the United States and Brief Descriptions of Their Functions

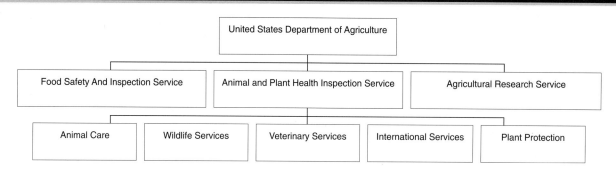

Food Safety and Inspection Service: FSIS is the public health agency responsible for ensuring that the nation's commercial supply of meat, poultry, and egg products is safe, wholesome, and correctly labeled and packaged, as required by the Federal Meat Inspection Act, the Poultry Products Inspection Act, and the Egg Products Inspection Act. Veterinary medical officers supervise and carry out inspection activities at licensed processing plants throughout the country. FSIS has an international policy division that ensures the safety and quality of imported meat, poultry, and egg products by working with foreign governments to establish equivalency in their food inspection and safety procedures (see http://www.fsis.usda.gov/index.htm).

Agricultural Research Service: ARS is the main in-house research arm of the USDA. It maintains numerous research and experimental stations around the country focusing on specific issues related to crop and livestock health and production. In veterinary medicine, ARS scientists work on issues of foreign animal disease at the Plum Island Animal Disease Center, off Greenport, Long Island, New York, and on existing livestock disease problems at the National Animal Disease Center in Ames, Iowa. There are several additional research facilities addressing specific production and disease issues at various locations within the United States, such as the Poisonous Plant Research Laboratory in Logan, Utah (see http://www.ars.usda.gov/).

Animal and Plant Health Inspection Service: APHIS is the principal agency for regulatory veterinary medicine in the United States (see http://www.aphis.usda.gov/). APHIS performs its varied services through the activities of five distinct operational services, described as follows.

Animal Care: Animal Care conducts inspections to ensure the proper stewardship of animals used in research, exhibition, or other regulated industries in compliance with the Animal Welfare Act and the Horse Protection Act.

Wildlife Services: Wildlife Services works to reduce wildlife damage to agriculture and natural resources and to minimize potential wildlife threats to human health and safety. It cooperates with other agencies in the protection of threatened and endangered species and cooperates with foreign governments and private organizations on issues of animal and bird damage and nuisance control.

Veterinary Services: VS protects the health of livestock and poultry resources by regulating the entry of imported animals and animal health products. VS coordinates emergency actions against foreign disease through its Emergency Programs Unit and, with the states, operates eradication programs for domestic animal and zoonotic diseases. The service provides health certificates for exported animals and animal products. It conducts diagnostic tests and issues licenses for veterinary biological products and manufacturers. VS also contains the Centers for Epidemiology and Animal Health, responsible for national animal health monitoring and disease reporting. The deputy administrator of APHIS Veterinary Services serves as the chief veterinary officer of the United States.

International Services: IS conducts activities outside the United States to protect American agriculture and to enhance U.S. exports. It maintains a worldwide information network on animal and plant diseases and pests. It assists foreign governments in combating plant and animal disease infestations and manages preclearance programs of agricultural products destined for the United States. IS also provides technical support for, and participates in, international trade negotiations related to agricultural products.

Plant Protection and Quarantine: PPQ protects the nation's agricultural resources from the international spread of plant and animal pests and diseases. The service conducts passenger and baggage port inspections at international airport terminals, seaports, and border stations and carries out surveillance of ship cargoes, rail and truck freight, and mail from foreign countries. PPQ certifies U.S. agricultural products for export to meet international requirements. During the outbreak of foot and mouth disease in the U.K. in 2001, the PPQ represented the front-line defense for keeping foot and mouth disease out of the United States by screening incoming travelers and commodities potentially contaminated with the virus.

species, sex, etc.); evaluation of prevailing management factors; documentation and tracing of any animal purchases, sales, and movements, including precise origins and destinations; interviews with animal dealers and transporters; and consideration of any other factors that may have played a role in the occurrence of the disease outbreak.

Clearly, for effective disease investigation to be carried out, a number of prerequisite conditions must prevail:

- Livestock owners must trust veterinary authorities enough to be willing to report the occurrence of unfamiliar diseases or disease outbreaks
- Sufficient numbers of regulatory veterinarians, trained in proper and thorough disease investigation, must be available to carry out investigations in a timely manner
- A functioning diagnostic laboratory must be available for accurate and timely performance of diagnostic tests for diseases of major concern in the country
- Communication and transportation infrastructure in the country must be adequate to facilitate a rapid investigative response
- Sufficient rule of law with adequate enforcement must exist to ensure compliance with disease investigations, especially when provisional quarantines are initiated while awaiting diagnostic confirmation

In the United States, preliminary disease investigation is usually a state function. When practicing veterinarians suspect cases of diseases that are on their state's reportable disease list, they notify the State Veterinarian/Bureau of Animal Health. A state veterinarian, usually accompanied by the reporting practitioner, will then visit the farm or premises where the disease has occurred and begin the disease investigation. If a foreign animal disease exotic to the United States is suspected by the state veterinarian following initial investigation, then the state veterinarian will call in a federal APHIS veterinarian trained as a foreign animal disease diagnostician (FADD) to participate in the investigation. Each state is assigned at least one APHIS veterinarian.

Emergency Response

If a disease investigation confirms the presence of a highly infectious, contagious animal or zoonotic disease, or if the disease is exotic to the country or region, then it is necessary for regulatory authorities to mount a rapid and effective emergency response to eliminate, or at least control, spread of the disease. An appropriate response depends to a large extent on a thorough understanding of the epidemiological character of the disease in question, including such factors as its incubation period, range of host species, mode of transmission, involvement of vectors, existence of wildlife reservoirs, patterns of shedding, development of carrier states, and climatic or ge-

ographical limitations to its spread. It also depends to some extent on the availability of certain technologies, tools, and equipment, for example, sensitive diagnostic tests that can detect subclinical infections, vaccines that offer strong, lasting immunity, or adequate spraying equipment to control highly contagious external parasites such as sarcoptic mange mites or disease vectors such as mosquitoes. The emergency response also requires adequate personnel with clearly defined responsibilities and authorities and a clearly established chain of command. Most importantly perhaps, an effective response requires the full cooperation of livestock owners and citizens in implementing the emergency response plan.

Emergency response to disease outbreaks is a public good with externalities. Some individuals may incur negative outcomes as a result of the overall effort to protect livestock owners collectively. This is because effective emergency response efforts sometimes call for the quarantine or the "stamping out" of disease through destruction of animals that have been in contact with, or in areas adjacent to, animals confirmed infected. As the reader might surmise, a farmer who is informed that his animals need to be destroyed or restricted from sale because his neighbor's animals are sick is not likely to greet such news with enthusiasm. To ensure cooperation for the sake of the public good, laws empowering regulatory authorities to undertake quarantine or destruction of animal for emergency disease control must exist and be enforceable. It also helps if the laws include mechanisms for economic compensation to livestock owners for economic losses incurred through cooperation with disease control efforts and the public treasury maintains adequate funds to pay out such compensations reliably.

In the United States, emergency responses to reportable diseases are coordinated by state veterinarians in cooperation with federal APHIS veterinarians when foreign animal diseases are involved. More details of this coordinated emergency response are provided in Chapter 9. When zoonotic diseases outbreaks occur, state public health officials, including public health veterinarians, become involved in the emergency response. In outbreaks of disease involving large numbers of animals or covering a wide geographical area, regulatory agencies may solicit the cooperation of veterinary practitioners and veterinarians at teaching and research institutions to participate in the emergency response effort. Large-scale emergency responses may quickly exhaust the staff, resources, and equipment of veterinary agencies at the state level. Therefore, planning for such emergencies is often coordinated through the state emergency management agency so that the resources of other governmental and nongovernmental entities can be drawn upon as needed. Such entities might include departments of fish and wildlife and environmental protection, law enforcement agencies such as the state police, and the National Guard, among others.

Animal Disease Control

Preventing the introduction and spread of foreign animal diseases and emerging zoonotic diseases is a major concern in international veterinary medicine. The challenges associated with the prevention and control of such diseases are increasing because of the globalization and expansion of international trade, increased international travel for recreation and business, global climate change, and increased movement of displaced people and livestock as a result of civil instability and environmental degradation, as discussed further in Chapter 9 and elsewhere in this book.

Mounting an emergency response to an acute epizootic or zoonotic disease outbreak is only one of several important aspects of disease control. Overall, the key objectives of a nation's disease control program are to

- Prevent the introduction, and control the spread, of foreign animal diseases

- Eliminate or control the spread of epizootic diseases that occur within the country

- Eradicate or limit the spread of enzootic animal diseases of economic importance and zoonotic diseases that already exist within the country

- Minimize the impact of noninfectious diseases on animal health and production

Epizootic diseases are those that are highly infectious and likely to spread rapidly through susceptible populations. Control of acute outbreaks of epizootic disease requires a coordinated emergency response as already described. However, mounting a "fire brigade" response to isolated disease outbreaks, even when performed successfully, is only one part of a fully developed disease-control strategy. In putting together a comprehensive national disease-control plan, a number of considerations must be taken into account, including

- Knowledge of the diseases already present, as determined from an operational disease surveillance system

- Accurate projections and estimates of the economic cost of each disease if left unchecked

- A benefit/cost analysis of effective control efforts versus potential economic losses from uncontrolled disease

- The existence of suitable methods (e.g., a reliable diagnostic test to identify subclinical cases) and tools (e.g., a vaccine offering lifelong immunity) to support successful implementation of disease control measures

- Adequate personnel, equipment, transport, lab support, and other resources to undertake an effective control program

- A reliable program for monitoring the effects of disease control following completion of a disease control campaign in order to protect the achievements of the campaign

- Adequate funding to implement and sustain the disease control program until its goals are reached

- Sufficient rule of law and appropriate legislation and funding in place to ensure compliance in disease control programs when negative externalities exist

Once these conditions are met, national and regional priorities can be established for disease control efforts. While each of these conditions is important in its own right, their relative importance and the ability to address them will vary among countries and for different diseases. Many developing countries face serious obstacles in establishing and implementing effective disease control programs, as discussed later in this chapter.

The strategy for control of epizootics will differ with each disease, depending on its epidemiological characteristics. A summary of different approaches to disease control with examples of the diseases appropriate for each approach is presented in Table 8-3. Note that some diseases can be completely eradicated, while others, because of either their epidemiological nature or a lack of adequate methods and tools to identify and control them, are more likely to be contained than eliminated.

Similarly, zoonotic diseases vary in their epidemiological characteristics, and different strategies are required to contain them. Often, successful programs for controlling disease in humans are aimed at eliminating the infection from the animal reservoir, as in the case of bovine tuberculosis eradication in the United States, which has succeeded through an assiduous program of testing and slaughter of infected animals. However, control of zoonoses that involve insect vectors or extensive wildlife reservoirs can be more problematic. Even when effective control measures are available, various constraints may limit their application in the control of zoonotic disease.

Rabies offers a good example. Island nations such as the United Kingdom, Japan, Australia, and New Zealand take advantage of their geographical isolation to prevent the introduction of rabies through strict control of the movement of susceptible species into their countries. In the United States, where rabies is endemic, it is not feasible to eliminate wildlife reservoirs of the disease, but the occurrence of rabies in humans has been minimized by mandatory vaccination of companion animals. In many developing countries, rabies is still prevalent, and human populations are very much at risk because resources are inadequate to mount large-scale vaccination campaigns to immunize dogs and cats, although some progress in now being made in selected countries through the use of oral bait vaccinations that do not require handling and injecting individual animals. Nevertheless, the World Health Organization reports estimates of over 40,000 human deaths annually from rabies, mostly in developing countries.

In the United States, national animal-disease control is a cooperative effort between APHIS at the federal level, state veterinary and public health agencies, and private practitioners. While government has direct authority and responsibility for

Table 8-3   Approaches to the Control of Various Types of Epizootic Disease

Approach to Disease Control	Techniques Used	Examples of Relevant Diseases
Isolation and elimination of foreign epizootics	Stamping out diseased, inapparently diseased, infected, and latently infected animals	African swine fever; exotic foot and mouth disease
	Slaughtering diseased and infected animals and vaccinating exposed and potentially endangered animals	Classical swine fever (hog cholera); endemic foot and mouth disease
Eradication of persistent epizootics using sanitation and control programs	Depopulation of whole herds by slaughtering; separate management of serological reactors	Bovine tuberculosis; bovine brucellosis; enzootic bovine leucosis in highly infected populations
	Permanent diagnostic monitoring of populations and removal of single serological reactors	Leptospirosis in swine; enzootic bovine leucosis in lightly infected populations
	Combination of hygienic measures and vaccination	Host-adapted salmonellae, e.g., *S. dublin* in cattle, *S. cholerasuis* in swine; *S. agalactiae* in sheep and goats
	Combination of hygienic measures and antibiotic treatments	Swine dysentery
Progressive reduction of the occurrence of epizootics for which means of total eradication are not available	Control of wildlife reservoirs and immunization of animals (and humans) at risk	Rabies
	Combination of hygienic measures and vaccination	Non-host adapted *Salmonellae*, e.g., *S. typhimurium*
	Permanent diagnostic monitoring, postexposure and prophylactic treatment, slaughter of animals that have become uneconomic	Atrophic rhinitis of pigs
	Preexposure vaccinations	Erysipelas of swine; myxomatosis of rabbits
Interruption of disease transmission process by zoosanitary measures	Control of animal movements, quarantine, and control of vectors and intermediate hosts	Babesiosis; liver fluke disease

Adapted from Blaha T, ed. Applied Veterinary Epidemiology. Developments in Animal and Veterinary Sciences, Vol. 21. Amsterdam: Elsevier, 1989.

much of the zoonotic and infectious animal disease control activity in the United States, only 1.4% of all the veterinarians in the country work directly for the federal government and 1.1% for state or local government. Given the relatively few veterinarians directly involved in regulatory veterinary medicine, the vast land area of the United States, the large size of its animal populations, and the diversity of its animal agriculture, the nation has been remarkably effective in controlling and even eliminating important epizootic and zoonotic diseases. Since the Bureau of Animal Industry (BAI), precursor to APHIS, was established by an act of Congress in 1884 to control contagious

bovine pleuropneumonia and other contagious animal diseases, many serious enzootic and foreign animal disease threats have been effectively contained or eliminated through the efforts of BAI/APHIS, supported by the rule of law and the cooperation of livestock owners, animal industries, and private practitioners.

Not all threats to the health and productivity of a nation's livestock resources are infectious. There are numerous noninfectious conditions that can occur regionally, conditioned by climate, geography, soil type, or other geophysical and management factors. Mineral deficiencies such as selenium or iodine constrain production in areas where forage plants cannot take up adequate mineral from deficient soils. In arid regions with long dry seasons, vitamin A deficiency is common in both livestock, and people because of prolonged periods without access to green forage or plants. Grazing animals in arid regions may also be subjected to plant toxicities when dry conditions reduce the availability of nutritious forage plants and animals are forced to consume excessive quantities of toxin-containing plants. In such situations, veterinary services must be directed at educating livestock owners about the causes and economic significance of noninfectious disease problems and dedicate some energy and resources to noninfectious disease control efforts. In some countries, the provision of selenium injections, vitamin A supplements, or iodized salt may do as much to improve overall productivity in national herds as provision of antibiotics or vaccines.

Control of Animal Movement and Quarantine

A key element in containing the spread of many important animal diseases is control over the movement of animals. Commingling of animals at sales, transport of animals to markets, mixing of different herds on common grazing lands, seasonal migrations of pastoralists with their herds, and sporadic movement of refugees who own livestock are some of the ways that diseases can be transmitted between animals by virtue of mobility. The risk of transmission through animal contact is increased for diseases in which a subclinical carrier state occurs. Since such animals do not show clinical signs of illness, their potential to spread disease by shedding infective organisms and infecting other naïve, susceptible livestock can easily go unrecognized.

Therefore, veterinary authorities recognize the importance of officially inspecting animals that move across defined political or administrative boundaries within a country. Depending on the diseases of concern, regulatory authorities will establish specific requirements that must be met before animals can be moved into a protected region. These requirements can include official inspections, detailed physical examination, specific diagnostic tests, retention of the animals for a fixed period of observation, a specific vaccine or prophylactic treatment, and the issuance of an official health certificate clearing the animals for movement. Such a certificate and the animals listed therein are then inspected by regulatory authorities in the area to which the animals are going and must be approved by these authorities before the animals are allowed entrance.

A similar process is undertaken in relation to the international transport of livestock. Importing countries have specific requirements that must be met before animals are allowed entry. In addition, the importing country maintains quarantine stations staffed by regulatory veterinarians where entering animals are held for observation to ensure that they are not in the incubation stage of some infectious disease. The length of observation will vary with the diseases of concern, which depend on the disease profile of the country of origin and the species

of animals being imported. The international movement of animals for trade is discussed further in Chapter 9.

Control of animal movement is a public good with externalities. In the United States, each state promulgates rules and regulations concerning the restrictions and requirements for movement of animals into the state. Enforcement of the rules and regulations resides with the State Veterinarian and Bureau of Animal Health. However, the private practitioner is responsible in most cases for inspecting animals, taking appropriate samples for diagnostic testing, filling out official health certificates for animals to be moved across administrative boundaries, and submitting copies of those certificates to the appropriate regulatory authorities for approval. The requirements for interstate transport of animals differ from state to state. All the state requirements for animal movement have been compiled by APHIS as a public service and can be accessed at http://www.aphis.usda.gov/vs/sregs/ on the internet. APHIS regulates the importation of animals into the United States and maintains quarantine stations at major ports of entry where imported livestock must be kept for an appropriate observation period as a prerequisite to completing the importation.

Regulation of Veterinary Drugs and Biologicals

The manufacture and sale of drugs and biologicals poses a potential moral hazard that requires regulatory oversight to protect the public. Because the consumer has no reliable way to test the purity, safety, or efficacy of a product offered for sale, unscrupulous manufacturers or distributors can easily misrepresent such products. When bogus vaccines, antibiotics, anthelmintics, and acaricides enter the market and their use becomes widespread, the risk of disease transmission is increased rather than diminished, because not only do the false drugs fail to produce the intended effects, they also engender a false sense of security with regard to disease control. This is not a theoretical concern. Frauds related to the misrepresentation and sale of bogus drugs are commonplace in many parts of the world.

To control abuses and ensure the safety and efficacy of veterinary drugs, government authorities use varying approaches to regulation, depending on country circumstances. Poor, developing countries, with little or no capacity for domestic production, may control the procurement of drugs and vaccines from abroad through the central government and then distribute supplies to government veterinarians at the district level. Such governments argue that state control of procurement and distribution of veterinary drugs is necessary to prevent inferior or counterfeit drugs entering the market. In practice, however, it has frequently produced the opposite effect. Government agencies charged with procurement and distribution of drugs are often extremely bureaucratic, and the process of ordering and delivery is much slower than can be accomplished in the private sector. When bureaucratic delays are added to general mismanagement, inadequate budgets for drug purchase, and transportation difficulties in delivering drugs to district veterinary offices, the net result is often that a black market in veterinary drugs emerges and flourishes as the demand for such drugs far exceeds the capacity of government to reliably supply them.

In countries with domestic production capacity, ethical drug production is controlled through a combination of legislation, inspection, testing, and licensing. Consistent, thorough implementation of such a complex regulatory program, however, can strain the budgets of many nations, and effective oversight may be compromised. In Pakistan, for example, it is reported that substandard and counterfeit drug production and sale is widespread, despite the existence of laws to prevent such practices. The trade in counterfeit and substandard drugs within the country exceeds US$160 million annually. It is estimated that less than half of the licensed drug manufacturers in the country comply with international production standards. Shopkeepers actually will ask customers if they want first-quality (authentic name brands), second-quality (licensed but substandard manufactured equivalents), or third-quality (totally fake counterfeits) drugs. Counterfeit drugs are produced that are exact replicas of well-known imported drugs, copying every detail of the packaging and labeling, but compounding the pills or capsules out of inexpensive and wholly ineffective inert ingredients, such as talc or corn flour While drug manufacture is officially regulated in the country, inadequate numbers of inspectors, corruption, legal loopholes, and excessive bureaucracy all contribute to the flagrant marketing of substandard and counterfeit drugs in both the veterinary and human health markets.

In the United States, regulatory oversight is shared by a number of agencies. The USDA has regulatory responsibility for reviewing the safety and efficacy of new vaccines and other biologicals such as diagnostic reagents as well as for licensing them. These oversight function are performed by APHIS through the Center for Veterinary Biologics. The Food and Drug Administration (FDA), through its Center for Veterinary Medicine, is responsible for licensing parenteral drugs following a rigorous process to evaluate their safety and efficacy in the specific animal species for which the manufacturer is seeking approval. The FDA is also concerned about the effects on humans of veterinary drugs that are used in animals raised for food, as discussed below under the heading of food safety. Topical drugs, such as insecticides applied to the skin for external parasite control, are regulated by the Environmental Protection Agency, mainly because topical agents used in dips and sprays present potential hazards to soil, water, wildlife, other domestic animals, and humans if improperly used or carelessly discarded.

Animal Welfare

Ensuring the humane treatment of animals is a societal responsibility that is usually fulfilled through the promulgation of laws and regulations that define at least minimum standards of acceptable animal care. The extent to which a society embraces and enacts animal welfare legislation is strongly linked to social, economic, cultural, and religious perceptions concerning the status, use, and role of different animals within that society. When animal welfare laws are enacted, such laws usu-

ally address one or more of the following groups of animals with regard to humane treatment:

- Laboratory animals used in research, in terms of housing, comfort, and alleviation of pain
- Livestock, in terms of comfort and welfare during transport, at markets, and at slaughter
- Companion animals, with regard to incidents of neglect, cruelty, or intentional mutilation
- Animals exploited commercially for sale, exhibition, or contest
- Wildlife, especially with regard to techniques used in trapping

Veterinarians in society have a professional obligation and moral responsibility to minimize, alleviate, and prevent animal suffering as an integral part of their everyday professional activity. In addition, most countries use veterinarians in some official capacity to ensure that laws regulating the humane treatment of animals are properly observed.

In the United States, at the federal level, government-employed veterinarians working within the Animal Care division of APHIS are responsible for ensuring compliance with the Animal Welfare Act. This law was first passed in 1966 and amended several times since. The act requires that minimum standards of care and treatment be provided for most warm-blooded animals bred for commercial sale, used in research, transported commercially, or exhibited to the public. The act also prohibits staged dogfights, bear and raccoon baiting, and similar animal fighting ventures. Details of the Animal Welfare Act and the activities of APHIS Animal Care can be found on the internet at the APHIS Animal Care website (http://www.aphis.usda.gov/ac/). In contrast to similar legislation in Europe, the Animal Welfare Act does not include farm animals used in agriculture under its jurisdiction.

Veterinary medical officers (VMOs) working for APHIS Animal Care conduct both scheduled and unannounced inspections of commercial and research facilities to ensure that all regulated facilities comply with the law. When deficiencies in animal care are noted and not subsequently corrected after official notification of the facility management, legal remedies are available, including fines and/or license suspensions or revocations. APHIS Animal Care is also responsible for enforcement of the Horse Protection Act, which prohibits the sale, exhibition, auction, or interstate transport of horses that have been sored. The Humane Slaughter Act sets out humane standards for the commercial slaughter of food animals and empowers veterinary inspectors working for the Food Safety and Inspection Service to shut down the slaughtering operation in plants when deficiencies in humane handling are noted.

In addition to the federal Animal Welfare Act, many state and local governments have passed animal welfare legislation on a wide range of animal issues, including, for example, bans on the. use of leghold traps for trapping wildlife. Enforcement of such legislation may be on the state or local level and may involve local humane organizations as well as various government agencies. Animal control officers are usually not veterinarians, though humane societies may have veterinarians on staff who investigate potential cases of animal cruelty.

Protection of Human Health

The control of diseases transmissible from animals to humans is an important function of veterinarians, in cooperation with physicians and other health professionals. There are at least 150 distinct zoonotic diseases known to occur in different places around the world, many with a worldwide distribution. They are caused by a variety of agents, including fungi, bacteria, rickettsia, viruses, protozoa, helminths, annelids, and arthropods. Zoonotic disease control is becoming an increasingly important aspect of overall public health efforts around the world as new zoonotic diseases emerge and known diseases, previously under control, find new expression.

Zoonotic diseases can be transmitted to people mainly by direct or close human contact with living animals, by contact with disease-transmitting vectors, or by consumption of foods derived from infected animals. Veterinary services are frequently structured so that control of infections in living animals and vectors are managed separately from control of contamination in foods of animal origin.

Control of Zoonotic Infections

A nation's veterinary services become most directly involved in zoonotic disease control when the epidemiology of the disease in question allows direct control of the infection within the animal reservoir itself. Factors that favor such an approach include the absence of vectors and wildlife reservoirs in the maintenance and spread of the disease and restriction of the agent to a limited number of animal species. In such circumstances, veterinarians use a variety of approaches to eliminate or control infections with zoonotic potential in animal populations. Testing and slaughter has been very effective in the control of bovine tuberculosis. Testing and slaughter plus the addition of vaccination in endemic areas has been effective in control of bovine brucellosis. Vaccination of domestic animals has been used to control rabies and recently, with the development of effective oral vaccines, is also being applied to wildlife reservoirs as well. For diseases that can be prevented by vector control or vaccination of human populations, primary responsibilities for management of zoonotic disease shifts away from the nation's veterinary service to agencies more directly involved in human or public health. Veterinarians are still likely to be involved, as veterinarians often have official positions within public health agencies in most countries, and interagency cooperation with veterinary services may be an important aspect of the overall success of the control program, as the recent outbreak of West Nile virus in the United States illustrated.

In the United States, national zoonotic disease control efforts, as for brucellosis and tuberculosis, are carried out through cooperative federal/state programs that use both government veterinarians and private practitioners. Through the national APHIS accreditation system, individual veterinary practitioners are accredited to carry out official functions in support of national disease control efforts (see, http://www.aphis.usda.gov/vs/nvap/). In the case of brucellosis control, for example, accredited veterinarians are authorized to administer official vaccinations, while in tuberculosis control, they are authorized to carry out, interpret, and report the results of intradermal tuberculin tests. The accreditation system is an innovation that allows federal regulatory authorities to deliver disease control services effectively without incurring the burdensome costs of maintaining a large cadre of veterinary employees in the field. Private practitioners, in turn, can charge clients for delivering these regulatory services, which gives veterinarians added incentive to participate in the accreditation scheme. In some states, practitioners may have contracts with, and be reimbursed by, the state to perform such services. This represents a cost-effective approach to the delivery of a veterinary service in the public good.

Food Safety Assurance

Historically, the main role of veterinarians in food safety has been in the area of meat inspection. Many important zoonotic conditions can be transmitted by consumption of, or even contact with, contaminated meat. Some of the major diseases of concern include anthrax, tuberculosis, brucellosis, trichinosis, listeriosis, campylobacteriosis, salmonellosis, other coliform infections, and most recently, transmissible spongiform encephalopathies. Most countries of the world have legislation requiring inspection of slaughterhouses and the slaughtering process, though compliance with such regulations varies considerably, since in many poorer countries, unsupervised slaughter in local butcher shops or even on the roadside is widespread (Fig. 8-1). Where meat inspection occurs, government-employed veterinarians are responsible. Veterinarians, or technicians supervised by veterinarians, are required to inspect animals both before and during slaughter. Antemortem examination is critical to ensure the humane treatment of animals destined for slaughter as well as to detect clinical signs of disease that might otherwise not be recognizable by visual examination of organs during the slaughter inspection, for example, rabies, listeriosis, or certain types of toxicity.

As discussed further in Chapter 9, food safety has emerged as a critically important issue in the realms of consumer protection and in international trade. As such, the responsibility for ensuring food safety now touches all veterinarians, not just those involved in meat inspection. The contamination of foods with drug residues and toxic agents and the issue of antibiotic resistance in microorganisms transferred from animals to humans have become major public health concerns in recent years. All veterinary practitioners who administer drugs to food-producing animals therefore are involved directly in issues of food safety and have a professional responsibility to follow regulations on the prescribed use of drugs in approved species and to observe the prescribed withdrawal or with-

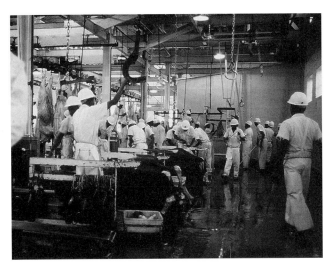

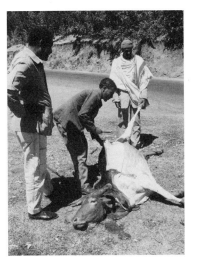

Figure 8-1. Much of the livestock slaughtering in developing countries remains outside established inspection channels. *Left,* The hygienic sheep and goat slaughter operation in Zimbabwe reflects the standards currently in force in most developed countries. *Right,* The more traditional approach is represented by a cow in Ethiopia being butchered on the roadside. This enterprising cow owner slaughtered his cow in the early afternoon of market day about a half-mile down the road from the market. When villagers who had sold produce at market earlier in the day returned down the road with money in their pocket, they were predisposed to indulging in the luxury of a cut of meat. By late afternoon, the carcass was gone. (Photos by Dr. David M. Sherman)

holding times before meat, milk, or other products from treated animals can enter the human food supply. Furthermore, there is a growing movement among policymakers and scientists to view food safety in a more holistic way, which recognizes that the goal of achieving pathogen reduction begins not at the slaughter plant, but at the farm, and extends to the consumer's dinner table. As such, veterinarians are increasingly involved in quality-management assurance programs at the farm level to ensure that healthy animals enter the food chain.

In the United States, meat inspection occurs at the federal and state levels. Veterinarians working in federally inspected plants are employed as veterinary medical officers by the Food Safety and Inspection Service of the USDA. Individual states have meat inspection divisions, usually within the state department of agriculture or the department of public health. The Center for Veterinary Medicine in the FDA, in conjunction with drug manufacturers, is responsible for establishing and approving the withholding and withdrawal times of parenteral drugs to ensure that the drugs have been eliminated from the living animal to a degree consistent with the protection of human health prior to slaughter or the sale of milk.

Clinical Service Delivery

Clinical services include diagnostic, therapeutic, prophylactic, and advisory activities aimed at maintaining the health and welfare or improving the productivity of individual animals or groups of animals. Clinical service is a private good, benefiting primarily, and often exclusively, the keeper or owner of the animal, with minimal direct benefit to others in society. Therefore, in many countries, veterinary clinical services are delivered in the private sector, with private veterinary practitioners providing their services on a fee-for-service basis.

However, this is not the case in all countries. The degree to which veterinarians are available in the private sector to provide clinical services is largely dictated by market forces. In many developing countries, the intensity of animal production is too low and the capitalization of animal owners too modest to stimulate the development of private veterinary practice. For these and other reasons, as discussed later in this chapter, clinical services in many developing countries are delivered, for better or for worse, by veterinarians in government employ.

In the United States, virtually all clinical veterinary service is provided by private veterinary practitioners. Over 86% of the nation's 57,259 professionally active veterinarians are in private practice, according to statistics reported by the American Veterinary Medical Association for 2000. As indicated above, private practitioners also assist government in activities related to animal disease control and public health through the national veterinary accreditation program administered through APHIS.

The forces of supply and demand have worked very well in the private sector to ensure the availability and appropriateness of veterinary clinical service delivery in the United States. The veterinary establishment has demonstrated notable flexibility over time in responding to the changing needs of the marketplace. At the beginning of the 20th century, the major thrust of private practice was equine practice, with draft animals representing the main source of agricultural power and local transportation in the country. Following the invention of the internal combustion engine, the development of the automobile, and the mechanization and intensification of agriculture, the emphasis on private practice moved from equine medicine to food-producing animals. This shift was reflected in the closing of numerous independent, urban-based veterinary colleges in the country that were geared primarily toward training equine practitioners and the emergence of veterinary schools at land-grant universities where the emphasis in training was related primarily to food-producing animals. Following the Second World War, with the consolidation of farms and major population shifts to urban and suburban areas, demand for companion animal practitioners increased, and the profession responded with changes in the veterinary curriculum and an increase in the number of veterinary schools in the late 1970s and early 1980s. Today, almost 70% of all private practitioners in the United States are involved in predominantly, or exclusively, small animal practice.

The moral hazards associated with private practice, namely, the assurance of professional competency and the safety and efficacy of the drugs and biologicals offered for sale, are controlled by government oversight. State veterinary medical or professional licensing boards monitor professional competence. The cost is met in part by taxpayer dollars and in part by the registration fees of veterinarians. Various federal regulatory agencies evaluate and approve pharmaceuticals and biological products. The costs are met in part by taxpayer dollars and in part by the industries bringing specific products to market. Veterinarians and livestock owners are obliged to use approved products within the allowed guidelines, under penalty of law.

Support Services

A number of ancillary activities are required in support of veterinary service delivery. These support services are important to ensure that a high standard of veterinary service is delivered by qualified providers, that the available veterinary services reflect both the needs of animal owners and the national objectives for animal agriculture and public health, and that citizens in general and animal owners in particular are kept apprised of new services, new technologies, emerging diseases, and new regulations concerning animal health and production. To provide these ancillary support services, societies must invest in veterinary education, animal health research, and extension efforts, as discussed below.

Education and Oversight

Well-educated and properly trained personnel are a fundamental prerequisite for effective veterinary service delivery. Veterinarians are a key element in delivering comprehensive animal health services, but a wide range of other professional, technical and support staff are also required. For instance, disease surveillance and diagnostic laboratory support services may require special expertise in epidemiology, statistics, economics, microbiology, parasitology, and entomology as well as a large cadre of specially trained laboratory technicians. Field service delivery, in addition to professional veterinarians, may require animal health assistants (veterinary technicians), vaccinators, artificial inseminators, tick dip station attendants, stock inspectors, and food inspectors. Overall operations of laboratories and surveillance programs require administrative and general support staff as well.

Determining the number of veterinarians needed to provide animal health services in a country is problematic. There is no standard formula for this, and the calculation differs for each country, depending on a wide variety of local considerations. Primary considerations include

- The overall importance of animal agriculture to the national economy

- The importance of export of livestock and livestock products to the national economy

- The general character of animal production, e.g., commercial, subsistence, intensive, extensive

- The number and types of animals and their ownership and distribution within the country

- The importance of animals in the daily lives of people for draft power, food, transport, etc.

- The prevailing animal disease situation

- The prevailing zoonotic disease situation

- Geographical and infrastructural constraints on mobility of veterinary personnel

- The prevalence and importance of companion animals in society

- The general level of education in the country and the capacity to train veterinarians

- The availability of financial and human resources to support veterinary education

- The extent to which veterinary assistants and other paraprofessionals can be trained and provide service under the supervision of veterinarians

Professional Education   A national commitment to train veterinarians should be linked to the overall needs assessment for professional veterinary services within the country. Not all countries need sufficient personnel to justify maintaining veterinary training institutions within the country. Others do not have the economic resources to commit to establishing and maintaining facilities and staff for veterinary education. While there are 189 member states in the United Nations, the *Membership Directory and Resource Manual of the American Veterinary Medical Association* lists only about 100 countries with schools or colleges that grant a professional degree in veterinary medicine. For countries without veterinary schools, veterinary personnel needs are met by arranging for qualified students to attend schools in other countries or by allowing veterinarians who are noncitizens the opportunity to seek employment within the country.

Postgraduate and continuing education are also important aspects of professional development. Veterinary expertise in epidemiology, microbiology, pathology, public health, and other disciplines is required to meet the diverse challenges of comprehensive national animal health and public health programs. Graduate veterinarians must also have access to refresher courses to remain up to date on emerging developments in their field.

The format of veterinary education varies around the world. In all places, prospective veterinarians must have completed high school and qualified for entrance into the university. In many countries, particularly those influenced by the British system of education, veterinary medicine is a bachelor's degree (e.g., BVSc), obtained in a 5-year course following high school, in contrast to North America where veterinary medicine is a professional course of study that follows completion of the bachelor's degree.

Veterinary education has traditionally been considered a public good, justified by the fact that the veterinarian's main function was to protect the national livestock resource from disease. As such, most veterinary schools were at public universities, the cost of veterinary education was subsidized by public funds, and in many cases, tuition was paid with treasury funds. The complexion of veterinary medicine and veterinary education is now changing, as increasing numbers of veterinarians, particularly in developed countries, move into the private sector, delivering veterinary services primarily to companion animals. Chile, which for a long time had only three veterinary schools, all at publicly funded universities, now has three new veterinary schools that all opened at private universities in the last decade. Veterinary schools in the European Union (EU) have increased from 39 in 1978 to 52 in the year 2000, and the Federation of Veterinarians of Europe has expressed great concern that many of the new schools are providing an inadequate level of training and that a surplus of veterinarians is being produced. Under the EU system, veterinary degrees from any specific country are recognized by all member countries, allowing free movement and employment of European veterinary graduates within the EU (see http://www.fve.org/index.html).

Paraprofessional Education   Paraprofessional staff are a valuable resource for augmenting veterinary service delivery, particularly in developing countries where there may be insufficient numbers of veterinarians to carry out the wide range of necessary functions inherent in a comprehensive national program of veterinary services.

Many countries offer a formal 2-year training course for animal health (veterinary) assistants at special technical training institutes developed for the purpose. It is usually required that candidates have completed high school. The position of animal health (veterinary) assistant is recognized as a specific class of civil service employment in the government veterinary service. Such staff is often responsible for a considerable portion of the hands-on clinical veterinary medicine that occurs in the field, participating in treatments and prophylactic interventions such as vaccination, deworming, and dipping. Some countries also recognize other formal categories of paraprofessional staff such as vaccinators and inseminators. These individuals also must undergo formal approved training, but the course of study is considerably shorter, usually 6 months or less.

In recent years, a new category of paraprofessional has been emerging, the community-based animal health worker (CAHW). The use of CAHWs has evolved as various agencies have attempted to resolve the issue of ensuring the availability of at least some rudimentary animal health care in situations in which routine delivery of veterinary services is problematic, such as in remote regions, during war, or for pastoralists who are frequently moving with their animals. The training period for CAHWs is generally much shorter than that for the traditional categories of paraprofessionals discussed above, and most training of CAHWs is carried out by nongovernmental organizations (NGOs). The issue of CAHWs is generating considerable interest around the world and is discussed in more detail later in this chapter.

Registration and Licensure   When veterinarians or animal health assistants offer to provide clinical veterinary services, a moral hazard is presented. The potential consumer has difficulty knowing whether or not the provider is qualified to deliver safe and effective services. The consumer also may not be able to judge whether or not the intervention provided has yielded the intended result. Therefore, it is customary in most societies to regulate the delivery of professional services, especially in the health field, through a system of examination, licensure, and monitoring.

In the United States, all graduate veterinarians must pass a nationally administered competency examination upon graduation as a prerequisite for entering practice. In addition, individual states may have their own examinations and requirements, including evidence of familiarity with state laws, which veterinarians must pass before they are permitted to practice in the state. Furthermore, each state has a board of veterinary medicine or its equivalent that will hear complaints about professional conduct and competence and that has the power to revoke the right to practice for some punitive period of time or permanently. The board also sets requirements for periodic relicensure, usually annually, often based on evidence that the veterinarian has undertaken a required number of hours of continuing education.

Research

The capacity to carry out research is an important supporting element of effective veterinary service delivery. Reducing losses from disease and improving animal productivity depends to a considerable extent on the development of new methodologies and technologies that can be adopted by veterinarians and livestock owners in the field. No two countries have identical animal health and production situations. The mix of livestock species, patterns of ownership, feed supplies, market opportunities, endemic disease patterns, scientific expertise, institutional research capacity, and funding base differs among countries. Therefore, each country must plan carefully to develop a research program that is realistic in scope and relevant to the country's needs and that will have the greatest overall impact for the amount invested.

Establishing a research plan and priorities can be a challenging exercise, as politics often enters the equation. In some developing countries for instance, commercial farmers may represent a small proportion of the livestock-owning public and even a relatively small percentage of the overall economic receipts generated through livestock production in the country. However, because of their relative individual wealth, they are often influential beyond their numbers. As a result, research activities may be directed toward the commercial sector, when the overall impact of a national research effort could yield far greater benefits if directed toward the problems of smallholders or pastoralists. For example, research resources might be directed toward addressing the problems of a new intensive poultry scheme, while the disease or productivity problems of village chickens receive little or no attention, even though thousands of villagers keep chickens and depend on them for supplemental income and a source of animal protein.

Similarly, there may be cultural biases at work both within the country and possibly from outside donor countries willing to support a research program within the country. In many countries, cattle are associated culturally with wealth or accomplishment, while sheep and goats are identified with poverty. As such, investment in cattle research may far exceed investment in sheep and goats, even though small-ruminant numbers exceed cattle numbers, and more people are directly involved in small-ruminant production than in cattle production. There is, however, growing recognition of the importance of noncommercial agriculture to economic growth in developing countries. Donors and governments are working together to develop research priorities that reflect the needs of the country accurately and maximize benefit to livestock owners.

For example, the Danish government, through its foreign aid agency, DANIDA, has committed to a 15- to 20- year project in Uganda in cooperation with Uganda's National Agricultural Research Organization (NARO) to develop the Livestock Systems Research Program. The program, which began in 1998, aims to encourage and support demand-driven and development-oriented research through close collaboration with farmers, community-based organizations, NGOs, and district-based extension services to ensure that research activities and outcomes reflect the perceived needs of livestock owners in the field. Five main research themes have been chosen, encompassing 18 subthemes. These themes are presented in Table 8-4 to offer the reader an example of the kinds of local issues that can and should be addressed in a national research program in a developing country where smallholder and pastoral livestock production are an important component of the overall economy, and large numbers of poor people depend directly on livestock for their livelihood.

In the United States, research in animal health takes place in both the private and public sectors, with considerable interaction between the two. Universities play a major rule, competing for both public and private funds to support animal health research and development. Producer groups (e.g., the beef cattle industry) may collectively agree to levy a small fee against their own sales, usually referred to as a "checkoff," to generate a fund for research to ensure that the research community addresses the needs of their industry. The federal government and state governments make research funds available for which university researchers can compete to carry out research for priority activities identified at the state or federal level. Private corporations, especially pharmaceutical companies, may contract research to universities, though most have

their own extensive in-house research capabilities as well, geared toward new product development.

At the federal level, the USDA, in addition to funding research activities at universities, maintains its own research capabilities through the Agricultural Research Service (ARS). Several institutions focus specifically on research related to animal health and production. The two main institutions are the Plum Island Animal Disease Center off Greenport, Long Island, New York, and the National Animal Disease Center (NADC) in Ames, Iowa. The Plum Island Center focuses on research related to animal diseases foreign to the United States, such as rinderpest and foot and mouth disease, to help ensure that the country has the diagnostic, therapeutic, and prophylactic tools necessary to contain an unexpected introduction of exotic disease. The NADC in Iowa conducts research on animal diseases that already exist within the United States and that are of national concern for economic and/or public health reasons. In addition the ARS supports a number of additional laboratories around the country that focus on specific disease problems or specific sectors of the animal industry. These laboratories include, among others, the Southeast Poultry Research Laboratory in Athens, Georgia, the Arthropod-borne Animal Diseases Research Laboratory in Laramie, Wyoming, the Poisonous Plant Research Laboratory in Logan, Utah, and the Fish Diseases and Parasite Research Laboratory in Auburn, Alabama.

Extension

Extension efforts are part and parcel of an effective research program directed at improving animal health and production. *Applied research*, as the term implies, is of limited value if useful research findings are not disseminated to the potential beneficiaries in an understandable form and then actively adopted and applied. *Agricultural extension* is the process by which new information and technology is transferred from the laboratory or agricultural experiment station to farmers and livestock producers in the field. Extension is generally recognized as a public good, and governments usually support and maintain an extension system, though it is increasingly recognized that extension activities often provide direct benefits to individual farmers. Thus there is a growing trend to charge a fee for extension services, to allow some cost recovery by government.

Extension programs, like research programs, have to be tailored to the prevailing circumstances within a country. The number of extension agents, their location in the country, and the methods they use to disseminate information or transfer new technologies and methodologies depend on factors such as communication and transportation infrastructure, accessibility to local communities, and the literacy level of farmers. For example, in countries with poor infrastructure, remote populations, and low levels of literacy, radio has been used effectively in extension efforts to present new information about disease risks and disease control through serialized weekly radio programs that use humor and drama about events in a fictional village to capture the attention of rural listeners. Dr. John Woodford, for instance, while working for the United

Table 8-4   Research Themes of the Livestock Systems Research Program in Uganda, a Cooperative Research Effort of Uganda's National Agricultural Research Organization (NARO) with Funding from the Danish Government and Technical Cooperation from the Danish Institute of Agricultural Sciences

1.	**Smallholder dairy production systems**
1.1.	Introduction and evaluation of forage legumes for improved dairy production
1.2.	Establishing a database of local feed resources
1.3.	Use of crop residues and agroindustrial byproducts
1.4.	Feed conservation technologies
1.5.	Nutrient recycling and household resource management
1.6.	Pasture seed characterization and production technology development
1.7.	Improvement of health delivery in the smallholder dairy production system
2.	**Small-ruminant production systems**
2.1.	Epidemiology of small ruminant diseases
2.2.	Feed resource evaluation and management in goat-feeding systems
2.3.	Performance and characterization of goats in Uganda
2.4.	Constraints and potentials of consumption and marketing of goat products
3.	**Free-range poultry systems**
3.1.	On-farm evaluation and improvement of free-range chickens
3.2.	Health management in free-range poultry
3.3.	Marketing of poultry and poultry products in the free-range system
4.	**Pastoral and Agropastoral Systems**
4.1.	Improvement of livestock health delivery in pastoral and agropastoral systems
4.2.	Improvement of range and natural resources management in pastoral and agropastoral systems
4.3.	Farm power development and dissemination for mixed crop/livestock systems
5.	**Diagnostic Tools**
5.1.	Development and improvement of diagnostic and analytical tools in livestock farming systems

Nations Development Programme, produced such a series of programs focusing on animal health care to be broadcast by the BBC in rural Afghanistan through their Pashtun language service.

In the United States, extension services are implemented at the state level, through a network of county agents linked centrally to the state university system. In fact, the creation of the Land Grant University System in the United States in the 19th century was driven to a large extent by recognition of the high social value derived from the rapid transfer of new agricultural discoveries from the laboratory and experiment station to farmers in the field. Extension specialists, with expertise in specific technical areas, have faculty appointments within relevant departments of the university such as crop agriculture, animal science, horticulture, entomology, and veterinary medicine. These campus-based extension specialists are the link between university research and the public. The number of specialists and the degree to which they are specialized reflects the intensity of various types of agricultural activity within the state. In veterinary medicine, for example, there may be separate extension specialists for swine, dairy, beef, and poultry, depending on the importance of these various livestock enterprises in the state. The extension specialists work closely with the county-based extension agents to deliver educational programs through meetings, demonstrations, workshops, publications, and electronic delivery methods. County agents, on their part, are listening posts for the concerns of the communities in which they work and can help to influence the research and service priorities of the university by communicating the needs of their communities back to the extension specialists on campus.

Constraints on Animal Health Care Delivery in the Developing World

When considering the building blocks of effective veterinary service delivery, it is important to recognize that technological advances in veterinary science are only a small part of successful disease-control programs. Clearly, highly trained and specialized personnel, accurate and sensitive diagnostic tests, potent therapies, and effective vaccines are all valuable tools for disease control. However, there are important social, cultural, and economic conditions that are prerequisite to the effective application of these tools to achieve effective veterinary service delivery. Such conditions include domestic tranquility; social stability; an informed, cooperative citizenry that respects the authority of its government; clearly written and evenly applied statutes and regulations; enforceable penalties for noncompliance with existing laws; and the capacity to enforce such penalties reliably and legally. Furthermore, there must be adequate financial resources to implement disease control efforts, and those funds must be distributed rationally to various aspects of the disease control effort, including salaries, transport, vaccines, laboratory testing, and owner compensation for destroyed animals, in the context of a clearly defined budget.

The absence of these predisposing conditions in many parts of the world allows the persistence of important and costly diseases even though the technological tools for controlling those diseases have become available. This is well illustrated by the example of contagious bovine pleuropneumonia (CBPP). This scourge of cattle was eradicated in the United States in the 19th century, before the causative agent was even properly identified. However, it still persists today as a costly enzootic disease of cattle with epizootic potential in much of Africa, despite the fact that considerably more is known about its causes and control (see sidebar "A Brief History of CBPP Control in the United States and Africa").

In many developing countries today, livestock continue to represent a critical element in the economic activity and daily life of the country. Yet, despite this central role of animals, animal health and productivity often remain suboptimal, many livestock owners have limited access to animal health care, new diseases are introduced through porous borders, enzootic diseases persist, zoonotic diseases are inadequately controlled, and lucrative export markets remain untapped because the disease-free status of the nation's livestock cannot be ensured. This situation is especially frustrating in countries where considerable numbers of trained veterinarians and veterinary technicians are present but are hampered in their ability to work effectively.

In the following sections, the constraints on veterinary service delivery in developing countries are discussed. These constraints are organized into four main categories: organizational and economic constraints, infrastructural constraints, disaster-related constraints, and animal management constraints. In practice, it is often difficult to separate these various obstacles to effective and economical veterinary service delivery, as many of the constraints may be simultaneously in effect in any given country at any given time.

Organizational and Economic Constraints

The countries of the developing world are not homogeneous. Differences exist in history, culture, resources, and geography that strongly influence the delivery of veterinary services. However, it is beyond the scope of this book to address every country situation in particular. Instead, general types of constraints are discussed and relevant examples offered to illustrate the situation. Many of these examples come from sub-Saharan Africa. A key reason for this is that a considerable amount of analysis has been made on the subject of veterinary service delivery in Africa, supported in large part through efforts by the World Bank, the European Community, and other major donors in order to improve the efficiency of veterinary services in the region. Much of the impetus for this focus on sub-Saharan Africa was the resurgence of rinderpest there between 1979 and 1983. This rinderpest pandemic killed millions of cattle and untold wildlife and called international attention to the fact that serious problems had developed in the delivery of veterinary services in many African nations. As a result, considerable data and documentation is available from sub-Saharan Africa to illuminate a discussion of constraints on veterinary service delivery as well as providing examples for its improvement.

The development of organized veterinary services in Africa is closely linked to the process of European colonization and began around the beginning of the 20th century. Colonial farmers and ranchers frequently shunned local livestock breeds in favor of more-familiar, higher-producing livestock, usually cattle, imported from Europe. These animals, expensive to purchase and transport, were more susceptible to local tropical diseases than indigenous animals and required considerable, sophisticated veterinary inputs to maintain their health and productivity. Furthermore, colonial livestock ranchers looked to Europe as a market for sale of livestock and livestock products. This required the implementation of disease control programs that could assure European importers that exported stock were free of highly infectious and contagious diseases not present in Europe. Thus, colonial administrations developed government veterinary services that emphasized disease surveillance and control programs primarily to protect the interests of commercial farmers and ensure that export markets were maintained. In some cases, considerable success was achieved, for example, in control of tick-borne diseases through regular dipping.

The 1960s heralded the end of colonialism and the emergence of numerous independent nations in sub-Saharan Africa formerly under the control of European powers, notably England in East Africa and France in West Africa. Existing veterinary service structures in the colonial administration generally were taken over intact by new national governments. In recognition of the importance of livestock in the national economies of many nations in sub-Saharan Africa, donor countries offered considerable support for strengthening veterinary infrastructure, helping to construct research stations, diagnostic laboratories, and veterinary faculties. Roughly between 1965 and 1985, the number of veterinary faculties in sub-Saharan Africa increased from 3 to 28, the number of veterinarians increased from 2,500 to 42,000, and the number of research workers from approximately 1,300 to 4,900. By the early 1980s, as much as 35% of the funds for livestock services in national budgets came from donor sources. While such extensive financial support stimulated useful expansion of indigenous capacity in the livestock sector, it encouraged complacency concerning the true cost of veterinary service delivery and discouraged actions that might have promoted self-sufficiency.

By the 1970s several key features came to characterize the structure of many national veterinary services in sub-Saharan Africa. While seemingly unusual from an American perspective, they reflect the political climate of Africa at the time, when the notion of African socialism strongly influenced governance in newly emerged nations. Those features were

- Virtually all graduates of veterinary faculties were guaranteed employment in the government veterinary service.
- Government veterinarians were responsible for all veterinary service delivery, including clinical interventions.

- Treatments and vaccinations were provided free of charge to livestock owners.

These characteristics, while they reflected a noble purpose, posed some serious structural challenges for sustainable veterinary service delivery in Africa. A commitment to hire all veterinarians in government service irrespective of current or projected personnel needs represented an inappropriate management of human resources. Linking veterinary school enrollments to projected government personnel needs would have helped to rationalize the system, but such links were not consistently applied. University enrollment itself was a politically charged issue, and politicians were often unwilling to reduce class sizes when influential constituents were seeking university admission for their children, even when veterinary personnel needs were exceeded.

In Africa, government veterinary services were usually vertically integrated from a central veterinary authority in the Ministry of Agriculture down to district and subdistrict veterinary posts (Fig. 8-2). The responsibilities of district veterinarians were twofold. They were intended to perform regulatory functions for government relative to disease surveillance and control but were also intended to provide clinical services to local livestock owners. This dual role blurred the distinctions between public and private goods and was costly to government, as it obliged government to pay salaries and expenses of veterinarians to provide clinical services, including medicines, that would likely have been paid for, at least in part, by livestock owners.

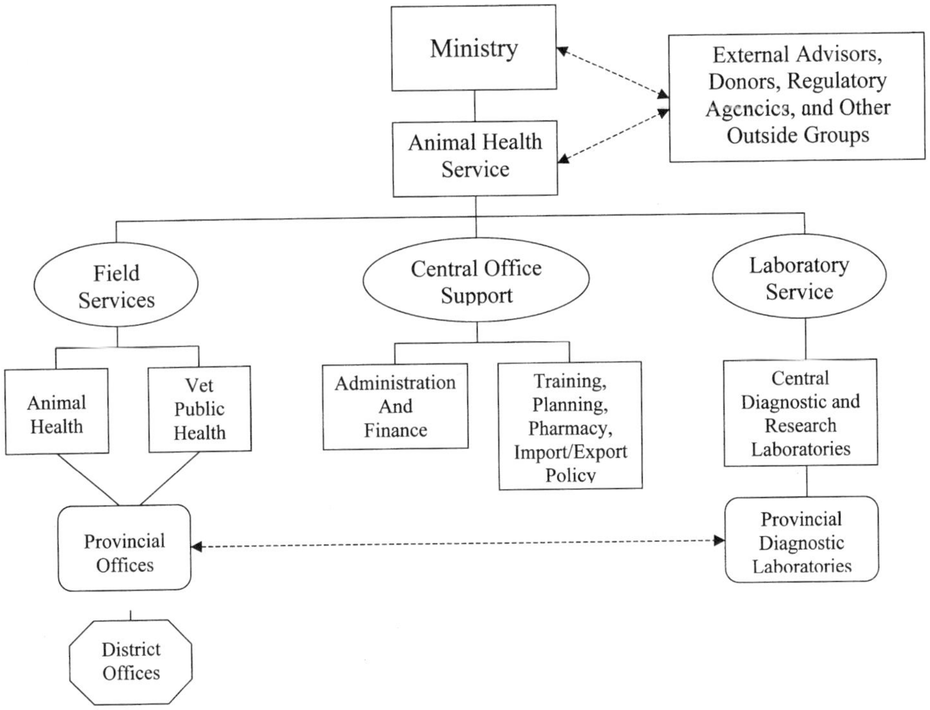

The sustainability of what amounted to nationalized veterinary services was sorely tested during the extended economic recession of the late 1970s and early 1980s that followed the OPEC oil embargo of 1974 and the subsequent increase in world oil prices. Deep recession and mounting foreign debt led to reduced government revenues and major budgetary readjustments throughout Africa. In the veterinary service sector, budgets consisted essentially of two principal components: staff salaries and operating costs. The latter category included all the tools, equipment, medicines, vaccines, transportation, and other provisions necessary for veterinarians to carry out their professional duties.

Figure 8-2. Generic structure of a national government veterinary service typical of many African countries. District veterinary offices are often responsible for clinical services as well as regulatory veterinary medicine. *Solid lines* represent management and functional links; *dotted lines,* functional links. (Derived from FAO. Guidelines for Strengthening Animal Health Services in Developing Countries. Rome: FAO 1991.)

As it was not politically expedient to release veterinarians from government service, staff salary allocations remained intact, and virtually all budgetary savings came primarily from cuts

A Brief History of CBPP Control in the United States and Africa

CBPP is a highly infectious and contagious respiratory disease of cattle now known to be caused by the mycoplasma *Mycoplasma mycoides* subsp. *mycoides*, small-colony type. In 1843, however, when the disease was first introduced into the United States from Europe, the germ theory of disease had not yet been proposed or validated by Pasteur, and the infectious etiology of CBPP was unknown. By the 1880s, CBPP had become such a significant constraint on the United States cattle industry that the Bureau of Animal Industry (BAI), precursor to the Animal and Plant Health Inspection Service, was established by act of Congress on May 29, 1884. The BAI was created, in large part "to provide means for the suppression and extirpation of pleuro-pneumonia." Dr. Daniel Elmer Salmon, the first veterinary graduate of Cornell University and a leader in the emerging field of microbiology, was appointed head of the BAI. At that time, CBPP occurred only east of the Allegheny mountains, but by August of 1884, outbreaks of CBPP were reported from Illinois, Kentucky, and Ohio. The possibility of CBPP becoming endemic in the whole continental United States was a serious threat. Dr. Salmon and his staff of 20 at the nascent BAI immediately had their hands full of challenges.

Though Salmon had no way to recognize or isolate the causative agent, no laboratory diagnostic tests for identifying subclinical cases, and no commercial vaccines to protect susceptible animals reliably, he and his veterinary colleagues did have a keen understanding of the epidemiology of the disease, based on careful observations. It was clear that CBPP was highly contagious and that it was transmitted not only by sick animals, but also by clinically recovered animals that persisted as difficult-to-detect carriers and transmitters of the disease. Salmon recognized that the disease would be best controlled by slaughter of all sick and exposed animals. Since no tools existed to detect latently infected cattle and recovered carrier animals, all exposed animals had to be considered potentially diseased. Unfortunately for Salmon, the original BAI legislation authorized quarantine of sick and exposed cattle, but did not authorize slaughter of, or owner compensation for, affected or exposed animals. In 1885, the futility of effective control under these circumstances was brought home to Salmon when he was unable to prevent the shipment of exposed (and subclinically infected) cattle from Kentucky to Texas. Miraculously, the shipment of these infected cattle did not result in establishment of CBPP in Texas, but the danger was so serious that it prompted Salmon to write in his 1885 annual report to the United States Commissioner of Agriculture that efforts to control CBPP were certain to fail unless the BAI was granted both stronger enforcement powers including the right to slaughter sick and exposed animals and a sufficient budgetary allocation to allow fair compensation to farmers whose cattle were slaughtered. Respectful of Salmon's advice, Congress, in 1887, gave BAI authority to purchase and destroy diseased animals and to carry out a national campaign to control CBPP by quarantine, slaughter, and disinfection. By September 26, 1892, just 8 years after the establishment of the BAI, Salmon was able to announce that CBPP had been eradicated from the United States at a total cost of US$1.5 million. Thus, CBPP, which, according to Dr. Salmon, would "cost our country hun-

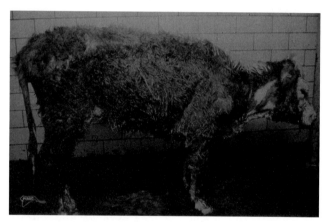

Cow with clinical signs of contagious bovine pleuropneumonia (CBPP). (Photo from USDA/APHIS)

in operating costs. Ratios of personnel costs to operating costs shifted from the 1960s to the late 1970s from an average of about 1.7:1 to 3:1 in West African countries. This meant that funds available for nonpersonnel expenditures dropped from one third to one quarter of the overall veterinary service budget. Similarly, in the East African nation of Kenya, the ratio of staff to nonstaff expenditures went from 0.7:1 in 1975 to 2.2:1 by 1982. By the 1990s, this ratio reached 9:1 in some East African countries.

This economic upheaval had a dramatic and deleterious effect on veterinary service delivery and the overall health and productivity of livestock. In essence, though veterinarians remained employed, they lacked the tools and resources to carry out their work. Central diagnostic laboratories lacked the reagents to conduct routine surveillance tests. Drugs and vaccines, ordinarily procured and distributed by government, became in short supply. Funds for fuel and vehicular maintenance dried up, so veterinarians were unable to go into the field for

dreds of millions of dollars, and make the rearing of cattle a precarious business for all time to come," was eliminated from the nation before its cause was even known-a genuine triumph of regulatory veterinary medicine.

Today, our scientific knowledge of CBPP and the technical tools we have to combat it are much advanced. The causative agent is well characterized. A complement fixation test can identify infected, subclinical carriers reliably. Reasonably effective live vaccines have been produced, with T1 strain vaccines providing at least 2 years of immunity, and avianized vaccines offering immunity of 3- to 4-years' duration. Yet in large areas of sub-Saharan Africa, the disease has persisted despite control efforts and continues to spread to this day. A variety of factors, unrelated to veterinary knowledge, contributed to this situation during the 1980s and 1990s. They included economic recession, reduced budgets for veterinary disease control efforts, declining transportation infrastructure, the existence of large numbers of mobile cattle maintained by pastoralists, and, perhaps most importantly, breakdowns in civil authority associated with droughts and wars. Wars, which have been plentiful in Africa over the past 20 years, are particularly damaging to disease control efforts. In the case of CBPP, numerous civil wars, notably in Ethiopia, Sudan, Uganda, Angola, and Rwanda have allowed the disease to become endemic in these countries, while mass movements of refugee populations along with their livestock have contributed to the spread of the disease to neighboring and even distant countries such as Kenya, Tanzania, Burundi, Zambia, eastern Congo, Namibia, and Botswana. By the late 1990s, as many as 27 countries in Africa were experiencing CBPP *(shaded areas on map).* There is real concern that South Africa, which has been free of the disease for close to a century, is once again in danger of becoming infected.

The persistence and spread of CBPP in Africa despite development of new technical tools and a history of effective control elsewhere in the world clearly underscores the fact that effective veterinary service delivery depends as much on social and economic factors as it does on science and technology. Peace, security, and the rule of law are critical prerequisites for sustainable disease control, perhaps more so even than the availability of vaccines, antibiotics, and diagnostic tests. Yet, disease control efforts cannot simply be abandoned when conditions become difficult. Rather, disease control efforts must be adapted to prevailing conditions. The Pan African Rinderpest Campaign, for example, has integrated CBPP control efforts into its multiple-country rinderpest control programs and is using community-based animal health workers to carry out both rinderpest and CBPP vaccination in remote and insecure areas. A comprehensive plan for CBPP control in Africa, which addresses local constraints, has been proposed by the FAO and is described in the publication *Prevention and Control of Transboundary Animal Diseases.*[6]

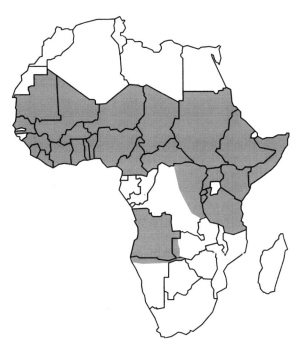

Map of Africa showing countries (shaded) in which CBPP is currently present.

disease investigations, vaccination campaigns, or maintenance of cattle tick dips. Morale became low as district veterinary officers remained stuck behind desks with little or no work to do. Livestock owners, in turn, lost confidence in veterinary services, believing that the district veterinarian had very little to offer.

The net effect of reduced operational funds was a breakdown in veterinary service and an increase in disease problems. Diseases that had been reasonably under control such as rinderpest and CBPP reemerged and spread because of inadequate vaccination campaigns and the inability to restrict animal movements effectively. For example, West Africa experienced 15 focal outbreaks of rinderpest in 1978, 41 focal outbreaks in 1981, and a generalized regional epizootic in 1982. Tickborne diseases, such as East Coast fever, which had been effectively controlled by regular dipping of cattle at government dip stations, also recurred. Large land areas that had been cleared of tsetse flies became reinfested, thus making the areas unavailable for cattle production because of the risk of trypanosomiasis. Cattle populations in sub-Saharan Africa, which had grown at a rate of 3.7% during the 1960s, slowed to a growth rate of 2.1 for the 1970s, partly at least because of increased mortality and decreased fertility associated with a breakdown in veterinary service delivery.

In much of sub-Saharan Africa, debt burden and a slow rate of economic growth continue to place burdens on national treasuries and hamper the effective delivery of veterinary services. Corruption, too, has sometimes reduced the resources available for government programs in the veterinary sector, as in other sectors. However, government policymakers and foreign donors have learned some important lessons from the experiences of the 1970s and 1980s, and some significant structural adjustments have been undertaken. These reforms have been stimulated largely through the activities of the Pan African Rinderpest Campaign (PARC), a program begun in 1986 with the goal of eliminating rinderpest from the continent. PARC is a cooperative, multinational effort coordinated by the Organization of African Unity with funding from the European Union and other international donors. Reforms linked to PARC include privatization of clinical service delivery, cost recovery on drugs and vaccines, and increased use of veterinary paraprofessionals, as discussed later in this chapter.

Infrastructural Constraints

Even when veterinary services are properly organized and reasonably well funded, numerous constraints on effective veterinary service delivery remain. Among the most significant of these constraints are problems associated with infrastructure, including transportation, communication, and public utilities.

Transportation

Inadequate transportation infrastructure can pose serious obstacles to veterinary service delivery. Reliable accessibility to the countryside is essential to organized disease surveillance, disease investigation, and emergency response. In much of the developing world, deficient highway systems and a shortage of vehicles represent significant impediments to veterinary work. East Africa provides some useful examples.

Kenya is approximately four fifths the size of Texas, and Ethiopia is twice the size of Texas. Texas has 124,126 km of state and federal highway, 100% of which are paved. Kenya has 63,798 km of major highway, only 13.9% of which are paved, while Ethiopia has 28,479 km of major highway, of which 15% are paved. Neighboring Sudan, which is equivalent in size to just over one fourth of the continental United States, has only 11,898 km of major highway, 36% of which are paved, while Uganda, roughly the size of Oregon, has 27,000 km of major highway, only 6.6% of which are paved. The highways that do exist, do not necessarily serve regions of the country where livestock are concentrated, as roads are planned primarily as intercity connectors. This is particularly true in East Africa, where large concentrations of cattle and other livestock are kept by pastoralists in semiarid areas of northern Kenya, southern Sudan, eastern Uganda, and southern Ethiopia. These are the "remote" areas of their respective countries and generally lack dependable, all-weather roads. This not only inhibits veterinary service delivery, but also impairs the marketing of livestock products from outlying areas to urban centers.

The extent to which roads are paved is an important consideration, as unpaved roads may be unpassable for long periods of time because of weather. East Africa, for example is characterized by a climate of alternating dry and rainy seasons, with substantial rainfall concentrated over a period of days or weeks. Many unpaved roads become unusable during these sustained periods of rain, which hampers veterinary activities. Veterinary departments must work around these obstacles, planning vaccination campaigns during dry periods and hoping that work is completed before rains begin (Fig. 8-3). When emergencies occur, the effectiveness of the response can be severely hampered by accessibility problems, as for example, in the outbreak of Rift Valley fever that recently occurred in northeastern Kenya (see sidebar "Kenya and El Niño, 1997-98. A Challenge for Veterinarians," in Chapter 6).

Availability of vehicles and their maintenance are additional transportation obstacles in many developing countries. Until recently, very few sub-Saharan countries had the capacity for motor vehicle production or assembly in-country, so virtually all vehicles had to be imported, at great expense. Similarly, spare parts had to be imported at considerable cost and were frequently in short supply. The result was that veterinary departments often had inadequate motor pools, and a notable proportion of vehicles were not in working condition(Fig. 8-4). This situation was exacerbated during periods of recession when there might not even be sufficient funds to provide fuel for vehicles. At the district level, local veterinarians were often without a motor vehicle, thus severely limiting their mo-

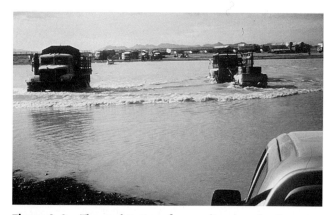

Figure 8-3. The combination of unpaved roads and a climate that delivers seasonal torrential rains can severely hinder mobility and impede veterinary field work. River beds that serve as roadways in dry season may become impassable during peak rains. (Photo courtesy of Dr. Mohammed Imam, Mercy Corps International, Quetta, Pakistan)

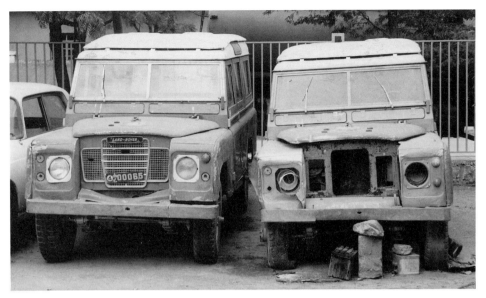

Figure 8–4. Lack of adequate transportation is a major constraint on veterinary service delivery. Inadequate budgets and the need to import parts from abroad for foreign-manufactured vehicles means that the motor pool often cannot provide the vehicles necessary to carry out field work. In many cases, ministry parking lots are filled with broken-down vehicles that are kept for cannibalization of parts to keep similar vehicles on the road. (Photo by Dr. David M. Sherman)

bility and usefulness in what might be very sizable districts. In recent years, more-practical minded administrators have seen the value of providing district veterinarians with motorcycles or even simply bicycles, to improve their mobility at a cost well below that associated with the importation of an imported four-wheel-drive vehicle.

Communication

Modern telecommunication has become a valuable adjunct to disease control efforts. Surveillance and monitoring data from multiple locations can be transferred electronically to central computers for rapid collation and analysis. Disease outbreaks in the field can be reported immediately to regulatory authorities, and emergency response efforts can be mounted and coordinated efficiently. Using satellite-assisted global-positioning systems, disease outbreaks can be located and mapped precisely through the countryside to assist in logistics and planning.

In the developed world, the simple telephone has become a basic fact of life. Yet, in much of the developing world, telecommunications remain inadequate. In the late 1990s, Kenya, with a population of over 28.8 million people, had about 384,000 telephones. Uganda, with 22.8 million people, had about 61,000 phones, while the Sudan, with 34.5 million people, had an estimated 77,215 phones. The disparity of phones to population tells only part of the story. The phones that exist are rarely distributed evenly throughout the country. Most phones are concentrated in urban areas, with many rural areas underserved, and some rural areas not served at all. Small

towns may have a single phone, at the Post and Telecommunications Office, which may be available to the community only during office hours.

Currently, wireless cellular phone technology is improving the overall situation in developing countries. However, equipping veterinarians in outlying rural areas is not always a national priority for governments on tight budgets. When the delay in reporting diseases due to inadequate communication is coupled with a delayed response due to inadequate vehicular transport and poor road conditions, the opportunity for unchecked disease spread and significant livestock morbidity and mortality is high. Even today, it is not extraordinary in some remote rural areas for a pastoralist herder to have to walk for a day or two to reach a district veterinary office to report a serious disease outbreak such as anthrax or CBPP and have many of his cattle dead by the time he and the veterinarian can return to the herd.

Electricity and Refrigeration

A reliable supply of electrical power is an important prerequisite for many aspects of veterinary work, particularly in research, laboratory diagnosis, and proper maintenance and storage of many types of medicines and vaccines. It is difficult, for example, to centrifuge large numbers of blood samples, properly incubate bacterial cultural specimens, autoclave surgical instruments, or provide consistent refrigeration to maintain viability of live vaccines when power supplies are intermittent or even absent. Inadequate power generation and unreliable power delivery remain serious general constraints to development in a number of African and Asian countries. For example, when the author lived in Quetta, Pakistan, in the mid 1990s, the power authority, to meet general demand, scheduled regular daily "load shedding" for different districts of the city during which no electrical power was available for several hours at a time. The scheduled load sheddings were matched in frequency by unscheduled and unexplained power losses that could sometimes occur several times in a week or even a single day. Some institutions and organizations had emergency gasoline-powered generators that automatically switched on when regular power went off, but such generators were expensive and not widely available. Consumers could never be sure if antibiotics, vaccines, and other pharmaceuticals purchased at local pharmacies had been refrigerated consistently and reliably, as required to maintain their efficacy.

Disease control campaigns that depend on mass vaccination with modified live vaccines are particularly constrained by lack of electricity and refrigeration, because of to the inability to maintain a reliable "cold chain" in the field. The *cold chain* is the capacity to keep vaccines reliably refrigerated through all phases of their lifetime from manufacture to administration. This capacity is sometimes unavailable in the very places where it is needed most. The case of rinderpest control in Africa offers a good example. An effective modified live vaccine against rinderpest was developed by Dr. Walter Plowright in the late 1950s, an accomplishment for which he was subsequently awarded the World Food Prize in 1999. The Plowright vaccine essentially produced lifetime immunity in cattle following a single dose, without the need for boosters. This made the vaccine extremely convenient to use in the field, as logistical campaigns did not require recollecting and revaccinating cattle with follow-up injections. The Plowright vaccine was used to great effect to control rinderpest in Africa during mass vaccination campaigns between 1962 and 1976 and again in the current PARC that followed the resurgence of rinderpest between 1979 and 1983.

Despite the availability of the Plowright vaccine, rinderpest has continued to persist in some countries of East Africa, usually in remote, arid regions with high ambient temperatures. The reasons for the persistence of rinderpest in these remote regions are complex and include such things as highly mobile pastoralist cattle populations, cattle rustling, civil instability, poor roads, and lack of adequate veterinary personnel. However, the inability to maintain a cold chain has been a critical factor. Even when other problems could be overcome, it still was difficult to maintain adequate stocks of vaccine under reliable refrigeration either at district veterinary offices or on ice in the field at the time of vaccination. With ambient temperatures exceeding 37°C during the day and vaccinators in the field at remote cattle camps for days at a time, the viability of Plowright vaccine could not be ensured.

Challenged by this problem, Dr. Jeffrey Mariner and colleagues at Tufts University, in collaboration with Dr. Charles Mebus and other scientists at the USDA's Plum Island Animal Disease Center, worked on the development of a modification of the Plowright vaccine that did not require refrigeration in the field to maintain immunogenicity.[11] This thermostable, lyophilized vaccine, called Thermovax, retained the minimum required potency for more than 20 weeks when held at a temperature of 37°C. As such, vaccinators can carry the vaccine to remote locations and still be confident that the vaccine will confer immunity when administered. Thermovax has been adopted by the PARC, and its application in difficult areas of East Africa has helped to make the eradication of rinderpest in Africa a realistic goal.

Product Availability and Reliability

In many developing countries, the selection and availability of veterinary drugs has not been a function of the marketplace. Instead, drug procurement and distribution has been a centralized function of government. Veterinarians within the Ministry of Agriculture generate a set list of antibiotics, anthelmintics, acaricides, and other pharmaceuticals considered to be required within the country. The list is tendered for bidding by commercial manufacturers or distributors, often out-side the country. Once bids are accepted and the commodities received, they are then distributed throughout the government veterinary system, with set amounts delivered to veterinary medical officers at district and subdistrict veterinary posts. Such a system is cumbersome and frequently does not allow the necessary flexibility to respond effectively to the needs of livestock owners. The quotas of different types of medicines may not reflect the profile of cases within a given practice. A district veterinary office for example may use up the antibiotic quota months before new shipments are to be released, while the storeroom remains full of unused acaricides. During the budgetary constraints of the 1970s and 1980s following the rise in world oil prices, some governments were unable to provide any quantities at all of certain key drugs, because suppliers were foreign and the governments lacked adequate foreign exchange.

Centralized procurement remains in effect in some developing countries, but increasingly, trade in veterinary drugs is shifting into the marketplace, controlled primarily by supply and demand. Private traders are increasing, and the variety of products being offered is expanding. This must be considered an important and valuable development. Along with expanded opportunities, however, come added risks. Unscrupulous manufacturers and middlemen may offer a wide variety of ineffective or counterfeit drugs. Smart livestock owners quickly become wary and cynical. Dr. Kit Flowers, of Christian Veterinary Mission, tells of observing a pastoralist herder purchasing a syringe full of injectable tetracycline from a local trader for use in his cattle. Before agreeing to the purchase, the herder squirted out a bit of the syringe contents and tasted the putative antibiotic to check for the characteristic bitterness of tetracycline. The sale of false tetracycline, in which cooking oil or some other oily substance is colored with cola or tea, was so commonplace in the area that the savvy herder had developed his own reasonably reliable system of quality control to screen drugs prior to purchase.

Disaster-Related Constraints

Natural and man-made disasters can severely hamper veterinary service delivery. Regrettably, both forms of catastrophe have been abundant in recent years, particularly in the developing countries of Asia and Africa.

War and Civil Instability

Warfare continues to be a disruptive and destructive force in human society. While wars between nations continue to occur, wars within nations, or civil wars, have emerged as the dominant form of armed conflict in the past 30 years. The trend toward civil war has been exacerbated by the collapse of the Soviet Union, which resulted in the reemergence of independent nations in central Asia and the reconfiguration of national entities in Eastern Europe. Political boundaries often do not coincide with the spatial distribution of distinct ethnic or religious groups, nor do such boundaries ensure an even distribution of natural resources within the nation. Conflicts arise as various peoples try to realign political boundaries or the populations within them to better reflect their common identities or to capture a greater share of natural resource wealth for their particular group. In recent years, this process has come into play in Croatia, Bosnia, and Kosovo in the former Yugoslavia, between Armenians and Azaris in Azerbaijan, between secularists and Islamists in Tajikistan, and in the Russian Federation, where armed conflicts during the 1990s have erupted in Ingushetia, Dagestan, and Chechnya, largely over ethnic claims to territorial independence or religious differences. Recurring news photos of displaced families fleeing villages in horse- or donkey-drawn carts remind us of the critical role that animals play in the daily lives of millions of people around the world, including Europe.

In Africa and Asia, a similar process of conflict has been going on for a longer period. Political boundaries drawn by colonial powers in the late 19th and early 20th centuries frequently divided tribal groups. This was often done intentionally to undermine the power and influence of tribal leaders and to encourage tribal conflicts. Following the liberation struggles of the 1950s and 1960s, many nations gained their independence but retained their colonial boundaries. This has led to considerable internal conflict, as various ethnic groups seek political autonomy or reunification with ethnic kin in neighboring countries. The secession of Biafra from Nigeria in 1967 and the horrendous civil war that followed focused international attention on the issue of ethnic self-determination in Africa. Since that time, the continent has been the scene of numerous similar conflicts in Liberia, Uganda, Zimbabwe, Ethiopia, Somalia, Burundi, Rwanda, Sierra Leone, the Congo (Kinshasa), and Sudan. In Asia, separatist movements have led to armed conflicts in Pakistan, resulting in the creation of Bangladesh; in Iraq and Turkey, where Kurdish populations seek autonomy; and in Afghanistan, where a war against Soviet invaders has evolved into a prolonged civil war fueled largely by ethnic rivalries.

Veterinary service delivery is severely compromised during civil wars. In countries where veterinary services of all types are in the hands of government, an untenable situation develops. Government employees, in this case veterinarians, represent the enemy and are no longer able to travel in the countryside held by the opposition. This situation existed to the extreme in Afghanistan during the years that the Soviet-supported government was in power. The government controlled only cities and towns, while the Mujahadeen opposition controlled the countryside. For close to a decade, veterinary services of any kind were essentially unavailable outside urban centers, where most district veterinary offices were located. A similar situation prevails in southern Sudan, where civil war has raged between the predominantly Islamic north and Christian/animist south for close to 20 years. Government-employed veterinarians in the south rarely venture outside the heavily garrisoned towns retained by government forces.

Not surprisingly, in prolonged conflicts, the health and productivity of national herds and flocks suffer tremendously, as do the people who own and depend on animals for their livelihood. Animals are seized indiscriminately and without compensation by soldiers for food or transport, and in the process, farmers lose valuable work animals required for plowing and other farm work. Grazing animals are maimed or killed by landmines. Feed supplies for livestock become scarce, and disease problems increase in nutritionally compromised animals. Clinical veterinary services become unavailable, and diseased animals that might otherwise recover, die instead. Without the rule of law, livestock rustling also increases, and animals carrying infectious diseases may be stolen and moved to new areas where such diseases are under control and indigenous populations are immunologically naive, increasing the risk of epizootics. Similarly, refugees displaced by fighting to new locations or returning to liberated territories may bring diseases along with them in their livestock.

In some situations, civil war is so prolonged that the normal framework for veterinary service is essentially destroyed, and major reversals occur in ongoing disease-control efforts. This process was documented in Zimbabwe following the 7 years of internal conflict between the white-controlled government and the black nationalist movement that led to the transition of Rhodesia to Zimbabwe.[9] The situation is even more extreme in Afghanistan, where fighting has persisted for over 20 years and the existing government veterinary service has essentially been destroyed. In Afghanistan, international agencies have entered the void to create a de facto veterinary service to fill the country's needs, using CAHWs and paraprofessional staff to good advantage. This approach to veterinary service delivery is discussed further, later in the chapter.

Even when overt war is not being waged, civil instability and lawlessness can still inhibit veterinary service delivery. In some countries, the presence of central government is neither felt nor respected in remote areas. It may be difficult to recruit veterinarians to staff district veterinary offices in such areas or to keep them very long if they do assume a post. The very real risk of carjacking by armed bandits on remote stretches of road discourages veterinary staff from carrying out field activities such as disease investigation or vaccination.

Natural Disasters

Natural disasters such as droughts, floods, and earthquakes can adversely affect animal health and veterinary service delivery in a manner similar to that seen in war. Widespread, prolonged droughts can be devastating, leading to wholesale crop failures, extensive loss of human and animal life, and serious disruption of established social order. Such terrible droughts have occurred often in recent times in sub-Saharan Africa, notably in 1972–1973, 1984–1985, and 1990–1992. In 1973, for example, in the countries of Senegal, Upper Volta, Mauritania, Mali, Niger, and Chad, it was estimated that prolonged drought had reduced the populations of cattle by 50%, sheep by 80%, camels by 95%, and horses and mules by 85%. It was also estimated that the calf crop from surviving cattle was reduced by half because of the debilitated state of cows.

Lack of feed in prolonged drought diminishes disease resistance. Animals that survive outright starvation are more likely to succumb to infectious and metabolic diseases. Scarcity of water forces herders to congregate livestock around known water sources such as wells and irrigation channels. This promotes commingling of herds and a density of animal populations that increases risk of transmitting infection. It also increases the risk of parasitic diseases, notably liver fluke infections, as animals are obliged to drink from contaminated irrigation ditches containing intermediate host snails. Herders also may move their animals into high-risk disease areas in search of food and water. This happened during Sahelian droughts when herders moved their cattle south into tsetse-infested areas, thus increasing the incidence of trypanosomiasis.

Floods can alter the frequency of certain diseases, particularly infectious diseases caused by spore-forming bacteria when spores are redistributed on low-lying grazing lands by floodwaters. Inadequate vaccination for anthrax and clostridial diseases can lead to high levels of morbidity and mortality following flooding. Earthquakes may destroy veterinary clinics and make roads impassable, thus hampering disease-control efforts. In all natural disasters, as in war, large refugee populations may develop as people flee affected areas with their livestock to seek safe haven. Commingling of animals from different areas under such circumstances can lead to epizootic disease outbreaks.

Animal Management Constraints

How animals are kept and who owns them influence the availability and effectiveness of veterinary service delivery. The mobility of pastoralists, the relative poverty of subsistence farmers, and the political influence of commercial farmers all present challenges for veterinary service providers.

Pastoralism

In semiarid regions of the world, notably in Africa, central Asia, south Asia, and the Middle East, animal grazing represents the only feasible economic use of nonarable lands. Pastoralists are nomadic animal herders who tend large, mixed herds of grazing animals and who move their herds regularly according to seasonal rainfall patterns and the local availability of forage. Pastoralism as a form of animal husbandry is discussed in more detail in Chapter 4.

In developed countries, semiarid regions are exploited for livestock production through the establishment of ranches. Pastoralism persists, both as a mode of animal agriculture and a way of life, primarily in developing countries. The demand for veterinary service among pastoralists is very high, since their very survival is directly linked to the well-being of their animals. However, the mobility of nomadic herders presents special problems for reliable delivery of curative and preventive veterinary services. Migrating herders may only intermittently pass district veterinary offices along their migratory routes and may be far from such veterinary posts when disease outbreaks strike. Herders may carry veterinary drugs and supplies with them in their travels as a safeguard, but the variety and quan-

tity of medicines and vaccines is limited by lack of refrigeration and storage space in traveling caravans. Even when herders have access to government veterinary services, they may not fully use them. More often than not the veterinarian who is assigned to the district veterinary office is from a different tribal group than the pastoralists in the area. Ethnic and cultural differences can lead to mistrust and misunderstandings that sour the relationship between veterinarians and the herders.

The existence of pastoralists in a country offers special challenges to regulatory authorities charged with the responsibility for disease control within the nation. Investigating disease outbreaks in mobile pastoralist herds in remote regions of the country with poor transportation and communication infrastructure is problematic to say the least. Mistrust between herders and government authorities can further aggravate the problem. In these situations, full-blown epizootics can become established before control measures can be instituted. One approach to improving disease-control efforts is to establish veterinary inspection stations along known migratory herding routes. Pastoralists, however, have been known to circumvent these stations, and because of budgetary constraints or civil unrest, some stations have been closed or destroyed (Fig. 8-5).

Subsistence Farmers

In developing countries, many rural people are subsistence farmers, producing food primarily for their own consumption and local sale rather than for commercial markets. Subsistence farmers usually follow a mixed farming system that includes a diverse mix of crops and animals that spreads out the risk of crop failure or animal disease and allows maximum use of farm outputs, allowing, for example, the feeding of crop residues to livestock and the application of livestock manure to croplands.

Subsistence farmers usually own a limited number of animals, perhaps a single ox, a few chickens, or a pig or two. Yet these animals can be vital to the farmer's success, as the ox, for example, may be essential for plowing fields, and the sale of a few eggs provides some necessary cash flow. Obtaining veterinary services may be difficult for subsistence farmers. They may live far enough from a district veterinary clinic that bringing a sick animal to the clinic is impossible without a motor vehicle, which more often than not is unavailable. Unable to transport the animal, they may also be unable to pay for the veterinarian to visit the farm, even if the cost is limited to reimbursing the veterinarian for fuel used on the trip. Subsistence farmers may also not be able to pay for needed medicines and vaccines in places where fees are charged. Private practitioners see little economic opportunity in establishing practices in areas dominated by subsistence farmers because they see little chance of recovering their investment in establishing and outfitting a practice. The end result is that subsistence farmers, who collectively may own most of the livestock in a developing country, individually are often unable to obtain adequate veterinary services.

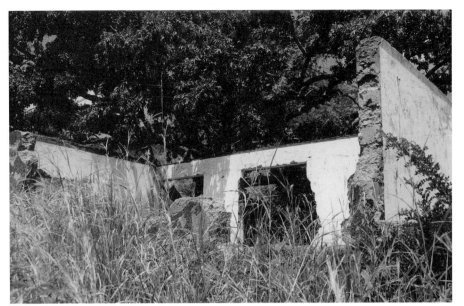

Figure 8-5. War has a crippling effect on animal disease control. The wrecked building shown in this picture was once part of a livestock inspection station in eastern Uganda, located on a major cattle market route. The facility was destroyed and abandoned during Uganda's protracted civil turmoil in the 1980s. The loss of such facilities and related inspection activities are contributing factors to the resurgence of CBPP and other livestock diseases in the country and region. (Photo by Dr. David M. Sherman)

Commercial Farmers

Commercial farmers are those who produce commodities for the commercial market. In the animal agriculture of developing countries, such farmers are likely to be beef cattle ranchers, dairy farmers, or intensive swine and poultry producers. As such enterprises usually require substantial capital investment, these farmers tend to represent the wealthier strata of animal owners in a developing country. As wealth often equals influence, such farmers may have disproportionate access to the resources available for veterinary service delivery in the country relative to their overall contribution to the agricultural economy of the nation. In many African countries, for example, it is not uncommon for politicians and elected government officials also to be cattle ranchers. Thus, much attention might be paid to eliminating diseases that inhibit a beef export market, while disease constraints that limit the health and productivity of draft cattle within the country are not addressed, even though their numbers and their contribution to the overall economy of the nation through field work and transport are much greater.

The need to balance the interests of commercial and subsistence farmers is well illustrated in the example of South Africa. During apartheid, commercial farmers contributed substantially to the overall economy of the country, and the training and activities of extension workers were geared primarily toward serving the needs of commercial farmers. Now, with the end of apartheid, land reform legislation is allowing many black Africans to return to the land as farmers, albeit subsistence farmers. Extension services in some regions of the country are essentially unprepared to address the needs of subsistence farmers, which differ substantially from those of commercial farmers, and a major overhaul of extension curricula and extension-worker training is now under way.

This is not to say that commercial farmers do not have legitimate animal health needs that require and deserve attention. As demand for livestock products continues to increase and as commercial farmers increasingly seek to take advantage of export markets, the challenges to regulatory veterinary medicine will also increase. Government authorities will have to be able to vigilantly monitor disease occurrence and control outbreaks, reliably conduct internationally recognized and approved laboratory diagnostic tests, and effectively oversee animal movements to guarantee regional or national disease-free status within their borders. All these things are necessary for competitive participation in export trade, according to international standards agreed upon by the OIE and the WTO. Many developing countries at present cannot consistently provide these services at the requisite level of performance. In the coming years there will be increasing opportunities for veterinarians in developed countries to provide technical consultation and cooperation to strengthen veterinary infrastructure and professional expertise in developing countries so that they may take advantage of the commercial opportunities offered by expanded world trade.

Opportunities to Improve Animal Health Care Delivery

Because the economies of many developing countries are largely undiversified and depend heavily on agriculture, livestock production remains an important contributor to the overall wealth of these nations. For example, in Asia, on average, 8.6% of the gross domestic product is derived from livestock. For Africa, the figure is 8.2%, and for Latin America, 8.1%. By comparison, the average contribution in Europe, North America, and Australia combined was only 2.8%, despite the greater overall productivity of the livestock sector in these developed regions. In addition, demand for livestock products is steadily increasing in developing countries. Thus, developing nations must improve the productivity and output of their livestock sectors to meet increasing consumer demand, rather than draining foreign currency reserves to import foods of animal origin.

It has been estimated by the Food and Agriculture Organization of the United Nations (FAO) that in developing countries, animal disease reduces potential livestock outputs by 30% annually, an amount more that twice that in developed countries. Sporadic, uncontrolled epizootics can reduce this productivity even further. For example, the widespread rinderpest outbreak in sub-Saharan Africa in 1983–1984 was truly catastrophic. Cattle valued at US$300 to 400 million, were lost in that period. Clearly, the economic health of developing nations requires that the capacity exists to effectively and reliably deliver basic veterinary services such as disease surveillance and control and the provision of curative services to livestock owners.

The major constraints on animal health care delivery in developing countries have already been discussed in this chapter. Some of these constraints, such as unreliable electricity, washed-out roads, and lawlessness in remote regions, are beyond the control of veterinary authorities. However, a number of constraints are intrinsically related to the existing structures and policies governing veterinary service delivery, and these constraints can be addressed by administrators and policymakers responsible for veterinary service delivery within a given country.

Several approaches for improving veterinary service delivery in developing countries have emerged over the past two decades. They include

- Altered patterns of veterinary employment that better reflect the delivery of services for the private good and public good
- Better management of limited resources by government veterinary services to carry out services for the public good
- Shift of clinical service delivery into the private sector
- Increased access of the rural poor to veterinary service

The principal tools that have been used to achieve these improvements have been cost recovery, privatization, greater reliance on community-based paraprofessionals, wider use of ethnoveterinary medicine, and changes in veterinary education. Each is discussed separately in the sections below.

Cost Recovery

The provision of government veterinary services, including drugs and vaccines, at no cost to the end user, has been a fairly widespread practice in developing countries. The situation in sub-Saharan Africa, as it existed in the early 1980s has been described by de Haan and Nissen.[3] Nine of 18 countries of West Africa provided all veterinary services free of charge. Five countries provided vaccinations, drugs, and treatment interventions free of charge. Five countries provided free vaccinations but charged for drugs and treatments. One country charged for all services except rinderpest and CBPP vaccines. Only 3 of 18 countries in the region (16.6%) charged for all vaccinations and treatments.

However, by the early 1980s many African governments were already facing a crisis in veterinary service delivery. A combination of factors was limiting the capacity of governments to reliably offer the free goods and services that they were committed to providing. These factors included global recession, shrinking budget allocations for veterinary service, and a disproportionate allocation of funds for personnel costs relative to operational expenses within those budgets. The failure to recover costs on drugs and vaccines dispensed further aggravated the budgetary problem, exhausting the capacity of government to reorder and maintain adequate supplies of needed biologicals and pharmaceuticals. It became increasingly clear that provision of free goods and services was untenable. The rinderpest pandemic that spread virtually unopposed through much of sub-Saharan Africa between 1979 and 1984, helped to focus attention on the problem.

The Pan African Rinderpest Campaign (PARC) was initiated in 1986 to address the issue of rinderpest control on the African continent. The program currently remains active under an expanded disease-control effort known as the Pan African Programme for the Control of Epizootics (PACE). The PARC effort involves the voluntary participation of 34 African countries. While the primary goal of PARC is to eradicate rinderpest from the continent, the active participation of 34 nations working toward a common and cooperative goal also offered an excellent opportunity to revitalize and reform national veterinary services on the continent. While PARC is not the only engine for reform of veterinary service delivery in the developing world, it serves as a good example.

Each participating country has its own national PARC program to address control of the disease within its borders. Each country also has access to external funds and technical expertise to introduce certain reforms and restructuring to its national veterinary service. Cost recovery and privatization are two of the main reforms that have been undertaken by PARC member nations. Most participating governments have come to accept, in principle, the concept that to deliver services effectively and sustainably, government must charge fees for veterinary goods and services to recover costs. By 1990, 16 of the 34 participating PARC countries were charging livestock owners for clinical service delivery; 23 countries were encouraging voluntary payment from livestock owners for compulsory vaccinations such as rinderpest, and 8 countries were requiring payment for compulsory vaccination from owners. By 1993, virtually all participating countries had some element of cost recovery built into their veterinary service programs, charging fees for any or all of the following: drugs, treatments, laboratory fees, noncompulsory vaccinations, compulsory vaccinations, inspections at abattoirs, border inspections, and issuance of health certificates.

One of the obstacles to more rapid acceptance of cost recovery has been a strong belief among old guard administrators and policymakers that livestock owners will not agree to pay for veterinary services because they are used to having them for free and see such free service as an entitlement. This attitude has been proven time and again to be misguided. A strong argument can be made that poor livestock owners in developing countries understand the notion that you do not get something for nothing. Owners in countries with so-called free service came to realize that too often, the district veterinarian could offer no useful service because the office shelves were devoid of useful or unexpired drugs.

Through its activities, PARC has demonstrated that herders are, in many cases, even willing to pay for compulsory vaccinations. While compulsory vaccinations, such as those carried out to control rinderpest, generally are seen to serve the public good by protecting the national herd, individual herders can recognize that their own personal animals are protected as well, which bolsters their willingness to contribute to covering the cost of vaccination. Similarly, many NGOs working with the rural poor in the development of community-based animal health programs have demonstrated that subsistence farmers and herders will pay for curative treatments for their animals with either cash or in-kind payments once it is explained to livestock owners that a proportion of the fee paid to the health care provider allows that provider to purchase more drugs from the project stores so that a reliable supply of drugs is available within the program. Such a claim of course must then be proven by example. The drug supply must be reliably sustained over time, or again, owners will become disillusioned and cynical. This concept of a revolving fund to maintain stores of drugs and vaccines is now being adopted by government veterinary services as well as by NGOs.

Cost recovery in a government veterinary service is not without its obstacles and challenges. One important constraint is lack of experience in establishing the real costs of veterinary services in a system that historically did not depend on cost recovery to generate revenue. The true costs of service delivery must be known to set adequate and realistic fees. Another challenge is accountability. In countries where government drug procurement and distribution is centralized, fees collected at the district level must find their way back to the federal coffers so that the funds can be directed toward additional drug purchase. This can be problematic, as sometimes money gets lost along the way, falling victim to sloppy bookkeeping or overt corruption. Even when the money does find its way back to central government, existing government accounting procedures may dictate that the money be turned over to the general treasury in the Ministry of Finance. In such cases, there may not be a procedural mechanism to ensure that the funds can be credited to, or used by, the veterinary department in the Ministry of Agriculture. Decentralization of drug procurement by government and internal reforms of government accounting systems can help to resolve these obstacles, but such institutional changes do not happen overnight.

Privatization of Clinical Veterinary Services

Another key reform being promoted through the PARC program, and supported by its international donors, is privatization of clinical veterinary service delivery consistent with the notions of public and private good discussed at the beginning of this chapter. At the time of PARC's inception in 1986, most countries of sub-Saharan Africa provided clinical veterinary service, a private good, through the public sector, at government veterinary clinics staffed by government veterinarians. As in the case of cost recovery, however, there was growing realization and acknowledgment that in many cases, farmers and herders were willing to pay for clinical services that were reliably available and effective and that some opportunities existed for private veterinary practice in a number of African countries.

In addition to potentially improving clinical service delivery to farmers, privatization offered some other advantages to government. It offered alternative employment opportunities for veterinarians, thus allowing government to reconsider their historical commitment to hire all veterinary graduates. It offered the opportunity to reduce personnel costs and some portion of the operational costs traditionally associated with clinical service delivery in the government sector. Most importantly, assuming that veterinary budgets were not further reduced by central authorities, it gave veterinary departments the opportunity to refocus their human and financial resources on the task of carrying out veterinary activities that are clearly in the public good, such as disease surveillance and control, meat inspection, and other public health activities.

To encourage government veterinarians to take up private practice, a number of incentives have been offered. These include

- A 1- to 2-year leave of absence from government service to test the feasibility of private practice
- Financial support in the form of low-interest loans or credits to help equip and establish a practice
- Assurance that government would cease providing competitive clinical services in an area once a private veterinarian established a practice in that area
- Assurance that government would subcontract some services to the private practitioner, such as meat inspection, compulsory vaccinations, tick dip supervision, and artificial insemination
- Subsidized use of government laboratory services

Some governments also have made it clear that they will no longer be guaranteeing employment to new veterinary graduates, so veterinary students must confront the prospect of alternative employment before graduation. This has a ripple effect on veterinary education, as discussed later.

Privatization is not without its challenges, and the process has not progressed as rapidly or widely as originally hoped. A number of constraints exist. First, it has been difficult to induce government veterinarians to leave government positions. Even though pay is low and the work often frustrating because of lack of equipment and supplies, government service does offer security in employment and the prospect of a pension at retirement. The relative risks of private practice, particularly the prospect of a debt burden through loans, has been a significant deterrent. Another factor has been government inability to enforce the competition ban in private practice areas. Many government veterinarians moonlight, albeit against regulations, at clinical practice to supplement their meager government salaries, and they are reluctant to stop moonlighting or give up their government positions in support of the private practice initiative.

Perhaps the most important constraint on privatization has been the relative lack of commercially viable opportunities for establishing a successful private practice. While there is considerable commercial livestock production in southern Africa, the livestock sector in the rest of sub-Saharan Africa remains largely in the realm of subsistence agriculture. Certainly, many countries have pockets of commercial livestock activity, for example, concentrations of moderate-sized herds of imported and crossbred dairy cattle near major urban areas, but most veterinarians willing to establish private practices seek out these areas first, and the market for veterinary service quickly becomes saturated. A few veterinarians have been able to establish small animal practices in capital cities and other major urban centers, where an emerging middle class and a growing community of foreign diplomats, development workers, and business people have created some market demand for companion animal medicine (Fig. 8-6). However, this market remains limited.

The major market for veterinary services in developing countries of Africa and the rest of the world remains subsistence farmers and herders. However, providing clinical service to subsistence farmers is often seen as a risky basis for establishing private practice. Subsistence farmers have fewer animals and less money to spend on veterinary services. To maintain income, practitioners must increase their points of service delivery and increase the overall size of their practice area. This

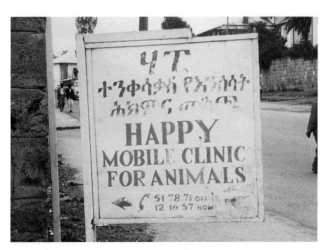

Figure 8-6.   Advertising signboard for a companion animal clinic and veterinary house-call service in Ethiopia's capital city, Addis Ababa. Note that the sign is written in both Amharic and English, as the clientele includes many foreigners living in the capital. There is a growing demand for small-animal practitioners in the major cities of many developing countries. (Photo by Dr. David M. Sherman)

in turn, increases transportation and other overhead costs. These considerations discourage veterinarians from establishing practices to serve subsistence farmers. The problem is magnified even further in relation to mobile pastoralists.

The subsidization of private practitioners by government to perform some services in the public good is one of the more useful tools for overcoming these problems. This can be accomplished by granting contracts to perform specific services, as shown in Figure 8-7. Contracting for services offers practitioners some incentive, through additional income, to serve the needs of subsistence farmers and pastoralists and, at the same time, reduces the financial burden to government, which can use the service of practitioners for a fee without having to pay their full-time salaries and pension. In some remote areas, private practice by graduate veterinarians simply remains nonviable. In these cases, clinical service delivery may remain in the hands of a government veterinarian, or alternative approaches to veterinary service delivery such as the use of community-based paraprofessionals must be considered.

While privatization efforts continue in Africa, with new approaches and innovations being tested and evaluated, a whole new region of the world has become a focus of interest for privatization of veterinary practice, namely the former Soviet Union. Under communism, animal agricultural enterprises were state owned and run. Veterinary service delivery, likewise, was a government function. The breakup and privatization of state farms and herds has created significant challenges for veterinary service delivery in the newly emergent nations of the former Soviet Union. Many developed nations with well-established traditions of private veterinary practice are providing technical assistance in the former Soviet bloc countries to assist in the transition from public to private sector service. For example, Land O'Lakes, the American dairy cooperative, through its international division, has a number of projects supported by the United States Agency for International Development (USAID) to facilitate dairy privatization in several eastern European countries and former states of the Soviet Union. Their training and technical assistance programs include activities related to veterinary service delivery (e.g., mastitis control programs) for privatized dairy farmers. American veterinary practitioners with strong private practice experience in dairy herd health have been employed as consultants in support of these project activities. (Also, see sidebar in Chapter 5, "Hard Times in Mongolia: American Veterinarians Help with a Difficult Transition to Private Veterinary Practice.")

Development of Community-Based Paraprofessional Services

While privatization is an important reform, the shift of veterinarians into the private sector to provide clinical service does not ensure that clinical services will become widely available. Success for private veterinarians means cultivating a clientele able to pay for their services. As such, the tendency is for privatized veterinarians to locate in areas with wealthier farmers and commercial livestock production. This means

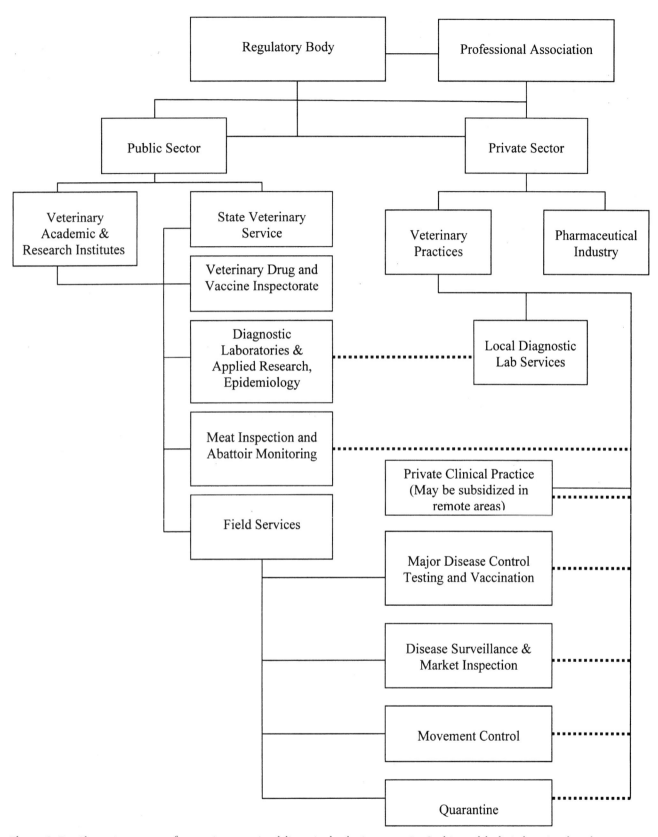

Figure 8–7. Alternative structure for veterinary service delivery in developing countries. In this model, clinical services have been privatized, and government can retain private practitioners as needed on a contractual basis to assist in the delivery of services for the public good (contracted and subsidized services represented by *dashed lines*). (From Food and Agriculture Organization of the United Nations. Prevention and Control of Transboundary Diseases. FAO Animal Production and Health Paper no. 133. Rome" FAO, 1997.)

that privatization, though a step in the right direction, has not, in most cases, directly helped the rural poor. It is estimated that livestock actively contribute to the livelihoods of 70% of the world's rural poor, or approximately 900 million people worldwide. Some may be landless villagers who tether a sheep or goat by the roadside, others are pastoralists grazing large, mixed herds of livestock along traditional routes, while still others are sedentary farmers engaged in small-scale, mixed-farming enterprises that include a variety of crops and animals.

An alternative approach to reaching the poor with clinical veterinary service has been to promote the use of community-based animal health workers (CAHWs). These are local people who are derived from, and serve, the animal health needs of their own communities after a period of training by an external agency, usually an NGO. Community-based animal health programs have become very popular and have been implemented by numerous agencies under various circumstances around the world, for example

- In Afghanistan and the southern Sudan, where war has eliminated any preexisting government veterinary services

- In arid northern Kenya and mountainous Nepal, where difficulties of geography and lack of infrastructure inhibit veterinary service delivery

- In Ethiopia, where the introduction of improved breeds of dairy goats required better animal health support

- In numerous other countries of Asia, Africa, and Latin America, where existing veterinary services, for economic or political reasons, are unavailable or unaffordable to livestock owners who are poor

The Purpose of a Community-Based Animal Health Program

When poor, livestock-owning communities are surveyed by development workers and asked to rank their needs for improving their well-being, such communities often name better access to animal health care as an important priority. For development agencies, this commonly expressed need offers an effective entry point for community development efforts through the implementation of community-based animal health programs to improve rural livelihoods.

The primary purpose of a community-based animal health program is to reduce morbidity and mortality, and thereby increase productivity in local livestock through improved access to affordable, basic, animal health services. This is accomplished by the selection and placement of community-based paraprofessionals who are trained to recognize, and equipped to treat or prevent, a selected and specific group of diseases and conditions previously determined to commonly affect local livestock.

The rationale behind the community-based animal health care concept is that while a wide range of diseases may *potentially* affect livestock, the overwhelming majority of disease-induced morbidity and mortality in any given locality is caused by a finite set of common and predictably occurring disease problems that are conditioned by local geography, climate, and animal-management systems. For community-based animal health programs to be effective, these common diseases must be accurately identified. Then, paraprofessionals must be trained to properly recognize and treat (or prevent) this finite set of common disease conditions, usually on a fee-for-service basis. Through the activities and interventions of these paraprofessional CAHWs, substantial improvements can be realized by the community in terms of better animal health and related ancillary benefits, even though sophisticated, full-service, professional veterinary services may still remain unavailable to the community.

The Elements of a Community-Based Animal Health Program

An overview of the necessary elements for the creation and successful implementation of a sustainable community-based animal health care program is presented in Table 8-5. Each element is discussed briefly in the following sections. The dis-

Table 8-5	Critical Elements in the Implementation of Sustainable Community-Based Animal Health Services
Site selection based on community support and needs assessment	
Review of existing veterinary legislation	
Cooperation/participation of veterinary authorities	
Ethnoveterinary studies and disease ranking	
Epidemiological and etiological studies	
Selection of drugs and supplies	
Establishment of drug procurement chain and realistic fee schedules	
Curriculum development, trainer selection, and training	
Selection of community-based animal health workers (CAHWS)	
Training of CAHWS	
Monitoring of CAHWS	
Disease surveillance activity	
Privatization of drug supply	
Continuing education	
Integration with professional veterinary services	

cussion assumes that the community-based animal health care program is not limited to a single village or community, but rather a group or network of similar communities in a district or region. It also assumes that the program is being developed or initiated by an NGO, which is usually the case.

Site Selection Based on Community Support and Needs Assessment Impetus for a community-based animal health program should come from the community itself. As sustainable programs usually require animal health care delivery on a fee-for-service basis, these programs are doomed from the start if they do not have the sincere support of the community members, who must see themselves as genuine stakeholders and clear beneficiaries, prepared to pay for the services provided through the program.

Review of Existing Veterinary Legislation This is an essential early step. Implementing agencies must know in advance if there are any legal restrictions on the diagnosis and treatment of disease by nonprofessionals in the targeted country. Virtually all countries have national legislation covering the conduct of veterinary practice. In many cases, these laws or regulations are restrictive, concerning clinical activities by non-veterinarians. Such regulations, for example, may spell out formal training requirements at specific institutions or disallow the dispensing of antibiotics by anyone other than a licensed veterinarian. Ignorance or flaunting of such regulations at the beginning of a project can result in serious legal complications and threaten the overall viability of the project.

Cooperation/Participation of Veterinary Authorities Even if training paraprofessionals to deliver veterinary services is legal, it should be expected that the introduction of CAHWs into a district will be resented by some professional veterinarians in the area. Every effort should be made to diffuse that resentment. It is critical to enlist the involvement and support of local veterinarians and veterinary authorities in the program development. Many opportunities exist for their participation throughout the entire implementation process, and these opportunities should be capitalized upon. Local veterinarians must be made to feel that CAHWs are not competitors but, rather, extensions of their own influence and importance within the community. Having veterinarians participate in supervisory and supportive roles, such as training, monitoring, and drug supply, can bolster the long-term prospects for success of the program and favorably influence the entire framework of veterinary service delivery in the country.

Ethnoveterinary Studies and Disease Ranking This is an important participatory phase of the project. Community livestock keepers need to have the opportunity to demonstrate their knowledge and experience with regard to local livestock-keeping practices, perceived production constraints, indigenous animal health interventions, patterns of animal morbidity and mortality, the most common causes of that morbidity and mortality, and their perceived needs with regard to livestock health and production. This information is essential, so that subsequent phases of project implementation, such as curriculum development for training and drug selection to out-

fit CAHWs, reflect the local situation accurately and adequately. It also sets the stage for ongoing community participation throughout the project's evolution. Such participation is critical when responsibility for the program is ultimately transferred to community control.

Epidemiological and Etiological Studies Inputs from livestock keepers concerning animal disease occurrence need to be validated by professional veterinary investigations to ensure the ultimate effectiveness of the program. Livestock keepers commonly identify major disease problems by the predominant clinical sign they routinely observe, for instance, labored breathing in young goats, especially following exercise. Professional veterinary investigations, backed up by sampling and possibly even laboratory confirmation, must determine the predominant underlying cause of these reported signs. For example, if the labored breathing is due to pneumonia, a diagnosis that can be confirmed by necropsy, the pneumonia could be of infectious or parasitic origin, with numerous possible causative agents in each category. The ultimate correct selection of drugs to be provided to CAHWs and their effectiveness will depend on understanding the etiological basis for the common signs considered important by livestock keepers. Accurate diagnostic assessments may be critical to the program. In the case of labored breathing in goats, the lungs may not even be involved in the disease process. Gastrointestinal parasitism, especially haemonchosis, can lead to signs of labored breathing by producing anemia, which reduces the oxygen-carrying capacity of the blood, thereby leading to labored breathing after exercise as animals struggle to take in more oxygen. In such a case, CAHW efforts must be directed toward gastrointestinal parasitism, not pneumonia. These critical diagnostic assessments, made during the planning phase of the program, require the active involvement of knowledgeable and experienced veterinarians.

Selection of Drugs and Supplies A portable kit of drugs and supplies must be developed for CAHWs. The kit inventory is based on the diseases ranked most highly by livestock keepers and the subsequent professional investigations that confirm the causes of those diseases. There are several considerations in preparing a CAHW kit. The number of items should be kept to a minimum so that CAHWs can physically carry their kits easily from household to household. As much as is practically possible, broad-spectrum drugs should be selected so that a single drug will cover a number of etiological possibilities. Drugs should be safe for the dispenser, the animal, the animal keeper, and the environment. They should be as inexpensive as possible (without sacrificing quality or efficacy) so that poor livestock keepers can afford to purchase them from CAHWs. The drugs and supplies should be obtainable reliably through existing supply networks so that availability can be ensured over the long term. Sometimes it is difficult to achieve all these goals simultaneously. For example, topical insecticides for pour-on application are potentially dangerous to use, but they are considerably cheaper than injectable medications capable of killing external parasites. Professional veterinary consultations are important for proper development of the drug and supply list.

Establish Drug Procurement Chain and Realistic Fee Schedules   The drugs and equipment selected for use must be regularly and reliably available. Dependable suppliers must be found, and contracts established. Sources will vary considerably depending on local situations. In countries with a strong commercial sector, private traders may be the best source of materials. In less-developed places, importation or ordering and distribution through the implementing agency of the project may be necessary, at least initially. The sustainability of CAHW projects depends on the willingness of the community to pay for services provided by the CAHWs. The costs of medicines must be recovered in the fees charged by CAHWs, so that additional medicines can be purchased without the repeated infusion of funds from external sources. Reasonable fees have to be established that are within the realm of affordability for service users but that also allow cost recovery and some minor profit for the CAHW, to serve as an incentive for continuing work. Implementing agencies may have to subsidize costs initially until the program is well established and service users are accustomed to paying. The failure of some users to pay can seriously threaten the overall program, and community pressure must be brought to bear so that all service users cooperate in the payment scheme (Fig. 8-8).

Curriculum Development, Trainer Selection, and Training   An appropriate training curriculum and enthusiastic, supportive trainers are necessary to develop a competent and effective cadre of CAHWs. Veterinary professionals must actively participate in the curriculum development. At the same time, the training course must not be turned into an intensified, condensed version of a full-blown veterinary school curriculum.

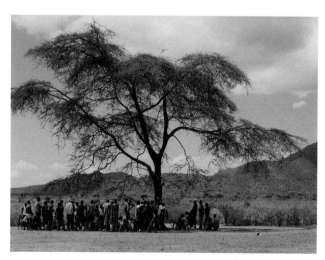

Figure 8-8.   Karimojong tribesmen gather under a "tree of men" to discuss the future of their community-based animal health care program. Some members of the community were pressuring CAHWs to provide service without payment, thus jeopardizing the overall viability of the program. Strong community involvement, including commitment of community leaders, in this case, tribal elders, is important for the sustainability of such programs, as is respect for the principle of fee for service. (Photo by Dr. David M. Sherman)

The challenge is to ascertain and capitalize on the indigenous knowledge that local livestock keepers already possess concerning anatomy, physiology and disease processes; to integrate that knowledge with some core principles of veterinary science, such as the germ theory of disease; and then to add specific, practical information concerning the proper identification, selection, and use of the particular set of drugs, vaccines, and equipment with which the CAHW will be provided. With a well-designed curriculum and supportive trainers, even nonliterate livestock keepers can be trained to perform successfully as CAHWs. One key element is to have respectful trainers who can put educational snobbery aside and build on the strong base of knowledge that livestock keepers have about their animals, derived not from books, but from years of close association and experience. Whenever possible, trainers should be local people, known and respected by the community.

Selection of CAHWs   Proper selection of trainees strongly influences long-term success. Potential CAHWs should be livestock keepers known to their communities and recognized for their animal husbandry skills or experience with traditional healing. They should be honest and responsible individuals. Some observers encourage selection of married individuals rather than single individuals, as they are considered more likely to remain in the community. Similarly, some agencies have had better experience with nonliterate trainees than literate ones because literate individuals have more employment options open to them and are less likely to remain CAHWs. Depending on local custom and project goals, either men or women or both can be trained as CAHWs. The selection and training of women as CAHWs can be a powerful tool for empowerment in development projects targeted toward poor rural women.

Training of CAHWs   CAHW training should be done locally whenever possible and should not be for too long a period, so as not to compromise the livelihoods of trainees by removing them from homes, families, and livestock. Training in a well-designed CAHW program should take between 2 and 3 weeks. The training program should include hands-on practical exercises as well as theoretical training. It is useful, when possible, to have trainees, supervised by competent instructors, participate in practical exercises (e.g., administration of anthelmintic boluses). These practical exercises can involve community livestock so that livestock keepers can begin to recognize the quality of the training being received and the potential value of the CAHW service to themselves and their livestock. Sustainable programs are usually built on the concept of fee-for-service and the need for CAHWs to buy more medicine using the funds they received from selling previously supplied medicine. Therefore, training should include lessons and practice on pricing, money and inventory management, simple accounting, and record keeping. Training must also include safety issues when potentially dangerous drugs are used.

Monitoring of CAHWs   Once CAHWs are trained and assume their responsibilities within their communities, a commitment to quality control is vital to the overall success of the program.

This means monitoring the technical and personal performance of CAHWs and soliciting feedback from their communities regarding their effectiveness and impact. This needs to be followed up by individual performance evaluations between CAHWs and qualified monitors and the possibility of retraining if necessary. Qualified trainers can also serve as monitors, so time away from training to do field evaluations should be built into the training schedule. The opportunity for trainers to see the performance of their graduates in the field will help them fine-tune their training program. The monitoring function is a valuable way to engage the participation and interest of local veterinarians in the community-based animal health program.

Disease Surveillance Activity One benefit of training CAHWs to recognize the most common diseases in local livestock reliably is that it increases their awareness of the appearance of disease that they have not been trained to recognize. Therefore, when a new, potentially epizootic disease appears in a community, CAHWs may recognize it sooner and seek the assistance of veterinary authorities. This sort of ad hoc disease reporting will occur spontaneously at first, but it can be formalized as a CAHW function and integrated with existing government disease surveillance and control activities. In developing countries with poor communication and transport infrastructure, the opportunity for government to have extra eyes and ears in the field for early detection of potentially costly disease outbreaks can be extremely valuable for improving the efficiency of national disease control programs.

Privatization of Drug Supply In most cases, the implementing agency, usually an NGO, initially takes responsibility for the CAHW drug supply, including the selection of sources, ordering, warehousing, distributing, and bookkeeping. For the drug supply to be sustainable and the project to be successful in the long term, the NGO needs to select or help develop an appropriate local organization to which this responsibility can be transferred. Such an organization may be, among others, a community cooperative, a district veterinary office, a commercial distributor, or other suitable group. It may fall to the NGO to assist in the development of appropriate business and management skills to ensure that the privatization of the drug supply is properly achieved, but this is a worthy and vital activity.

Continuing Education As the community-based animal health program takes hold and achieves success, the diseases and conditions originally ranked as important constraints by livestock keepers will come under control. Confidence in CAHWs will increase as will expectations about the services they can provide. New production constraints will emerge as important concerns of livestock keepers as earlier constraints are controlled. Upgrading of CAHWs through continuing education will be required to address these new challenges and demands. This will require an organized continuing-education effort based on solicitation of new community inputs about recognized needs and desired services, CAHW feedback, additional confirmatory investigations, and the development of new curricula.

Integration with Professional Veterinary Services If a sense of trust and cooperation has developed between CAHWs and local veterinary authorities during the development of the community-based animal health program, then every effort should be made by the implementing agency to capitalize on those gains and facilitate long-term cooperation. As mentioned, the local district veterinary officer may assume responsibility for drug supply to CAHWs, serve as a clinical consultant, and conduct continuing-education programs. In turn, CAHWs may provide valuable disease surveillance and reporting functions and can be hired or recruited by government, when circumstances demand, to assist in mass vaccination campaigns or quarantine efforts related to emergency disease control. Creating a sense of mutual reliance between the community-based program and government authorities may be the most significant way to ensure sustainability of the community-based animal health program (see sidebar "Delivering Veterinary Service in War-Torn Afghanistan").

The Benefits of a Community-Based Animal Health Program

Livestock keepers realize improved animal health through reduced morbidity and mortality, greater animal fecundity, the potential for more surviving progeny, and increased livestock productivity. This translates into broader diversification of risk for households, greater financial security, more potential cash income and purchasing power through sale of animals or animal products, better family nutrition, and more reliable access to draft power or animal transport for marketing farm products. Cash income may be utilized to reach personal household goals like payment of school fees for children, medicines for elders, or purchase of desired consumer goods to improve the quality of life, like a new roof, bicycle, or radio.

While it is generally assumed that poor livestock keepers realize considerable direct benefit from community-based animal health programs, there is, in fact, very little documentation of the tangible benefits. Among the few published studies, Schreuder et al. report on a program in Afghanistan in which the impact of paraveterinarians on animal mortality in districts receiving paraprofessional services was compared with that in similar, nearby districts in which paraprofessional services were not introduced and no veterinary service was available.[14,15] On average, districts with paraveterinary services had mortality reductions in calves, lambs, and kids of 25, 30, and 22%, respectively, and reductions in mortality of adult cattle, sheep, and goats of 30, 40, and 60%, respectively. Benefit-cost analysis showed returns between 1.8 and 4.8 times the amount invested in the program. More implementing agencies must build such performance data evaluation into their future programs so that the effectiveness of community-based animal health programs can be more broadly documented and appreciated. Such data, if consistently favorable, can serve as a persuasive argument when approaching donors for funding, or when asking governments to support or approve community-based animal health care initiatives.

Delivering Veterinary Service in War-Torn Afghanistan

Afghanistan is a culturally rich, but economically poor nation with a predominantly rural population whose principal livelihood is derived from agriculture. Animals play a critical role in the daily lives of Afghan people, providing agricultural power, transportation, food, fiber, fuel, and cash income. Maintaining animal health is critical to the well-being of the nation.

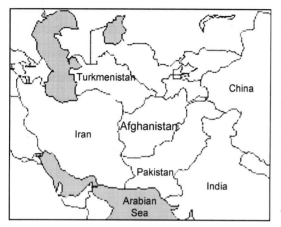

Map of Afghanistan.

Over the past 20 years, Afghanistan has experienced a prolonged period of invasion, occupation, war, and civil strife that has produced great human suffering and social disturbance. Many basic services and civil institutions have been degraded or disrupted. Veterinary service delivery was an early casualty of this long period of social instability that began in 1979. Early on, many veterinarians and veterinary assistants were obliged to leave the country as refugees. Those professionals who remained were unable to work effectively in the countryside because of the breakdown of the centralized veterinary service, degraded infrastructure, ongoing hostilities, and lack of drugs and equipment.

Recognizing the existing vacuum and the urgent need for veterinary services in rural Afghanistan, a number of private voluntary organizations, such as the Dutch Committee for Afghanistan, in association with international relief and development agencies, such as the United Nations Development Programme (UNDP) and FAO, came forward to fill the void in animal health care. Using expatriate technical advisors, but staffed mostly by Afghans, these organizations began to develop a system of paraprofessional veterinary clinical service delivery to serve the Afghan countryside. The system was based on several key elements:

- Short, intensive, training programs for paraprofessional veterinary staff, including paraveterinarians and basic veterinary workers (BVWs). Paraveterinarians were trained for 5 to 6 months and required a high school diploma to be eligible for the training program. BVWs were trained for 2 to 3 weeks and required no formal education to be eligible. Instead, they required first-hand animal husbandry experience as farmers, herders, or traditional healers. Paraveterinarians served as the trainers in BVW training programs.

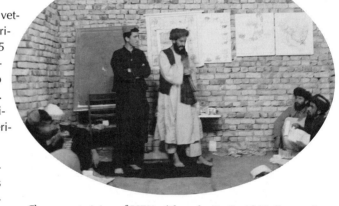

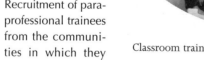

Classroom training of BVWs. (Photo by Dr. David M. Sherman)

- Recruitment of paraprofessional trainees from the communities in which they would ultimately work. It was thought that for paraprofessionals to work effectively, they must possess knowledge of local people, language, customs, geography, and husbandry practices. Most importantly, the community should accept the animal health care provider as one of its own. Therefore, the community itself, in consultation with program representatives, selected their candidates for BVW training.

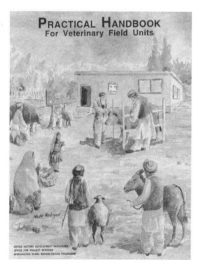

UNDP Practical Handbook for Veterinary Field Units. (Photo by Dr. David M. Sherman)

- Establishment of district-based veterinary field units (VFUs) and village-based subunits to provide locally accessible clinical veterinary services. Paraveterinarians staffed the district-based VFUs, providing management of drug and equipment inventories, coordination of area vaccination efforts, and technical support and monitoring of the network of BVWs located in villages around the district. The UNDP, which initially financed and coordinated the district-based VFUs, in turn provided technical support to staff paraveterinarians. The Practical Handbook of necessary veterinary knowledge pictured at left is an example of the support UNDP provided.

- Establishment of veterinary clinical service delivery on a fee-for-service basis to promote sustainability of the system and motivation for the staff. Basic veterinary workers had to purchase replacement drugs at district-based VFUs with cash. Therefore, BVWs had to charge community members for medicines, vaccines, and treatments. Fees had to be sufficient to cover the cost of resupply and also provide some small income to the BVWs. The distribution of BVWs in villages promoted local use of clinical services, as BVWs with backpacks containing their medicine and supplies were able to reach many clients on foot, horseback, or bicycle.

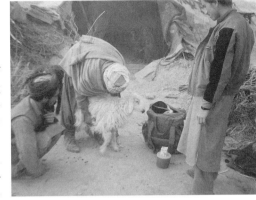

BVW examining sheep in the field in Afghanistan. (Photo provided by Dr. David M. Sherman)

- Development of a privatized system for resupply of veterinary drugs, vaccines, and equipment. The program actively sought the involvement of pharmaceutical companies and commercial distributors in neighboring Pakistan, so that ultimately, international agencies could remove themselves from the chain of drug distribution and VFU management and turn them over to the private sector.

The VFU/paraprofessional system in Afghanistan has had considerable success. Over 300 district VFUs have been established, staffed by over 500 paraveterinarians and supporting a large network of village-based BVWs. This program, initially managed by UNDP and transferred to the FAO in 1994, has made animal health care service available throughout virtually the entire country in spite of tremendous logistical obstacles and security threats, including full-scale civil war. Though such paraprofessional activities cannot provide the full range of necessary services possible with graduate veterinarians, the program has had a positive impact in the daily lives of farmers and herders. This impact has been measured in prospective, case/control studies carried out by the Dutch Committee for Afghanistan.[14,15] These studies showed that provision of veterinary services by paraprofessionals at the village level resulted in significant reductions in livestock mortality and improved the welfare and livelihood of animal owners in rural Afghanistan.

In 1998, the Taliban government in Afghanistan, having consolidated their control over most of the country, began to address issues of governance. Officials in the Ministry of Agriculture noted that the existing laws of Afghanistan, as promulgated prior to the Soviet invasion of 1979, only allowed graduate veterinarians and certified veterinary assistants to practice veterinary medicine. Some within the ministry proposed that the prevailing VFU/paraveterinary system was therefore illegal and should be stopped. In February 1999, a workshop was convened by the Dutch Committee for Afghanistan, which has been the principal agency involved in training paraveterinarians in Afghanistan. At the workshop, representatives of the Taliban government, the FAO, and other interested parties discussed the future of veterinary service delivery in the country. After much frank and thoughtful deliberation, the representatives of the Taliban government agreed that paraveterinarians should be legally recognized as animal health care providers in Afghanistan and that paraveterinarians should continue to be allowed to work in the private sector to provide clinical services at the village and district level. This agreement was based on the condition that some form of certification examination would be developed and that existing and future paraveterinarians would have to pass the examination to be permitted to work. It was further agreed that the Taliban government and the FAO would work together to prepare a fair and reasonable examination.

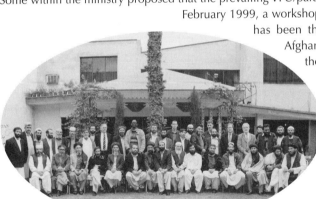

Meeting in Peshawar, Pakistan, with representatives of the Taliban government to discuss the future of community-based animal health service in Afghanistan, 1999. (Photo provided by Dr. David M. Sherman)

Ensuring a future for paraprofessionals in the provision of clinical veterinary services does not imply that there is no future role for veterinarians in Afghanistan. The scientific training and professional expertise of graduate veterinarians is sorely needed in that nation to restore important functions and services that protect the public welfare. These activities include, among others, public health education and zoonotic disease control, meat inspection and other food safety monitoring, regional and national disease investigation and control, and import/export regulation. By transferring basic clinical service delivery to paraprofessionals in the private sector, the government of Afghanistan will help to ensure that the limited financial resources available to the Ministry of Agriculture for veterinary services can be focused on those activities that need to be carried out in the national interest by qualified veterinary professionals. The VFU/paraprofessional system of Afghanistan serves as a useful and instructive model for all developing nations seeking to decentralize their clinical veterinary services while improving the availability and reliability of animal health care delivery to their rural populations.

Readers who seek out additional information on community-based animal health programs will quickly note a variety of ways in which CAHWs are identified. There is no agreed upon standard, though *community-based animal health worker* seems to be emerging as the preferred term. Other terms in use, either currently or historically, include *barefoot veterinarians, basic veterinary workers, key men, veterinary auxiliaries, veterinary scouts, primary animal health care workers,* and *paraveterinarians* or *paravets.* The two terms *veterinary assistant* and *veterinary technician* are usually reserved for paraprofessionals who have undergone extended formal training for a year or more and are recognized, certified, or licensed by government authorities.

Use of Ethnoveterinary Medicine

Community-based animal health networks certainly have the potential to reach large numbers of poor, rural livestock owners. However, certain obstacles to achieving universal coverage still remain. Though the situation is evolving, many governments and national veterinary associations continue to resist community-based animal health programs, and some may prohibit them outright through veterinary practice legislation. Secondly, many community-based animal health programs rely upon and promote the use of commercial medicines and biologicals, often of foreign origin. While unquestionably effective, some difficulties are associated with reliance on commercial drugs and vaccines. One difficulty is the supply line itself. In many cases, the drugs being introduced are not already available locally, so that existing trade channels of wholesalers, traders, transporters, and retailers do not exist. While suppliers can be located and trade channels created, their persistence is not ensured. Withdrawal of a foreign pharmaceutical company from the national market, seasonally impassable supply roads, or a lower-than-expected volume of sales with a concomitant loss of interest among traders can all result in an unreliable supply of the drugs that participating communities have come to accept and depend on. Such disruptions in drug supply can seriously undermine the credibility of a community-based animal health care program, resulting in a loss of community support that can kill the program.

The inherent risk in creating dependency on foreign drugs and innovations underscores the importance of identifying, acknowledging, and incorporating ethnoveterinary medicine into efforts to improve rural animal health care in developing countries. All over the world, in societies with a long tradition of livestock keeping, accumulated knowledge, proven husbandry practices, and indigenous medicines exist that can contribute significantly to overall efforts of animal disease control.

Ethnoveterinary medicine can be defined as local people's knowledge pertaining to animal health and production. It is a knowledge derived over time from the intimate association between people and animals and the landscape they inhabit and share. It is rarely informed by book learning. Rather, it is born out of multigenerational experience, keen powers of observation and deduction, and repeated acts of trial and error. Policy-makers, aid organizations, and technical consultants need to develop a greater awareness of, and respect for, such indigenous knowledge and practices.

Consider, for instance, the matter of tick-borne diseases in Africa. Traditional herders may never have heard of the rickettsia that causes cowdriosis or the protozoa that cause babesiosis and East Coast fever. Yet their cumulative experience has taught them that heavy tick burdens on cattle are associated with the occurrence of such diseases in their cattle herds. Thus, a number of indigenous practices have evolved throughout Africa that are at least partly associated with efforts to control ticks on cattle. In some cultures, cattle are inspected daily, and ticks are hand-picked from them and destroyed by burning or feeding to poultry. In others, grazing in shrubby grasslands is avoided during the rainy season because it is known that tick numbers are higher during rains and the ticks congregate on shrubs to drop on passing livestock. Still others practice controlled burning of grasslands to kill ticks. Elsewhere, herders may apply extracts of local plants to cattle at the predilection sites of ticks such as the ears, to chemically or physically deter tick attachment. Other groups have identified local strains of cattle that are resistant to tick infestation or the diseases they carry and have selected for these strains through breeding. When such practices are abandoned in favor of new technology that is introduced but then not sustained, the results can be damaging and harmful.

The African landscape is littered with abandoned cattle dips (Fig. 8-9) that were introduced through various development schemes to promote livestock health and production on the advice of outside technical experts and with funding provided through foreign aid from developed countries. Such dips may be abandoned for a number of reasons: the technical expertise is not available locally to manage and maintain them properly; government budgets cannot support them once donor funds have terminated; acaricides become too expensive or difficult to obtain; sites become contaminated because of improper disposal of toxic acaricides; security cannot be maintained, and equipment and supplies are stolen or destroyed; or local people are unwilling or unable to pay for the service and stop coming to the dip. This situation begs the question whether the construction of dips was the most appropriate approach to the problem in the first place and whether local livestock owners were ill-served or well-served by the effort.

To outsiders, indigenous knowledge can, on first impression, sometimes seem foolish. A disease problem that the outsider recognizes immediately as bacterial or protozoal in origin may be attributed by local people to evil spirits or magic spells, causing the outside "expert" to dismiss local knowledge as backward or useless. Yet, if the expert continues to listen and question further, these same local people can perfectly detail the epidemiological pattern of the disease, describing its seasonal occurrence; the conditions under which outbreaks are most likely to occur; the age, breeds, and species of animals most likely to be affected; and the likelihood of disease recurrence in animals once exposed. They may also be able to describe management practices that reduce the risk of disease occurrence, the use of local medicines that are effective in

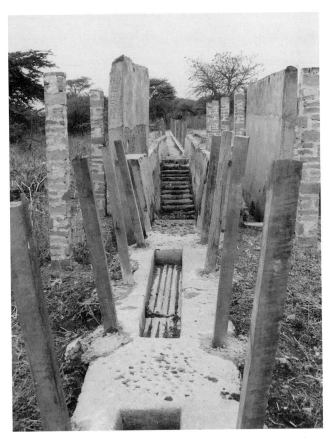

Figure 8-9. Many tick dipping stations have been abandoned in Africa. In this case, the dip was found to be unworkable because of poor construction design. Among other things, the walls of the dip were too far apart, allowing cattle to turn around in the dipping tank and impede the flow of oncoming cattle. (Photo by Dr. David M. Sherman)

ameliorating the clinical signs, and possibly even some rudimentary form of vaccination that is practiced to prevent the disease. Knowing about bacteria, protozoa, and other etiological agents is a luxury of formal education and access to microscopes. On the other hand, the information that the herders provide on the local pattern of disease occurrence and their approaches to treatment and therapy may be invaluable in developing sustainable strategies for disease control (see sidebar "Ethnoveterinary Medicine: To Spray or Not to Spray? That is the Question").

Interest in ethnoveterinary medicine has expanded greatly in recent years, prompted by a variety of factors. First, there is the concern that much ethnoveterinary knowledge and practice may be lost before they are ever recorded. This is a real possibility, as traditional societies become increasingly disrupted or fragmented from the pressures of population growth, economic development, landscape transformation, and the increasing influx of foreign cultural influences brought about by global telecommunications and trade.

Secondly, there is recognition that existing knowledge and practices that have already been recorded need to be studied and validated so that their true value and potential for wider

application can be determined. Beliefs or practices that have been derived by trial and error and careful observation must be differentiated from beliefs and practices based on outright superstition or faulty observation. In south Asia, for instance, a traditional anthelmintic is used widely by herders and farmers in their sheep and goats for control of gastrointestinal parasites. The medicine is derived from the powdered fruit capsule of the plant *Mallotus philippinensis* and goes by several local names in different tribal languages, *kamala* being the name used in English. Interviews with herders in western Pakistan suggested a strong belief in the efficacy of this drug for internal parasite control, since sheep and goats are seen to void tapeworm proglottids in their feces following oral administration of the powdered preparation in water. While herders stated that their animals also seemed clinically improved following treatment, careful veterinary examinations suggested that the animals were still experiencing the clinical effects of significant helminth infestation. Jost et al., therefore, set up a controlled trial in which worm-free goats were experimentally infected with nematode larvae and then treated with either the commercial anthelmintic, fenbendazole, or with kamala at four doses that bracketed the dose range usually administered by herders.[8] Postmortem studies and fecal egg counts indicated that while fenbendazole completely eliminated nematode infestations, the kamala had virtually no effect on nematode burdens.

These results do not discredit the herder observations that tapeworms are expelled by kamala, as the drug does produce a peristaltic/purgative effect that will clear unattached tapeworm proglottids from the alimentary tract. However, kamala had no direct effect on nematode burdens, which are much more responsible than tapeworms for the serious clinical parasitism that occurs in small ruminants. Controlled studies such as this are quite valuable in determining the true usefulness of local medicines. Such studies provide guidance for preparing rational recommendations for the integration of traditional medicines and management practices into comprehensive animal health care programs that reflect the local situation.

A third interest in ethnoveterinary medicine relates to refining the field research methods used to gather information about ethnoveterinary medicine. Much of the work of collecting and documenting indigenous knowledge and practices involves the exchange of oral information from community members to scientists from outside the community. Community organization, social hierarchies, wealth distribution, work assignments, cultural attitudes, and gender differences within the community are just a few of the variables that outsiders must consider when gathering information and interpreting the meaning and the validity of data. For example, men who tend animals in the countryside may have good knowledge about management practices and environmental factors that predispose to disease in their livestock, while women, who may be responsible for cleaning the entrails of animals slaughtered for food, may have greater knowledge of the pathological aspects of disease or the occurrence of subclinical disease, as a result of regular handling and inspection of organs. Speaking to men alone or

Ethnoveterinary Medicine: To Spray or Not to Spray? That Is the Question

The export of cattle hides and sheep and goat skins used for finished leather goods is the second most important source of foreign exchange for Ethiopia, after coffee. However, the Ethiopian tanning industry has faced serious problems in recent years due to a decline in the availability of high-grade raw material from small ruminants and an associated decline in the proportion of processed skins that meet international standards for export. As a result, Ethiopia is in danger of losing international markets through its inability to supply the required quantity and quality of skins for export. The Ethiopian hides and skin export in-

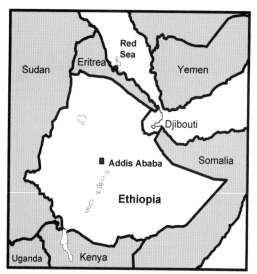

dustry earned nearly US$65 million in 1995-1996. Data for these same years from six of eight commercial tanneries in the country indicate that 20 to 24% of purchased sheep and goat skins were classified as rejects because of various defects and were therefore unavailable for export, resulting in an industry loss of US$6.9 million.

Defects in hides and skins can be categorized as occurring during different phases of production, namely, preslaughter, perislaughter, or postslaughter. Preslaughter defects represent damage that occurs to the skin while the animal is still alive. In Ethiopia, it is estimated that 65% of the defects found in skins are preslaughter defects occurring in the live animals. The predominant preslaughter cause for downgrading sheep and goat skins in Ethiopia has generally been identified as *ekek,* the Amharic word meaning itch. Ekek in live sheep is manifested by itching and sometimes loss of hair or wool. While the specific causes of ekek are not known with certainty, it is generally believed that the condition is associated with external parasites.

In skins processed at Ethiopian tanneries, the so-called ekek lesion appears as multiple, small, circular defects about 5 mm in diameter. These circular lesions may be raised above the skin surface, and they also may have a pit or depression in their center that represents a defect in the grain surface. These lesions may affect anywhere from 1 to 100% of the skin surface. They significantly affect the finished quality of the leather produced and reduce its market value.

The problem of ekek for the tanning industry is profound. The ekek defect is not detectable in the raw skin. The raised, paler, circumscribed defects appear only after processing of skins at the tannery to the pickled state. Thus, the tanning industry loses three times with regard to each ekek-affected skin: first, by the purchase of raw skins of undetectable inferior quality; second, by the cost of processing these inferior skins; and third, by the fact that such skins are then downgraded after processing and are therefore unsuitable for sale in the more profitable export markets.

Since late 1995, Ethiopian veterinary researchers, with financial and technical assistance from an FAO Technical Cooperation Project, investigated the causes of parasitic skin diseases in sheep and the effects these parasites have on processed skin quality and grading.

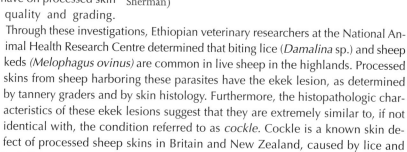

Processed sheep skin showing damage associated with ekek. Note pale circumscribed defects. (Photo by Dr. David M. Sherman)

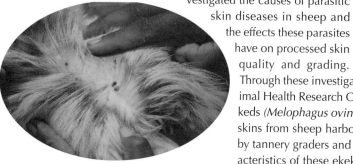

Hair parted to reveal keds (*melophagus ovinus*) on a sheep in Ethiopia. (Photo by Dr. David M. Sherman)

Through these investigations, Ethiopian veterinary researchers at the National Animal Health Research Centre determined that biting lice (*Damalina* sp.) and sheep keds *(Melophagus ovinus)* are common in live sheep in the highlands. Processed skins from sheep harboring these parasites have the ekek lesion, as determined by tannery graders and by skin histology. Furthermore, the histopathologic characteristics of these ekek lesions suggest that they are extremely similar to, if not identical with, the condition referred to as *cockle.* Cockle is a known skin defect of processed sheep skins in Britain and New Zealand, caused by lice and keds.[7]

Based on these findings, the Ethiopian veterinary team, in conjunction with their FAO international consultants from the USA, South Africa, and England, worked up a series of experimental treatment trials to determine if elimination of keds and lice on live animals would reduce or eliminate ekek lesions in skins derived from treated animals. All the veterinarians involved, regardless of origin,

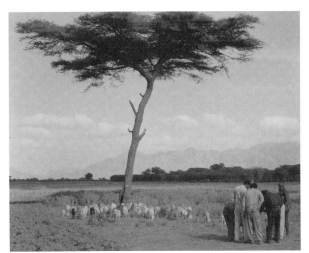

Ethiopian veterinarians and FAO consultants examining sheep in the field. (Photo by Dr. David M. Sherman)

readily agreed that it would be useful to evaluate at least two topical acaricides. Amitraz was selected for evaluation because it was currently imported into Ethiopia by the veterinary authorities. Diazinon was also selected for evaluation, even though it was not currently available in Ethiopia. The reasoning was that diazinon was potentially less expensive than amitraz and had been proven effective in New Zealand trials for control of cockle.[7] In addition, however, the Ethiopian team suggested that shearing be included in the trials as an alternate treatment, since many Ethiopian herders, even though there was a poor market for their low-quality wool, regularly sheared their sheep because they recognized that shearing led to a reduction in ked numbers and improved the general condition of the animals. The Ethiopians wanted to evaluate this traditional practice as another potential approach to the control of ekek.

Shearing was included in the treatment trials along with diazinon and amitraz, and the results were startling. In sheep sacrificed 30 days following treatment, the results were similar in the insecticide-treated groups and the shearing group, as compared with untreated controls. Ked numbers were reduced to zero in all three treatment groups. Louse numbers were reduced to zero in the two insecticide-treated groups and were reduced dramatically in the sheared group, though not completely eliminated. Based on visual inspection scores made by professional tannery graders as well as by histological examination of skin samples, there was a major reduction in ekek lesions in the sheared group of the same magnitude as that in the two insecticide-treated groups. By 90 days posttreatment, the reduction in severity of ekek lesions was again similar in the sheared and two insecticide-treated groups. By 90 days, keds and lice had begun to reinfest sheared sheep and amitraz-treated sheep, although they were still completely absent from diazinon-treated sheep.

The inclusion of a traditional ethnoveterinary practice in the FAO field trial produced interesting and, to the foreign technical advisors, surprising results. It appeared that the mechanical shearing of sheep, using a simple knife blade, as traditionally practiced by Ethiopian herders, had the potential to reduce ekek lesions and improve the quality of skins for international trade if animals were slaughtered and skins marketed within 90 days of shearing. While insecticide applications using pump sprayers were also effective, and in the case of diazinon, provided ectoparasite control of longer duration, serious consideration needs to be given to shearing as a method of ekek control. Ethiopian herders, such as the shepherdess shown in the photo at right are generally cash poor. The purchase of diazinon or amitraz for ectoparasite control would

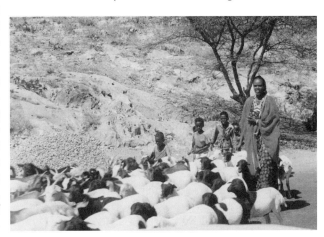

A woman herding sheep in Ethiopia. (Photo by Dr. David M. Sherman)

be beyond the means of many herders. In turn, the Ethiopian veterinary service, with financial constraints of its own, would not be in a position to provide free treatments nationwide and would require some means of cost recovery. Furthermore, widespread application of insecticides would require the additional purchase of many hand pumps or the creation of dip sites. The promotion of widespread insecticide use might also open the door to significant environmental and public health problems. Therefore, serious consideration must be given to traditional shearing as a means of ekek control and the promotion of this practice in extension efforts. Clearly, the value of ethnoveterinary medicine should not be underestimated, and expert consultants working outside their own cultures need to be prepared to listen as well as advise.

women alone or not understanding the division of labor within the community would provide the outsider with a less than complete view of local knowledge about animal health and disease.[2]

Finally, a great deal of the new interest in ethnoveterinary medicine is motivated by the prospect of commercial exploitation. While modern pharmacology has become to a large extent a laboratory science, a great many of our most effective and widely used drugs, such as aspirin, were originally derived from plants or animals. Recognizing that we now live in a period of drastically accelerated degradation of rainforests and other natural landscapes, pharmaceutical firms and universities are sending their botanists, anthropologists, pharmacologists, and other interested scientists to remote regions of the world to identify potential new products with natural origins. Not surprisingly, this "bioprospecting" often involves seeking out local traditional healers in the hopes that they will reveal their indigenous knowledge and practices, thus identifying local plants and other materials that have real medicinal value and can serve as the basis for new classes of drugs.

A more detailed presentation of the field of ethnoveterinary medicine is beyond the scope of this volume. A number of useful publications have become available in recent years on the subject. Two volumes in particular provide valuable summaries and overviews of this complex and interesting field. The first is *Ethnoveterinary Medicine: An Annotated Bibliography*.[12] The second is *Ethnoveterinary Research and Development*.[13] Extensively referenced, these two volumes provide readers with numerous sources of additional information on specific aspects of ethnoveterinary medicine as practiced and studied in different locations around the world. They will help veterinary students appreciate the wide range of research challenges and field opportunities that exist in this interesting province of international veterinary medicine.

Linking Veterinary Education to Local Needs

While many factors can influence the delivery of veterinary services, the proper training of veterinarians and veterinary paraprofessionals is a critical element in ensuring the overall quality of veterinary service within a nation. At least 100 nations of the world have their own schools of veterinary medicine. It is not always clear what factors determine the number of schools within a nation, though national pride, local politics, and international donor influence probably play as significant a role as livestock numbers and needs assessments. In general, smaller, less-developed countries tend to have a single faculty, while larger, more-developed countries tend to have multiple schools.

In many developing countries, the budgetary constraints that have undermined veterinary service delivery also have affected veterinary education. Low faculty salaries and inadequate operational budgets produce low morale and can adversely affect the quality of education. Many schools in developing countries have highly motivated and well-educated faculty with postgraduate degrees attained abroad. Nevertheless, poorly

equipped laboratories, inadequate and antiquated library collections, and lack of sufficient vehicles to take students on field exercises all contribute to a diminished educational experience for veterinary students. Class sizes may also be a factor. In some countries of Latin America, for example, there may be more or less open enrollment in veterinary schools, with poor academic performers weeded out after admission, rather than before, as in the United States. As such, graduating classes may be one tenth the size of entering classes because of academic attrition. This places undue teaching and financial burdens on schools to teach first-year classes and run laboratory courses such as anatomy for large groups of students, 90% of whom may never graduate.

In some cases, however, the use of rigorous academic screening as the sole indicator of eligibility for veterinary school admission may not serve the best interests of the nation's veterinary service. In many African countries, for example, public education is not guaranteed. Families must pay for elementary and secondary schooling. As a result, affluent urban children are proportionately more likely to complete school than poorer rural children and ultimately gain entry to the university through a competitive admissions process. The result for veterinary schools is a largely urban-raised, urban-educated student body with relatively little knowledge of, or connection to, the problems or challenges of rural life. When these students graduate from veterinary school, they are not inclined to seek employment in rural areas and, if posted to a distant rural district veterinary office as a government employee, in some cases, may simply count the days until they can be reassigned closer to home. Even if they are professionally committed to their posts, tribal differences, language barriers, a lack of knowledge of local management practices and disease problems, and a possible lack of acceptance by the local community, can greatly inhibit their effectiveness as veterinary officers. For these reasons, a strong case can be made that geographical distributions and ethnic background need to be considered along with academic record as criteria for admission to veterinary school for the nation's veterinary service needs to be adequately met.

The number of veterinarians to be trained also needs to be rationalized according to carefully conducted needs assessments and removed as much as possible from political consideration. The limited resources of veterinary teaching institutions should not be further diluted by having to train more veterinarians than the country can use effectively. Planning projected personnel requirements should include not only veterinarians, but also technical and paraveterinary support staff. Such planning exercises should take into account potential changes in responsibility for clinical service delivery that could occur as a result of greater use of paraprofessionals to serve the basic veterinary needs of subsistence farmers and herders. Existing traditional programs that invest in training veterinary technicians for a full 2 years following high school need to be reexamined in light of the recent successes of some nongovernmental paraveterinary training programs that produce competent veterinary paraprofessionals in periods as short as 6 months.

A major challenge for veterinary schools is adapting curriculum to local needs while ensuring a solid grounding in the basic principles of veterinary medicine. In the developing countries of Africa, as discussed throughout this chapter, the need for effective national disease control remains a top priority. Yet many schools initially adopted curricula from developed countries that emphasize clinical management of individual animals over issues of population medicine, including epidemiology, herd health, food safety, and zoonotic disease control. The growing trend toward international standards of livestock health as a prerequisite for participation in international trade of livestock and livestock products makes the need for veterinarians well trained in disease control even more urgent in countries with abundant livestock resources that wish to exploit export opportunities.

At the same time, however, the trend toward privatization in developing countries means that at least some veterinarians will need to be trained in clinical medicine and production medicine as well as population medicine. This multiplicity of demands offers great challenges to many veterinary schools, especially in light of their limited resources. One emerging approach for dealing with the need for curricular diversity is to allow flexibility in course selection and career-path tracking following completion of a standard basic curriculum in the beginning years of the veterinary training program. This approach has been applied widely in the United States and other developed countries in recent years to good effect. Students are able to develop specialized proficiencies while still being able to pass national accreditation tests that evaluate general veterinary knowledge. In the African context, for example, tracking would be a useful tool for preparing prospective graduates for private practice by developing a privatization track that included relevant accounting and management courses at the university's business school, as well as extra time for clinical rotations and farm visits to prepare for clinical practice.

Course work should reflect local needs. For example, Uganda has a considerable length of coastline along Lake Victoria as well as numerous other sizable lakes within its borders. Fishing has long been a source of income for both subsistence and commercial fisherman, and in recent years, aquaculture has also emerged as a commercial venture. The Faculty of Veterinary Medicine at Makerere University (MUFVM) in the capital city of Kampala, has added an aquatic veterinary specialist to the faculty and has incorporated fish diseases and fish-farm management into the curriculum. Similarly, Uganda has abundant wildlife resources and an extensive national park system that were significantly degraded during the years of civil unrest that ended in 1986. The veterinary faculty recognized that the health of wildlife is an appropriate concern for the nation's veterinarians for a number of reasons. First, it is understood that wildlife tourism will be extremely important to the future economic development of the country. Second, the consequences of widespread wildlife-livestock interactions must be understood and taken into account when planning and implementing national disease-control programs. Finally, there

has been a growing interest in wildlife use in commercial enterprises such as ostrich farming, crocodile farming, and game ranching within the country. These initiatives, to be successful, will require the research and clinical inputs of veterinary science and, in turn, can offer employment opportunities for veterinary graduates.

In response, MUFVM has created a new Department of Wildlife and Animal Resource Management (WARM) to focus faculty interest and resources on wildlife education for veterinary students. Fourth-year veterinary students are required to take an 80-hour lecture course in wildlife medicine and conservation and, at the end of the fourth year, to participate in a 2-week field exercise in conservation medicine that takes the students and faculty into the Uganda National Parks to interact with National Parks staff and local communities. In addition, MUFVM has also developed a postgraduate 1-year Diploma Course in Wildlife Health and Management for veterinary graduates who wish to specialize in wildlife-related fields.

The important role of veterinary education in effective veterinary service delivery is recognized by international agencies committed to improving animal health and production around the world. Since the 1970s, the FAO has convened a number of expert consultations on the state of veterinary education, aimed at evaluating the prevailing situation and developing recommendations for improvement. The fifth expert consultation convened in 1995.[5]

Conclusion

Organized veterinary medicine performs many important functions in the social and economic life of a nation. These include the provision of public goods such as control of epizootic diseases, food quality assurance, and prevention of zoonotic diseases as well as private goods such as the diagnosis, treatment, and prevention of disease in companion animals and livestock owned by individual citizens.

The delivery of veterinary service is not a "one size fits all" proposition. The veterinary needs of different countries vary considerably, as do the constraints on delivery of veterinary services. In developed countries, large numbers of livestock are managed intensively by small numbers of people as a livelihood, while the vast majority of citizens who keep animals do so as a personal choice, electing to keep a companion animal in their home. In many developing countries the situation is reversed, large numbers of citizens keep livestock as an essential part of their livelihood, while companion animal ownership is comparatively uncommon. In developed countries, a small proportion of veterinarians are directly employed by government in regulatory veterinary medicine and are able to control notifiable diseases effectively, while in many developing countries, large numbers of veterinarians are employed by government in a regulatory capacity, but important notifiable diseases persist unchecked. This is less a reflection on the professional capability of veterinarians in developing countries than on the physical conditions, financial limitations, and organizational structures under which they must work.

The value and importance of improving veterinary service delivery in developing countries cannot be overemphasized. It is in everyone's best interest to see the developing nations of the world become self-reliant and economically secure. Many developing countries still have predominantly rural populations and economies based on agriculture, with livestock as a critical element of the nation's agricultural productivity, as well as growing urban populations demanding a diverse diet that includes foods of animal origin. The need for effective veterinary services in such countries is essential to ensure that

- Otherwise nonproductive grazing lands can be used by herds of grazing livestock and wildlife free from the dangers of disastrous epizootic disease outbreaks

- Farmers have ready access to veterinary advice and ethical drugs so they can maintain healthy animals to work their lands productively and bring their produce to market

- Domestic animal production can be increased to meet growing demands for food of animal origin in expanding urban centers, without having to resort to importation

- New and novel commercial livestock enterprises can find the technical support they need in the area of health management to succeed and contribute to both the nation's food supply and economic development

- Governments and businesses can expand export markets for their livestock and livestock products abroad, confident that trade will not be impeded by uncontrolled outbreaks of notifiable disease or failures to ensure a standard of food quality that meets international trade requirements

- Consumers can purchase meat and other animal products confidently, without fear of food poisoning;

- All citizens can be free of the risk of exposure to chronically debilitating zoonotic diseases such as brucellosis and hydatid disease or acutely fatal ones such as rabies

- Wildlife resources can be effectively managed, and, where appropriate, commercially exploited in a sustainable fashion

- Veterinarians can derive satisfaction, a strong sense of accomplishment, and a comfortable livelihood from their professional activities

Considerable opportunities exist for veterinarians from developed countries to assist in efforts to reform and improve veterinary service delivery in developing countries, offering, for example, administrative and organizational experience in regulatory medicine, technical expertise in disease surveillance methodologies and laboratory diagnostic techniques, professional and business experience in support of the privatization process, and training and clinical advice for the establishment of community-based animal health programs. Numerous international organizations such as the FAO; governmental foreign aid agencies such as USAID; and NGOs such as FARM Africa, Heifer Project International, Vet Aid, and others have all recruited and used expatriate veterinarians in consultative roles related to veterinary service delivery in developing countries.

Readers interested in additional information on the issues of veterinary service delivery in developing countries are encouraged to refer to *Improving the Delivery of Animal Health Services in Developing Countries,* by the British research and consulting group Livestock in Development.[10] This small volume offers a concise overview of the subject, identifying the problems that exist, the efforts that have been made to address them, and needs for the future. It includes an extensive list of references that can lead readers to source materials on a wide array of relevant field activities, including community-based animal health projects carried out by various foreign aid agencies and NGOs around the world.

Discussion Points

1. What are the reportable or notifiable veterinary and public health diseases in your state? How does this list compare with the list A and B diseases of the OIE? Should all diseases on the OIE lists be notifiable in your state? Discuss why or why not.

2. As discussed in the text, several different federal agencies are involved in oversight of safety and efficacy of drugs and biologicals used daily by veterinarians. Critically evaluate this oversight system. What problems do you find? What changes would you suggest to improve or simplify this oversight? Hold a class forum on this subject.

3. In the sidebar on CBPP, the persistence of the disease in Africa was highlighted. However, CBPP also continues to occur in parts of southeast Asia and, sporadically, in Portugal. What factors contribute to the occurrence of CBPP in these other places? How would you assess the risk of CBPP being reintroduced into the United States?

4. Can you find any research data on the efficacy of castor bean for external parasite control? Design a research trial that would critically evaluate its safety and effectiveness. Pick any other traditional medicine or practice that you have heard of and find out how much objective scientific data exist on its efficacy and safety.

5. In general terms, how might the content of a veterinary curriculum in a developing country such as Vietnam, Tanzania, or Peru differ from the veterinary

curriculum offered in the United States? Pick a specific country in the world, obtain their veterinary curriculum and analyze its relevance to the country. Do this in consultation with veterinary students, faculty, and/or graduate veterinarians from that country, some of whom may be faculty members or graduate students at your own university.

6. Do you believe that a CAHW can be properly trained in a 3-week period to identify and safely and correctly treat common livestock diseases that are prevalent in animals in that community? What prerequisites are necessary to accomplish this?

7. Pick a country anywhere in the world that has recently experienced war. Determine what effect the war has had on the animal disease situation in that country and the delivery of veterinary services. What can be done to improve the situation?

References

1. Blaha T, ed. Applied Veterinary Epidemiology. Developments in Animal and Veterinary Sciences, Vol. 21. Amsterdam: Elsevier, 1989.

2. Davis DK. Gender-based differences in the ethnoveterinary knowledge of Afghan nomadic pastoralists. Indigenous Knowl Dev Monit 1995;3(1):3–5.

3. de Haan C, Nissen NJ. Animal Health Services in Sub-Saharan Africa. Alternative Approaches. World Bank Technical Paper no. 44. Washington, DC: World Bank, 1985.

4. Food and Agriculture Organization of the United Nations. Guidelines for Strengthening Animal Health Services in Developing Countries. Rome: FAO, 1991.

5. Food and Agriculture Organization of the United Nations. Veterinary Education. Fifth Joint FAO/WHO Expert Consultation. FAO Animal Production and Health Paper no. 125 Rome: FAO, 1995.

6. Food and Agriculture Organization of the United Nations. Prevention and Control of Transboundary Animal Diseases. Animal Production and Health Paper no. 133. Rome: FAO, 1997.

7. Heath ACG, Cole DJW, Bishop DM, et al. Preliminary investigations into the aetiology and treatment of cockle, a sheep pelt defect. Vet Parasitol 1995;56:239–254.

8. Jost CC, Sherman DM, Thomson EF, et al. Kamala (*Mallotus philippinensis*) fruit is ineffective as an anthelmintic against gastrointestinal nematodes in goats indigenous to Balochistan, Pakistan. Small Ruminant Res 1996;20:147–153.

9. Lawrence JA, Foggin CM, Norval RAI. The effects of war on the control of diseases of livestock in Rhodesia (Zimbabwe). Vet Rec 1980;107:82–85.

10. Livestock in Development. Improving the Delivery of Animal Health Services in Developing Countries: A Literature Review. Crewkerne, UK: Livestock in Development, 1996.

11. Mariner JC, House JA, Sollod AE, et al. Comparison of the effect of various chemical stabilizers and lyophilization cycles on the thermostability of a Vero cell-adapted rinderpest vaccine. Vet Microbiol 1990;21:195–209.

12. Mathias-Mundy E, McCorkle CM, eds. Ethnoveterinary Medicine: An Annotated Bibliography. Ames: Iowa State University Research Foundation, 1989.

13. McCorkle CM, Mathias E, Schillhorn van Veen T, eds: Ethnoveterinary Research and Development. London: Intermediate Technology Publications, 1996.

14. Schreuder BEC, Moll HAJ, Noorman N, et al. A benefit-cost analysis of veterinary interventions in Afghanistan based on a livestock mortality study. Prev Vet Med 1996;26:303–314.

15. Schreuder BEC, Noorman N, Halimi M, et al. Livestock mortality in Afghanistan in districts with and without a veterinary programme. Trop Anim Health Prod 1996;28:129–136.

Suggested Readings

Catley A. Methods on the Move. A Review of Veterinary Uses of Participatory Approaches and Methods Focussing on Experiences in Drylands Africa. London: International Institute for Environment and Development, 1999.

Food and Agriculture Organization of the United Nations. A manual for the primary animal health care worker. Rome: FAO, 1994.

Hugh-Jones ME, Hubbert WT, Hagstad HV. Zoonoses: Recognition, Control and Prevention. Ames: Iowa State University Press, 1995.

Leonard DK, ed. Africa's changing markets for health and veterinary services; the new institutional issues. Houndmills, UK: Macmillan, 2000.

Office International des Epizooties. The economics of animal disease control. Sci Tech Rev 1999;18(2):276 pp.

Schwabe CW. Veterinary Medicine and Human Health. 3rd Ed. Baltimore: Williams & Wilkins, 1984.

Chapter 9
International Trade, Food Safety, and Animal Disease Control

OBJECTIVES FOR THIS CHAPTER

After completing this chapter, the reader should be able to

- Recognize the impact that globalization is having on free trade and the increased importance of animal disease control and food safety in this new world order
- Understand the economic and social consequences of inadequate international animal disease control
- Identify contemporary challenges to international animal disease control
- Identify the international organizations involved in animal disease control and food safety and their functions
- Know how to respond to a suspected foreign animal disease outbreak in the United States

Introduction

We live in the era of globalization, an ongoing process characterized by the integration of markets, nations, and technologies to create an interdependent, worldwide economy. The driving force behind globalization is free-market capitalism. The operative principle of globalization is that the more willing a nation is to open its economy to free trade and unfettered markets, the more efficient and productive its economy will become, creating new opportunities for prosperity and improved standards of living where they did not exist before.

Opportunities however, are often coupled to risks. This is certainly true in the area of free trade. When you offer your products in the global marketplace, cultural differences come into play, and the quality and desirability of your products may be called into question. Or, when the doors are opened for others to bring their products to you, they may bring more than you bargained for, in the unwelcome form of disease and pestilence. This is certainly true in the area of agriculture, where global free trade has raised serious concerns about how animal pests and diseases can be controlled effectively and how the safety of food can be ensured.

This chapter begins with a brief overview of the modern process of globalization and the development of the free trade movement, followed by a discussion of the current situation regarding international trade in livestock and livestock products. Then, contemporary challenges to effective animal disease control are examined, and current concerns about food safety are discussed. The final sections deal with the challenge of safeguarding the United States from incursions of foreign animal disease and the mechanisms by which this is accomplished.

Throughout the chapter, the important role of veterinary medicine and veterinarians is emphasized.

Globalization and Free Trade

The notion of a global economy is not new. The age of sail, beginning roughly in the 15th century, created a global network for European traders that led ultimately to the era of European colonization and empire building that persisted well into the 20th century. However, the scope and volume of goods, services, and capital that are currently exchanged across national borders are unparalleled in human history.

Thomas L. Friedman, in his insightful guide to understanding globalization, *The Lexus and the Olive Tree*, lists three key developments, which he refers to as democratizations, that have fueled the accelerated growth of today's global economy.[10] These are the democratization of technology, the democratization of finance, and the democratization of information. This process of democratization has made the tools of technology, finance, and information accessible to ordinary citizens in countries around the world on a scale previously unimagined. In turn, these tools have empowered ordinary citizens to participate directly in economic development and to influence social policy both at home and abroad.

Developments in technology that have facilitated such democratization in the last quarter of the 20th century include computerization, advanced telecommunication, miniaturization, compression technology, and digitalization. Closely linked to these technological developments are developments leading to the democratization of information, which include the emergence of the internet and e-mail, cellular phones, satellite technology, and the associated expansion of multi-channel TV. The availability of television has had a profound effect on how the world conducts its affairs. When everyone can see how "the other half lives," pressure mounts on local politicians and officials to develop and implement policies that improve the local standard of living. At the same time, the internet and email allow citizens to mobilize public opinion against unresponsive politicians with a force and immediacy previously unimagined.

Contemporary developments leading to a democratization of finance include a sharp increase in the number and variety of financial instruments available to investors; the expansion of capital markets; emergence of employee control of pension fund investments; the end of fixed currency exchange rates and the emergence of foreign exchange markets; and relaxation of controls and restrictions on foreign investment. These changes have allowed greater participation of investors worldwide and transformed the operation of financial markets. A multitude of investors, armed with an abundance of inexpensive and timely information about the status of companies and countries, can, in the global marketplace, shift their investments out of a suspect corporation or country at virtually a moment's notice. The significance of this enhanced investor power is not lost on corporate executives, investment fund managers, and even high government officials, who all feel the pressure to improve production efficiency, provide adequate returns on investment, and outperform their competition. Friedman notes that the personal computer and the internet have undermined all top-down institutions that have tried to control decision making, whether they are corporate conglomerates or totalitarian governments.

While the democratization of technology, finance, and information had been steadily progressing through the latter half of the 20th century, it was the end of the Cold War, symbolically represented by the fall of the Berlin Wall in 1989, that created the conditions that allowed globalization to surge forward and redefine international relations in politics and commerce. From the end of World War II until the collapse of the Soviet Union, the world was divided into two ideological camps, the Free World and the Communist World, each intent on global hegemony. In pursuit of this global dominance, each side actively enlisted allies among the world's nations, wooing them with economic aid. Many developing countries received significant aid from the West or the Soviet Union. This flow of funds served first and foremost to buy allegiance and/or strategic support from third-world governments. Often, there was little expectation that such aid would be used to reform government, promote economic development, or promote social welfare, even though these payments were often publicly identified as development aid. In fact, both the West and the Soviet Union at one time or another supported repressive, corrupt, and incompetent governments in their efforts to maintain or influence the balance of power around the globe. The leaders of so-called nonaligned nations in the developing world were frequently adept at playing both sides against the middle in the Cold War and were able to reap substantial rewards from both ideological camps. Regrettably, much of that money ended up in the private bank accounts of corrupt officials.

Suddenly, with the Soviet Union dismantled, world affairs were no longer defined principally by political ideology, but rather by economic opportunity. Free-market capitalism emerged as the dominant and defining engine of world affairs. Many client states that had survived on the largesse of the superpowers suddenly found themselves bereft of outside aid, floundering economically, and left to stand on their own. Former republics of the Soviet Union such as Georgia, Uzbekistan, and Khazakstan; Warsaw Pact nations of Eastern Europe such as Rumania, Bulgaria, and Albania; and Soviet allies such as Mongolia and Cuba experienced significant declines in economic activity and standard of living when the Soviet Union was no longer purchasing their goods or subsidizing their fragile economies. Similarly, many Central American, African, and Asian countries that had enjoyed American financial support as bulwarks against communism suddenly found that the flow of aid had diminished drastically and they were essentially on their own.

Since the collapse of communism, it has become clear that while other systems might be able to distribute wealth more equitably throughout society, no system other than free-market capitalism has been so successful at generating wealth.

The nations that have been most successful in transforming themselves from client states to prosperous independent nations, such as Poland, Czechoslovakia, Taiwan, and South Korea, are those that have most fully and effectively embraced free-market capitalism. These nations have successfully adopted the social, political, and economic changes, referred to as *structural adjustments,* that are necessary to attract foreign investment and foster the entrepreneurial spirit of their own citizens (Table 9-1). Less-successful countries (e.g., Russia) are those that have been reluctant to give up on the old ways, clinging to protectionist regulations, top-down decision making, secret dealings, privilege, and corruption. Increasingly, the world's nations are hearing the globalization message and fine-tuning their economic and political institutions to become active players in the global marketplace. As this trend continues and global investors continue to search the globe for the best return on investments, competition will become increasingly important in defining investor attractiveness. The countries and corporations that can most reliably provide the highest-quality goods at the best prices in the most efficient manner will be the ones who retain investor interest and confidence and continue to prosper. This includes the production and marketing of livestock and livestock products, the global demand for which continues to expand dramatically.

Trade in Livestock and Livestock Products

Who would have ever thought that concerns about the value of the local currency in Thailand could trigger a series of global financial events that could lead directly to the risk of bankruptcy for grain and hog farmers in America's heartland? Yet that is exactly what happened in 1997–1998 when overall farm receipts dropped by as much as 20% following a drop off of orders from financially troubled Asian nations.

Who could imagine that a leg of lamb shipped all the way from Australia or New Zealand could be offered at a lower price in an American supermarket than a leg of lamb from sheep finished on a feedlot in Colorado? That lamb from "down under" can probably be found in your own local supermarket, as sheep imports now have over 30% of American market share, up from just 7% in 1993. This influx, a direct result of free trade, is driving some American sheep farmers out of business.

Did you ever wonder what happened to all the chickens' legs when you purchased a package of chicken breasts? The Minister of Agriculture in Haiti would be glad to tell you. He has complained to the U.S. government that a flood of frozen chicken legs from the U.S. into the Haitian markets under new free-trade agreements has essentially destroyed the indigenous Haitian poultry industry, which was just beginning to establish itself.

Guess who has lobbied hard to support China's entry into the World Trade Organization (WTO)? The National Cattlemen's

Table 9-1 Structural Adjustments Required for Nations to Attract and Keep Foreign Investment
Make the private sector the primary engine of economic growth
Maintain a low rate of inflation and price stability
Reduce the size of state bureaucracy
Maintain a balanced or close to balanced national budget
Eliminate or reduce tariffs on imported goods
Eliminate restrictions on foreign investments
Eliminate quotas and domestic monopolies
Increase exports
Privatize state-owned industries and utilities
Deregulate capital markets
Make the local currency convertible
Promote domestic competition through deregulation
Allow foreign ownership of industries and foreign investment in stock and bond markets
Eliminate corruption, kickbacks, and subsidies
Open up pension fund systems to foreign investment options
In the age of globalization, nations wishing to participate in the new global economy by attracting foreign investment as a stimulus for economic growth often have to radically transform their economic and political structures to present minimal risk to investors. A number of structural adjustments have emerged as prerequisite for entering the global economy. In his informative book on understanding globalization, *The Lexus and the Olive Tree,* Thomas L. Friedman refers to these structural adjustments as the "Golden Straightjacket" because they put conforming nations on the path to prosperity, while constraining their political, economic, and often, cultural flexibility.

Beef Association, that's who. The NCBA along with other agricultural groups is keen to gain access to the Chinese market of over 1 billion people but wants to be sure that fair trading practices are ensured under WTO rules. In 2000, as a prelude to the prospect of WTO membership, the U.S. Congress approved permanent normal trading relations status with China, and the U.S. and China signed a fair trade agreement wherein China would lower tariffs on American beef from 45 to 12% over a 5-year period. The NCBA estimates that this agreement can add $9/head to the value of fed cattle and that exports of beef and beef products to China will likely triple in volume and quadruple in value from a level of $60 million at the time of the agreement to $240 million. At the same time, American beef producers recognize that once the Chinese market is open, they will have to compete with Australia, Argentina,

Canada, New Zealand, and other beef producers for market share. American consumers may find that the shift of beef supplies to the Chinese export market leads to higher beef prices at home.

As these examples suggest, international trade is an integral part of modern agricultural production and marketing. International trade affords both risks and opportunities to producers willing to enter the global marketplace. In recent years, liberalization of the rules of international trade in agriculture, along with increased market demand have brought many producers into the global marketplace through trade. This was not always the case. As recently as 50 years ago, trade in agricultural products was comparatively insignificant by today's standards of activity. Following World War II, many countries that had experienced acute food shortages preceding and during the war focused on becoming self-sufficient in food production, reluctant to depend on foreign imports.

This is not to say there was no interest in international trade. The General Agreement on Tariffs and Trade (GATT), for instance, which represents the first contemporary effort to expand and codify global trade, was first established in 1947. However, GATT initially had little focus on agriculture. In fact, signatories agreed to a waiver in 1953 to keep agriculture out of GATT negotiations. Also, the first steps toward the European Union (EU) began as early as 1957, when West Germany, France, Italy, the Netherlands, Belgium, and Luxembourg joined together as a trading block. By the 1960s, integration of global capital markets had begun, with international capital flow influencing foreign exchange markets. Taking advantage of fluctuations in exchange rates can serve as a considerable impetus for countries to engage in international trading activities. Agriculture finally became an issue in GATT negotiations during the Kennedy round of GATT talks from 1962 to 1966. There was a concerted effort to liberalize agricultural commodity trading which led to some tariff reductions on selected agricultural products and prompted some trade agreements between individual countries.

International trade in agriculture expanded rapidly in the 1970s for a number of reasons. In the early 1970s, reduced food harvests worldwide, and especially in the Soviet Union, created demand for grain, particularly American grain. Between 1972 and 1973, U.S. grain exports jumped 67%, to over 3 billion bushels. Throughout the decade, world demand remained high for U.S. grain, as the value of the dollar remained low, global economic growth advanced, and average incomes and buying power around the world increased. By 1979, the U.S. had a 60% share of the world grain trade.

The 1980s were an era of contraction and turmoil in international agricultural trade. The decade started off with a punitive embargo of U.S. grain exports to the Soviet Union as a response to the Soviet invasion of Afghanistan. Then, recession caused grain exports to fall and prices dropped. Other nations began to increase production and export of grains in the face of a stronger U.S. dollar. The mid-1980s was a rare period in which trade in agricultural products failed to expand faster than agricultural output. Trade competition became fierce, and the period was marked by the appearance of numerous nontariff barriers to trade. When the Uruguay round of GATT talks began in 1986, fair trade policies for agricultural commodities and products finally emerged as a major agenda item, leading to removal of quotas, reduction in tariffs, decrease in export subsidies, and a proposed gradual decrease of domestic subsidies, which had long distorted international trade.

During the 1990s, international trade regained some vigor and emerged as an important element in the overall trend toward globalization. The decade was marked by both the formation of the WTO and the signing of the North American Free Trade Agreement (NAFTA) in 1994. Liberalization of agricultural trade and strengthening of fair trade policies received greater attention. It was recognized that considerable price distortions existed for agricultural products, and that nearly 80% of these price distortions were accounted for by practices and policies of developed economies. Japan, for example, remained notably protectionist with regard to agricultural imports, while European governments continued to resist the elimination or reduction of producer subsidies, at least in part because of fear of the political fallout from antagonizing the continent's well-organized, outspoken, and demonstration-prone farmers. Nevertheless, some progress on fair agricultural trade was made. During the period 1995-2000, a number of important reform commitments were implemented by developed-country WTO members, including reduction of tariffs by 36%, conversion of most nontariff barriers to tariffs or to tariff-rate quotas, reduction of aggregate levels of domestic support by 20%, and implementation of declining ceilings on the value and volume of subsidized exports.

The impact of trade liberalization on the growth of agricultural exports from America has been positive. In 1990, U.S. agricultural exports were approaching $40 billion annually. By 1996, agricultural export sales from the U.S. reached $60 billion and represented the largest category of U.S. exports. By the end of the decade, about 1 million jobs in America, both on and off the farm, were linked to agricultural exports, and one third of productive land, approximately 40.5 million hectares, was linked to production for export, 40% specifically for Asian markets. Farmers and ranchers in general have become twice as reliant on foreign trade as the U.S. economy as a whole.

While this expansion of agricultural trade can bring profits to American producers, it also can bring peril. When the Asian financial crisis of 1997 occurred, creating economic turmoil in Thailand, Indonesia, Korea, Malaysia, and Japan, these events had a direct affect on the income and well-being of American farmers. Demand for American farm products in Asian markets fell abruptly, inventories piled up, and prices plummeted. Between 1997 and 1998, wheat prices dropped by 30%, corn prices by 24%, soybeans by 26%, and cattle by 9%. Many American farmers were forced to sell their harvests at a loss, with rock bottom prices not even covering production costs.

Increased Demand for Livestock Products

Not only has the volume of international trade in agriculture changed considerably since World War II, so has the character of that trade. Historically, agricultural trade involved transfer of bulk commodities, primarily cereal grains, for direct human consumption. Over time, as global incomes improved and demand for food products increased, changes began to occur. An increasing proportion of cereal grain trade was earmarked for livestock feeding, and commodities used for animal feed, such as soybeans and alfalfa meal, grew in importance. For instance, in 1961, total global export of alfalfa meal and pellets was a mere 49.5 thousand metric tons, but it had increased almost 30-fold, to 1.48 million metric tons, by 1999. There has also been an increase in the demand for, and export of, value-added processed food products. Currently, processed foods account for about two thirds of all international trade in the food and agriculture sector and have exceeded the trade in bulk agricultural commodities since 1991. On average, over the past 25 years, the value of total world trade in processed foods has increased at a rate of about 10.5% annually. Technological advances in processing, preservation, shipping, and storage have allowed the expansion of global markets for perishable or hard-to-handle products such as cut flowers, fluid milk, fresh cheeses, and boxed meat. The capacity to ship meat long distances in a chilled rather than a frozen state, for instance, facilitated expansion of export markets as consumers tend to perceive chilled meat as a higher-quality product.

Rising incomes worldwide have led especially to an increase in demand for livestock products. In 1961, total exports for meat products of all categories, including both bulk and processed foods, were 3.50 million metric tons. By 1999, this trade had increased almost sevenfold, to 23.36 million metric tons. Dietary change and the demand for livestock products can be linked statistically to income growth. In the poorest countries, with subsistence economies and national average per capita incomes below $500, the diet often contains little animal protein, except for pastoralist communities that have animal herding as the basis of their livelihood. This is the situation in much of sub-Saharan Africa. Economists have observed that when national per capita incomes reach levels of approximately US$500 to $1000 per annum, there is a slowing in the demand for dietary staples such as food grains and tubers, which begin to be replaced by meat and other animal products. Countries such as China, Egypt, Indonesia, and the Philippines are at this stage. While cultural, religious, and geographical factors influence choice, usually poultry meat and egg demand rises first and most rapidly, because of the relatively low cost and easy availability of such products.

When national per capita incomes reach the range of $1,000 to $10,000 per annum, demand for staples is in obvious decline, and demand for livestock products has accelerated. Countries reaching this level of prosperity often are not producing the range and quantity of livestock products domestically to meet the surge in demand, and thus they become active importers of animal protein. Many countries in central Europe, southeast Asia, North Africa, and Latin America are at this stage of development. In countries where annual per capita income exceeds $10,000 (i.e., the industrialized or developed countries), domestic production of livestock products is usually high. In these countries, import demand for livestock products stabilizes, but at a high level, as strong purchasing power and consumer preference demand a diverse range of high-quality and specialized products, often from overseas markets.

The United States has turned from being a net importer of meat to being a net exporter in the last 15 years, largely because of improved access to foreign markets achieved through agreements that liberalized trade, such as NAFTA and GATT. By the end of the 1990s, about 10% of total U.S. beef output, 17% of U.S. broiler meat output, 6% of U.S. pork output, and 56% of U.S. hides and skins were destined for export markets. Meat imports are growing very rapidly in Mexico, Saudi Arabia, the Republic of Korea, Egypt, and Hong Kong, and many analysts believe that demand for imported livestock products will continue to grow in China, which represents an enormous potential market. Overall, it is estimated that demand for livestock products in Asian countries will continue to grow at an average rate of 7% per year. At the start of the 21st century, the United States held 48% of the world share of poultry exports, a 19% market share of world beef exports, and a 19% share of world pork exports. While the United States should be able to remain dominant in the expanding world market for livestock products, the country will also face increased competition. In the poultry sphere, Brazil is seen as the major competitor. In the marketing of pork, the EU is the major U.S. competitor, and for beef, Australia and Canada represent the major competitors, with Brazil and Argentina showing considerable potential as competitors in the world beef trade.

As buying power around the world continues to increase, so likely will the demand for livestock products. International trade will continue to expand to meet growing demand. Even though economically advancing nations tend to expand their own livestock production, in many cases, they may still not be able to meet internal demand. Many analysts believe that is the case with Asia, where the fastest economic growth is occurring, and demand for imports will remain high. One reason for this is that many Asian nations have very high population densities and limited land resources, leaving relatively little opportunity to expand agricultural production, particularly in the area of livestock production. Japan, Singapore, Hong Kong, Taiwan, and South Korea are obvious examples. Less obvious is China. While China has a large land area, it also has a huge population to support, and much of the Chinese land area is not arable. Furthermore, some observers note that expansion of cropland is being severely constrained by expansion of urban areas and lack of sufficient water, with water resources being diverted for industrial and urban use.

The Impact of Disease on Trade

As international trade in livestock products grows, so will competition. In recent years, it has become evident that livestock disease can be a very important factor in developing and retaining new markets for livestock products. Hence, animal disease control has become a critical factor in retaining a competitive edge. Countries that can keep their national herds and flocks free of infectious and contagious disease enjoy distinct market advantages over those who cannot. Countries that have established export markets and then are cut off from them because of a serious disease outbreak may have great difficulty reestablishing their markets for several reasons. First, international agreements may require thorough documentation of disease eradication and a mandated waiting period before exports can resume. Second, the disease outbreak, especially if it involved a zoonotic disease, may result in a loss of consumer confidence in the wholesomeness and safety of products supplied by the exporting country (Fig. 9-1). Third, former markets may shrink or disappear because competitors have filled the void during the exporter's absence.

Countries that have not been able to control infectious and contagious disease within their own borders may be cut off from export markets altogether, even though livestock represent a major resource within the country. For example, many poorer countries with large national herds of sheep and goats in sub-Saharan Africa and south Asia are cut off from exporting small ruminants to lucrative markets in nearby Middle Eastern countries where demand is high, because of failure to effectively control endemic contagious small-ruminant diseases such as foot and mouth disease, contagious caprine pleuropneumonia, and peste des petits ruminants.

Concerns about disease as a barrier to trade are not merely theoretical. Billions of dollars have been lost to exporting countries in recent years because of disease situations, as the following examples illustrate.

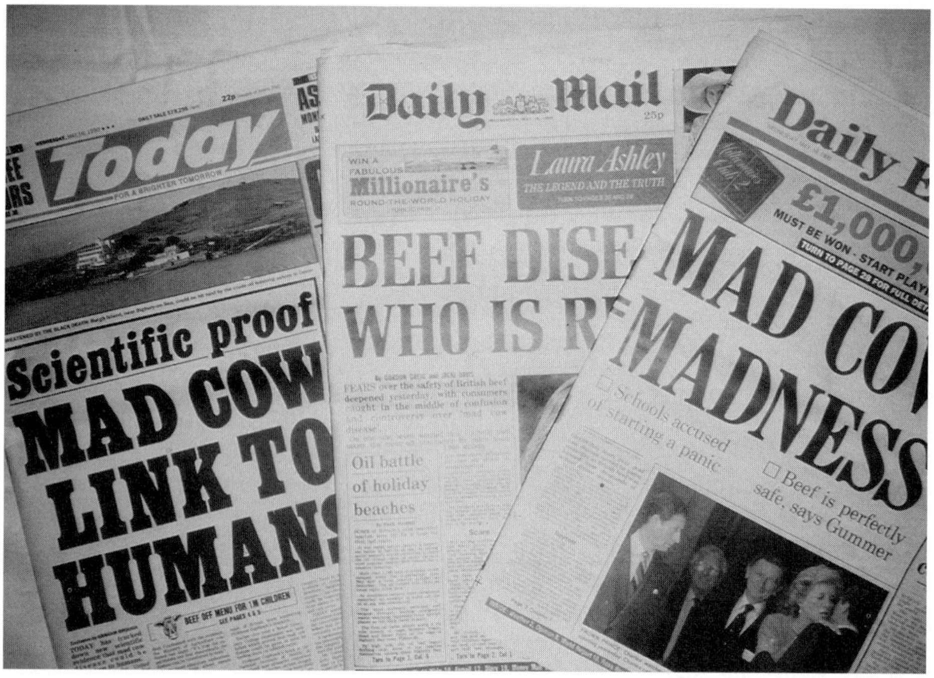

Foot and Mouth Disease in Swine in Taiwan   Starting in March 1997, foot and mouth disease (FMD) swept rapidly through the hog farms on the island of Taiwan, affecting between 200 and 300 new farms a day. By mid-June, 6144 farms were affected, involving 1,011,421 FMD-infected pigs and 184,231 dead pigs. In addition, close to 4 million pigs were killed as part of the subsequent disease control effort through depopulation and disposal. Before the outbreak, Taiwan was the third largest exporter of pork products worldwide. Some 40% of the country's population of 14 million hogs was earmarked for export markets. Taiwan exported 30% of its overall pork production to Japan, mostly as fresh, chilled pork. As a result of the outbreak, Japan shut off importation of Taiwan pork. Within Taiwan, pork consumption fell off sharply as domestic consumers expressed their fears about the wholesomeness and safety of the pork supply. Within 1 week of the start of the outbreak, the price of pork fell by 60%, dropping below production costs, so that even farmers who were not directly affected by the disease outbreak were economically affected. Though a national control program was immediately implemented, including vaccination, the disease flared up again in December 1997, partly because of the reluctance of farmers to pay for vaccinations when hog prices were already depressed. The December outbreak raised the prospects that Taiwan would not be cleared to begin exporting fresh chilled pork to Japan again until 2003, since Japanese import requirements prohibit importing unprocessed pork from an area infected with FMD unless the disease has been eradicated and vaccines have not been used for at least 2 years. In the meantime, the United States, Canada, and Denmark have replaced Taiwan in the Japanese market. The financial cost of the epidemic was estimated at US$378.6 million, including indemnities, vaccines, carcass disposal, environmental protection, and loss of market value. The ban on ex-

Figure 9-1.   Consumer confidence in beef products was seriously undermined by the emergence of bovine spongiform encephalopathy (BSE) in the United Kingdom in the 1980s. When it became evident that so-called mad cow disease was also likely infecting humans and could cause a fatal neurological disease, the public reaction bordered on hysteria. Even though quantitative risk assessments indicate the chance of contracting variant Creutzfeldt-Jakob disease from eating beef is only about 1 in 10 billion, anxiety about BSE remains front and center in the public's mind as these British headlines suggest. Veterinarians must play an active role in promoting science-based efforts to improve food safety, reliably identify and report genuine risks, and restore public confidence in foods of animal origin. (Photo courtesy of Lieutenant Colonel Jeffrey E. Melander, United States Army Veterinary Corps)

ports of pork to Japan is projected to have a total economic cost to Taiwan's pig industry of about US$1.6 billion.

Avian Influenza in Hong Kong In May 1997, a 3-year-old boy died in Hong Kong. By August, the cause of the boy's death had been determined to be the avian influenza virus strain H5N1, which was first discovered in birds in 1961 and had never previously been known to infect human beings. The same strain of influenza virus had been isolated from an outbreak of poultry disease on farms in the New Territories of Hong Kong 2 months earlier. Health officials expressed considerable concern about the potential transmission of the virus from birds to people. By the end of December, there had been 16 confirmed human cases, including several deaths. A general alarm swept through the citizenry, and shopkeepers reported a 40% drop in sales of poultry products. To address public concern, the government of Hong Kong ordered the destruction of all poultry within its jurisdiction on December 29, 1997. In a 36-hour period, a complete depopulation was carried out, involving over 1.2 million chickens on 160 chicken farms and in a thousand markets. All ducks, geese, quail, and other edible birds were also destroyed and buried under seal in landfills. As a result of the emergence of this apparent zoonosis, the poultry industry of Hong Kong was virtually eliminated overnight.

Nipah Virus in Swine and Humans in Malaysia A human viral encephalitis outbreak began in Malaysia in September 1998. By June 1999 when the outbreak subsided, there had been approximately 200 cases, with 80 deaths. Epidemiologists noted something very unusual in the pattern of disease. In predominantly Muslim Malaysia, virtually all the affected individuals were ethnic Chinese, and virtually all of these people owned or worked on pig farms. In addition, slaughterhouse workers in neighboring Singapore were also affected. Though the cause was initially thought to be Japanese encephalitis, the leading cause of viral encephalitis in Asia, further investigation revealed that the etiological agent was in fact a previously unknown paramyxovirus, subsequently named Nipah virus. It became clear that pigs were the principal source of the virus and that humans were most likely affected by direct contact with infected swine. Sudden death was observed in infected pigs, and antibodies to Nipah virus were found in horses, dogs, cats, and fruit bats. Identification of pigs as the source of virus was devastating to the swine industry. The government initially ordered the slaughter of 350,000 pigs in the two worst affected states, but subsequently, at the end of March 1999, expanded the slaughter effort to include 1.3 million swine. Import of Malaysian pork to Singapore was banned, and Indonesia quickly stepped in as its principal supplier. Though no additional cases in pigs have been observed since May 1999, consumer confidence in Malaysian pork in neighboring countries was severely shaken by the emergence of this dangerous zoonotic disease, and it may be many years before the Malaysian swine industry can fully recover. Between 1997 and 1999, the export value of all Malaysian pork products declined from US$6.24 million to 2.50 million.

Foot and Mouth Disease in Cattle in Argentina For almost 70 years, fresh Argentine beef was banned from the United States because of concern about FMD. So there was considerable satisfaction on the pampas when in May 2000, the Office International des Epizooties (OIE), the international animal disease-monitoring agency, declared Argentina "an FMD-free country in which vaccination is not practiced," thus clearing the way for expanded export. Argentine beef quickly became popular in American steakhouses and supermarkets with consumers interested in choosing low-fat beef from grass-fed, free-ranging cattle. However, the export trade was short-lived. In August 2000, the United States reinstituted a ban on import of beef from Argentina following the discovery that 10 head of cattle smuggled into the country from neighboring Paraguay were antibody positive for the FMD virus. Though no clinical cases were observed in the smuggled bovines, Argentina promptly destroyed over 3500 cattle that had come into contact with them. Then, after assessing the risk of incursions of infected cattle from neighboring countries, Argentina decided as of March 2001 to establish a border buffer zone and restriction zone in which vaccination would be carried out. As a result, the OIE rescinded its declaration of Argentina as an FMD-free country where vaccination is not practiced, and beef exports from the country remain depressed.

Hog Cholera in the Dominican Republic The swine industry in the United States is a multibillion-dollar enterprise, associated with over 600,000 jobs and an export market valued at more than 1 billion dollars annually since the late 1990s. One important factor in the success of American pork in export markets is freedom from diseases such as classical swine fever, also known as hog cholera. The United States has been free of hog cholera since 1978, following an intensive 16-year effort by state and federal government in cooperation with the swine industry. Therefore, considerable alarm was raised in the United States when hog cholera was reported on the nearby Caribbean island of Hispanola, first in Haiti in October 1996 and then in the Dominican Republic in June 1997. The Dominican Republic is only about 600 miles from Florida, and there is considerable traffic into the United States from that country, with over 200,000 visits a year by Dominican nationals. The U.S. Department of Agriculture (USDA) felt compelled to intercede in the control of hog cholera in the Dominican Republic to minimize the risk of introduction of the disease to the United States. By October 1997, USDA Animal and Plant Health Inspection Service (APHIS), at the request of the government of the Dominican Republic, was providing technical assistance and equipment to bring the outbreak under control and establish surveillance activities. Despite these efforts, serious concern remained that hog cholera could enter the United States, most likely as a result of contaminated pork products being carried in the luggage of air passengers entering the United States from the Dominican Republic. In March 1999, the secretary of agriculture declared an emergency relative to the risk of hog cholera entering the country and allocated US$5.3 million to efforts to reduce that risk. The money was earmarked for supporting increased surveillance of airline passengers and their luggage at embarkation points within the Dominican Republic and included $400,000 for the purchase of improved x-ray equipment to scan the luggage of departing passengers and hiring and training of at least 40 additional inspectors.

Bovine Spongiform Encephalopathy (BSE) in the UK and then Europe The previously unknown disease BSE in cattle, first identified in the United Kingdom in 1986, has emerged as the defining example in our time of how livestock disease can adversely affect trade and undermine consumer confidence in the wholesomeness of foods of animal origin. The subsequent identification of BSE as a potentially zoonotic disease linked to the human neurological condition variant Creutzfeldt-Jakob disease (vCJD), in 1994 further undermined trade prospects and created new public health concerns. A ban on the importation of British beef by EU nations between 1996 and 1999, triggered by concern about the spread of vCJD, cost the British beef industry an estimated US$3.3 billion. By the year 2000, BSE had been diagnosed in native cattle in Ireland, Portugal, Switzerland, France, Belgium, Germany, the Netherlands, and Denmark and appeared to be on the increase in continental Europe. At the beginning of 2001, the Food and Agriculture Organization of the United Nations (FAO) warned that virtually any country in the world that had imported cattle, meat, or bone meal from the UK and western Europe for use as livestock feed during or since the 1980s was potentially at risk for BSE and also possibly vCJD. As if on cue, Japan announced its first case of BSE in a cow in September 2001. Keeping BSE out of the United States has been a major focus of industry, government, and health officials. At the time of this writing, the effort has so far been successful. BSE-free status means enhanced international trade opportunities for American cattle producers and the beef industry as well as considerable peace of mind for consumers protected from the threat of vCJD.

Nontariff Trade Barriers and Animal Disease

Clearly, all nations have legitimate reasons for setting high standards for the health of animals and wholesomeness of animal products being imported into their countries. However, setting standards of acceptance and enforcing them can lead to conflicts between importing and exporting nations. Questions may arise about whether or not the objections raised on matters of health and wholesomeness are legitimate and fair concerns or whether they really represent the use of disease and safety issues as nontariff barriers to trade. Consider the following two examples.

- *Canada versus Brazil:* On February 2, 2001, the Canadian government abruptly announced that it was halting the importation of canned corned beef and beef extract from Brazil. This trade is worth over $9 million annually to Brazil and represents 10% of its meat export market. The reason given by Canada for the sudden ban was growing concern over the potential introduction of BSE into Canada from Brazil. The previous week, Brazilian officials had acknowledged that Brazil had been importing live

cattle from Europe as recently as 1999. Canada claimed it had been asking Brazil for 2 years to provide complete information on its importing activities, domestic animal health status, and BSE surveillance efforts to assure Canada that Brazil is free of BSE. Canada declared that the information was never fully provided and did not include documentation of imports of live cattle from Europe. To add further to Brazil's troubles, both Mexico and the United States joined Canada in the ban by virtue of their partnership with Canada in NAFTA.

Brazilians were incensed. Brazilian citizens held demonstrations outside the Canadian Embassy. Brazilian bar owners poured their Canadian whiskey in the street. Brazilian longshoremen refused to unload Canadian ships. Brazilian officials decried the ban, declared it unjustified and outrageous. Officials pointed out that virtually all Brazilian beef is derived from range-fed cattle that receive little or no grain supplement, let alone concentrate feed that contains animal protein potentially contaminated with the BSE agent. The Brazilian officials suggested that alleged concern about BSE by Canada was in fact a retaliatory trade action, using health concerns as a nontariff barrier to trade. At the time of the ban, Canada and Brazil were already engaged in a heated trade dispute involving the nations' respective airplane manufacturing industries The Brazilian airplane manufacturer, Embraer, was presenting formidable competition to the Canadian airplane manufacturer, Bombardier, and the Canadians felt that Embraer had an unfair market advantage, since Embraer received considerable subsidies from the Brazilian government allowing them to undercut the price of Canadian-built passenger planes on the world market. Canada had already filed a grievance with the WTO about the airplane manufacturing debate and had received permission from the WTO to impose trade sanctions against Brazil. Brazilian officials claim that the beef ban is directly linked to the airplane issue and that the BSE concern is simply a smokescreen, serving as a nontariff barrier to trade. So, was the Canadian decision to block Brazilian exports on the basis of concerns about BSE warranted or justified? How can the true risk of BSE in Brazil be established? Where and how would such disputes involving disease and trade in livestock products be resolved?

- *The European Union versus the United States:* In 1989, the EU initiated a ban on importation of beef from animals that had been treated with growth-promoting hormones. As most commercial cattle feeders in the United States use an FDA-approved hormonal implant in their management programs, this ban effectively cut off U.S. beef from the European market, a loss estimated at approximately US$100 million annually to the American beef industry. The Europeans justified this ban on the basis of public health concerns, citing the carcinogenic potential of the hormones contained in growth-promoting implants in the United States. In response, U.S. producers and their advocates point out that all of the hormones used in cattle are carefully regulated and approved by the federal government and that by the time cattle reach market age, the concentration of hormone in implanted cattle is virtually indistinguishable from the concentration of hormone detectable in beef from untreated cattle. Furthermore, they point out that many other foods contain estrogenic hormones in much higher concentration than beef from implanted cattle. Ninety grams of untreated beef, for example, may contain about 1.0 ng of estrogen, while 90 g of beef from an implanted steer may contain 1.9. In contrast, 90 g of peas contains about 336 ng of estrogenic hormone.

Is the use of FDA-approved hormonal growth implants in feeder cattle a legitimate public health issue or does it simply represent an attempt by the Europeans to reduce competition through use of a nontariff barrier to trade? The United States government thinks the latter and in 1996 formally requested the WTO to arbitrate the dispute. In 1998, the WTO issued a finding that the EU hormones directive violated multilateral trade rules and ordered the EU to come into compliance with WTO rules by May 1999. When the deadline passed and the EU failed to lift the ban, the United States retaliated with sanctions on a wide variety of EU agricultural exports to the United States, valued at $117 million. At the time of this writing, the conflict remains unresolved. Are FDA-approved growth promotants used in cattle production dangerous? Can an objective scientific decision be made on this issue? How will the problem ultimately be resolved?

These two stories underscore how important health and disease issues have become in the arena of international trade in livestock and livestock products. They also reveal the critical, central, and emerging role that veterinary science must play in informing matters of trade related to health and disease. In each of the cases described, trade negotiators have to rely on information provided by veterinary diagnosticians, epidemiologists, and researchers to help understand the issues at hand and develop their negotiating strategies. Among the veterinary matters represented in these two scenarios are matters of risk assessment, disease diagnosis, and disease monitoring as well as research on the metabolism of growth hormones in cattle and the carcinogenic potential of growth hormones and their metabolites.

Before the liberalization of trade, nations that wished to protect their own beef producers from foreign competition or to punish trading partners for perceived unfair trading practices would simply attach a heavy import duty or tariff on the targeted product to accomplish the protection or punishment they intended. However, in the age of multinational free-trade agreements, the dismantling of trade barriers, and the prospect of arbitration at the WTO, the use of tariffs for protection or punishment has largely become unacceptable. Human nature being what it is, some nations will continue to resort to nontariff barriers to trade to achieve their goals. Domestic producers in various sectors may put considerable pressure on politicians and policymakers to maintain some form of trade protection against foreign competition with their own particular products in domestic markets. Governments in turn can make their regulatory agencies feel this pressure, leading to actions that are based more on expediency than on good science. For agricultural trade in general and livestock products in particular, there is great potential for manipulation of regulations imposed in the name of food safety and disease control to be exploited as nontariff barriers to trade. Veterinarians will play increasingly important roles in keeping science in the forefront to ensure that food safety and disease concerns are legitimate and not simply smokescreens for protectionism.

Fair Trade and International Disease Control

Recognizing the growing importance of disease matters on the conduct of international trade, nations that are signatories to international trade agreements have sought to develop standards, practices, and procedures that help to ensure that the regulations and requirements set for disease control are transparent, reasonable, and fairly applied. They have also sought to minimize the use of animal health issues as nontariff barriers to trade and to create avenues of redress when such barriers are suspected.

In both the GATT and NAFTA, participating nations agreed to establish rules to control the use of technical health issues as barriers to trade. Toward this end, the GATT Uruguay Round Agreement on the Application of Sanitary and Phytosanitary Measures was formulated and adopted by the WTO when it succeeded GATT in 1995 as the principal world body concerned with international trade. NAFTA essentially replicated the same sanitary and phytosanitary (SPS) rules and principles reached under GATT. The GATT/WTO Agreement on the Application of Sanitary and Phytosanitary Measures is more commonly and more easily referred to as the SPS Agreement.

The SPS Agreement

The full text of the SPS Agreement can be found on the WTO website (www.wto.org) under the heading "Trade Topics." The aim of the SPS Agreement adopted by the WTO is to protect human, animal, or plant life and health from risks associated with animal or plant pests and diseases, food additives, or contaminants that might occur as a result of international trade. The agreement strives to achieve this protection by setting codes of conduct on the development, adoption, and enforcement of SPS measures. These codes of conduct are designed to prevent the use of SPS measures as disguised restrictions to trade, while protecting each member's right to implement SPS standards within their own country to protect human, animal, and plant life and health. The key provisions of the SPS Agreement are as follows:

Assurance of Basic Rights The agreement confirms the right of each WTO member to establish the level of SPS protection that it considers appropriate and provides that a member may achieve that level of protection through SPS measures that

- Are based on scientific principles and scientific evidence

- Are applied only to the extent required to provide a member's chosen level of protection

- Do not result in unfair discrimination or disguised restrictions on trade

- Conform to the obligations outlined throughout the agreement

Acceptance of International Standards To avoid creating unnecessary barriers to trade, the agreement encourages WTO members to use relevant international standards in the development of their SPS measures. However, it permits each member to adopt more stringent, scientifically based measures when necessary to achieve its chosen level of protection.

In the area of food safety, international standards are developed and approved through the Codex Alimentarius Commission, discussed in more detail later in this chapter. Standards for control of pests and disease in plants and plant products are the purview of the International Plant Protection Convention (IPPC). The IPPC is a multilateral treaty signed by 113 governments that is administered through the IPPC Secretariat located in the Plant Protection Service of the FAO.

With regard to matters of animal health, the WTO has designated the OIE as the reference agency for international scientific standards on matters of animal health and disease control and the principal scientific consulting body on such matters as they relate to international trade in livestock and livestock products (See sidebar on the OIE). The main functions of the OIE are

- To inform governments of the occurrence and course of animal diseases throughout the world and of ways to control these diseases

- Coordinate, at the international level, studies devoted to the surveillance and control of animal diseases including research on the pathology, diagnosis, treatment, and prevention of such diseases

- Harmonize regulations for trade in animals and animal products among member countries by providing guidelines and standards for health regulations applied to international trade

As the SPS Agreement explicitly calls for the use of standards, guidelines, and recommendations developed under the auspices of the OIE, the OIE has developed a set of publications to guide countries in the implementation and harmonization of their regulations applicable to the international trade in animals and animal products. These publications include the *International Animal Health Code* for mammals, birds, and bees; the *Manual of Standards for Diagnostic Tests and Vaccines*; and a comparable code and manual for aquatic animals. The full text of these publications is available on the OIE website (www.oie.int) under the heading "Standards." The OIE does not certify the animal health status of member countries, rather it serves to validate the documentation submitted by member nations against the established and agreed-upon procedures and standards embodied in the OIE codes and manuals.

Acceptance of Equivalence If requested, members will accept the sanitary or phytosanitary measures of other countries as equivalent, even if they are different. This will occur if the exporting member can demonstrate that its measures achieve the level of protection chosen by the importing country. The equivalence provision of the SPS Agreement encourages importing countries to recognize that different procedures can be used to achieve the same desired level of protection.

An example of such matters of equivalency involves a poultry dispute between the United States and the EU in 1997. The problem stemmed from fundamentally different approaches to poultry hygiene. The EU banned poultry imports from the United States because of differences in chilling and decontamination of poultry and poultry products. The EU mandates high standards of cleanliness at all stages of production, while the United States approves the use of chlorinated water as a decontaminant at the end of the production process. As a result of this dispute and other conflicts related to the notion of equivalency and to avoid protracted trade wars, the United States and the EU worked cooperatively to develop an equivalency agreement, jointly signing the United States-European Community Veterinary Equivalence Agreement in July 1999.

The agreement provides the framework for the United States and the EC to work together on various public health and animal health issues related to trans-Atlantic trade in animals and animal products. It identifies specific areas in which the United States and EU recognize that their different regulatory and legislative requirements can achieve an equivalent level of protection for public and animal health. In practical terms, this means that producers in the United States or the EC can meet the standards of the importing country in different but equivalent ways. Thus, the agreement is intended to reduce compliance costs for producers, associated with different public and animal health regulations between the two sides, while ensuring the protection of public and animal health. Annual exports of U.S. animal and animal product exports to the EU are approximately $1.5 billion, with a similar value of annual EU exports to the United States.

The Use of Import Risk Analysis The SPS Agreement establishes that WTO members must base their SPS requirements for controlling the introduction of diseases and pests through imports on scientifically based risk assessment. Such evaluations must include a range of relevant information including, among others, disease incidence in the exporting country, species susceptibilities, sampling and testing methods, animal production and processing methods, ecological and environmental conditions, the veterinary capacity of the exporting country, and economic factors in disease control.

Risk analysis is a process that involves hazard identification, risk assessment, risk management, and risk communication. *Hazard identification* is the process of cataloging the pathogenic agents that could potentially be introduced with the importation of a specific animal or animal product. It also requires establishing which of these pathogens are present in the exporting country but absent in the importing country. *Import risk assessment* is the process of scientifically estimating the probability that an importation event would result in the introduction of a disease agent and the exposure of that disease agent to susceptible domestic animal populations. The assessment also includes an evaluation of the consequences of such an adverse event occurring.

Risk management is the rational selection of appropriate actions that can reduce the risk of disease importation identified in the risk assessment to an acceptable level. The risk management toolbox includes such things as quarantine, diagnostic testing, use of sentinel animals, additional processing of products (e.g., pasteurization or irradiation), restricted use or distribution of imports, or outright prohibition of importation.

Risk communication is the process of effectively transmitting information about risk assessment and management to consumers, decision makers, and other interested parties and receiving relevant information from those same groups. For risk analysis to be accepted as an effective means of controlling the spread of disease, risk communication must be unambiguous and transparent.

Import risk analysis depends on scientific investigation but also frequently requires making assumptions about disease transmission potential, since the specific incidence of a disease, the pathogenicity of various strains, and other similar variables cannot always be determined precisely. Since assumptions are inherently subjective, import risk analysis can be controversial. As part of the effort to promote harmonization of disease control efforts in trade, the OIE sets out specific guidelines for WTO members to follow in developing import risk analyses.

These guidelines are found in the International Animal Health Code. For readers especially interested in a global perspective on the role of risk analysis of animal health in international trade, a special issue of the OIE journal, *Scientific and Technical Review* (volume 12, number 4, December 1993) contains a compendium of articles on this particular subject.

Recognition of Regionalization The concept of regionalization is based on recognition of the fact the disease risk associated with animals or animal products imported from any part of the world may be influenced more by climatic, geographical, and biological factors than by national or political boundaries. The SPS Agreement acknowledges this and allows the identification and delineation of regions and zones determined to be pest-or disease-free or to have low pest or disease prevalence. An exporting member nation must provide objective evidence whenever it claims that goods from its territory originate from such a region.

For the United States, regionalization is an important concept relative to trade in livestock because it allows disease control to be addressed with more flexibility than would be possible if disease-free areas were defined strictly on the basis of national borders. The United States is a physically large country, encompassing a wide range of climatic regions from the tropical to the near arctic. Insect vectors that carry disease may thrive in some regions and be absent in others. Take for instance, the case of bluetongue, a viral disease of ruminants, transmitted by biting midges. The occurrence of bluetongue is limited to areas where the midge can overwinter. If import/export regulations are based on political boundaries, then countries free of bluetongue might disallow the importation of livestock from anywhere in the United States because bluetongue is endemic in the southwestern United States. However, with regionalization, the United States can export cattle, sheep, and goats from bluetongue-free regions once the distribution of the vector and the disease can be adequately documented.

A current example of the potential impact of regionalization involves the occurrence of the foreign animal disease infectious salmon anemia in farmed salmon in coastal waters of Maine at the beginning of 2001, presumed to have been introduced from Canada, where the disease has affected farmed salmon in the Maritime provinces for some time. In response to the outbreak in Maine, Chile announced it would no longer purchase salmon brood stock from the United States. However, virtually all of the brood stock regularly purchased comes from suppliers in the Pacific Northwest. As it is highly unlikely that the Maine outbreak would reach across the continent to that distant area of the country, regionalization would allow continued trade with the northwest while the disease problem is being addressed in the northeast.

Commitment to Transparency The SPS Agreement states that members shall promptly notify other members about changes in sanitary or phytosanitary measures, providing both the reasons and the objectives for the changes. The International Code of Animal Health of the OIE, which serves as the reference for standards relating to animal health in international

Office International des Epizooties - OIE - International Office of Epizootics

The OIE was established in 1924 following a diplomatic conference in Paris convened by the French government. The conference was catalyzed largely by an outbreak of rinderpest that occurred in Belgium in 1920 following the introduction of infected zebu cattle from Pakistan through the port of Antwerp. This event emphasized that greater international cooperative effort was required to detect the occurrence of highly contagious animal diseases and to communicate information about such diseases in a timely fashion. By improving international cooperation, governments could take more effective steps to avert devastating epizootics or harmful zoonotic diseases moving into or out of their countries. On January 25, 1924, 28 countries signed the international agreement to create and participate in the OIE. The OIE office is in Paris, France, in the building shown at left, at 12 rue de Prony. The organization has grown considerably in size and importance since its inception. In 1995 the WTO named the OIE as the recognized technical reference agency for matters of animal health arising in relation to international trade under the Agreement on the Application of Sanitary and Phytosanitary Measures, discussed in more detail in the section on the SPS Agreement. In March 2001, membership in the OIE reached 156 nations when Nicaragua and North Korea announced their accession to the organization.

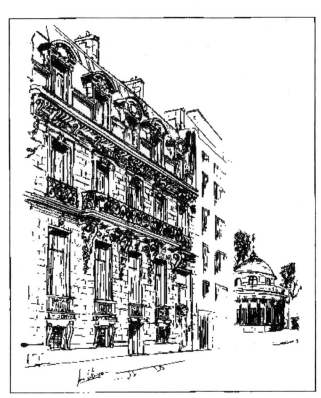

Headquarters of the OIE in Paris, France. (With permission of the OIE)

Disease reporting remains an essential function of the OIE. Member states are obliged to report any actual or suspect in-country occurrences of list A diseases (Table 9-2) or any other diseases with potentially serious repercussions on public health or the economy of animal production to the OIE within 24 hours of their detection and then file weekly reports on the evolution of the disease situation until it is resolved. In the absence of list A disease activity, monthly reports are required, and an annual report is required documenting the status of both list A and list B diseases. For its part, the OIE disseminates disease information to member states in several ways. A weekly report, Disease Information, is issued that includes the official reports member states submitted during the previous 7 days. The report is available in hard copy and electronically by email or on the OIE website (www.oie.int). A second publication, the Bulletin, is published every 2 months

trade, specifically calls for transparency with regard to animal disease status in member nations. It states that an exporting country should be prepared to supply information on its animal health situation and national animal health information systems so it can be determined whether that country is free of, or has free zones of, the OIE's list A and list B diseases (Table 9-2). The exporting country must also declare the regulations and procedures in force to maintain its disease-free status. In addition, the code requires provision of regular and prompt information on the occurrence of transmissible diseases, as well as details of the country's ability to apply measures to control and prevent list A diseases and, where appropriate, list B diseases.

For the United States, transparency has proven to be somewhat problematic. With a well-developed veterinary regulatory in-

frastructure, a well-trained force of private practitioners, strong institutional diagnostic capabilities, and a strong commitment to freedom of information, the occurrence of disease in the United States is well documented, and the information freely shared. As a result, other nations have used such freely available information to block entry of animals or animal products from the United States for relatively common diseases that may in fact be present in their own countries but which are not routinely detected or reported. Examples include infectious bovine rhinotracheitis, bovine viral diarrhea, salmonellosis, and porcine reproductive and respiratory syndrome. However, forward-thinking policymakers do not suggest that the United States should retreat from transparency. The net effect of openness is enhanced disease control and an international reputation for wholesomeness and quality of American livestock products. This offers a marketing edge that far outweighs the

and serves as a less urgent summary of accumulated information received from national veterinary services concerning new outbreaks of list A diseases and also provides a list of countries that have reported the absence of these diseases. The Bulletin also functions as a newsletter, providing information on activities of veterinary services and the OIE and calendars of forthcoming international events.

OIE also publishes an annual compendium of disease events, World Animal Health, which summarizes the year's outbreaks of disease on a country-by-country basis. It also provides relevant information on related topics. The 1999 volume, for example, included information on emerging diseases of wildlife, changes in the missions and organization of various national animal health services, and the effectiveness of new approaches to disease control. OIE also publishes a scientific journal, Revue Scientifique et Technique (Scientific and Technical Review), three times a year. Two of the issues focus on specific themes relevant to animal disease or public health. For example, the first issue of 2001 was on mycobacterial infections in domestic and wild animals.

Another important function of the OIE is to promote technical expertise related to matters of animal disease control. This is accomplished through a network of specialist commissions, working groups, collaborating centers, and reference laboratories. The specialist commissions study problems of epidemiology and control of animal diseases and issues related to the harmonization of international regulations. The Foot and Mouth Disease and Other Epizootics Commission, for example, assists in identifying the most appropriate strategies and measures for disease prevention and control and convenes groups of experts, particularly in emergencies. The Standards Commission works on establishing standards for methods of disease diagnosis and for testing biological products such as vaccines. OIE working groups are created as needed to collect, analyze, disseminate, and assess progress in knowledge relative to emerging issues or matters of sudden concern. The output of working groups is used to inform the OIE in the formulation of policy relative to the matters under study. At present, OIE has working groups addressing matters of biotechnology, veterinary drug registration, informatics and epidemiology, and wildlife diseases. Collaborating centers provide technical expertise to the OIE in specific areas of competence. They provide expert advice, research, and training and assist in the development, standardization, and dissemination of relevant techniques to promote harmonization of international disease control efforts. Examples of OIE Collaborating Centers are the USDA/APHIS Center for Epidemiology and Animal Health in Fort Collins, Colorado, which advises on animal disease surveillance systems and risk analysis, and the Centre for Environment, Fisheries and Aquaculture Sciences in Weymouth, UK, which advises on aquatic animal diseases. The reference laboratories are recognized and selected for their expertise in the diagnosis of specific animal diseases. They maintain reference reagents for the disease in question and are involved in the development and standardization of improved diagnostic techniques. They also provide training for technical staff from member countries and are available for expert consultations. Examples of reference laboratories are the Institute for Animal Health at Pirbright, UK, for foot and mouth disease, the Onderstepoort Veterinary Institute in South Africa for African horse sickness, and the USDA National Veterinary Service Laboratory in Ames, Iowa, for equine infectious anemia. A full list of OIE collaborating centers and reference laboratories around the world is available on the OIE website. This website is an excellent resource and repository of information for any reader interested in international aspects of animal disease control.

costs of having transparency occasionally used as a weapon against U.S. exports.

Dispute Settlement The SPS Agreement addresses the matter of resolving conflicts when disputes arise between trading nations on matters related to the terms of the agreement, such as differences in interpretation of equivalency or the perception that technical requirements are being used as trade barriers. In disputes involving scientific or technical issues, the parties in conflict are first encouraged to work out their differences bilaterally and voluntarily. If no resolution is achieved, the parties to the dispute can bring the matter to the Committee on Sanitary and Phytosanitary Measures, which is the administrative body of the SPS Agreement. The committee can facilitate and encourage ad hoc negotiations between the disputing parties but has no legal or binding authority to issue a judgment on the matters in dispute. If the negotiations facilitated by the

committee fail to bring the disputing parties to a voluntary agreement, the aggrieved party can bring the dispute to the Dispute Settlement Body of the WTO. The Dispute Settlement Body will then select a panel from existing rosters of qualified officials in the area of international law or trade policy to consider the dispute.

When technical matters are involved, the panel will draw on the advice of experts chosen by the panel in consultation with the disputing parties to form an advisory technical experts group. These technical advisory groups may include representatives of the relevant international organizations overseeing technical aspects of trade such as the OIE or the Codex Alimentarius Commission. Based on testimony of the disputing parties and input from the expert advisory group, the panel will issue a ruling on the dispute that is then voted upon by the entire WTO membership. If a party is found to be in violation

Table 9-2   List A and List B Diseases as Designated by the Office International des Epizooties (OIE)

List A Diseases (15) [a]

Foot and mouth disease
Vesicular stomatitis
Swine vesicular disease
Rinderpest
Peste des petits ruminants
Contagious bovine pleuropneumonia
Lumpy skin disease
Rift Valley fever
Bluetongue
Sheep pox and goat pox
African horse sickness
African swine fever
Classical swine fever
Highly pathogenic avian influenza
Newcastle disease

List B Diseases [b]

Multiple species diseases
Anthrax
Aujeszky's disease (pseudorabies)
Echinococcosis/hydatidosis
Heartwater
Leptospirosis
Q Fever
Rabies
Paratuberculosis (Johne's disease)
New World screwworm (Cochliomyia
    hominivorax)
Old World screwworm (Chrysomya
    bezziana)
Trichinellosis

Cattle diseases
Bovine anaplasmosis
Bovine babesiosis
Bovine brucellosis
Bovine genital campylobacteriosis
Bovine tuberculosis
Bovine cysticercosis
Dermatophilosis
Enzootic bovine leukosis
Haemorrhagic septicemia
Infectious bovine rhinotracheitis
Infectious pustular vulvovaginitis
Theileriosis
Trichomonosis

Trypanosomosis (tsetse-transmitted)
Malignant catarrhal fever
Bovine spongiform encephalopathy

Sheep and goat diseases
Ovine epididymitis (Brucella ovis)
Caprine and ovine brucellosis
    (excluding B. ovis)
Caprine arthritis/encephalitis
Contagious agalactia
Contagious caprine pleuropneumonia
Enzootic abortion of ewes (ovine
    chlamydiosis)
Ovine pulmonary adenomatosis
Nairobi sheep disease
Salmonellosis (S. abortusovis)
Scrapie
Maedi-visna

Equine diseases
Contagious equine metritis
Dourine
Epizootic lymphangitis
Equine encephalomyelitis (Eastern and
    Western)
Equine infectious anaemia
Equine influenza
Equine piroplasmosis
Equine rhinopneumonitis
Glanders
Horse pox
Equine viral arteritis
Japanese encephalitis
Horse mange
Surra (Trypanosoma evansi)
Venezuelan equine encephalomyelitis

Swine diseases
Atrophic rhinitis of swine
Porcine cysticercosis
Porcine brucellosis
Transmissible gastroenteritis
Enterovirus encephalomyelitis
Porcine reproductive and respiratory
    syndrome

Avian diseases
Avian infectious bronchitis

Avian infectious laryngotracheitis
Avian tuberculosis
Duck virus hepatitis
Duck virus enteritis
Fowl cholera
Fowl pox
Fowl typhoid
Infectious bursal disease
    (Gumboro disease)
Marek's disease
Avian mycoplasmosis
    (M. gallisepticum)
Avian chlamydiosis
Pullorum disease

Lagomorph diseases
Myxomatosis
Tularemia
Rabbit haemorrhagic disease

Fish diseases
Viral haemorrhagic septicaemia
Spring viraemia of carp
Infectious haematopoietic necrosis
Epizootic haematopoietic necrosis
Oncorhynchus masou virus disease

Mollusc diseases
Bonamiosis
Haplosporidiosis
Perkinsosis
Marteiliosis
Mikrocytosis

Crustacean diseases
Taura syndrome
White spot disease
Yellowhead disease

Bee diseases
Acariosis of bees
American foulbrood
European foulbrood
Nosemosis of bees
Varroosis

Other List B diseases
Leishmaniosis

[a] List A diseases are defined by OIE as transmissible diseases that have the potential for very serious and rapid spread, irrespective of national borders, that are of serious socioeconomic or public health consequence, and that are of major importance in the international trade of animals and animal products.

[b] List B diseases are defined as transmissible diseases that are considered to be of socioeconomic and/or public health importance within countries and that are significant in the international trade of animals and animal products.

*Under the terms of the International Animal Health Code, OIE member countries are obliged to report occurrence of list A disease to OIE within 24 hours of occurrence, while the occurrence of list B diseases is generally reported on an annual basis.

of the SPS Agreement, that party has the option of correcting the inappropriate measure, of retaining the measure and compensating the other party, or otherwise being subject to sanctioned trade retaliation. The WTO dispute settlement system also includes a procedure for appeal. The dispute between the United States and the EU on the exclusion of growth hormone-treated American beef in European markets was largely played out through the SPS and WTO dispute settlement process and was evaluated and judged essentially on the basis of the relevant obligations contained in the SPS Agreement. Details of the growth hormone/beef dispute between the United States and the EU including technical aspects of interest to veterinarians have been described by Leighton.[19]

Developing Country Compliance Issues There is a paradoxical aspect to the SPS Agreement with regard to the trade prospects of developing countries. The principal objectives of the SPS Agreement are to ensure that first, high standards are maintained in matters related to animal and plant health and food safety in international trade and, second, that technical matters related to maintaining high standards of quality are not themselves used as inappropriate barriers to trade. To comply with the SPS Agreement, exporting nations need to possess a high level of technical capability and infrastructural capacity to achieve reliable disease control and ensure food safety. However, many developing countries and certainly the least-developed countries do not have the financial and human resources, infrastructure, or institutional capacity to eliminate endemic animal diseases or ensure disease-free status. Therefore, the very rules intended to prevent technical matters of disease control from becoming barriers to trade may themselves be the ultimate barrier to trade, effectively shutting out many poorer nations from international trading opportunities because they cannot maintain the technical capacity to control disease reliably. This is particularly burdensome for the many developing countries in which livestock represent a major domestic resource with the potential to earn foreign exchange and promote economic development through international trade.

To their credit, the framers of the SPS Agreement, during the Uruguay Round of GATT, recognized this paradox and included some provisions in the agreement to address the discrepancies between developed and developing nations in their capacity to abide by its terms. Article 9, for instance, calls upon member states to facilitate the provision of technical assistance concerning SPS to other members, especially developing-country members, either directly or through appropriate international standardizing organizations. Article 10 allows special and differential treatment of developing countries, calling for member states to take into consideration the special needs of developing countries by granting, for example, time-limited exceptions, or longer time-frames for compliance, to maintain opportunities for their exports. Finally, the SPS Agreement, in Article 14, allows least-developed member countries to delay implementation of the agreement for up to 5 years, while other developing countries may delay for up to 2 years, when they experience problems with their technical infrastructure, resources, or expertise.

U.S. Agencies and International Animal Trade

Government plays an active role in the promotion and regulation of trade. The United States Department of Agriculture (USDA) is the federal agency primarily involved in trade matters related to agricultural products. Within the USDA, the Foreign Agricultural Service (FAS) bears the primary responsibility for USDA's overseas activities. FAS actively participates in export market development. FAS also collects and analyzes statistics and market information, which are disseminated to the public in a variety of publications and databases (see the FAS website at www.fas.usda.gov/). In addition, the FAS administers USDA's export credit guarantee and food aid programs and helps strengthen agriculture and agribusiness in developing nations through development, training, and technical assistance programs. FAS deals with a broad range of agricultural commodities. Activities related to livestock trade issues and export opportunities are specifically addressed through the FAS Dairy, Livestock, and Poultry Division.

FAS also coordinates and directs USDA's involvement in international trade negotiations, working closely with the U.S. Trade Representative's office. Trade policy experts in FAS help identify and alleviate foreign trade barriers and other practices and policies that hinder U.S. agricultural exports. As the inquiry point for WTO SPS issues and technical barriers to trade, FAS serves as the official conduit for notifications and comments about these measures. When specialized technical input is required, FAS will draw on expertise from other sources. For example, with regard to matters pertaining to animal disease diagnosis and control measures and regulatory policies relative to trade in livestock and livestock products, FAS will call upon veterinary expertise within various branches of USDA's APHIS to advise on technical details and participate in negotiated resolutions.

APHIS is the principal veterinary regulatory agency of the federal government, charged with the overall mission of protecting the nation from the introduction and spread of animal diseases and zoonoses from any source, including, but not limited to, international trade. The overall structure and activities of APHIS are discussed in more detail in Chapter 8 and a descriptive organizational chart is shown in Table 8-2. Within APHIS, several branches and units address matters specifically related to international trade in livestock and livestock products. The main branches are International Services and Veterinary Services

International Services (IS) is the overseas arm of APHIS, with over 300 employees stationed at over 27 locations on six continents. IS carries out a variety of functions, including the following:

- Bilateral cooperation with host countries on surveillance and control of plant and animal diseases and pests that pose a risk to U.S. agriculture. Examples of animal-related activities include screwworm eradication in Mexico and Central America, tropical bont tick control in the Caribbean Islands, and FMD eradication in Colombia.

- Support of U.S. export opportunities through consultation with foreign agricultural officials to clarify technical issues that might otherwise unnecessarily impede trade, for example, extended quarantines imposed on imported livestock for diseases not present in the United States. Related activities include certification of sanitary requirements through local negotiation and resolution of trade retention problems when U.S. export shipments are delayed at ports or terminals on procedural grounds.

- Collection and exchange of information on disease occurrence, survey techniques, and control methods in foreign countries to reduce the risk of disease introduction to the United States.

- Representation of the U.S. government on technical matters relative to plant and animal disease issues in dealings with a variety of organizations including the WTO, OIE, FAO; World Health Organization (WHO); Codex Alimentarius Commission, and IPPC

An important unit within the APHIS IS is the Trade Support Team, which provides analytical and strategic guidance to help APHIS in its efforts to facilitate agricultural trade while maintaining the nation's biosecurity. The Trade Support Team is the central APHIS office for tracking pending trade issues and initiatives. The team also serves as liaison with other U.S. government agencies on matters of biosecurity as those agencies develop and implement broader trade policies, ensuring that matters related to disease control are not neglected during the course of exceedingly complex negotiations on trade agreements.

The Veterinary Services (VS) branch of APHIS is directly responsible for efforts to prevent the incursion of animal diseases into the United States. VS protects the health of livestock and poultry resources by regulating the entry of imported animals, animal products, and biologicals. With regard to importation of livestock, APHIS maintains four animal quarantine stations in the United States: at Newburgh, New York; Miami, Florida; Los Angeles, California; and Honolulu, Hawaii. VS also coordinates emergency actions against foreign disease and, with the states, operates eradication programs for domestic animal and zoonotic diseases.

Another important aspect of preventing the introduction of foreign animal disease is interdiction of travelers at ports of entry around the United States. Foreign visitors and returning travelers may carry plant or animal products that harbor insect pests or infectious agents that, if introduced into the United States, can lead to the establishment of foreign animal disease. Plant Protection and Quarantine (PPQ) is the branch of APHIS responsible for screening passengers at more than 90 ports of entry into the country. PPQ agents work closely with

U.S. Customs agents at airline and passenger ship terminals. The uniformed agents walking the baggage claim areas at these facilities with beagle dogs are PPQ inspectors. The beagle dogs are trained to detect food items in luggage. APHIS also uses other larger breeds of dogs at distribution centers for international mail arrivals to check packages for meat and other agricultural products with the potential for introduction of pests or disease. PPQ is also responsible for screening incoming, commercially traded goods at ports of entry by land, sea, or air to detect animal and plant pests and pathogens.

The National Center for Import and Export (NCIE), a unit of VS, provides information, forms, guidance, and regulatory activity relative to the importation and exportation of animals and animal products. For instance, NCIE is involved in the process of regionalization as discussed above in the section on the SPS agreement. To have a region declared disease free for the purpose of exporting animals or animal products to the United States, a country must submit formal documentation to the NCIE establishing that the proposed region is free and can be kept free of disease. The criteria that NCIE considers for approval of a regionalization request are presented in Table 9-3.

Veterinary practitioners may find themselves in direct contact with the NCIE when they have clients wishing to export livestock to foreign countries. Local practitioners may be called upon by clients to give advice or may be involved as USDA-accredited veterinarians in the testing and examination of livestock intended for export, to complete appropriate and necessary export certificates relative to animal health. The NCIE maintains a list of import requirements of foreign countries for different species of livestock. This information is available on the internet at www.aphis.usda.gov/export/vsindex.html.

The Food Safety and Inspection Service (FSIS) of the USDA is the agency primarily responsible for the wholesomeness and quality of the nation's meat, poultry, and egg supply. The quality of these livestock products is ensured largely through inspection activities carried out at licensed processing plants nationwide. These inspections are carried out directly or under the supervision of veterinary medical officers employed by the agency. However, FSIS also has an active role in international trade in livestock products. Its international policy division ensures the safety and quality of imported meat, poultry, and egg products by working with foreign governments to establish equivalency in their food inspection and safety procedures.

Many industry, trade, and professional groups related to animal agriculture are actively involved in international trade issues, providing trade-related information to their constituents and making their collective voices heard in Washington on matters of trade policy that affect their respective industries. Groups such as the National Beef Cattlemen's Association, the National Pork Producers Council, the United States Meat Export Federation, and the United States Animal Health Association have developed policy positions relative to key international trade issues such as the entry of China into the WTO or have done market research to identify new or expanded export opportunities for American producers. However, not all sectors of agri-

Table 9-3   Factors Considered by the National Center for Import and Export in Evaluating Requests to Export Animals or Animal Products to the United States from Distinct or Definable Regions[a]

- The authority, organization, and infrastructure of the veterinary services organization in the region

- The type and extent of disease surveillance in the region-e.g., is it passive and/or active? what is the quantity and quality of sampling and testing?

- Diagnostic laboratory capabilities

- Disease status: Is the disease agent known to exist in the region? If "yes," at what prevalence? If "no," when was the most recent diagnosis?

- The extent of an active disease control program, if any, if the agent is known to exist in the region

- The vaccination status of the region. When was the last vaccination? What is the extent of the vaccination if it is currently used, and what vaccine is being used?

- Disease status of adjacent regions

- The degree to which the region is separated from regions of higher risk through physical or other barriers

- The extent to which movement of animals and animal products is controlled from regions of higher risk, and the level of biosecurity regarding such movements

- Livestock demographics and marketing practices within the region

- Policies and infrastructure for animal disease control in the region-i.e., emergency response capacity

[a] The National Center for Import and Export of the USDA Animal Plant and Health Inspection Services (APHIS) is responsible for reviewing documentation from foreign applicants wishing to have imports approved from selected regions of their territories on the basis of pest- and/or disease-free status as permitted under the SPS Agreement of the World Trade Organization. The list identifies the various factors that the NCIE considers in determining whether the applicant has indeed documented the pest- or disease-free status of the region and the ability to maintain such status in the region.

From website of the National Center for Import and Export, http://www.aphis.usda.gov/vs/reg-request.html.

culture are equally enthusiastic about free trade in agricultural products. Those sectors with less opportunity for export or those facing increasing competition at home (e.g., the sheep industry) may take a very different view from government and industry groups actively promoting free trade.

The American Veterinary Association is increasingly recognizing the importance of international trade and international disease control matters for its constituent veterinary members. In 1998, the American Veterinary Medical Association (AVMA) Executive Board took action to have the AVMA represented within the U.S. delegation to the OIE, and in May 1999, the AVMA president-elect was invited by the USDA to join the eight-member U.S. delegation to the 67th annual meeting of the International Commission of the OIE. The delegation also included representatives of APHIS and the U.S. Animal Health Association.

Current Challenges in Animal Disease Control

Dunlop and Williams provide interesting background on the history of animal epizootics and early scientific efforts at animal disease control.[5] They cite Virgil's observations in the 1st century BC of devastating cattle plagues around Rome so severe

that "the peasants themselves had to take the place of draft oxen and . . . tug the creaking wagons over a towering hillside." While animal disease has been noted and feared through the millennia, there was very little scientific understanding of animal epizootics or approaches to controlling them until the 15th century, when the Paduan physician Hieronymus Fracastorius took a keen interest in a cattle plague occurring in northern Italy. Though it is not clear if the disease was rinderpest or FMD, Fracastorius, through careful observation and long before the germ theory of disease was established, recognized and reported that the disease appeared to arise from some "infectious matter" that was spread from sick to healthy animals either by direct contact between animals, by contact with contaminated materials, or via exhaled air.

At the beginning of the 18th century, Bernadino Ramazzini, a medical professor in Padua, developed a systematic approach to epizootic disease investigations, using pathological evidence from postmortem examinations to dispel common astrological explanations of disease occurrence. He demonstrated that the rinderpest panzootic that was sweeping through Europe in the early 1700s had been introduced into Europe and spread from sick to healthy animals. He even made some efforts at protecting cattle through vaccination, drawing a thread soaked in material from affected cattle through and under the skin of healthy animals. A second physician, Giovanni Lancisi, collaborating with Ramazzini, supported the notion of contagion as an underlying factor in the spread of the rinderpest outbreak and proposed several radical notions to control the disease, which today represent the fundamental principals of epizootic disease control, namely, restricted movement of animals from the sites of disease outbreaks, burial of affected animals, and inspection and approval of meat from healthy animals. By following these recommendations, the rinderpest outbreak around Rome was controlled within 9 months, whereas it persisted elsewhere in Italy and Europe for years where these measures were not adopted.

The insights of the Italians were not quickly or universally accepted. Another panzootic of rinderpest swept through Europe from Russia in the 1850s and arrived in England in 1865. British veterinary authorities who proposed a policy of slaughter for affected animals and restriction of trade were severely criticized by many medical professionals and church and political leaders, who resisted the notion of contagion and still held firm to the miasma theory of disease causation. This resistance ultimately faded with the emergence of microbiology in the second half of the 19th century. The germ theory of disease and the bold experiments of Pasteur finally provided the scientific basis for understanding contagious animal disease and set the groundwork for modern epizootic disease control involving careful clinical examination, laboratory diagnosis of infectious agents, identification of vectors, vaccination, and the various controls on movement of animals and animal products that Lancisi had reasoned out so brilliantly over a century earlier.

Such advances have clearly improved the capacity of the veterinary community to recognize and control epizootic disease outbreaks. In the United States alone, for example, numerous important epizootic diseases were eradicated in the late 19th and 20th centuries, including contagious bovine pleuropneumonia, FMD, glanders, dourine, and hog cholera. Nevertheless, at the beginning of the 21st century, a number of trends have been identified that challenge the capacity of veterinary authorities to continue to effectively prevent or control epizootic diseases with the same success that they have enjoyed in the past. For disease control efforts to remain effective into the future, the impact of these newly emerging risk factors must be recognized, analyzed, and addressed. In the following discussion the emerging risk factors challenging animal disease control are discussed. They include increased international trade, increased international travel, downsizing of government, modern agricultural practices, wildlife-livestock interactions, civil instability, emerging diseases, and developing-country issues.

Increased Trade in Animals and Animal Products

As the global economy grows and consumer demand for animal protein in the diet expands, the volume of animals and animal products entering international trade continues to increase. Table 9-4 shows the growth of export trade in selected live animals and animal products over the last 3 decades of the 20th century. During that period, the increase in export of live pigs was over fourfold, and in live chickens, over fivefold. For animal products the increase in export of chicken meat was over 15-fold, and for fresh milk, over 17-fold. This increase in trade and the emergence of new trading partners present great challenges for regulatory authorities responsible for disease control. Trading agreements must be established that take into account international SPS standards. The animal disease situation and disease control capacity of exporting countries must be deemed acceptable. Equivalency of acceptable standards must be established for disease diagnosis and control in live animals and for processing and sanitary procedures in food products. Health certificates need to be issued and examined, and in the case of live animals, quarantines may need to be observed. National governments vary enormously in their capacity to address these issues, with tremendous differences in human resources, training, investigative capacity, technical expertise, and infrastructure. Even the best-prepared may be daunted by the challenge of maintaining effective oversight when budgetary and staffing increases fall short of expanded workload.

To complicate matters, the movement of livestock and livestock products around the world is not limited to legal trade. Illegal movement is a growing concern. As mentioned earlier, the reintroduction of FMD into Argentina in 2000 was most likely associated with smuggled cattle brought from neighboring Paraguay. Epidemiological investigations suggest that the FMD outbreak in the UK in 2001 resulted from illegally imported and uninspected meat brought in from Asia for the ethnic restaurant trade. It is believed that scraps of this infected meat found their way into UK pig swill feeding operations.

Nor is the international trade in animals limited to livestock. As discussed in more detail in Chapter 7, millions of fish, birds, reptiles, amphibians, and mammals enter legal trading channels every year for the pet trade, for use in research, for education, and for other purposes. Countless others are traded illegally. While legal trade in wildlife is regulated in the United States by the U.S. Fish and Wildlife Service (USFWS), controlling the introduction or spread of disease from wild animals offers special challenges, if for no other reason than that our collective knowledge of the range and behavior of diseases that affect wild animal species and the disease vectors they may carry is much more limited than our knowledge about disease and disease transmission in domestic animals. The potential spillover of livestock disease from the pet trade was illustrated in March 2000 when APHIS announced the ban on importation of certain species of land tortoises that harbor exotic ticks known to be vectors of heartwater disease, an acute, infectious disease of ruminants, including cattle, sheep, goats, white-tailed deer (*Odocoileus virginianus*), and antelope (*Antilocapra americana*).

The fact that people are traveling more frequently with their pets is another challenge for disease control authorities. Dogs and cats can not only be a source of disease for other pets, but may also serve as mechanical or biological vectors for livestock and zoonotic diseases. Take for example the case of screwworms. New World screwworms (*Cochliomyia hominivorax*), a

Table 9-4a.   Worldwide Trends in Export of Livestock 1969-1999[a]

Live Animals Exported (head)	1969	1979	1989	1999
Pigs	3,971,789	8,223,820	13,306,178	16,060,186
Chickens	132,866,000	320,613,000	361,161,000	698,907,000
Cattle	6,354,417	7,374,375	7,260,964	9,464,263
Sheep	8,167,416	13,324,703	20,622,061	17,923,607
Goat	1,592,406	1,761,503	1,955,092	2,853,179

b.   Worldwide Trends in Export of Livestock Products 1969-1999[a]

Commodities Exported (Metric tons)	1969	1979	1989	1999
Beef and veal	1,405,422	1,826,577	2,164,713	1,416,269
Chicken meat	406,352	1,093,503	1,962,862	6,301,334
Pig meat	1,538,169	2,415,993	3,975,976	6,980,341
Eggs in the shell	356,827	655,916	811,440	967,450
Fresh milk	390,531	2,118,021	3,621,594	6,640,982

[a]These numbers are for all country exports combined. Information for live animals is total head per year. Information for animal products is metric tons per year.

Data obtained from the FAOSTAT agricultural database of the Food and Agriculture Organization of the United Nations (FAO) (http://apps.fao.org/).

scourge of the cattle industry and a potential zoonosis, were eradicated from the United States in 1982, and APHIS remains active in keeping the disease out of the country, prohibiting the importation of livestock infested with screwworm larvae. Nevertheless, in 1997 a Basset hound entering the United States from Panama cleared customs in Miami to continue onward to its home in Texas. The owners noticed it limping soon after arrival and took it to the local veterinarian's office. Fortunately, that veterinarian was astute and thorough. She located a wound on the paw, identified screwworm larvae in the wound, and promptly notified APHIS personnel in the area so that the risk of disease spread was effectively contained. More recently, in response to the outbreak of FMD in Europe, APHIS felt compelled to issue specific recommendations for the decontamination of pets returning from Europe (see www.aphis.usda.gov/oa/fmd/fmdpets.html).

International equestrian events are also a concern for disease control officials. The 2000 Olympics were especially problematic for animal health officials in Australia, which has some of the tightest controls on animal importation in the world. Every horse going to Sydney for the Olympics had to spend a fortnight at a prequarantine stable before traveling to Australia and also had to possess a lengthy certificate detailing its whereabouts for the 46 days preceding that prequarantine stabling.

Horses were only allowed to be shipped to Australia from Europe, North America, Japan, and New Zealand, so horses from other countries first had to be transferred and kept in one of these approved places for an additional 46 days before the prequarantine. Once arriving in Australia, all imported horses were subject to an additional 14-day quarantine. Despite the regulatory challenges, 266 horses from 35 countries were flown into Sydney to compete.

Increased International Travel

Whether traveling with pets or not, the world's citizens are increasingly mobile. According to information available through the World Tourism Organization, world tourism grew by an estimated 7.4% in 2000, spurred by prosperity and special interest in millennial observances. This was the highest growth rate in nearly a decade, with the total number of international arrivals in the year 2000 reaching a record 698 million. All regions of the world hosted an increased number of tourists in 2000, with the fastest developing areas being East Asia and the Pacific. International arrivals to the United States were up by 8.7% because of continuing growth from major overseas markets, especially Japan and the UK, leading to a total of 52,690,000 passengers arriving in 2000. An approximately equal number of Americans traveled to overseas destinations and returned home to the United States, the vast majority by airplane.

The volume of air travel and the speed with which travelers can be transported around the globe are serious concerns relative to disease control, not only for animals, but also for plants and humans. The duration of many international trips is shorter than the incubation periods of many infectious diseases. With approximately 1.5 million air passengers crossing international borders every day, the capacity for responsible officials to identify passengers at risk of introducing disease is severely stretched. Of course, not every flight or passenger is a potential source of any or every disease, but the risks are significant enough that they deserve some consideration here.

Bridges and Cummings of the USDA/APHIS Centers for Epidemiology and Animal Health have evaluated the potential for international travelers to transmit foreign animal diseases to U.S. livestock and poultry.[1] They point out that depending on the disease in question, travelers may present no risk of disease spread or may serve as either biological vectors, mechanical vectors, or both. The risk of transmission for a particular disease depends on a number of intrinsic factors including the level of contagion of the infectious agent, its survival time outside its natural host(s), influences of temperature and humidity, and its ability to be transmitted by mechanical means. Extrinsic factors include the occurrence of a particular disease where the traveler has traveled and the likelihood that the returning traveler would have contact with susceptible mammalian or avian hosts. With those extrinsic factors in mind, it is clear that veterinarians, agricultural consultants, farmers, ranchers, and others likely to have livestock contact pose a greater risk than the typical urban or suburban traveler with regard to the spread of animal disease. The relative risks of transmission of OIE list A diseases by travelers returning to the United States by either biological or mechanical means is presented in Table 9-5.

Note that the risk of biological transmission of FMD by travelers is ranked negligible, but the risk of mechanical transmission of FMD is ranked moderate. This is because the amount of FMD virus on shoes or clothes may be an infective dose, particularly if travelers have had direct contact with infected animals within 5 or so days of returning to the United States. Thus, passengers themselves represent a potential threat for transmission of FMD in addition to any potentially contaminated food or farm products that they may carry with them. The importance of this potential route of transmission became most evident in February 2001 when FMD broke out in the United Kingdom. APHIS inspectors in the Plant Protection and Quarantine division who work at international arrivals terminals in the nation's airports were under heightened alert and hard pressed to screen the myriad passengers returning from the UK and Europe.

The scope of the challenge facing APHIS inspectors is reflected in the statistics available from the agency for fiscal year 1999, when 16.4 million passengers arrived in the United States on

Table 9-5 Relative Risks of Transmission of List A Diseases of the OIE by Travelers Returning to the United States

Risk of Biological Transmission of List A Diseases by International Travelers

Risk Rating	Disease
High	None
Moderate	None
Low	Avian influenza Newcastle disease
Negligible	Rift Valley fever Food and mouth disease Swine vesicular disease Vesicular stomatitis
None	Classical swine fever (hog cholera) African horse sickness African swine fever Bluetongue Contagious bovine pleuropneumonia Lumpy skin disease Peste des petits ruminants Rinderpest Sheep and goat pox

Risk of Mechanical Transmission of List A Diseases by International Travelers

Risk Rating	Disease
High	Newcastle disease Swine vesicular stomatitis
Moderate	Avian influenza Foot and mouth disease African swine fever
Low	Vesicular stomatitis
Negligible	Rift Valley fever Classical swine fever Lumpy skin disease Peste des petits ruminants Rinderpest Sheep and goat pox
None	African horse sickness Bluetongue Contagious bovine pleuropneumonia

Data derived from Bridges V, Cummings D. The potential for international travelers to transmit foreign animal diseases to U.S. livestock and poultry. Fort Collins, CO: USDA:APHIS:VS, 1998. (Available on the internet at www.aphis.usda.gov/vs/ceah/cei/health.htm#travelers)

direct flights from the UK. A total of 20,515 passengers from the UK were sampled as part of the APHIS monitoring program, representing about 0.125% of the total passenger volume. Of these inspected passengers from the UK, 462, or 2.3%, were carrying a total of 919 kg of potentially hazardous items such as meat products, cheese, or hides. Some 22 of the sampled passengers who were carrying potentially hazardous items revealed an intention to visit or work on a farm or ranch while in the United States. Destinations reported by these passengers included Maryland (6), Georgia (4), New York (4), Virginia (4), California (2), and Texas (2). These data of course beg the question of how many passengers representing a potential disease transmission hazard were not identified by APHIS inspectors.

Downsizing of Government

Privatization of public institutions, deregulation of industries, and downsizing of government are important trends that emerged in the 1970s and continue to shape public policy today. While these approaches to governance have had some positive effects, their impact on animal disease control is a cause for concern. At the same time that international trade in livestock and livestock products has increased and global travel has expanded, resources available for disease surveillance, monitoring, regulation, and interdiction often have decreased in either relative or absolute terms. This is occurring not just in the United States but in many countries around the world.

In the United States, the control of animal disease is a joint state and federal process. Regulatory veterinarians at the state level cooperate with APHIS veterinarians on the eradication of existing diseases such as tuberculosis and brucellosis as well as on the prevention and elimination of foreign animal diseases that may enter the country. The National Association of State Departments of Agriculture (NASDA), which generally include the state agencies involved in animal disease control, issued a policy statement in September 2000 expressing serious concern that funding cuts and other resource constraints might hamper the ability of the federal animal disease control agency, APHIS, to finalize several important disease control programs that are near successful completion, notably cattle and swine brucellosis eradication, bovine tuberculosis control, and swine pseudorabies control. Furthermore, they noted that government infrastructure for emergency disease preparedness in the event of a foreign animal disease outbreak has decreased significantly at both the state and national levels. NASDA expressed serious concern that the capacity for the United States to control and eradicate foreign disease may be compromised. In particular, the organization cited the need for increased funding to upgrade the facilities and diagnostic capacities of the National Animal Disease Laboratory in Ames, Iowa, and the Plum Island Animal Disease Center in Greenport, New York. The Iowa laboratory is the principal national diagnostic laboratory for diseases already present in the United States, while the New York laboratory is the principal diagnostic laboratory for foreign animal diseases.

In the era of downsizing, government agencies and services of all kinds are susceptible to cutbacks, so a funding shortage in itself does not constitute a basis for special pleading. Advocates for a strengthened effort in animal disease control recognize this and have responded by developing convincing economic arguments that can be used by politicians and policymakers to secure funding for animal disease control efforts. A whole area of specialization in veterinary epidemiology and economics has emerged to address the cost-benefit analysis of various interventions and approaches to animal disease control at the local, national, and international levels. Such analyses not only provide ammunition to defend the importance of supporting animal disease control programs, but also can identify more-efficient, less-costly approaches to disease control, thus improving disease control efforts without necessarily increasing budgets. A special 1999 issue of the OIE's *Scientific and Technical Review*, entitled *The Economics of Animal Disease Control*, offers a diverse selection of papers on this subject, including case studies from around the world and is an excellent source of additional information for the interested reader.[23]

Cost sharing is another innovation that is gaining acceptance in the face of downsizing. Keeping foreign animal disease outside a country's borders has traditionally been seen as a public good (i.e., a service provided to society in general because it benefits everyone in society equally). However, in the context of international trade and export opportunity, it is becoming clearer that certain segments of society may benefit specifically from protection against certain diseases. For example, keeping a zoonotic disease out of the country protects the general public and is thus a public good. Keeping a swine-specific disease out of the country whose presence might shut off export markets to swine producers clearly provides targeted benefits to the swine industry. In recognition of the principle that beneficiaries should pay for benefits according to their proportional advantage, Australia has embarked on government/industry partnerships to finance emergency disease control responses. Through Animal Health Australia, a government/industry association not unlike the U.S. Animal Health Association, Australia is working on detailed cost-sharing agreements for national and state governments and various livestock industry groups to control a comprehensive list of economically important animal diseases. Details on this plan and its progress are available on the internet at www.aahc.com.au/eadp/funding.htm.

The Creation of Populations at Risk

The very capacity to control disease effectively may put developed countries at risk of serious consequences should a lapse in disease control occur and a highly contagious disease enter the country. FMD offers a good example. In much of Asia and Africa, FMD is endemic, and in some countries, little effort is made to control it. Since much livestock raising in these countries is at the subsistence level and since so many other constraints on livestock production exist, the economic impact of FMD in these countries is, relatively speaking, minimal. In addition, as discussed in Chapter 8 and later in this section, many developing countries lack the veterinary infrastructure and resources necessary to control highly contagious diseases such as FMD, even if they have the will to do so. So, FMD remains endemic.

At the other end of the spectrum however, are countries of Europe and North America with highly developed, intensively managed livestock production systems and equally well developed veterinary service capacity. Livestock operations in these countries are run as commercial enterprises, with much attention paid to overhead costs and profit margins. There is essentially zero tolerance for a debilitating condition such as FMD, which, though not a highly fatal disease, would be devastating in its capacity to depress productivity in affected enterprises such as cow dairy operations. The presence of FMD would also interfere with export sales of livestock and livestock products, which have become an important source of income for animal agriculture and the food-processing industries in developed countries. Countries free of FMD will not accept animals or potentially contaminated animal products from countries with FMD. Complicating this situation is the fact that trade restrictions also exist for animals with evidence of antibody to FMD virus. Until now, no reliable way existed to distinguish between antibody due to natural infection and antibody due to vaccination. Therefore, countries that want to maximize their export marketing opportunities do not vaccinate for FMD. As a result, the entire national herd of cloven-hoofed animals is at risk of infection if FMD enters the country. Such nations depend on the capacity of their regulatory services to keep such exotic diseases out of the country. However, under such circumstance, if FMD actually does get into an FMD-free country that does not carry out vaccination, the results can be catastrophic in naive herds, as the FMD outbreak in the UK in 2001 clearly demonstrated (see sidebar "Foot and Mouth Disease in the United Kingdom, 2001").

Intensive animal agriculture offers distinct advantages for producers in terms of economies of scale, improved management of production variables, and greater quality control. However, housing large numbers of animals in close proximity also clearly contributes to the risk of rapid dissemination of highly contagious disease, particularly those such as FMD, easily spread by aerosol transmission. This is not to say that confinement of animals is intrinsically unhealthy. In fact, a major impetus for the confinement of grazing stock was to reduce problems associated with parasitism, a major constraint in extensive grazing systems. Many intensive commercial livestock operations, particularly swine and poultry production systems, practice a high degree of biosecurity and preventive medicine involving restricted access, shower in-shower out policies of hygiene, sophisticated ventilation systems to control the airborne distribution of fomites and pathogens, and all in-all out management of stock through the production cycle. They also implement comprehensive herd or flock health programs, including extensive vaccinations and regular diagnostic testing. The degree of care is reflected in the fact that many such enterprises are specific-pathogen free.

Nevertheless, should a highly contagious infection like FMD in swine, rinderpest in cattle, or avian influenza in birds gain entry to such an operation, it would move through animals and birds in close contact with grim efficiency. With feedlots maintaining cattle populations in the tens of thousands and poultry units containing birds in the hundreds of thousands, the economic impact of foreign animal disease outbreaks can be enormous. An outbreak of highly pathogenic avian influenza centered in Pennsylvania from November 1983 to April 1984 resulted in over US$225 million in losses to the egg, broiler, turkey, and chicken industries. Over 17 million birds were destroyed in efforts to control the outbreak, and the retail price of eggs increased by more than 30%.

Wildlife-Livestock Interactions

Concerns about transmission of diseases between wildlife and livestock are not new. In Africa, for example, in association with European settlement and the expansion of commercial animal agriculture, considerable and often draconian measures were taken to minimize the risk of diseases being transmitted from wildlife to cattle. Wild ungulates, for instance, were recognized as reservoirs for trypanosomiasis, and extensive areas were cleared of wild species to make the areas safe for cattle grazing. Plowright chronicles the early history of rinderpest control in Africa and emphasizes the importance that veterinary authorities placed on the elimination of ungulate species known to be susceptible to rinderpest, to control rinderpest in cattle.[24] The elimination of game and establishment of wildlife-free buffer zones were frequently used tools to protect livestock from this virulent cattle plague. Today, a greater body of research and improved epidemiological data suggest that wildlife, though susceptible to rinderpest, are not an important reservoir for the disease when extensive vaccination of cattle is practiced. Once the disease is eliminated from cattle, it dies out naturally in wildlife.

Problems associated with disease interactions are not restricted to Africa or to the past. In fact, some major wildlife-livestock disease interactions have emerged as serious, ongoing challenges for veterinary scientists and regulatory authorities in the United State in recent years. Problems that have received the most attention and concern include the occurrence of bovine brucellosis in bison in Yellowstone Park in Wyoming and their perceived potential to transmit it to proximate cattle, and the occurrence of bovine tuberculosis in Michigan and its reintroduction into cattle herds in the state. These new developments threaten the longstanding, largely successful efforts by federal and state authorities to eliminate these two important diseases of cattle. In addition, chronic wasting disease (CWD), a transmissible spongiform encephalopathy in farmed and wild elk and deer in the western United States has emerged as a serious disease-control challenge, raising concerns, as yet unproven, that the disease may represent a risk of infection of susceptible ruminants and possibly humans. Nor are such problems limited to the United States. A resurgence of tuberculosis in Cape buffalo (*Syncerus caffer*) in South Africa, for example, threatens the cattle industry there. Regulatory officials in New Zealand are confronted with bovine tuberculosis in brushtail possum (*Trichosurus vulpecula*), while British and Irish authorities are seeking ways to deal with a reservoir of bovine tuberculosis in badgers (*Meles meles*).

These problems reflect trends and developments concerning wildlife-livestock interactions that are affecting the disease dynamic in many places around the world. Such trends and developments include:

- Greater contact between wildlife and livestock as wildlife habitat diminishes and human settlement encroaches on remaining habitat

- An evolving conservation ethic that does not readily accept the elimination of wildlife to protect livestock interests, particularly when threatened or endangered wildlife species are involved

- Increased density of some wildlife populations tied to human activity and possibly climate changes that favor survival of larger populations

- Expanded use of wild species in commercial enterprises, such as deer and elk farming

There is a real need and opportunity for veterinary scientists to play an expanded role in elucidating the behavior of diseases that affect both wildlife and domestic animals. As the bison brucellosis controversy in Yellowstone National Park revealed, some very basic information about the natural history of brucellosis in wild species was lacking. No one could say with any certainty just how much of a risk infected bison wandering out of the park boundaries actually posed to grazing cattle. Yet control efforts involved killing buffalo that left the park. For such interventions to be acceptable to the public, they must be based on sound science. In the case of the transmissible spongiform encephalopathies, substantial research efforts are still required to characterize the natural history of the diseases in various wild and domestic species, to develop improved diagnostic capability, and, possibly, to develop preventive measures. Some preliminary studies by Hamir et al suggest that CWD is transmissible from mule deer to cattle.[12] Detailed epidemiological studies are necessary in many cases to identify important risk factors associated with disease spread. In Michigan, for instance, investigations revealed that deer feeding or baiting with supplemental feed by hunting clubs drew deer to common feeding areas that became contaminated with the causative agent, increasing the risk that tuberculosis would spread among the deer population. The practice has been subsequently banned.

Regional War and Civil Disturbance

International disease-control efforts can be seriously compromised or even reversed by war and civil disturbances, either political or natural. The effect of civil war on veterinary service delivery and the control of animal disease in Zim-babwe are discussed in some detail in Chapter 8. Africa in general has been the site of numerous armed conflicts in recent decades, and these have been associated with the spread of disease. Contagious bovine pleuropneumonia has extended its range in eastern and central Africa in recent years, often in association with civil unrest and movement of livestock and refugees, notably in Uganda, Rwanda, the Congo, and Tanzania.

As discussed in Chapter 8, a concerted effort to eliminate rinderpest from the African continent has been under way since 1986, first through the Pan African Rinderpest Campaign (PARC) and more recently through the Pan African Programme for the Control of Epizootics (PACE). Despite these largely successful efforts, a few foci of rinderpest resisted eradication. Not surprisingly, the areas where rinderpest has persisted the longest are places where political instability, local insurrections, or outright civil war have occurred. Through the 1990s, these pockets included southern Sudan, northern Uganda, Somalia, and Ethiopia. By the year 2000, with some regional conflicts resolved, the disease remained only where conflict persisted, namely Somalia and southern Sudan. Technical advances such as heat-stable rinderpest vaccine and novel approaches to vaccination such as the use of community-based animal health workers in remote areas have made the possibility of rinderpest eradication real. The major constraint remains the absence of the rule of law in certain remote areas plagued by conflict. Similarly, coordinated international efforts to control rinderpest in south Asia may be constrained by the persistent political instability of war-torn Afghanistan, which continues to serve as a reservoir of the disease, with sporadic epizootics having occurred in recent years. The movement of U.S. military personnel and equipment into the region in 2001 following the terrorist attack of September 11 increases the risk that rinderpest or other exotic animal diseases could be introduced into the United States unless strict sanitary measures are observed when equipment and personnel are returned to the United States.

Closer to home, developments in Latin America may also have implications for disease control in the United States. APHIS has worked closely and cooperatively with Mexico, with various countries in Central America, and with Colombia to keep the geographical corridor between South and North America free of FMD. The current civil instability in Colombia, with armed insurgents expanding their activity in the Colombian countryside does not bode well for maintenance of rigorous animal disease surveillance activities and reliable control of livestock movements. As FMD remains active in other Latin American countries south of Colombia, increased vigilance is required to ensure that the political situation in Colombia does not increase the risk of FMD to the north.

On a more positive note, there is evidence that progress can be made in the midst of conflict. In the Middle East, where long-standing enmity between nations continues to undermine normal diplomatic relations and economic ties, the European Commission and the United States Agency for International

Foot and Mouth Disease in the United Kingdom in 2001

After a 34-year hiatus, FMD returned to the United Kingdom with a vengeance. On Monday, February 19, 2001, a veterinary inspector at an abattoir in Brentwood, Essex, suspected FMD in pigs being held for slaughter. The virus was identified the next day as subtype O PanAsiatic, a highly virulent strain of the FMD virus. By Friday, February 23, there were six confirmed cases: four more in Essex, near the Brentwood abattoir, and two in Northumberland, some 400 km away. Thus, it became apparent that the first confirmed case at the Brentwood abattoir did not in fact represent the primary outbreak and that considerable movement of infected animals had already occurred prior to the original diagnosis. An examination of records indicated that there had been over 2 million sheep movements alone in the 3 weeks leading up to February 23. This was especially troubling, as FMD in sheep does not usually manifest severe clinical signs, and it was very likely that infected sheep had been moving around the country undetected. Therefore, on February 23, the Minister for Agriculture introduced a total ban on animal movements nationally, and the government began to mobilize for what was to be a long, difficult, and costly eradication campaign.

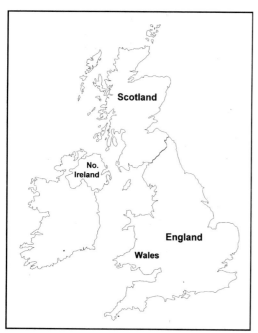

The eradication campaign was carried out on a massive scale, using the basic disease control tools of case identification, traceback, quarantine, movement control, and destruction and disposal of infected and exposed animals. From February 10 through the end of March, the number of newly identified cases grew daily, reaching a peak of 50 per day and remaining at this high level through April. The number of animals destroyed reached into the millions, and delays were encountered in disposing of dead animals. The military had to be called in to provide additional manpower and equipment for carcass disposal and for the cleaning and disinfection of infected premises. By May 2, over 2000 military personnel were directly involved, and an additional 1417 veterinarians had been mobilized to help, including veterinarians from the United States, Australia, Canada, New Zealand, Sweden, and other countries.

The logistical challenges were so complex that Prime Minister Tony Blair was prompted to observe that the scale of combating FMD disease exceeded the logistical demands even of the Gulf War. The world's television screens were filled with macabre images of bovine funeral pyres and limp carcasses dangling from the teeth of backhoe buckets. Grim-faced stockmen who worked the farms of their forefathers for generations past were suddenly deprived of their livelihood and faced an uncertain future. The National Farmers Union in the UK estimated that farmers were losing $360 million a month during the FMD outbreak. With the FMD outbreak following so closely on the heels of the BSE crisis in the UK, many analysts expressed open concern about whether animal agriculture in the nation could survive these dual catastrophes. In addition, with much of the countryside off-limits because of quarantines, the attractive image of a bucolic, rural England, so compelling to countless tourists and so lucrative for the tourist industry, was badly tarnished, a perception confirmed by a sharp drop in tourism revenues.

About May 1, the daily number of new cases fell below 10 per day and remained at that lower daily rate through most of September. The last FMD case was seen Sunday, September 30, 2001, and on January 22, 2002. The OIE declared that the UK had returned to "FMD free status without vaccination" for the purposes of international trade. By this time, however, some dramatic statistics had been recorded. The outbreak had raged for over 7 months and had spread over much of the nation. There were 2030 confirmed FMD cases. The total number of animals slaughtered to effect eradication was 4,073,000; including 593,000 cattle, 3,334,000

Development have been successfully promoting efforts at regional cooperation in animal disease control and harmonization of regulations for the movement and trade of livestock between neighboring nations. Through these efforts, Egypt, Israel, Jordan, and the Palestinian Authority have been working together on a number of projects including a regional veterinary information system, regional brucellosis and rabies control, control of major poultry diseases in the area, and joint

efforts in improving diagnostic capability. Details about this notable regional cooperation are available at the website http://www.move-in.org/.

The Situation in Developing Countries

The highly transmissible diseases included in the OIE list A diseases (Table 9-2) remain endemic in many developing

sheep, 142,000 pigs, 2,000 goats, 1,000 deer, and 1,000 other animals. The cost of eradication alone, independent of spillover effects on the general economy is estimated to have exceeded US$3.1 billion.

As the outbreak unfolded and the response was formulated, disease control officials came under a great deal of criticism from the public and the press. One particular area of controversy was the criteria used for destruction of animals. Disease control officials decided to slaughter animals on premises contiguous to infected farms, even if direct contact with infected animals could not be definitively established, and also to slaughter animals on suspicion of FMD based on clinical signs, without awaiting laboratory confirmation. Officials claimed that these actions were necessary because the disease had become so widely disseminated before disease control efforts were initiated. They believed that waiting for contiguous animals to manifest disease or for laboratory results to be returned would weaken the effectiveness of the control effort. The second area of controversy was the decision not to use vaccination. The public was very uncomfortable with the idea that animals were being killed when a vaccine was available but was not being used, especially since FMD was widely reported in the media to be a disease of low mortality. Officials responded by explaining the long-term implications of vaccination on disruption of international trade, as discussed elsewhere in this chapter.

The excessive slobbering associated with the painful oral lesions of FMD, as seen in this cow, are often lacking in sheep, making clinical diagnosis difficult in the latter species. (Photo by USDA, APHIS)

Interestingly, there is already evidence that these decisions by disease control officials were wisely considered and defensible. In August 2001, Morris et al. published a paper in the Veterinary Record describing a computer-based spatial simulation of the FMD outbreak while the outbreak was still in progress.[22] This paper not only vindicates the disease control strategy chosen by the decision-makers, it also clearly illustrates the power of computer modeling applied to the discipline of disease control. The model was first run using the actual disease control policies initiated by the Ministry of Agriculture, Fisheries and Food (MAFF) at the start of the outbreak. These included the slaughter of animals on infected farms within 24 hours, slaughter of about one to three of the surrounding at-risk farms per infected farm within a further 48 hours, and minimal interfarm movements of susceptible animals. The model indicated that under these conditions, there would be a total of 1800 to 1900 cases, and the epidemic would be eradicated between July and October 2001. These predictions turned out to be remarkably consistent with the actual outcome and appear to validate the accuracy of the model. When the model was run to exclude the much-criticized practice of preemptive slaughter on an adequate number of at-risk farms, the size of the epidemic increased substantially. Most strikingly, when the model was run so that the control policy was based on vaccination in buffer zones instead of the control policy that was actually implemented, the epidemic was predicted to run out of control, with over 6000 cases by October 2001 and no prospect of immediate eradication. This was most likely because the outbreak was already widely disseminated before control efforts were initiated. Under these circumstance, ring vaccination would not be effective because it would not be possible to create distinct buffer zones of immunized animals around discrete foci of infection, which is necessary for ring vaccination to create a "firebreak" against the spread of disease. For more information on the FMD outbreak in the UK, see the FMD home page at the website of the Department of Environment, Food and Rural Affairs, http://www.defra.gov.uk/animalh/diseases/fmd/default.htm

countries where numerous constraints on effective disease control may be present. Such constraints include shortages of trained personnel, inadequate budgets for disease surveillance and control, poor transportation and communication infrastructure that impede disease monitoring and response efforts, and a weak rule of law that makes animal testing requirements, livestock movement restrictions, and disease quarantines difficult or impossible to enforce. The problems facing developing countries in veterinary service delivery, including regulatory activities, are discussed in greater detail in Chapter 8.

Some of these constraints are being overcome by international cooperation and support. The PARC is mentioned in Chapter 8 as one example of a cooperative effort that has made progress toward elimination of the OIE list A disease rinderpest from the African continent. The PARC program officially ended in 1999 and has since been incorporated into a new, expanded program, the PACE. The 5-year PACE program covers 32 sub-Saharan countries and, like PARC before it, is coordinated through the Organization of African Unity, with substantial financial support from the EU and other donor agencies. PACE is the first continentwide epidemiology program of its kind. The main aim of PACE will be surveillance of epizootic diseases in Africa to accurately determine their prevalence and impact on livestock production. Such surveillance is critically important for countries that have successfully eradicated rinderpest through PARC but need to document their disease-free status continually to receive official recognition from the OIE as rinderpest-free countries. In addition to rinderpest, PACE surveillance activities will be focused on other important animal disease constraints in Africa, including contagious bovine pleuropneumonia, African swine fever, and Rift Valley fever.

In 1994, the FAO established a special program called the Emergency Prevention System for Transboundary Plant and Animal Diseases (EMPRES). The livestock disease component of the program resides within the FAO Animal Production and Health Division. The goal of EMPRES is to promote effective containment and control of the most serious epizootic transboundary livestock diseases by progressive elimination on a regional and global basis through international cooperation. EMPRES defines *transboundary diseases* as disease with significant economic, trade, and/or food security importance for a considerable number of countries; diseases that can easily spread to other countries and reach epidemic proportions; and diseases whose effective control and management requires active cooperation between several countries. Diseases of particular concern to EMPRES include rinderpest, contagious bovine pleuropneumonia, FMD, Rift Valley fever, lumpy skin disease, peste des petits ruminants (PPR), Newcastle disease, African swine fever (ASF), and classical swine fever.

EMPRES provides expert consultation, training, and technical support to veterinary authorities concerning national and regional disease control efforts, focusing on four key areas: early warning, early reaction, enabling research, and coordination. Several EMPRESS initiatives are described below:

- *The Regional Animal Disease Surveillance and Control Network* (RADISCON): Initiated in 1996, RADISCON is a joint initiative of the FAO and the International Fund for Agricultural Development (IFAD) and involves 29 nations located in North Africa, the Sahel, the Horn of Africa, the Middle East, and the Arab Gulf. The project helps each individual country establish its National Animal Disease Surveillance System (NADSS) and promotes information exchange through electronic communication with the overall goal of increasing the efficiency of national and regional animal disease control programs.

- *The Transboundary Animal Disease Information System* (TADinfo): TADinfo is a database management system for the storage and analysis of information on livestock diseases, aimed at improving disease management in developing countries. TADinfo software has been developed to use traditional forms of livestock demographic and disease information such as passive observation of disease occurrences by veterinary and paraveterinary staff, active disease surveys, abattoir/slaughter data, and livestock census and vaccination data.

- *Good Emergency Management Practices (GEMP) Program:* EMPRES defines *good emergency management practices* in animal health as the sum total of organized procedures, structures, and resource management that lead to early detection of disease or infection in an animal population, prediction of the likely spread, prompt limitation, targeted control, and elimination, with subsequent reestablishment of verifiable freedom from infection in accordance with the International Animal Health Code of the OIE. EMPRES has developed a GEMP multimedia program, available on CD and the FAO/EMPRES website, to promote the concept of a code of practice in dealing with animal disease emergencies in developing countries. The program provides information on the planning, recognition, response, and recovery phases of animal disease control efforts and also offers descriptive information and visual aids on the various list A diseases of the OIE. Any reader with further interest in animal disease control in developing countries should review the GEMP program at the EMPRES website, http://www.fao.org/waicent/faoinfo/agricult/aga/agah/empres/.

Emerging Diseases

Another challenge in animal disease control and public health are the so-called emerging diseases. Advances in medical science in the 20th century, such as the development of antibiotics and safe and effective vaccines, led to a generally optimistic view that human society had the power to control, or even eliminate, infectious disease as a cause of human and animal suffering. Indeed, for many decades, this seemed to be the case, until some very dramatic and disturbing developments undermined that optimism. Consider the following:

- The WHO reports that during the 1980s and 1990s, there were 29 new organisms linked to newly emerging communicable diseases in humans and that well-known diseases such as plague, dengue fever, diphtheria, meningococcal meningitis, yellow fever, and cholera are reemerging as serious public health concerns.[36]

- Acquired immunodeficiency syndrome (AIDS), a previously unknown viral disease emerged in the mid-1980s as a worldwide epidemic causing close to 22 million deaths by the end of the year 2000, with as many as 5 million new infections still occurring each year, most in Africa. The causative virus has been shown to have originated in chimpanzees and crossed into human populations.[11]

- Tuberculosis (TB), a traditional killer thought to be reasonably well under control, has returned with a vengeance over much of the world, aided by development of drug-resistant strains and human hosts whose immune systems are debilitated by the human immunodeficiency (HIV) virus. As many as 70% of active TB victims worldwide also have AIDS.

- Two new filoviruses have emerged—Marburg virus in the 1960s and Ebola virus in the 1970s—which cause epidemic, fatal hemorrhagic fevers in humans. These viruses are believed to have natural reservoirs in animals in the rainforests of Africa, but precise knowledge remains elusive. A third filovirus, Reston virus, was responsible for human exposures in Virginia, having been imported in infected cynomolgus monkeys from the Philippines.

- BSE emerged in the 1980s as a cattle disease in the United Kingdom caused by prions transmitted from scrapie-infected sheep to cattle that were fed meat and bone meal feeds containing neurological tissue from rendered sheep. The prion is a unique class of infectious agent, a protease-resistant protein with no associated genetic material. The world was horrified to learn in the mid-1990s that human beings may contract a fatal brain disease, variant VCJD, from eating prion-infected foods derived from prion-infected cattle.

- In 1993, a new group of rodent-transmitted hantaviruses in the family Bunyaviridae were identified in the United States, which were responsible for an acute respiratory disease in humans called hantavirus pulmonary syndrome. Since then, scientists have discovered or catalogued over 22 distinct hantaviruses around the world, at least 10 of which are linked to either hantavirus pulmonary syndrome or a separate hemorrhagic fever/renal syndrome.

- A new paramyxovirus, the Hendra virus was discovered in 1994 to cause severe respiratory disease in horses and humans and resulted in the deaths of stable workers in Australia. This virus is related to the Nipah virus responsible for disease in pigs and humans discussed earlier in this chapter

- In the mid-1990s, canine distemper virus crossed over into wild felines in the plains of East Africa. Almost a third of the lion population in Serengeti National Park in Tanzania and the Maasai Mara National Reserve in Kenya died as a result of the ensuing encephalitis. It is thought that the virus moved from domesticated dogs in local villages to spotted hyenas and then into the lion population.[26]

- Chronic wasting disease, a transmissible spongiform encephalopathy of elk and deer, first seen in captive cervids in Colorado and Wyoming in the late 1960s, is now known to infect wild elk and three species of deer in those states. The source of this prion disease remains unclear, though there is speculation that it crossed over from scrapie-infected sheep.

- Leptospirosis is reemerging as an important infection of dogs in the United States and has also been associated with a number of well-publicized human outbreaks, in Nicaragua in 1995 and in Ecuador and Illinois in 1998

- Porcine reproductive and respiratory syndrome (PRRS) was unknown before it was first reported in the United States in 1987. The disease, now known to be caused by an arterivirus, occurs in swine throughout North America and Europe.

- Neosporosis, a protozoal infection caused by *Neospora caninum*, was first identified as a cause of abortion in dairy cattle in 1989 and has since been recognized as a major cause of abortion in dairy cattle in the United States, the Netherlands, New Zealand, and at least 13 other countries. In California alone, neosporosis is estimated to produce $35 million in dairy production wastage annually due to abortion, low milk production, and early culls. It is now known that dogs are the definitive host of this protozoan and transmit the organism to cattle by fecal contamination of animal feeds.

There is no single, agreed-upon definition of *emerging disease*. The term is generally applied to previously unknown diseases that are newly recognized, known diseases that are spreading from endemic areas to new geographical areas where they were not previously seen, and to known diseases that are now infecting new target populations or even new species not previously recognized to be hosts. In addition, diseases that were thought to be under control but are once again more prevalent, such as tuberculosis, are sometimes referred to as *emerging diseases*, though more precisely, they are referred to as *reemerging or resurgent diseases*.

A wide variety of factors, individually or in concert, contribute to the evolution of an emerging disease. The WHO cites a number of these factors, including[36]:

- The ease of spread of disease from endemic to new areas through rapid and intense international travel
- Increasingly overcrowded cities with poor sanitation
- Changes in the handling and processing of food
- Deteriorating public (and animal) health laboratory and surveillance services
- Loss or shift of public funding, at least in human medicine, from infectious disease to neoplastic and cardiovascular diseases
- Microbial evolution and adaptation
- Ecological changes exposing humans to disease vectors and reservoirs in nature

Epstein,[7,8] Chivian,[3] and many other physicians and scientists draw particular attention to ecological factors as important determinants in the growth of emerging diseases. They cite global warming, extreme weather events, ozone depletion, loss of biodiversity, habitat encroachment, and environmental degradation with toxins and pollutants as important contributors to the increase and dispersal of disease vectors and microbial agents leading to increased risk of disease in humans and animals. Recent cholera epidemics, for instance, have been linked to coastal algal blooms in the world's oceans, which in turn are influenced by coastal pollution with agricultural runoff, climate change, and extreme El Niño weather events such as monsoons. The algal blooms provide nutrient substrate for active proliferation of *Vibrio cholerae* and increase the risk of transmission to humans along the coast.

The occurrence of hantavirus infections in humans in the southwestern United States has been linked to several environmental factors including large-scale incursion of human habitation into desert landscapes, loss of predators preying on infected rodent populations, and extreme weather events. First, unusually heavy rains promoted an abundant food supply for rodents, leading to increased rodent populations. Then, rains were followed by severe drought and a decreased food supply, which subsequently drove rodents into people's homes in search of food and water. This increased the risk of hantavirus transmission to humans. Similarly, the emergence of Lyme disease, a disease of animals and humans caused by *Borrelia burgdorferi* and transmitted by deer ticks, is thought to be related to increased deer populations associated with loss of predators and increased presence of humans and domestic animals in forested areas, where contact with the tick vector is increased.

There is enormous scientific interest in emerging diseases at present, and a thorough discussion of the topic is beyond the scope of this volume. Veterinary aspects of the emerging disease situation are now being discussed and investigated more widely. The University of Georgia hosted a conference "Emerging Diseases: Veterinary Medicine, Agriculture and Human Health," in August 1999, and a new textbook, *Emerging Diseases of Animals*, was published in 2000.[2] These and other useful resources related to emerging diseases are listed in Table 9-6.

Bioterrorism

Since the end of the Cold War, the risk of large-scale nuclear war between superpower nations has diminished. Now, national security analysts are increasingly concerned about hostile actions from state-sponsored terrorists, extremist political groups, fundamentalist religious sects, and other individuals or organizations with malevolent intent. Such groups can inflict damage on the United States by a variety of means. Explosive devices are commonly used, as attested by the horrific incidents at the World Trade Center in New York in 1993, the Alfred P. Murrah Federal Building in Oklahoma City in 1995, the U.S. Embassies in Kenya and Tanzania in 1998, and the World Trade Center again in 2001. However, other weapons pose a considerable threat, including so-called suitcase or dirty nuclear bombs wherein radioactive material is combined with conventional explosives; chemical agents such as nerve gas; and, the focus of this discussion, biological agents, including highly infectious organisms and lethal toxins.

Bioterrorism is defined as the intentional use of microorganisms or toxins derived from living organisms to cause death or disease in humans, other animals, or plants. Bioterrorist acts may be intended primarily to produce death in humans on a large scale or be targeted at specific individuals or groups. Bioterrorist acts may also be intended to produce large-scale economic disruption. One key target for economic disruption could be agriculture, aimed at interrupting food production and trade. Agriculture overall contributes $1 trillion annually to the U.S. gross national product, or 13% of the total GNP. Agricultural exports are valued at $140 billion annually, and 17% of the U.S. workforce is involved directly or indirectly in agriculture-related activity. The U.S. livestock industry alone is valued at $100 billion annually, including producers, suppliers, food processors, wholesalers, retailers, and international trade.

Animal agriculture in particular is now recognized as an important and vulnerable target for agriterrorism. The high value of the animal industry to the general economy, the increasing trend toward concentration of animals in intensive production units, the widespread movement of animals through auctions and markets by road, and the existence of a wide variety of highly contagious and deadly organisms and toxins affecting domestic livestock species all contribute to make animal agriculture a potential target for terrorist actions. Among agents of particular concern to security analysts are the viruses causing FMD, African swine fever, classical swine fever, highly pathogenic avian influenza, and Newcastle disease as they are easily

Table 9-6 Current and Useful Resources/Materials on the Subject of Emerging Diseases

Emerging Diseases: Veterinary Medicine, Agriculture, and Human Health. A conference held at the University of Georgia, College of Veterinary Medicine, Athens, GA, August 13-14, 1999. A wide variety of topics was covered, among them, emerging and reemerging diseases and disease agents of domestic animals, wildlife, and humans including *Salmonella typhimurium* DT 104, *E. coli* 0157H7, tuberculosis, leptospirosis, transmissible spongiform encephalopathies, avian influenza, Hendra virus, Nipah virus, and erlichiosis. Abstracts of papers presented at this conference are available on the internet at http://www.idreview.co.uk/content/pages/vol1/vol1-3.htm#vmah as published in the *Infectious Disease Review* 1999;1(3).

Emerging Diseases of Animals. This recent book presents information on specific emerging diseases including leptospirosis, bartonellosis, brucellosis, plague, avian influenza, tuberculosis, and transmissible spongiform encephalopathies. It also has chapters on general topics and policy issues related to emerging diseases of particular relevance to veterinary medicine, including xenotransplantation, biosafety, multiple drug resistance, and agricultural bioterrorism. Brown C, Bolin C, eds. Emerging Diseases of Animals. Washington, DC: American Society for Microbiology Press, 2000.

Emerging Infectious Diseases. *Emerging Infectious Diseases* is a peer-reviewed journal published by the Centers for Disease Control and Prevention in Atlanta, Georgia. The journal was initiated in 1995 as a forum for information on the tracking and analysis of disease trends. The journal is now published monthly in hard copy but is also available in full text on the internet at http://www.cdc.gov/ncidod/eid/index.htm. Articles of interest to veterinarians are commonly included in the journal, covering such topics as bovine spongiform encephalopathy, tuberculosis in humans due to *Mycobacterium bovis* in developing countries, B virus infections from pet macaque monkeys, and epidemiology of West Nile virus.

The Center for Health and the Global Environment. The Center for Health and the Global Environment (CHGE) was founded at Harvard School of Medicine in 1996 to improve environmental education in the medical community and to explore the human health consequences of global environmental change. The center administers a course at Harvard Medical School entitled "Human Health and Global Environmental Change." It also publishes an online journal, *The Quarterly Review,* which presents current knowledge on a variety of environmental topics with health implications, such as climate change, biodiversity loss, and pollution. The center also serves in an advisory capacity to government on policy matters relating to the health consequences of environmental change. More information about CHGE is available at their website at http://www.med.harvard.edu/chge/

Under the Weather: Climate, Ecosystems and Infectious Disease. The National Research Council was called upon by the federal government to organize a study of the relationship of climate change and disease and address three specific goals: to conduct a critical review of the relationship between climate variation and the transmission of infectious disease agents, to determine the potential for establishing early warning and surveillance systems for important climate related disease developments so that appropriate control interventions can be implemented, and to identify future research activities to study and quantify connections between climate variability, ecosystem transformation, and the transmission of infectious diseases and their impact on human health. The results of this comprehensive study are published in book form by National Academy Press. National Research Council. Under the Weather: Climate, Ecosystems and Infectious Disease. Washington, DC: The National Academy Press, 2001. The full text of this volume is available on the internet at http://www.nap.edu/books/0309072786/html/

The Center for Emerging Issues. The center is a unit of USDA, APHIS, Veterinary Services, located in Fort Collins, CO. The mission of the center is to identify and analyze both emerging animal health issues and emerging market conditions for animal products. The center's work on emerging animal health issues keeps key agency and industry decision makers and interested members of the public informed regarding health issues that may affect the United States. The CEI website at http://www.aphis.usda.gov/vs/ceah/cei/index.htm describes CEI projects on emerging animal health issues and posts updates on outbreaks of emerging diseases of animals around the world.

ProMED-Mail. ProMED-Mail is a global electronic reporting system for outbreaks of emerging infectious diseases sponsored by the International Society for Infectious Diseases. The system functions as a list serve and is open to anyone by on-line subscription. It is an excellent resource. There are daily updates on emerging diseases of humans, animals, and plants, and the site is carefully supervised and monitored to ensure the reliability of information. The ProMED-mail website is located at http://www.promedmail.org/pls/promed/promed.home

spread by aerosol transmission once introduced into susceptible populations.

While the role of veterinarians in detecting and responding to acts of agriterrorism is obvious, veterinarians will also serve a less obvious role in detecting acts of bioterrorism aimed at human populations. Analysts have identified a number of important zoonotic pathogens that are considered likely agents for a bioterrorist attack. In the event of such attacks, and depending on the mechanism of introduction, domestic animals may serve as sentinels for a human disease outbreak. It will be critical in disaster response for veterinarians to diagnose such diseases swiftly and accurately, recognize that they may be the result of a bioterrorist attack, and alert and cooperate with public health and disaster response officials. Among the bioweapons of particular concern as zoonotic threats are anthrax, tularemia, Q fever, plague, brucellosis, botulism, and equine encephalomyelitis viruses.[9]

An anthrax situation in the former Soviet Union in 1979 illustrates the role of animals as sentinels. An outbreak of anthrax occurred in humans in the town of Sverdlovsk, affecting 96 people and killing 64. Soviet officials declared that the unfortunate episode was related to the consumption of tainted meat. U.S. intelligence officials thought otherwise, suspecting that a factory located in the town was actually a bioweapons research and production facility. Investigation revealed that numerous sheep and cattle downwind from the factory in the same direction as the affected humans had also died of anthrax about the same time. As these herbivorous animals were unlikely to have consumed tainted meat, it became clear that the outbreak was related to an accidental release of anthrax spores from the bioweapons factory that traveled by aerosol to infect both animals and humans.

As awareness of the risk of bioterrorism grows, so do concerns that the nation is not fully prepared to deal with it. In the area of veterinary medicine there have been calls for improved funding of diagnostic laboratories with the capacity to detect foreign animal disease agents rapidly and increased training of veterinarians in the recognition of foreign animal diseases. The veterinary profession has pointed out that while federal and state governments have emergency management agencies and disaster plans, many agencies have failed to include a response to agriterrorism in their overall planning. This is now changing, and the outbreak of FMD in the UK as well as the terrorist attack of September 11 in 2001 have been strong catalysts for responsible officials to look at U.S. preparedness and increasingly include veterinarians in the planning process. Opportunities for veterinarians in relation to foreign animal disease control are likely to increase considerably in coming years, spurred in large part by concerns about bioterrorism. For more information, the Centers for Disease Control and Prevention (CDC) maintain an informative website on bioterrorism preparedness and response at http://www.bt.cdc.gov/. A full issue of the online journal *Emerging Infectious Diseases* dedicated to the subject of bioterrorism is available at http://www.cdc.gov/ncidod/eid/vol5no4/contents.htm.

New Tools for Disease Control

While the risks of animal-disease epizootics and the introduction of foreign animal diseases have been increasing in recent years, so have the tools available to understand, track, and control such disease events. Among the key areas of technological advance are molecular epidemiology, computer modeling of disease, and vaccine technology.

Molecular Epidemiology

Broadly speaking, molecular epidemiology is the application of molecular biology techniques to studies of the ecology and epidemiology of disease. Molecular epidemiology is finding wide application in human medicine to study genetic diseases, neoplasias, and diseases associated with environmental toxins, as well as infectious diseases. In veterinary medicine, the principal application has been in infectious and parasitic disease, to define the evolutionary history of organisms and their relationships to other organisms, to look for differences between attenuated vaccine strains and virulent field strains, and to study the dynamics of disease transmission in a population. Molecular epidemiology is also being used to track the evolution of antibacterial resistance in bacteria associated with food-producing animals.

Among the techniques applied in molecular epidemiology are amplification of defined fragments of viral genomes, using the polymerase chain reaction, followed by nucleotide-sequencing analysis to characterize, or "fingerprint," distinctive viral strains. Such techniques help clarify the source, evolution, and movement of viruses through animal populations and provide useful information for characterizing and controlling disease outbreaks. Molecular epidemiology has proven to be far more sensitive and informative than previous methodologies for the characterization of disease-causing viruses and thus provides a better understanding of epidemiological relationships, as the following examples illustrate.

Genetic analysis of FMD virus strains isolated from disease outbreaks is now a routine procedure at the OIE/FAO World Reference Laboratory for FMD at Pirbright, England. Analysis of the virus involved in the UK outbreak of FMD in 2001 identified it as the Pan Asian strain of serotype O, with the topotype ME-SA. Topotypes represent genetically and geographically distinct evolutionary lineages. This isolate is the same as the pandemic strain of FMD virus that was first identified in northern India in 1990 and that spread westward into Saudi Arabia in 1994 and then throughout the Near East and into Europe (Turkish Thrace, Bulgaria, and Greece) in 1996. When FMD first hit the UK, speculation and rumors regarding the source of the virus ran rampant. At one point, the British Army was accused of being responsible for the outbreak by importing meat contaminated with FMD from Uruguay and then carelessly allowing mess hall scraps to find their way into swine swill feeding establishments. Evidence of the genetic topotype of the virus argued against this, as the virus responsible for FMD in Uruguay was serotype 0, topotype Euro-SA, not ME-SA.

Peste des petits ruminants (PPR) is a serious infectious disease of goats, caused by a morbillivirus closely related to the rinderpest virus of cattle. Previously unknown outside of Africa and the Middle East, the disease began to be observed commonly in India and other countries of South Asia in the 1990s. There has been considerable concern about the emergence of PPR in South Asia, where goats are economically important in both commercial production and subsistence agriculture, and there has been a good deal of questioning about where the disease came from. Sequencing data for the NP gene of the PPR virus indicate four distinct lineages for the virus, with lineages I, II, and III occurring in Africa, lineages III and IV occurring in the Middle East, and lineage IV occurring in South Asia. These findings indicate that PPR was not introduced from Africa to South Asia. On the contrary, Diallo suggests that PPR is likely to have existed independently in South Asia for a long time before it was recognized as a distinct disease entity in the 1990s,[4] probably being misdiagnosed as either pasteurellosis, because of the respiratory manifestations of PPR, or as rinderpest, because of its gastrointestinal manifestations. While PPR and rinderpest virus are closely related, DNA probes are now available to readily distinguish between infection with these two agents. Recognition that PPR in South Asia is due to a distinct genotypic lineage of the PPR virus can help with development of better field identification, improved diagnostic capability, targeted vaccine production, and more-effective control efforts overall.

The Society of Tropical Veterinary Medicine devoted a considerable portion of their annual meeting in Montpelier, France, in 1997 to the issue of molecular epidemiology. Topics discussed included monitoring bovine babesiosis and anaplasmosis when moving cattle to risk areas; improving diagnosis of trypanosomiasis, theileriosis, and anaplasmosis; detecting pathogens in low-level carriers; and characterization of vaccine strains of *Theileria parva* and *Mycoplasma mycoides*, the respective causes of East Coast fever and contagious bovine pleuropneumonia, in the field. The proceedings of this meeting have been published.[17]

Computer Modeling

Computer modeling has proven to be a powerful epidemiological tool, and computer applications for disease control are now routinely integrated into academic and research programs in epidemiology and are being applied by government agencies responsible for disease control. The EpiCentre in the Institute of Veterinary, Animal and Biomedical Sciences at Massey University in New Zealand, for instance, is home to the EpiCentre Software Development Group, which, under the direction of Dr. Roger Morris, has developed a wide range of decision support systems for application in animal disease control. Some examples of EpiCentre programs and their use are as follows:

- *EpiMAN TB* is a decision support system designed to assist veterinarians and agricultural consultants in the management of TB control in cattle and deer in New Zealand, at a farm level and nationally.

- *EpiMAN FMD* is a powerful decision support system for the national control of an outbreak of FMD, designed to be operational quickly at a national emergency disease-control headquarters to provide effective, comprehensive support to the control effort. The program integrates spatial analysis and mapping, expert systems, simulation models, and databases.

- *EpiMAN SF* is based on the concepts and elements of EpiMAN FMD, for use by veterinarians,

epidemiologists, and disease-response managers in response to an epidemic of classical or African swine fever.

- *EpiMAN FS* is a food-safety modeling program that integrates spatial data about the location of farms with historical data about each farm. It provides the core requirements to trace food products "from farm to table" and protect the safety of food products. It uses a risk-based system for minimizing health hazards associated with food products.

- *HandiRISK* is a software package designed to help countries produce transparent, repeatable, and methodologically valid risk analyses relative to importation of livestock and livestock products. The program can guide the user through the construction of a quantitative or qualitative risk-analysis model and the subsequent simulation of an import scenario

- *DiseaseSpread*, a generic computer model of disease control in a national livestock population, was developed under contract to the British government for investigation of BSE.

While many programs are becoming available to assist in the management of disease outbreaks, computer analysis has also been successfully combined with other new technologies such as geographical information systems (GIS) and satellite remote sensing to predict disease outbreaks, thus allowing greater preparedness and response. For example, Linthicum et al. showed that by tracking sea surface temperature anomalies of the Pacific and Indian oceans and combining these data with vegetation changes detected by remote sensing satellites, Rift Valley fever epidemics could be forecast 5 months in advance of actual outbreaks[20] (see sidebar in Chapter 6, "Kenya and El Niño, 1997–1998: A challenge for Veterinarians").

Software designed for other purposes has also proven useful for application in veterinary epidemiology. In 2001, government epidemiologists in the UK dealing with the outbreak of FMD drew upon a computer model designed to track nuclear fallout in the aftermath of the Chernobyl nuclear power plant disaster in 1986. This model was based on an analysis of wind patterns to determine the airborne dispersal of radioactive material from the point source of the damaged reactor. As FMD can be spread by wind as an aerosolized virus, epidemiologists used the program to define the "footprint" of aerosol plumes. This allowed them to determine the size, shape, direction, and location of infection and surveillance zones to be established around point source outbreaks of FMD.

Vaccine Technology

Vaccines have proven to be enormously valuable instruments for disease control in both human and veterinary medicine. Smallpox was eradicated worldwide largely through global vaccination efforts, and polio is on the verge of elimination as a result of extensive vaccination campaigns. Vaccination is the cornerstone of rabies control in domestic animals and may prove instrumental in the ongoing global effort to eliminate rinderpest from cattle populations worldwide. However, vaccines are often imperfect tools. Modified live vaccines, for instance, are often more effective than killed vaccines but require more careful handling in the field to ensure their potency. Lack of infrastructure, such as a reliable cold chain, can render such vaccines ineffective. Most vaccines produce a humoral antibody response that plays a role in protecting the vaccinate from disease. However, such antibodies, when detected by serological testing methods may be impossible to differentiate from naturally occurring antibodies associated with infection. The inability to distinguish between the two can present significant obstacles to disease control efforts, interstate movement of animals, and international trade. For instance, while vaccines for FMD are available to assist in disease control, they are frequently not used by livestock-exporting countries because of restrictions imposed by importing countries concerned that existing serological tests cannot distinguish between vaccination and infection.

Some recent technological advances have helped to overcome these inherent problems associated with traditional vaccine production. Mariner et al., for example, successfully developed a heat-stable rinderpest vaccine that could retain the minimum required protective dose for more than 20 weeks at a temperature of 37°C.[21] This allowed vaccination teams to work in hot, remote areas of eastern Africa where reliable vaccination had not previously been possible because of lack of roads, refrigeration, electricity, and other logistical requirements necessary to maintain a cold chain to protect traditional vaccine.

The longstanding effort to control pseudorabies in swine in the United States was aided considerably by the development of genetically modified vaccines. Vaccines were developed in which the gene for expression of thymidine kinase is deleted, which blocks the vaccine virus's ability to infect and replicate in neurons. Specific ELISA tests were developed that could accurately discriminate between antibodies due to vaccination with gene-deleted vaccine and those due to infection with natural field strains of the virus. As a result, federal and state regulatory programs were revised to eliminate the use of conventional vaccines and allow the use of gene-altered vaccines. Interstate movement of vaccinated animals then became feasible, because vaccination could be reliably differentiated from infection.

There is considerable interest in the insertion of genetic markers in vaccines for a wide variety of animal diseases and the development of tests to accurately distinguish between infection and vaccination. As mentioned, FMD garners a great deal of interest in this regard because it is dangerous and costly to control FMD without vaccination, but it is also costly to vaccinate with traditional vaccines because of the implications for interference with trade. At least five different tests, such as the use of monoclonal antibody-based ELISA for antibodies to

nonstructural proteins of FMD virus, have been developed in the 1990s to discriminate cattle infected with FMD from noninfected vaccinates. An entire issue of the *Veterinary Quarterly* was dedicated to research papers on this subject (volume 20, supplement 2, 1998). Standardization and adoption of such tests could revolutionize FMD control efforts worldwide, allowing more widespread use of vaccines and perhaps eliminating the horrific spectacle of mass destruction and burning of cattle that played on the world's television screens during the UK FMD outbreak of 2001.

The newest and most exciting frontier of vaccine technology is the development of genetic vaccines. As described by Weiner and Kennedy, the most common type of genetic vaccines under development are plasmids containing double-stranded DNA derived from bacteria.[35] These plasmids have been altered to carry genes specifying one or more antigenic proteins normally made by a selected pathogen, but they exclude genes that would enable the pathogen to reconstitute itself and cause disease. These plasmid vaccines can be delivered by intramuscular injection, which puts genes directly into some cells and also leads to uptake by cells in the vicinity of the inserted needle. Recombinant plasmids that make their way into host cell nuclei enable the cell to synthesize the encoded antigenic proteins. Thus the injected animal can produce an antibody response when the encoded proteins are released from cells and a cell-mediated response when the proteins are broken down and properly displayed on the cell surface. Such vaccines would, theoretically at least, provide lifelong immunity, eliminate the need for boosters, and thus simplify long-term disease control efforts.

Already a wide range of veterinary applications are under development. Sagodira et al., for instance, have demonstrated protection of kid goats against cryptosporidiosis after their dams were vaccinated intranasally with a recombinant plasmid encoding for a surface sporozoite protein of *Cryptosporidium parvum*.[27] Other veterinary scientists are working on genetic vaccines against equine arteritis virus, bovine herpesvirus-1, *Corynebacterium pseudotuberculosis*, infectious bursal disease, bovine virus diarrhea, viral hemorrhagic septicemia of trout, rabies, equine influenza virus, and *Chlamydia psittaci*, among others. A useful website for information about developments in genetic vaccination can be found at http://dnavaccine.com/

Contemporary Issues in Food Safety

The risk of human beings becoming ill from the foods they eat is not a new phenomenon. No doubt the first ancient hunter-gatherer to sample a poisonous mushroom developed some opinions about the subject. However, in recent years concern has grown dramatically about the healthfulness of foods. This heightened concern has been punctuated by highly publicized events of food contamination and lapses in food safety practices. Consider the following events:

- *Hamburgers and Escherichia coli O157:H7 in the northwestern United States.* In 1993, several hundred people in four states in were sickened by consuming hamburgers purchased at various outlets of a fast-food restaurant chain. Over 200 people were hospitalized, and 4 died. Most victims were children. *E. coli* O157:H7 is a particularly dangerous food-borne pathogen that produces a potentially fatal hemolytic-uremic syndrome (HUS) in some victims, in addition to the gastroenteritis commonly associated with food poisoning. The ground beef used in the hamburgers was already contaminated when obtained from a single supplier in California. The procurement and distribution system of the nationwide restaurant chain resulted in distribution of the tainted meat over a wide geographical area, thus putting a large group of people at risk of exposure. That Americans increasingly are eating a greater proportion of their meals outside the home is also considered an increased risk factor for food poisoning.

- *Beef consumption and variant Creutzfeldt-Jakob disease in the United Kingdom.* In 1996, it was reported that BSE, commonly referred to as "mad cow disease," was transmissible to human beings consuming products derived from infected cattle and could cause vCJD. By the end of 2000, 84 confirmed human cases of the fatal neurological disease had been identified, mostly in the United Kingdom. While the CDC in the United States estimates that the risk of contracting vCJD from consumption of beef is only 1 in 10 billion, the horrific nature of the progressive brain disease and its fatal outcome have sent a shock wave of fear through consumers and have badly damaged consumer confidence in the safety of meat. Many critics contend that modern industrial cattle feeding and slaughter practices are responsible for the emergence of this frightening disease. They cite the "unnatural" feeding of animal-source protein to ruminants and the practice of cattle slaughter by captive bolt. The latter practice carries the potential of introducing contaminated brain and spinal cord tissue into portions of the beef carcass destined for human consumption. The BSE pathogen is only one of several important food-borne pathogens that have emerged in recent years that will require additional research to develop and implement appropriate preventive and control measures throughout the entire chain of food production and processing.

- *Dioxin in foods from Belgium.* In 1999, dioxin-contaminated waste machine-oil was accidentally incorporated into animal feed. This accident, coupled with an official delay in announcing the occurrence and extent of the ensuing problems, resulted in one of the most highly publicized food safety crises in recent years. The incident prompted the closure of more than 1200 farms because of slaughter of contaminated animals and the destruction of over 115,000 tonnes of pig, poultry, and beef products. A major crisis in consumer confidence ensued concerning government regulation of food safety, resulting in a loss of export markets to Belgian farmers, a major national economic loss, and the fall of the Christian-Democratic government. The episode began when farmers began to observe sick and dying chickens. When the cause was traced back to contaminated feed, it became apparent that the tainted feed had also been distributed for cattle and swine use and had been exported to Spain, the Netherlands, and France as well. Ultimately, 30 countries, including the United States, ended up posting temporary bans on Belgian food products, from veal to chocolate, which might contain tainted constituents of animal origin. The crisis is estimated to have cost Belgian farmers approximately US$225 million, with at least equal losses to the country's food processors. The EU initiated legal proceedings against Belgium for waiting a month before warning the EU about the contamination. Though the amount of potentially cancer-causing dioxins contained in the feed was less than originally feared, public health officials will have to monitor the human population for years to determine if any adverse effects resulted from the delay in identifying dioxin contamination in animals and animal products destined for the human food supply.

- *Salmonellosis from ice cream in the United States.* In 1994 a nationwide outbreak of *Salmonella enteriditis* occurred from consuming ice cream. While several hundred people actually reported diarrheal disease to health authorities in association with the consumption of ice cream, epidemiologists estimated that as many as 224,000 people may have been sickened. The ice cream, distributed widely, was prepared from an ice cream premix that had been transported in tanker trucks that had previously been used to haul raw liquid eggs and had not been properly sanitized. The eggs were the original source of the *S. enteriditis*. This episode points out that no phase in the food production process, in this case, truck transportation of an intermediate product, can be excluded from consideration in tracing the evolution of a food-borne outbreak.

- *Food poisoning from sources other than foods of animal origin*. In 1996, almost 6000 Japanese schoolchildren contracted diarrhea from consuming food contaminated with E. *coli* O157:H7, and 101 of them developed the complication of HUS. Epidemiological investigations pointed to radish sprouts as the principal contaminated food. That same year, an outbreak of enteritis from the protozoal parasite *Cyclospora cayetanensis* on raspberries imported from Guatemala affected approximately 1450 people in various locations in the United States and Canada. In 1994, outbreaks of gastroenteritis due to *Shigella sonnei*, affecting hundreds of people in the United Kingdom, Sweden, and Norway, were linked to consumption of contaminated iceberg lettuce, most likely originating in Spain. It was suspected that fecal-contaminated water was used to irrigate the lettuce or to cool it after packing. These incidents illustrate that food poisoning outbreaks are increasingly associated with foods other than foods of animal origin. However, there may still be indirect links to animal production associated with the direct application of animal manure containing pathogens to vegetable crops as fertilizer or the unintended contamination of soil and water sources with manure runoff from livestock production units as discussed in more detail in Chapter 6.

These events underscore the dramatic changes that are taking place in food production, processing, and marketing in our contemporary, globalized society. These changes include: increased international trade and travel; intensification and industrialization of livestock agriculture; greater global demand for food products; altered eating habits; changes in the structure and control of food processing, distribution, and retailing industries; and, increased challenges for regulatory agencies and industries to ensure the safety of food products.

Some specific concerns about ensuring food safety in the United States have emerged. These include:

- Increased importation of foods from countries that may have less-stringent SPS regulations than the United States

- The emergence of new pathogens with adaptations that promote survival, broaden the spectrum of foods that may be contaminated, and are difficult to treat as a result of antibiotic resistance as discussed below

- Changing eating habits that include increased consumption of fresh and raw fruits and vegetables, an increase in the number of meals eaten outside the home, and reduced awareness in some segments of society about hygienic practices for food purchase, preparation, and storage

- A greater proportion of the population at higher risk of illness from food-borne pathogens, including the elderly, persons with immunosuppressive diseases, and patients taking immunosuppressive drugs for cancer or other illnesses

- Centralized food production, processing, and distribution networks that facilitate the widespread dissemination of contaminated food to multiple locations from a point source of contamination, resulting in high levels of exposure

- Intensification of animal agriculture, which presents new challenges for waste management, sanitation, and hygiene in animal production systems and potentially increases dependence on the use of antibiotics for disease control

- A food service industry workforce that is frequently transient, poorly paid, lacking health insurance, and non-English speaking, all of which may contribute to a failure to recognize or report potentially contagious illnesses such as hepatitis or to understand and follow hygienic food preparation practices[28]

- A fragmented food safety inspection system in the United States involving multiple agencies and different standards of inspection, particularly in relation to imported foods in different categories

Foods may be contaminated or adulterated with a wide variety of materials that pose challenges to food safety and the public health. These include: infectious organisms and biological toxins; antibiotics, hormones, and other production-related additives; agricultural chemicals including pesticides; and, industrial chemicals including heavy metals and other pollutants. Concerns about the unwelcome presence of such materials in foods have driven public calls for greater regulation of food production, processing, trade, and marketing.

These concerns also have stimulated growing interest in organic agriculture and greater demand by consumers for organic products. European consumers have been vocally demanding organic food products for quite some time, and producers have been responding accordingly. In the United States, the organic movement, though not as well developed as in Europe, also has gained considerable momentum. Between 1992 and 1997, the area of certified organic cropland in the United States doubled to 1.3 million acres, though this still represents only 0.2% of the total cropland available. Production of organic eggs and milk grew even faster in the same period. Certified organic dairy cow numbers increased from 2,265 to 12,897, while organic laying hen numbers jumped from about 44,000 to about 540,000. In December 2000, after 10 years of debate and consideration of over 300,000 public comments, the USDA issued detailed guidelines for the production and marketing of agricultural products and set up the National Organic Program, which will accredit agents to certify organic producers. The subject of organic livestock farming has been critically reviewed.[30]

A newer food safety issue arises from advances in biotechnology. In recent years, the development and distribution of genetically modified foodstuffs has shaken consumer confidence in regard to food safety, public health, and environmental health. In some cases, consumer activism has resulted in withdrawal of genetically modified foods from the marketplace. While cultural and regional attitudes towards the acceptability of genetically modified foods vary, it is already clear that consumers in general expect rigorous regulatory oversight and transparency in the production and marketing of genetically modified food products. To date, most genetically modified foods have been of plant origin, but genetically modified foods of animal origin are under development. The intense public controversy that resulted from the use of bovine growth hormone to increase production in dairy cows provided a preview of the heated debate that is likely to accompany the development of genetically modified animals for food production. Veterinarians will be increasingly involved in the development and evaluation of such products and will assume a great deal of responsibility for informing the public that such products are safe, wholesome, and beneficial or otherwise.

Societal attitudes are also influencing public perceptions about the acceptability of certain foods that extend beyond the issue of food safety. Increasingly, consumer are expressing concerns about the well-being of the animals used to produce food. Animal welfare issues have begun to influence purchasing decisions, with consumers demanding information about the management of animals from which products such as eggs, meat, and milk are derived. There is increased expectation that food-producing animals receive acceptable standards of care. These consumer concerns are beginning to directly influence decisions among processors and retailers about animal management on the farm and decisions about procurement sources for livestock and livestock products.

A thorough and detailed discussion of all salient aspects of food safety merits a text of its own and is beyond the scope of this book. A number of excellent and timely resources are available for additional information about the topic (Table 9-7). The discussion here is limited to a general overview of food safety issues, emphasizing aspects of food safety related to international trade, new technologies, and emerging problems, challenges and opportunities for veterinarians, viewed from a global perspective.

Global Overview of Food-Borne Illness

Food-borne illness is a global public health problem of considerable magnitude. It affects citizens in developed countries as well as in developing countries, though the scope of the problem and the underlying causes differ notably in the two spheres. A key difference is the widespread lack of access to clean, safe drinking water in many developing countries. Water is the most fundamental of all nutrients and can serve as a vehicle for both communicable and noncommunicable diseases when it becomes contaminated with raw sewage, toxic metals, or agricultural and industrial chemicals. The most widespread pollutant and the one most associated with communicable disease and acute illness is domestic sewage. The extent of the problem is underscored by data from international organizations such as UNICEF and the WHO which indicate that more than half the world's population, about 3 billion people, do not have access to a sanitary toilet. Instead, human waste is deposited in farm fields, on roadsides, in waterways, and in other public areas where it can easily and readily contaminate groundwater supplies. In urban areas, rapid population growth leads to dense concentrations of people in shantytowns with no plumbing infrastructure, further aggravating inadequacies of public hygiene and sanitation. Homes may not only lack toilets; they may also lack clean running tap water, because municipal water systems are not well developed and water treatment facilities may be inadequate, overloaded, or nonexistent. Even in the industrialized nations, where water treatment infrastructure is well developed, the risk of communicable disease from the public water supply has not been completely eliminated, as the major epidemic of cryptosporidiosis from tap water in Milwaukee illustrated in 1993.

Illiteracy and lack of public awareness concerning fundamental principles of sanitation and hygiene further exacerbate the worldwide problem of disease spread through food and water. While in Pakistan in 1993, the author was flabbergasted to observe a roadside vegetable vendor dip a rusty bucket into an open sewer running in front of his vegetable stand and then carefully splash the water over his entire produce display to remove the road dust and make the vegetables appear clean and shiny. In Afghanistan, it is common practice after slaughtering a sheep or goat to cut the skin circumferentially above the hoof on each limb and then blow air under the skin to separate it from the underlying connective tissue. The hide can then, after a couple of additional strategic cuts, be easily removed by pulling it from the carcass rather than painstakingly dissecting it away (Fig. 9-2). If the butcher has TB, however, the whole carcass can be contaminated by the act of blowing under the skin. The fact that drug-resistant TB in on the rise in many countries around the world makes this a legitimate public health concern. Lack of public awareness or appropriate training in food handling is not limited to the developing world. In the United States, it is not unusual to see a counter worker in a fast-food restaurant wear gloves while preparing sandwiches. But when that same worker takes your money and makes change without removing those gloves and then goes back to preparing the next order, the function of

Table 9-7 Current and Useful Resources/Materials on the Subject of Food Safety

Food Safety and Quality Assurance: Foods of Animal Origin. This textbook provides good, detailed, technical information on food safety from a veterinary perspective, emphasizing the central role of veterinarians in ensuring food quality. The newer 2nd edition includes a distinct international perspective, comparing food inspection practices in Australia, Canada, the United Kingdom, and the United States. Hubbert WT, Hagstad HV, Spangler E et al., Food Safety and Quality Assurance: Foods of Animal Origin. 2nd Ed. Ames: Iowa State University Press, 1996.

Microbial Food Borne Pathogens. This March 1998 issue of *The Veterinary Clinics of North America, Food Animal Practice* presents discussions of specific food-borne pathogens of current concern as well as articles offering overviews of antibiotic resistance and food-borne disease surveillance and prevention programs. Tollefson L, ed. Microbial food borne pathogens. Vet Clin North Am Food Anim Pract 1998;14(1).

Chemical Food Borne Hazards and Their Control. This March 1999 companion volume to "Microbial Food Borne Pathogens" presents discussions on a variety of noninfectious agents that adversely affect food safety, including drug residues, pesticides, mycotoxins, heavy metals, and various industrial chemicals. It also discusses some of the regulatory programs and initiatives in place to address these food safety problems. Tollefson L, ed. Chemical food borne hazards and their control. Vet Clin North Am Food Anim Pract 1999;15(1).

Food Safety Symposium-Post Harvest. A symposium on food safety postharvest was held in conjunction with the annual meeting of the American Veterinary Medical Association in 1998. Excellent presentations from this meeting on various food-borne pathogens, chemical hazards, and their control were published collectively in the *Journal of the American Veterinary Medical Association.* J Am Vet Med Assoc 1998;213(12).

Contamination of Animal Products: Prevention and Risks for Animal Health. The OIE has dedicated two special issues of its journal *Scientific and Technical Review* to the topic of food safety in relation to trade. The first focuses on the prevention of risks of transmission of animal disease by importation of livestock and livestock products. The issue contains 26 articles with the discussion presented on a species-by-species basis. Sci Tech Rev 1997;16(1). (Abstracts available on the internet at http://www.oie.int/eng/publicat/RT/A_RT16_1.htm)

Contamination of Animal Products: Prevention and Risks for Public Health. This second, companion special issue of the *Scientific and Technical Review* focuses on the potential hazards to human health from the consumption and use of animal products. The issue contains 42 articles on the microbial food-borne pathogens associated with the major categories of animals that provide food for people around the world, with reports from a variety of countries and regions. Contaminants of nonbiological origin are also discussed as well as the food-borne zoonotic risks associated with microorganisms present in animal manure. Sci Tech Rev 1997;16(2). (see http://www.oie.int/eng/publicat/RT/A_RT16_2.htm)

Food Safety: Federal Efforts to Ensure the Safety of Imported Foods Are Inconsistent and Unreliable. This report by the federal government's General Accounting Office looks specifically at problems associated with ensuring the safety of imported foods entering the United States. It is quite frank in its criticism and provides a good analysis of the challenges and difficulties associated with efficient and reliable regulatory efforts. General Accounting Office: Food Safety: Federal Efforts to Ensure the Safety of Imported Foods Are Inconsistent and Unreliable. Washington, DC: GAO, May 1998. (Full text available on the internet by searching the GAO documents archive by title at www.access.gpo.gov/su_docs/aces/aces160.shtml)

Ensuring Safe Food: From Production to Consumption. This congressionally mandated report prepared by the Institute of Medicine and the National Research Council provides a detailed analysis of the structure and function of the United States' food safety system as it existed at the end of the 20th century and addresses issues of food safety for both imported and domestically produced foods. The report identifies problems and suggests approaches for improvement, emphasizing a science-based approach for reducing risks of food borne disease. Ensuring Safe Food: From Production to Consumption, Washington, DC: National Academy Press, 1998. (Full text available on the internet at http://www.nap.edu/books/0309065593/html/index.html)

The Use of Drugs in Food Animals: Benefits and Risks. This study commissioned through the National Research Council provides a detailed analysis of the controversial subject of the use of drugs in food-producing animals. This extensive, detailed work addresses the role of drugs in food-animal production, summarize available knowledge on human health effects of drug use in food animals, evaluates the approval and regulatory process and delivery systems for animal drugs, and assesses emerging trends, technologies, and alternatives to drug use in food animal production. National Research Council. The Use of Drugs in Food Animals: Benefits and Risks. Washington, DC: National Academy Press, 1999. The full text of this volume is available on the internet at http://www.nap.edu/books/0309054346/html/index.html

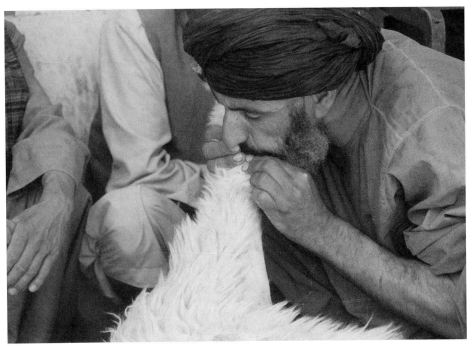

Figure 9-2. An Afghan man separating the skin of a slaughtered sheep from the carcass by blowing air into a knife cut made above the coronary band. While this clever technique makes removal of the hide easier, it can result in contamination of the carcass with infectious agents such as the tubercle bacillus. (Photo by Dr. David M. Sherman)

the gloves as a barrier to disease transmission is effectively overridden.

In the developing world, even when people understand about hygiene and the importance of boiling water to prevent infection, they are often too poor to afford the soap they need to wash their hands before handling food or to purchase the fuel they need to boil their daily water supply and so are obliged to consume contaminated water themselves and provide it to their children. Refrigerators to keep foods fresh and control bacterial proliferation are often unavailable and/or unaffordable. Too often, there is also no strong, effective government to firmly regulate food-processing industries, monitor agricultural pesticide residues on foods, or control the dumping of industrial chemicals into public waterways.

For all these reasons, it is not surprising that worldwide, an estimated 1.5 billion episodes of diarrhea occur annually, resulting in an estimated 3 million deaths, primarily in children under 5 years of age. Most of these illnesses and deaths occur in the developing countries. As many as 70% of diarrhea cases are believed to be due to gastroenteritis from biologically contaminated food. In the developing world, cholera, due to the bacterium *Vibrio cholerae*, continues to be a major cause of disease and death and is associated with both contaminated water and contaminated food, particularly rice, vegetables, millet gruel, and various types of seafood. Other viruses and bacteria, such as caliciviruses, hepatitis A virus, Norwalk-like viruses, *E. coli*, *Staphylococcus aureus*, *Salmonella* spp., and *Campylobacter* spp. are also important in epidemic outbreaks of food-borne

illness. In the developing world, trematode infections associated with ingestion of contaminated food continue to be an important public health problem, with 10% of the world's population at risk of infection

Developed countries are not immune to food-borne illness, though communicable disease problems associated with contaminated drinking water are far less common. Some estimates suggest that up to 30% of citizens in developed countries may experience a food-borne illness each year. In the United States, there are as many as 9,000 deaths and 325,000 hospitalizations due to food-borne illness annually, making it a major public health issue. The overall annual estimate of cases of food-borne illness in the United States is between 6.5 and 81 million. Estimates vary so widely because the main clinical expression of food-borne illness is diarrhea. Many individuals experiencing diarrhea do not seek medical attention and when they do, culture for specific pathogens with follow-up epidemiological investigation to determine the source of infection are not routinely conducted. However in recent years, the emergence of new pathogens, increases in the size of populations at special risk, and the development of more-serious clinical sequelae have raised concerns about the impact of food-borne disease, as discussed in the section below.

Food-Borne Pathogens

Thorns has recently reviewed the food-borne zoonotic diseases.[32] In many countries, bacterial food-borne zoonotic infections are the most common cause of human intestinal disease, with *Salmonella* spp. and *Campylobacter* spp. accounting for over 90% of all reported cases of bacteria-related food poisoning worldwide. Poultry and poultry products are most often incriminated in traceable food-borne illnesses caused by these bacteria, though all domestic livestock are potential reservoirs of infection. Most *Salmonella* and *Campylobacter* infections are enzootic. However, *Salmonella enteritidis* has been pandemic in both poultry and humans during the last decades of the 20th century. *Salmonella typhimurium* and *Campylobacter* spp. are more ubiquitous in the environment and colonize a greater variety of hosts and environmental niches.

From the 1980s onward, verotoxin-producing *E. coli* O157, notably *E. coli* O157:H7, has emerged as a major food-borne zoonotic pathogen. While ground beef was the vehicle for a number of highly publicized outbreaks, the organism is also associated with foods not of animal origin, such as sprouts and apple juice, though contamination of such foods with animal manure is sometimes implicated.

Listeriosis due to *Listeria monocytogenes* also emerged as an important food-borne zoonosis in the late 20th century, frequently associated with dairy products, particularly cheese. In developing countries, particularly in the Mediterranean region, and Central and South America, brucellosis associated with the consumption of unpasteurized dairy products is increasing, especially in association with *Brucella melitensis* from sheep and goats. At the beginning of the 21st century, the world was confronted with a new and frightening food-borne illness, vCJD, associated with consumption of products derived from cattle infected with the causative agent of BSE. An expanded list of contemporary food-borne pathogens and the foods they are most commonly associated with is provided by Headrick and Tollefson.[13]

One troubling aspect of the emerging food-borne pathogens is that their effects on human beings often are not limited to gastroenteritis, the most common clinical manifestation historically associated with food-borne illness. While most food-borne pathogens do produce diarrhea and are sometimes fatal, some of the emerging pathogens result in other life-threatening or debilitating sequelae:

- Campylobacteriosis due to *Campylobacter jejuni* can result in reactive arthritis or Guillain-Barré syndrome (GBS), an autoimmune reaction affecting the nervous system. Approximately 1 in 1000 cases of reported campylobacteriosis cases leads to GBS, and up to 40% of GBS cases in the United States may be triggered by campylobacteriosis.

- Listeriosis can produce septicemia and meningitis and, in pregnant women, can result in abortion, stillbirth, or premature birth, with signs of septicemia and meningitis sometimes observed in surviving newborns.

- Infection with *E. coli* O157:H7 and other verotoxin-producing *E. coli* can result in hemorrhagic colitis, hemolytic uremic syndrome (HUS), and thrombocytopenic purpura, as a result of systemic toxin absorption that produces epithelial damage and microthrombi affecting the kidneys and other organs. Infants, children, and the elderly are especially susceptible to these sequelae. Up to 40% of patients who survive HUS have chronic renal insufficiency.

- Brucellosis results in a chronic infection characterized by general malaise with recurrent fevers. Additional complications and organ involvement may include lymphadenitis, hepatitis, osteomyelitis, bursitis, orchitis and epididymitis, and abortion.

- vCJD is unlike any other food-borne illness. There are no acute signs. After an incubation period of years, the disease manifests as a progressive debilitating encephalopathy with psychiatric symptoms, prominent incoordination, an extended course, and ultimately death.

As these examples suggest, severe clinical disease associated with emerging pathogens may be due to inherent characteristics of the organisms themselves and their enhanced capacity to produce disease. In other cases, the more dramatic sequelae are associated with the increased susceptibility of certain segments of the human population to infection and an impaired capacity to control it. These would include infants, children, pregnant women, the elderly, and immunocompromised individuals such as AIDS patients or cancer patients on immunosuppressive drugs. In the latter cases, pathogens with the potential to produce septicemia and localize in organs outside the gastrointestinal tract are more likely to do so.

Another important characteristic of emerging food-borne pathogens is that many of these organisms have developed or exhibit adaptations that increase the likelihood that they may survive processing, become involved in disease, or resist treatment, as indicated in the following examples:

- By 1990, *S. enteriditis* had emerged as the most common serotype involved in salmonellosis in the United States. Shell eggs have become an important source of *S. enteriditis*, and the consumption of raw or undercooked eggs is a major cause of human infection. This pattern reflects the organism's ability to successfully infect the ovaries or oviducts of laying hens, thus allowing eggs to become internally contaminated before they are laid. This adaptation is presumed to be a recent development, mirroring the rise of the agent as the most common type of food-borne salmonellosis. Rabsch et al. suggest that effective regulatory programs to eliminate *S. gallinarum* in commercial poultry has created a niche for *S. enteriditis* to successfully colonize poultry.[25]

- *L. monocytogenes* is a cold-tolerant organism that can multiply in foods stored at standard refrigeration temperatures if the foods are contaminated. According to the CDC, an estimated 2500 persons become seriously ill with listeriosis each year, and 500 of them die. Pregnant women are 20 times as likely to fall ill than nonpregnant healthy adults, and AIDS patients are 300 times more likely to become sick than people with normally functioning immune systems.

- Verotoxigenic *E. coli* are essentially considered a "new" pathogen. *E. coli* O157:H7 causes virtually no illness in the animals it infects, making it difficult to detect, but it causes serious illness in humans who ingest it, in contrast to the hundreds of strains of E. coli that reside in the human gut with no adverse effect. The capacity for E. coli O157:H7 to tolerate low pH makes it difficult to control in unheated and unpasteurized foods. The epidemiology of E. coli O157:H7 remains poorly understood, although ruminants, especially cattle and sheep, appear to be the major source of infection.

- Strains of Salmonella spp. associated with food-borne illness have emerged that posses multiple drug resistance. S. typhimurium DT104 is the most widely reported and has been involved in epidemics in the UK in the 1980s and more recently with outbreaks in other European countries and the United States, where the organism has been isolated from a wide variety of animals. This strain, R-type ACSSuT, encodes chromosome-related resistance to ampicillin, chloramphenicol, streptomycin, sulfonamides and tetracycline. More recently, a strain of Salmonella enterica serotype newport with a similar multiple resistance pattern has been causing human illness in the United States The strain has been isolated from ground beef and, in preliminary epidemiological investigations, from cattle, horses, and dogs.

- Enterobacter sakazakii shows exceptional tolerance to drying. Though an uncommon food-borne pathogen, the organism has been associated with brain abscesses in infants fed a dried, powdered infant formula contaminated with the bacteria.

Much remains to be learned about the epidemiology of these food-borne pathogens. As many of them are resident in livestock or the livestock environment, advances in food safety must begin with research into the host-parasite relationships that exists in livestock species under contemporary animal husbandry conditions. For instance, S. gallinarum and S. pullorum have been successfully controlled in the United States because research indicated that the organisms were vertically transmitted and that elimination of these organisms from breeding flocks effectively eliminated the condition in laying and broiler flocks. On the other hand, the newer pathogen, S. enteriditis, though egg-associated, does not appear to be vertically transmitted and is recognized as an environmental contaminant in laying flocks. Therefore control efforts must be aimed at cleaning and disinfection, rodent control, and ongoing monitoring in commercial laying flocks. There are numerous and varied opportunities for veterinarians to get involved, both in research and in clinical settings, to better understand and control food-borne pathogens. The resources listed in Table 9-7 provide more detailed background on food-borne pathogens and offer a larger framework for understanding the challenges that exist in controlling food-borne illness.

Drug Residues and Antibiotic Resistance

The use of drugs, particularly antibiotics, has become an integral part of many intensive, commercial animal-production systems. Antibiotics especially are used for a variety of purposes, including the treatment and prevention of infectious disease, the promotion of growth, and the improvement of feed efficiency. All of these uses are considered cost-effective tools for raising animals profitably. However, the widespread use of antibiotics and other drugs has raised concerns among consumers about the wholesomeness of foods as well as in the public health community concerning human health risks associated with the use of drugs in animal production.

One key public health concern relates to the presence of drug residues in foods derived from animals. When drugs are administered to animals, residues of the drug or its metabolites may persist in various tissues and excretions for variable lengths of time. The amount and duration of persistence depends on a number of factors including the health status of the animal, the species of animal, the metabolic pathways of the drug, its pharmacokinetic distribution, and the dose, formulation, and route of administration. If people consume animal products containing drug residues they may experience a number of adverse effects, though again, many variables influence the potential for an adverse outcome. Possible adverse outcomes of major concern include allergic reactions to drug residues in individuals with drug hypersensitivity or overt clinical effects directly associated with the drug's mode of action.

Antibiotic resistance is another important issue related to the use of antibiotics in animals. This is of direct concern to food-animal producers and veterinarians because it may limit the effectiveness of proven, cost-effective therapies in livestock and poultry. It is a matter of importance to public health officials because of the risk that antibiotic-resistant organisms can complicate or thwart the successful treatment of human patients with bacterial infections. There are two aspects to this problem. First, organisms pathogenic to people can be contained in foods of animal origin, and some may be antibiotic resistant, such as the multiply drug-resistant S. typhimurium DT104 mentioned above. Secondly, antibiotic resistance, often associated with plasmids, can be transferred between organisms, so that exposure to antibiotic-resistant organisms in foods of animal origin can lead to the development of antibiotic resistance in human pathogens not directly derived from animal sources. The inability to control infections with a wide range of antibiotics can lead to greater treatment costs, more-severe disease, and increased mortality.

In the United States, the U.S. Food and Drug Administration (FDA) is the principal agency involved in the regulation of antibiotics and other drugs used in food animals, mainly through its Center for Veterinary Medicine (CVM). Through rigorous, science-based programs, CVM carries out safety and efficacy testing for premarket approval of new veterinary drugs, establishes acceptable withholding times for animals and animal products treated with approved drugs before they can enter the food chain, conducts postmarket surveillance of approved drugs, and carries out compliance activities to ensure proper and legal use of drugs in the field. More details on the CVM and its activities are available on its website at www.fda.gov/cvm/.

The FDA is also increasingly involved in activities related to monitoring and controlling the development of antibiotic resistance. In 1996, for example, the National Antimicrobial Resistance Monitoring System (NARMS) was established. NARMS is a collaborative effort between the CVM, the USDA, and the CDC. As described by the FDA, the NARMS program monitors changes in susceptibilities of human and animal enteric bacteria to 17 antimicrobial drugs. Bacterial isolates are collected from human and animal clinical specimens, healthy farm animals, and raw product from food animals in 17 states around the country. The goals are to provide descriptive data on trends of antimicrobial susceptibility in salmonella and other enteric organisms from human and animal populations, to facilitate the detection of resistance in humans and animals as it arises, and to provide timely information to veterinarians and physicians. The ultimate purpose of these activities is to prolong the life span of approved drugs by promoting prudent and judicious use of antimicrobials and to define areas for more detailed investigation. More information on NARMS and other programs related to antimicrobial resistance such as FoodNet can be obtained from the CDC website at www.cdc.gov/ncidod/dbmd/narms/.

The international scope of contemporary veterinary medicine and the power of modern global communications are well illustrated by recent developments related to drug residues and antibiotic resistance. Incidents that have occurred in Europe have had a notable effect on policymaking in the United States. In the case of drug residues, clenbuterol is an example. The primary clinical use for this beta-agonist drug is to dilate airways in asthma and other obstructive pulmonary diseases, and FDA has approved a syrup formulation of the drug for use in horses with lung disease. However, clenbuterol is also of great interest to beef cattle producers as the drug is a good repartitioning agent that improves lean tissue deposition. When administered to growing beef cattle, more of the animal's weight gain becomes muscle instead of fat. However, clenbuterol has never been approved by the FDA for use in food-producing animals, resulting in some illicit use of the drug. In the mid-1990s, there were several incidents of human illness in Spain, France, and Italy associated with the consumption of calf liver and other food animal products. Affected individuals showed signs consistent with the action of a beta-agonist, including muscle tremors, heart palpitations, nervousness, myalgia, and fever. Clenbuterol was found in calf liver at concentrations of 0.16 to 0.30 ppm. These episodes heightened FDA vigilance concerning the illegal use of clenbuterol in food animals in the United States. An aggressive public education and compliance campaign was undertaken to deter its use, and in 1998, an Oklahoma veterinarian was indicted by a federal grand jury for smuggling $68,000 of clenbuterol into the United States from Canada.

In the case of antibiotic resistance, developments in Europe relative to fluoroquinolone antibiotics again influenced U.S. policy. The fluoroquinolones enrofloxacin, ciprofloxacin, and orbifloxacin represent one of the newer classes of synthetic antibiotics. They have a novel bactericidal mode of action and a very broad spectrum of antimicrobial activity. They are particularly useful in human medicine to treat intractable enteric infections involving drug-resistant bacteria, especially *Salmonella* and *Campylobacter* spp. In 1995, the FDA approved the use of the fluoroquinolone enrofloxacin for use in poultry and, in 1998, approved an injectable form for use in beef cattle with respiratory disease. However, during this same period, public health officials in the Netherlands observed that the approved use of fluoroquinolones in poultry in that country was followed by a significant increase in the number of human and poultry isolates of *Campylobacter* spp. that were resistant to enrofloxacin. A similar pattern was observed in the United Kingdom after enrofloxacin was approved for use in animals there. Scientists and policymakers grew increasingly concerned that drug-resistant bacteria that were developing in poultry and other livestock were contaminating foods of animal origin and transferring enrofloxacin-resistant bacteria to the human population. Physicians and public health officials were greatly concerned about the development of resistance to this new class of drugs that was so important in clinical human medicine. In 1997, the WHO issued a report proposing that the subtherapeutic use of antibiotics in animals be phased out and that antibiotics used to treat human infection should never be used subtherapeutically in animals.

These developments stirred great debate in the United States among veterinary scientists, the pharmaceutical industry, the various animal agriculture industries, public health officials, physicians, and the general public. In August 1997, the CVM formally prohibited the extra-label use of fluoroquinolones in food-producing animals, citing concerns that some extra-label uses of these drugs could increase drug-resistant strains of zoonotic pathogens in food-producing animals at the time of slaughter. In the case of enrofloxacin use in cattle, it was emphasized that the drug was approved only for use in beef cattle for the control of respiratory disease and was not to be used at all in dairy cattle or veal calves. The CVM has vowed to take regulatory action against anyone using these drugs in this extra-label manner. In October 2000, the FDA went a step further and announced plans for a total ban on the use of fluoroquinolones in poultry, including withdrawal of approval on the two fluoroquinolone products already in use..

Other Food-Contaminating Substances

Microbial agents, their toxins, and veterinary drug residues receive considerable attention relative to food safety, but these are not the only agents that can contaminate food. On a global basis, numerous chemical agents pose serious risks to human health through the food supply, which can result in either acute or, more often, chronic disease problems. These agents can enter the food-processing chain at numerous points, from crop and animal production through postharvest processing, handling, and preparation.

Several broad categories of chemical agents can be involved. One major category is agricultural chemicals, including organophosphate or organochloride herbicides and pesticides, and some fertilizers. Another major category is industrial pollutants such as polybrominated biphenyls (PBBs), polychlorinated biphenyls (PCBs) and dioxins. A third important category is heavy metals, such as lead, cadmium, and mercury. Though heavy metal contamination is usually associated with industrial pollutants, heavy metals may be associated with agricultural product use as well. For example, cadmium, an important food contaminant, is found in relative abundance in rock phosphate, a major raw material for agricultural fertilizers.

Agricultural chemicals may be applied directly to animals and crops or to the soil in which food crops grow, and improper use can increase the risk of food contamination. Industrial pollutants are often dispersed into the air and waterways where they end up in soil, are taken up and concentrated by growing plants, and then possibly concentrated even further in the tissues of animals that consume such contaminated crops. Ultimately these contaminants can then enter the human food chain through meat, milk, or eggs. Environmental contamination by agricultural and industrial pollutants and its relation to animal agriculture and human health is discussed further in Chapter 6.

The risk to food safety posed by different chemical agents varies considerably in different countries around the world, based on a number of factors including, among others, the degree of industrialization, the level of economic development, the extent of government regulation of environmental hazards, and cultural differences in food preferences and preparation. Identifying these differences and their impact on food contamination was the focus of an extended international effort through the Global Environment Monitoring System (GEMS), a collaborative effort of the WHO in association with the United Nations Environmental Programme (UNEP), and the FAO. The GEMS-Food Contamination Monitoring and Assessment Programme was established in 1976. The program monitored an established list of food contaminants in a wide range of food commodities and products in selected countries around the world, representing both economically developed and developing nations. The monitoring effort included extensive analytical testing conducted through a global network of WHO Collaborating Centers for Food Contamination Monitoring. The United States participated in the network through the FDA's Center for Food Safety and Applied Nutrition.

In a report published by UNEP, GEMS/Food reported trends in food contamination from data collected over a 17-year period.[33] They concluded that the trend in food contamination in developed countries is generally downward, primarily because of strong governmental regulations that ban or restrict the use of certain toxic chemicals and also because of aggressive measures to reduce lead pollution from motor vehicles and other sources. In the United States, for instance, strict guidelines introduced in the early 1970s led to a reduction in the amount of mercury released into water from 540,000 kg per year to less than 9,000 kg per year within a few years. In contrast, many developing countries, continue to face higher risks of food contamination with chemical agents, as their levels in food remain high. This is due to a failure to ban persistent pesticides, such as the organochlorine DDT, and a general lack of strong governmental regulations or enforcement authority to limit industrial pollutants. GEMS/Food data have also been useful in establishing international standards for tolerance levels of various contaminants in food. More information about the GEMS/Food program is available at http://www.who.int/fsf/gems.htm.

In the United States, three federal agencies share responsibility for keeping foods safe from excessive pesticide residues. The Environmental Protection Agency (EPA) carries out preapproval assessments on the health and environmental effects of new pesticides, reviews and registers older pesticides to ensure that they continue to meet current health and environmental standards, and sets tolerance levels for pesticide residues permissible in the food and feed supply. The USDA's FSIS is responsible for monitoring for pesticide residues in meat, poultry, and egg products. The FDA monitors for residues in feeds and other foods and has enforcement authority to deal with violations. General information about federal government efforts in the area of food safety is available on the internet at http://www.foodsafety.gov/.

Genetically Modified Foods

Advances in molecular biology toward the end of the 20th century have led to the development of genetically modified plants and animals in which genetic material from one species of organism is incorporated into the genome of a target organism to express certain useful characteristics that the target organism does not posses naturally. This transgenic technology has been applied extensively to develop genetically modified plants commonly used as human food and animal feeds. Examples include soybeans tolerant to a specific herbicide, corn and cotton plants that produce bacterial toxins that resist important insect pests, and papayas with a viral gene that makes them resistant to a specific viral infection.

In some cases, a plant's own genes have been manipulated to modify gene expression in ways deemed useful by producers and marketers; for example, genetically altered tomatoes with delayed ripening, which reduces damage or spoilage during transport from farm to market. In the case of animals, exogenous gene constructs have been incorporated into embryos of rabbits, sheep, and goats so that the female animals that mature from these altered embryos can manufacture specific proteins in their mammary gland secretions that can then be extracted from the milk for use as human pharmaceuticals, for example, antithrombin III, an anticlotting agent with clinical application for coronary artery bypass patients. Such transgenic animals have been referred to commonly in the media as "pharm" animals.

While the scientific innovation behind transgenics is undeniably impressive and exciting, the transfer of transgenic technology to the consumer marketplace in the form of genetically modified foods and animal feeds has been fraught with conflict and turmoil on a global scale. The United States has been at the center of this controversy and has served as a mirror reflecting differences in culture and perception about science, trade, power, and choice. Many of the early developments and applications of genetic engineering for agricultural purposes occurred in the United States, largely through the scientific and commercial efforts of private corporations. Most of the early product developments involved innovations primarily directed toward farmers and only indirectly, consumers. Farmer acceptance of transgenic crops was high, and by 2000, it was estimated that more than 40% of American cropland was sown with genetically engineered corn, soybeans, cotton, and other genetically modified crops.

From the beginning, voices in American society expressed concerns about the potential dangers of genetically engineered crops and their use as food and animal feeds. These concerns were associated primarily with the fact that transgenic technology was so new and novel. It was argued that many questions about the safety and long-term implications of its use were not fully investigated and satisfactorily addressed before the genetically modified crops were introduced into the environment. What if herbicide-resistant genes found their way into weed species related to agricultural crops? What if proteins expressed in genetically modified foods functioned as allergens in people eating those foods? What if insect pests targeted by genetically modified crops became resistant to the insecticide expressed by the genetically modified crop plants? Despite these valid concerns, the marketing of genetically modified foods and animal feeds initially met with little resistance in the United States.

According to animal scientist John Hodges, this general acceptance of genetically modified (GM) crops and foods in the United States stemmed in large part from this country's proud historical tradition of government support of science in the name of improved agricultural production through land grant universities and agricultural experiment stations.[14] Despite the fact that GM foods were being developed largely by private corporations, a prevailing trust in agricultural science and the scientists who worked in agriculture largely allayed initial concerns. Hodges points out, however, that the situation was quite different in Europe. The emergence of mad cow disease in the 1980s undermined people's confidence in the wholesomeness of food. When mad cow disease, or BSE, was linked to the fatal human disease vCJD in 1996, public trust in agricultural scientists reached its nadir.

For years, many in the scientific community had reassured the public that BSE was not a risk to human health because no traditional infectious agents were identified with the disease in

cattle. This turned out to be a grave misjudgment of the potential "infectivity" for humans of the prion protein responsible for BSE, which was, at the time, not well understood. When it became clear to Europeans that GM foods and animal feeds from the United States were entering Europe with no identifying labels to distinguish them from non-GM foods, there was a powerful and widespread public backlash, fueled in part by understandable fears about what dangers might be lurking in these GM products and in part by anger at the United States for the perceived arrogance of introducing these products into European markets without any identifying features. When American producers countered that the GM foods were safe and virtually indistinguishable from non-GM foods, this only added to consumer skepticism. If there were no discernible differences in quality or price, then why were corporations tampering with the genome? Why were the products not clearly labeled, thus denying the traditional right of consumers to choose in the marketplace?

Resistance to GM foods also emerged in developing countries, for somewhat different reasons. Many developing countries, with a long and painful history of colonization, harbored longstanding resentments against the economic and political hegemony of powerful western nations. These countries were skeptical of the claims by American transgenic seed manufacturers that their products heralded a new green revolution that would create abundant harvests to feed the rapidly growing populations of the world's poorest nations. This skepticism turned to outright cynicism when it became clear that American corporations were seeking to market seeds containing transgenic genes known as terminator genes that prevented harvested seed from germinating unless treated with a chemical sold by the same company that sold the seed. In the subsistence farming systems of developing countries, it is fundamental practice for farmers to hold back seed from each harvest to plant the following year. The notion that cash-poor farmers would not be able to sow GM seed without purchasing a new supply each year or buying the chemical to activate the old seed was seen as both rapacious and repressive. When it was revealed that the USDA held a joint patent with one company on its terminator gene, this only strengthened the conviction in developing countries that GM crops were a tool for the United States government and business interests to exert their control and domination of agricultural production and markets worldwide. In response to the revelation about the USDA, India ordered that no seeds with terminator genes could be imported into the country.

Debate about GM foods remains heated and is becoming increasingly polarized. Violent demonstrations at international trade meetings, such as the Ministerial Conference of the WTO in Seattle in December 1999 have, at least in part, been catalyzed by the GM foods issue, with protesters seeking to block international trade in GM foods. For its part, the United States has, to a large extent, framed the GM foods debate as a trade issue, suggesting that refusal of other countries to accept GM foods on safety grounds is in fact a nontariff barrier to free trade. At this writing, the situation remains largely unresolved.

The matter of GM food is likely to remain in the headlines for some time to come. The issue will become increasingly important to veterinarians as transgenic technology is applied more broadly to livestock and foods of animal origin. Veterinary and animal scientists are involved in a wide range of potential applications of genetic modification such as incorporation of disease resistance, accelerated growth characteristics, and modification of marketing characteristics such as leaner meat, higher protein and reduced fat in milk, or the addition of vitamins. Veterinarians must learn from the GM food debate thus far. For transgenic science to be deemed acceptable, scientists must be transparent about their work, and they must take cultural, political, and economic considerations into account when determining which transgenic products to develop and where to market them.

Welfare of Animals Raised for Food

Societal concern about the welfare of animals is not a new phenomenon. The United States, a young nation by European standards, has a strong tradition of concern for the well-being of animals, the American Society for the Prevention of Cruelty to Animals having been founded in 1866. Concerns about the welfare of farm animals, however, came into sharp focus in the mid-1970s with publication of the book, *Animal Liberation*.[29] The book received wide attention and, in the context of the present discussion, it had two significant results. First, the book focused a predominantly urban public's attention on the husbandry practices of modern intensive animal agriculture systems and projected the view that by and large, animals managed in these so-called factory farms suffered inhumane treatment. Second, the book publicized author Peter Singer's notion of "speciesism" as a form of discrimination, suggesting that animals have rights on a level with those of humans.

The net result was that for a considerable segment of society, the concept of animal rights became intertwined with the historical concept of animal welfare, and a new era of activism concerning the well-being of animals emerged. For better or for worse, depending on your point of view, this activism has focused an intense spotlight on the practices of modern animal agriculture. Nevertheless, farm animals in the United States remain, in the legal sense, property. The principal federal law governing the treatment of animals is the Animal Welfare Act, passed by Congress in 1966 and subsequently strengthened through amendments in 1970, 1976, 1985, and 1990. The Animal Welfare Act requires that minimum standards of care and treatment be provided for certain animals bred for commercial sale, used in research, transported commercially, or exhibited to the public. However, to date, the Animal Welfare Act still exempts farm animals used for food, fiber, or other agricultural purposes from its jurisdiction. There is also no federal law regulating modern truck transportation of livestock, since the so-called 28-hour law of 1906 applies to railway and barge transport only.

In Europe, by contrast, protections for farm animals are more explicitly and formally acknowledged. In 1976, the member states of the Council of Europe (www.coe.int) signed the European Convention for the Protection of Animals Kept for Farming Purposes. This agreement applies specifically to animals in modern intensive stock-farming systems and requires that "animals shall be housed and provided with food, water and care in a manner which—having regard to their species and to their degree of development, adaptation and domestication—is appropriate to their physiological and ethological needs in accordance with established experience and scientific knowledge."

Even with this convention in place, animal welfare activism remained intense in Europe through the 1990s, and in 1997, acknowledging popular sentiment, the 15 member states of the EU agreed to a legally binding annex to the original treaty that established the EU. This new Protocol on the Protection and Welfare of Animals specifically refers to animals as sentient beings and commits the EU to pay full regard to the welfare requirements of animals when formulating and implementing community policies on agriculture, transport, research, and internal trade. Thus, animal welfare became a legitimate issue in matters of trade relating to livestock. In 1998, the animal welfare group Compassion in World Farming (www.ciwf.co.uk/) challenged the right of the British government to export veal calves to continental Europe because of the conditions under which those calves were raised after leaving the UK. The case was heard in the European Court and it was determined that Britain would be acting illegally if it imposed a unilateral ban on veal calf exports. At the time of the ruling, the issue was moot, as all cattle exports from the UK had been banned as a result of BSE. However, before the ban, the UK exported over one half million calves per year to Holland, Belgium, France, and Italy. Activists hoped to have a ban on veal calf exports in place for that future time when export prohibitions related to BSE were lifted.

Public concerns about the welfare of farm animals are being registered not only in the courtrooms, but in the marketplace. Ultimately the buying habits of consumers may have the greatest influence on what forms of animal husbandry are acceptable in society. Traditionally, Americans have been content to have access to an abundant and diverse supply of good food at low cost and have not been very concerned about the details of how such food is produced. However, activism concerning animal welfare has gained considerable momentum in the United States, and animal agriculture in recent years has found itself on the defensive. The power of the animal welfare constituency to influence the marketplace could not be better illustrated than by the recent actions of McDonald's Corporation, the largest and best-known food service retailer in the world, with more than 28,000 restaurants serving more than 43 million people a day in 120 countries. In August 2000, McDonald's announced that it would require producers who supply it with 1.5 billion eggs annually to adopt more humane methods of raising hens. Specifically, McDonald's is requiring suppliers to house hens in cages at least 465 cm^2 (72 in^2) per bird, to terminate forced molting by withdrawing feed and water, and to follow their scientific guidelines for the practice of debeaking.

Even though McDonald's accounts for only 2% of the table egg market in the United States, the fact that a company as visible as the leading hamburger giant would take a corporate stand on animal welfare issues for laying hens indicates the extent to which animal welfare concerns have become integrated into mainstream American society. Producers are feeling compelled to respond. The United Egg Producers, for instance, the leading industry group representing egg producers, convened a scientific advisory committee for animal welfare in 1999 to develop industry guidelines for animal welfare based on the best scientific information available and to identify areas in which additional scientific information is required to determine if current practices are consistent or inconsistent with welfare concerns. This pattern is being repeated in the swine and cattle industries as well, and opportunities for veterinarians to participate in efforts to improve and verify animal welfare in food-producing animals will continue to expand significantly for years to come. When Burger King announced in January 2001 that it too was instituting its own program to ensure the humane treatment of food animals by its suppliers, the corporation cited several sets of guidelines developed by producer groups to address animal welfare including the Good Management Practices of the American Meat Institute for handling and stunning cattle and swine, the Animal Husbandry Guidelines for U.S. Egg Laying Flocks of the United Egg Producers, and the Animal Welfare Guidelines for Broilers of the American Chicken Council.

International Trade and Food Safety

The sources and diversity of foods available in the United States has increased dramatically in the last 20 years. Previously seasonal foods are now available year round, brought in from distant countries where local climate allows off-season production not possible at home. As a result of expanded international trade, exotic fruits previously enjoyed only while on vacation in the tropics are now routinely available in the local supermarket, as are regional gourmet foods like French goat cheese, goose liver pate, and perhaps the most unique regional food in the world, the Australian concentrated yeast extract, Vegemite. Foods that were once costly and reserved for special occasions, such as shrimp and smoked salmon, are now routinely consumed at moderate prices due to global expansion of aquaculture and dramatic increases in imports.

Currently, more than half of all seafood, one third of fresh fruits, and 12% of all fresh vegetables eaten in America come from abroad. Some 70% of the fruits and vegetables imported into the United States pass through the winter produce port of Nogales, Arizona. In recent years, the local American supermarket has been transformed into an exotic, international bazaar, and the same wary caution that a nervous tourist might exercise about food poisoning before sitting down to a meal in a foreign land is now considered by some observers and critics to be equally justified here at home. This skeptical view of the risk of food-borne disease in the United States was bolstered by several severe food-related disease outbreaks in the country in the 1990s involving imported foods. These included the aforementioned outbreak of *Cyclospora* enteritis linked to

raspberries imported from Guatemala in 1996, which affected 1450 people; an outbreak of hepatitis A in 1997 linked to frozen strawberries imported from Mexico, which involved 270 people in five states; an outbreak of gastroenteritis due to *Salmonella enterica* serotype *Newport* in a shipment of alfalfa sprout seeds imported from the Netherlands in 1995, which sickened more than 130 people in Oregon and British Columbia; and an outbreak of gastroenteritis due to *Salmonella poona* traced to cantaloupes imported from Mexico in 1991, which affected 400 people in 23 states and Canada.

These events and others involving imported foods focused national attention on the structure and function of the federal programs in place to monitor and inspect imported foods and prompted policy reviews and legislative actions to make inspection of imported foods more efficient, science-based, and uniform. In 1998, two key reports were issued. The first, produced by the U.S. General Accounting Office (GAO), looked specifically at the federal government's efforts to ensure the safety of imported foods. The report found that in general, the overall effort was inconsistent and unreliable and that the federal agencies involved cannot ensure that the growing volume of imported foods is safe for consumers.

The GAO noted a significant discrepancy between the practices of the two key agencies involved in the regulation of imported foods, the FSIS, which has jurisdiction over meat, poultry, and some egg products, and the FDA, which regulates all other categories of imported foods. The FSIS places the burden for product safety on the exporting countries by allowing imports only from those countries with food safety systems that it deems to be equivalent to the U.S. system. FSIS has such equivalency agreements with about 37 countries and may periodically inspect meat-processing facilities in these countries to ensure that they continue to meet equivalency standards for importation to the United States.

In contrast, the FDA lacks such legal authority. As a result, it allows food imports from almost any country and takes on the burden of ensuring the safety of imported foods as they arrive at U.S. ports. To accomplish this, port-of-entry inspections are conducted. However, the GAO deemed such port-of-entry inspections ineffective for three reasons: (1) port-of-entry inspections do not guarantee that foods are produced under adequately controlled conditions, (2) FDA inspected less than 2% of all foreign shipments, and (3) some organisms of concern (e.g., *Cyclospora*) are not amenable to detection through inspection. In addition, GAO concluded that the FDA's procedures for ensuring that unsafe imported foods do not reach U.S. consumers are vulnerable to abuse by unscrupulous importers. In the case of both FSIS and FDA, the report also noted that inspection resources are not targeted at the imported foods posing the greatest risk of danger as determined by scientific, risk-based analysis.

A second report on food safety, mandated by Congress in 1997, was released in 1998. This detailed study on the system of food safety in the United States addressed both domestic and imported food products. The study was carried out by the National Research Council in conjunction with the Institute of Medicine. A panel of experts, which included two distinguished veterinarians, Dr. Lonnie King of Michigan State University and Dr. Harley Moon of Iowa State University, was convened to undertake the study. Their report, *Ensuring Safe Food: From Production to Consumption* (see Table 9-7), like the GAO report, identified a number of problems with the current food safety system.

While the overall standard of food quality assurance in the United States must be considered comparatively high in an international context, there is considerable room for improvement. The current safety system is a patchwork quilt of laws and multiagency participation assembled over the past century in reaction to ongoing changes in the nation's food supply. At least 12 primary federal agencies plus numerous additional subagencies are involved in the overall food safety system along with myriad state and local agencies such as departments of agriculture and public health (Fig. 9-3). Responsibilities are divided among a complex

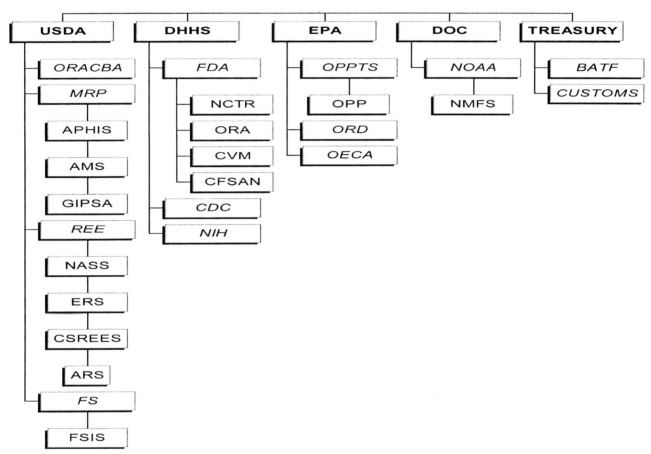

AMS - Agricultural Marketing Service
APHIS - Animal and Plant Health Inspection Service
ARS - Agricultural Research Service
BATF - Bureau of Alcohol, Tobacco and Firearms
CDC - Centers for Disease Control and Prevention
CFSAN - Center for Food Safety and Applied Nutrition
CSREES - Cooperative State Research, Education, and Extension Service
CUSTOMS - United States Customs Service
CVM - Center for Veterinary Medicine
DHHS - United States Department of Health and Human Services
DOC - United States Department of Commerce
EPA - United States Environmental Protection Agency
ERS - Economic Research Service
FDA - Food and Drug Administration
FSIS - Food Safety and Inspection Service
FS - Under Secretary for Food Safety

GIPSA - Grain Inspection, Packers and Stockyards Administration
MRP - Under Secretary for Marketing and Regulatory Programs
NASS - National Agricultural Statistics Service
NCTR - National Center for Toxicological Research
NIH - National Institutes of Health
NMFS - National Marine Fisheries Service
NOAA - National Oceanic and Atmospheric Administration
OECA - Office of Enforcement and Compliance Assistance
OPP - Office of Pesticide Programs
OPPTS - Office of Prevention, Pesticides, and Toxic Substances
ORA - Office of Regulatory Affairs
ORCABA - Office of Risk Assessment and Cost-Benefit Analysis
ORD - Office of Research and Development
REE - Under Secretary for Research, Education and Economics
TREASURY - United States Department of Treasury
USDA - United States Department of Agriculture

Figure 9-3. The fragmented character of the national food safety system in the United States is highlighted by this schematic listing of the federal United States Government agencies involved in food safety. The particular functions, responsibilities and authorities of each agency are discussed in the report *Ensuring Safe Food: From Production to Consumption.* Washington, DC: National Academy Press, 1998. (Full text available on the internet at www.nap.edu/catalog/6163.html?onpi_newsdoc082098)

number of categories, allowing both overlaps and gaps in authority. The main categories include

- Source of food (domestic or foreign)
- Commodity type (meat, dairy, eggs, seafood, fruits and vegetables, grain staples)
- Contaminant type (pesticides, drug residues, food-borne pathogens)
- Function (monitoring and surveillance, risk assessment, research, inspection and enforcement, outbreak management, and education)

The report concluded that outdated food safety laws and a fragmented federal structure serve as barriers to improving protection of the nation's food supply from contamination or other hazards and proposed a number of key recommendations:

- *The food safety system should be based on science.* Given the limited resources available to address safety issues, regulatory priorities and activities should be determined by strong scientific evidence that aims at prevention of food contamination and food-borne illness. Risk assessment should serve as the scientific basis for identifying and addressing the greatest threats to food safety, including microbiological pathogens, naturally occurring toxins, allergens, food additives, agricultural chemicals, environmental contaminants, animal drug residues, and improper methods of handling and preparing food. The Hazard Analysis and Critical Control Point (HACCP) monitoring system is identified as an important tool for science-based regulation of food safety. The principles of HAACP should be applied at every phase in the food-production process to determine at which steps food contamination is likely to occur and block it before it happens. HACCP is discussed in more detail later in this chapter.

- *The food safety system should be unified and centralized.* Congress should establish a unified, central framework to manage food safety programs, headed by one official with control of resources for all federal food safety activities. This person would be responsible for management of food-borne disease outbreaks, setting standards for food safety, inspection, monitoring, disease surveillance, risk assessment, regulation enforcement, research, and education. Several other industrialized nations, including Canada, Great Britain, Denmark, and Ireland have recently consolidated their organizational responsibilities for

food safety activities either in response to public concerns about food-borne illness or to promote effectiveness and cost savings. As different structural and administrative approaches were developed in each country, their experiences offer useful models for revamping the United States system.

- *The legal framework for food safety should reflect a science-based approach.* Congress should change federal statutes so that inspection, research, and enforcement are based on scientifically supportable assessments of risk. Some safety statutes are outmoded and represent inefficient use of resources. For example, the visual (organoleptic) inspection system for meat and poultry may actually detract from protection efforts by diverting resources from implementation of science-based inspection reforms such as the design, implementation, and enforcement of HAACP monitoring systems at slaughterhouses and processing plants. At a minimum, Congress should no longer require inspection of each animal carcass, as required by laws controlling meat and poultry inspection. Congress should also mandate that foods be imported only from countries with food inspection systems deemed equivalent to that of the United States.

- *A comprehensive national food-safety plan should be developed.* The plan should support research aimed at prevention and detection of risks and include surveillance activities to identify new risks as food supply or consumption patterns change. Federal efforts should be better integrated with state and local activities. Any such plan should recognize and address America's increasing use of imported foods and the distinctive hazards associated with them.

New Tools for Managing Food Safety

The increasing intensification of animal-production systems, the trend toward centralization of food processing and manufacturing activities, and the expansion of international trade in food products dictate the need for new tools to ensure the safety of foods of animal origin in the global marketplace. Such tools are already being developed and successfully applied. Some of these tools represent conceptual innovations; others represent technical advances, as discussed below.

Conceptual Advances

Conceptual tools include new approaches to managing risk in food production, food processing and distribution, and international trade. The cornerstone of all these new approaches is science-based risk management. In the area of food production, producer quality assurance programs are being developed to reduce the risk of food contamination while animals and animal products are still on the farm. HACCP plans represent an approach to detecting and controlling food contamination during processing. Equivalency is a means of ensuring adequate management of food safety in the arena of international trade.

Producer Quality Assurance Programs Producer quality assurance programs are voluntary efforts coordinated mainly through livestock commodity trade associations to promote on-farm practices among their members that advance the goal of food safety and increase consumer confidence in foods of animal origin. The initial impetus for quality assurance programs, which began about 20 years ago, was regulatory concern about a high frequency of violative antibiotic residues in meat and milk. Industry groups, acknowledging consumer discomfort with residues and wary of the risk of stricter regulation, began to develop producer awareness, training, and certification programs under the rubric of quality assurance, to reduce the occurrence of drug residues in foods of animal origin.

Over the years, quality assurance programs have been broadened to respond to a wide range of evolving consumer concerns and may now include efforts aimed at controlling preharvest contamination with zoonotic pathogens, enhancing animal welfare, and improving environmental stewardship.

Quality assurance programs are designed to devise and implement proactive intervention strategies to enhance the quality and consumer acceptance of farm products in a manner that is cost-effective to the producer and that provides a competitive edge in the marketplace. From the veterinary perspective, these programs extend the concept of herd health management beyond maintaining the health of animals primarily for the economic benefit of the farmer, to include the expanded goal of maintaining the health and well-being of the public at large who consume foods of animal origin. Table 9-8 presents a list of quality assurance programs currently in operation for various producer groups in the United States. Kla and Tollefson have recently reviewed the role of quality assurance programs in overall food safety efforts and provide details about such programs involving swine, cattle, and poultry products.[18]

Veterinarians play a central role in the development, implementation, and monitoring of quality assurance programs. Commodity groups call on veterinary expertise to identify production problems, evaluate risks, and aid in the development of interventions and practices aimed at reducing those risks. These are frequently referred to as *best management practices* (BMPs) or *good production practices* (GPPs). Veterinarians may also be involved in creating training materials for producers participating in quality assurance programs and conduct such training programs. Once programs are established in the field, veteri-

Table 9-8 Producer Quality Assurance Programs in the United States[a]		
Program Name	**Sponsoring Organization**	**Further Information**
Pork Quality Assurance	National Pork Producers Council	http://www.porkboard.org/Prod/Pqa/pqa.html
Beef Quality Assurance	National Cattlemen's Beef Association	http://www.bqa.org/
Milk and Dairy Beef Residue Prevention Protocol	National Milk Producers Federation	http://www.dqacenter.org/
Veal Quality Assurance Certification Program	American Veal Association	http://www.vealfarm.com/vqa/
New York State Cattle Health Assurance Program	Cornell University and the NY State Department of Agriculture and Markets	http://nyschap.vet.cornell.edu/
5-Star Total Quality Assurance Food Safety Program	United Egg Producers	http://www.unitedegg.org/uep5star.htm
Quality Assured Farm Raised Finfish and Shellfish	National Aquaculture Association	http://www.natlaquaculture.org/QA.htm
Trout Producer Quality Assurance Program	US Trout Farmers Association	http://www.ustfa.org/industry/quality.html
Catfish Quality Assurance Program	Catfish Farmers of America	http://msucares.com/aquaculture/catfish/qualityassurance.html

[a]Many of these programs are coordinated nationally but managed on a state-by-state basis, so information relevant to local industry conditions and local training programs may be available from state producer groups, agricultural universities, veterinary schools, extension services, or regulatory agencies. See, for example, the New York State program listed in the table. Some programs are structured to actually certify participating producers. Others provide information to producers on best management practices and quality assurance but do not have a formal certification program.

nary practitioners work closely with producers to help implement the program on their premises. This involves on-site evaluation of the farm and its activities, and development of a farm management plan. For programs that involve certification of producer compliance, the local veterinarian may be the person responsible for validating that the farmer is faithfully carrying out the quality assurance program. Almost all industry quality assurance programs require that the producer establish and maintain a bona fide client-veterinarian-patient relationship with a practicing veterinarian.

There are also numerous research challenges related to quality assurance programs, as the risk factors for certain emerging food-borne pathogens are not fully elucidated. Veterinarians must participate in epidemiological studies to determine these risk factors so that appropriate prophylactic measures and management interventions can be established. For instance, when multiple-drug-resistant S. typhimurium DT104 began to show up in food animals in Great Britain, researchers carried out epidemiological studies on farms to identify risk factors associated with occurrence of the organism and disease in cattle. Hollinger et al. identified several factors that increased risk of disease occurrence.[15] These included cattle passing through the premises of cattle dealers, introduction of newly purchased cattle into existing herds, confinement housing of cattle, lack of an isolation facility on the farm, and access by wild birds and cats to feed stores. This research suggests that maintaining a closed herd, raising all replacement animals on the premises, and screening feed stores would be appropriate management factors not only to reduce the occurrence of S. typhimurium within the herd, but also to reduce the risk that foods derived from these animals would be contaminated with the organism. Such analysis and action serves as the basis of quality assurance programs to improve food safety.

Hazard Analysis Critical Control Points (HACCP)   In the early 1960s, in collaboration with the Pillsbury Company and the U.S. Army Natick Laboratories, the National Aeronautics and Space Administration (NASA) developed a revolutionary quality control program to ensure food safety on NASA manned space missions and to reduce the chance of product defects entering the commercial food chain. This quality control program has been widely adopted in the food-processing industry and has come to be known as the HACCP system. The thrust of the HACCP system applied to food safety is to prevent contamination of foods throughout the food production chain, rather than to detect it after it occurs, as has been done under traditionally prevailing food safety inspection systems. Implementation of a HACCP system involves adherence to seven basic principles. While the particulars will vary among food-production systems and the products processed, the seven principles are universally applicable. Hogue et al. describe them as follows[16]:

- **Conduct a hazard analysis.** All potential hazards associated with the production of a particular food product are assessed. A comprehensive HACCP system encompasses the entire food production chain from farm to table and, therefore, producer quality-assurance programs, as discussed above, can and should use HACCP principles in establishing best-management practices for the farm operation. In addition, HACCP is applied to processing, manufacturing, distribution, marketing, and preparation for consumption of the food.

- **Identify critical control points.** In any food production process, there are elements, steps, or procedures at which some form of control can be applied and, as a result, a food safety hazard can be eliminated, prevented, or reduced to a tolerated level. Tolerable levels must be scientifically determined based on analysis of risk.

- **Establish critical limits for each critical control point.** Each critical control point will require interventions or measures that must be properly controlled to ensure the prevention, tolerable reduction, or elimination of the hazard(s) identified. Each preventive measure will have critical limits associated with it that serve as boundaries of safety for each critical control point. Such critical limits must be scientifically established.

- **Establish critical control point monitoring requirements.** Regular monitoring activities are necessary to ensure that the process is properly managed at each of the critical control points identified and that possible deviations are recognized in a timely fashion.

- **Establish corrective actions.** These are actions taken when monitoring indicates a deviation from an established critical limit.

- **Establish record-keeping procedures.** Adequate, structured, systematic records must be kept to document that the HACCP plan is established and clearly defined. Data related to monitoring must also be maintained to document that critical limits remain within boundaries, that verification activities are carried out, and that processing deviations are being handled appropriately.

- **Establish procedures for verifying that the HACCP system is working as intended.** Validation ensures that the critical control points and associated critical limits are adequate and sufficient to control likely hazards. Verification ensures that the HACCP plan is functioning acceptably with the intended result of ensuring food safety.

The FSIS Final Rule As mentioned earlier in the chapter, there was a large *E. coli* O157:H7 disease outbreak in the northwestern United States in 1993, associated with contaminated ground beef served at a fast-food restaurant chain. The negative publicity surrounding this disease outbreak prompted a strong governmental response. The USDA FSIS undertook a major effort to revamp the national food-safety inspection process. The result, initiated in 1996, was "The Final Rule on Pathogen Reduction and Hazard Analysis and Critical Control Point (HACCP) Systems." Implementation of the Final Rule has been phased in over several years. Very small slaughter and processing plants, defined as having fewer than 10 employees or less than $2.5 million in sales, were given until January 2000 to come into compliance.

Under the Final Rule, all slaughter and processing plants are required to adopt the HACCP system. To verify that HACCP systems are effective in reducing contamination with harmful bacteria, FSIS set pathogen-reduction performance standards that slaughter plants and plants that produce raw ground meat and poultry must meet in regard to *Salmonella* spp. In addition, slaughter plants are required to conduct microbial testing for generic *E. coli*, to verify that their process-control systems are working as intended to prevent fecal contamination, which is recognized as the primary avenue of contamination of carcasses by harmful bacteria during slaughter. FSIS has also required plants to adopt and follow written standard operating procedures (SOPs) for sanitation, to reduce the likelihood that harmful bacteria will contaminate the finished product. These SOPs apply to all daily sanitation procedures that a facility would carry out, such as cleaning equipment, food handling, and the personal hygiene of working staff.

The FSIS decision to implement HACCP at slaughterhouses and meat-processing plants was intended to accomplish a number of goals:

- Shift the emphasis of FSIS safeguarding activities from detection of contamination to its prevention
- Use risk assessment principles to improve the likelihood of identifying sources of contamination and controlling them
- Focus scarce inspection resources in areas of greater risk potential
- Adjust to the new reality that greater numbers of animals are being slaughtered and processed in progressively fewer and larger establishments

While the Final Rule has the ultimate objective of improving food safety, it also serves to enhance America's competitive position in the international trade in foods of animal origin. As discussed earlier, the GATT requires that countries ensure that their sanitary measures are based on science and use principles of risk assessment. Adoption of the HACCP system, establishment of performance standards with verification mechanisms, and careful documentation of SOPs help the United States objectively demonstrate a high level of science-based protection for food safety that meets or exceeds foreign equivalency requirements.

The Codex Alimentarius Commission and Food Safety The Codex Alimentarius Commission, generally referred to as the Codex, was established in 1962 by the WHO and the FAO to develop international food standards to protect consumer health and to facilitate fair trading practices in foods. This was done in part to rationalize the prevailing, chaotic, and ineffective system involving over 135 different organizations working on various aspects of international food standards. When the Agreement on the Application of Sanitary and Phytosanitary Measures was formulated and adopted by the new WTO in 1995 (see section on the SPS agreement, earlier in this chapter), the Codex Alimentarius Commission was designated the international reference organization for health and safety measures relating to trade in food. While individual nations may seek to impose higher standards than are spelled out by the Codex, the commission's standards represent the acceptable minimum. Today, 165 nations participate in the Codex and essentially agree to abide by its standards.

The Codex Alimentarius itself, as the Latin name indicates, is a food code. The commission administrating this code consists of 21 designated committees that focus on different areas of food safety such as food labeling, food additives and contaminants, pesticide residues, veterinary drug residues, analytical and sampling methods, and inspection systems. It also includes committees addressing specific commodity groupings such as fish and fishery products, fats and oils, milk and milk products, and meat. There are also task forces dealing with special issues such as foods derived from biotechnology, and there are five regional coordinating committees for Asia, Europe, Africa, Latin America/Caribbean, and North America/South West Pacific. More information about the commission, its functions, and details of the standards of the food code are available on the internet at http://www.codexalimentarius.net/. Today, the Codex has become, as its website declares, "the single most important international reference point for developments associated with food standards."

One aspect of the Codex of particular interest to the veterinary profession and the veterinary pharmaceutical industry are issues related to the use of veterinary drugs in animals and animal products entering international trade as food. The Codex Committee on Residues for Veterinary Drugs in Foods (CCRVDF) addresses concerns in this area. Among the responsibilities of the CCRVDF are to:

- Determine priorities for the consideration of residues of veterinary drugs in food
- Recommend acceptable maximum residue levels (MRLs) of such substances
- Develop codes of practice as may be required, e.g., in the manufacture and administration of drugs

- Determine criteria for analytical methods used for the control of veterinary drug residues in food
- Develop risk-analysis policy for veterinary drugs
- Provide a coordinating role in developing a policy on antimicrobial resistance

Thompson presents a good overview of the activities of the CCRVDF and provides insight into the workings of the Codex in setting veterinary standards, using the controversial drug recombinant bovine somatotrophin as an example.[31] This article also provides a good discussion of the important international trade issue, harmonization of technical requirements for registration of veterinary medical products. As pharmaceutical companies become multinational and expand their marketing efforts into an increasing number of countries, they often encounter a paralyzing array of variable and inconsistent standards for acceptance of drugs into different national markets. The harmonization effort described by Thompson seeks to address this problem and underscores the international complexities of doing business in the global village.

Technical Advances

Conceptual advances such as HACCP, risk analysis, and international standard-setting aimed at improving food safety have been accompanied by technical advances that provide new tools for quality control. These tools fall into two main categories: techniques for improved detection of food contaminants and new techniques for reduction of contaminants. In the latter category, irradiation of food has been a focus of controversy.

Tools for Detection of Contaminants Two key concerns in food safety are antibiotic residues and bacterial contaminants of foods of animal origin. Traditional methods of antibiotic assay and bacterial culture are generally costly and time consuming. Real time results that allow decision-making and corrective action during food production and processing have been needed and, increasingly, are available. On the farm, for instance, there are now simple, one-step test kits available that producers can use to determine if β-lactam-associated antibiotic residues in meat have been cleared, which use a few drops of the animal's urine. Similarly, dairy farmers have quick cowside tests that indicate rapidly if antibiotic residues have been cleared in milk.

A variety of assays have been developed to detect bacterial contamination of meat during slaughter and processing, which can provide answers from within 10 minutes to 24 hours. These assays fall into two main groups, depending on their foundation technology. One group contains antibody-based immunoassays to detect bacterial antigens. Techniques used include latex agglutination, immunoprecipitation, enzyme-linked immunosorbant assay (ELISA), immunodiffusion, immunosensors, and immunomagnetic separation. The other group contains nucleic acid-based assays such as DNA probes, polymerase chain reaction, and ligase chain reaction, which rely on the uniqueness of the pathogen's DNA or rRNA for identification.

Tools for Reduction of Contaminants Competitive exclusion represents a new technical approach to reducing pathogen loads in animals in the preharvest phase of food production. For instance, treatment with a bacterial culture that contains normal bacteria from the intestinal tract of adult chickens can protect newly hatched chicks from antibiotic-resistant salmonella. A similar product given to day-old chicks not only reduces salmonella excretion in chickens, but also reduces Clostridium perfringens in the gut, thus lowering the risk of necrotic enteritis and offering the possibility of eliminating the use of antibiotics in the feed usually required to control this disease. Competitive exclusion is also being evaluated in cattle for reduction of harmful E. coli O157:H7 by inoculation of the rumen with nonpathogenic strains of E. coli.

Postharvest technologies for reducing pathogen contamination span a variety of approaches, including chemical baths, rinses, or sprays. Low-concentration chlorine baths or trisodium phosphate sprays or dips are being used to eliminate bacteria during poultry processing. Ozone, which has been used for water treatment and sanitation for over a century is now being used in food processing as a food safety technique. After the cryptosporidiosis outbreak in Milwaukee in 1993, the city shifted from chlorine water purification to ozone purification, as cryptosporidia proved to be chlorine resistant. Similarly, in food-processing applications, ozone may cover a broader range of pathogens than chlorine.

Irradiation has emerged as a new and important approach to postharvest decontamination, but not without controversy. While the scientific community in general supports irradiation as safe and effective when properly conducted and monitored, there is a notable level of discomfort among consumers about using radiation as part of routine food processing. It has already been 20 years since the WHO concluded that irradiation of food up to an overall dose of 10 kiloGray (kGy) produced no toxicological hazard and introduced no special nutritional or microbiological problems. The USDA has permitted the irradiation of poultry since 1992. In 1997, the FDA approved irradiation for red meat in the United States, and in 1999, the USDA established rules for irradiation that went into effect in February 2000. The text of this USDA final rule on irradiation of meat food products is on the internet at http://www.fsis.usda.gov/OPPDE/ rdad/FR-Pubs/97-076F.htm. Irradiation of food to improve food safety is endorsed by the Codex Alimentarius Commission, the American Medical Association, the American Dietetic Association and health officials in over 40 countries worldwide.

Contemporary thinking about food safety emphasizes that science-based evaluation of risk must be applied at every point in the production chain from the farm to the table. There are opportunities for veterinary participation every step of the way. Practitioners must encourage farmers to see themselves not just as livestock producers, but also as food marketers and then work with farmers to develop best-management practices that reduce the risk of food contamination. Veterinarians must also be involved in the research and development of new technologies for enhancing food safety. Perhaps most importantly, veterinarians must take an active role in government and industry to ensure that policy decisions regarding livestock production and food processing are informed by sound scientific thinking and practices.

Foreign Animal Disease Control in the United States

Animal agriculture is a vital component of the nation's social and economic fabric. Keeping foreign animal diseases out of the United States is essential to maintaining a vigorous and prosperous animal industry. Failure to prevent the incursion of foreign animal disease can have tremendous economic and social consequences. It is estimated, for instance, that a large FMD outbreak confined to California alone could have overall economic consequences of $13.5 billion for the state, including costs of disease control, production losses, impact on the state economy, and loss of trade.[6] It would also affect the price and availability of food and would seriously disrupt the livelihoods of people and communities, even those only indirectly linked to the beef, dairy, and swine industries.

The task of controlling foreign animal disease and preventing such catastrophes falls primarily upon the veterinary community. That foreign animal disease control remains an important and challenging priority in the United States was evidenced in the recent past by the unexplained occurrence of an outbreak of exotic rabbit calicivirus in Iowa in 2000 and the introduction of West Nile Virus into the northeastern United States in 1999. West Nile virus is a significant, vector-borne, zoonotic agent affecting humans, horses, and birds that continues to spread through the eastern half of the country at the time of this writing.

In earlier sections of this chapter, factors leading to an increased risk of foreign animal disease are discussed and key agencies involved in preventing the introduction of foreign animal disease are identified. The following discussion specifically address the mechanisms by which a foreign animal disease is detected and controlled if it does gain entry into the United States.

History of Disease Control in the United States

Organized, government-supported, science-based animal-disease control efforts emerged in Europe in the mid-19th century. Great Britain established a state veterinary service in 1865 in response to an ongoing rinderpest crisis. In the United States, the Bureau of Animal Industry (BAI) was created by act of Congress in May 1884, and Dr. Daniel Elmer Salmon became its first chief. The need to control contagious bovine pleuropneumonia in the United States gave major impetus to a reluctant Congress to support the creation of the bureau (see sidebar in Chapter 8 "A brief history of CBPP Control in the United States and Africa"). However, Congress's favorable decision was ultimately rewarded by a string of BAI successes in animal disease control.

Overall, the BAI and its successor agency, the USDA/APHIS, have successfully eliminated 13 serious livestock and poultry diseases from the United States, including contagious bovine pleuropneumonia, FMD, fowl plague, glanders, dourine, Texas cattle fever, vesicular exanthema, screwworms, Venezuelan equine encephalitis, sheep scabies, exotic Newcastle disease, classical swine fever (hog cholera), and highly pathogenic avian influenza. Currently, ongoing programs for the eradication of bovine brucellosis and bovine tuberculosis are nearing successful completion, and considerable progress is being made on the elimination of swine pseudorabies. These and other significant milestones in the history of BAI/APHIS are provided in Table 9-9.

Currently, the principal federal government agency responsible for animal health in the United States is USDA/APHIS, established in 1971. The overall structure, function, and duties of various APHIS units are discussed in more detail in Chapter 8 (also, see Table 8.2). The APHIS unit responsible for responding to an incursion of foreign animal disease in the United States is Veterinary Services (VS). A special unit within VS, known as Emergency Programs (EP), was established in 1972, following back-to-back foreign animal disease outbreaks in this country—Venezuelan equine encephalomyelitis in 1971 and exotic Newcastle disease in 1972. These events focused attention on the need for specially trained personnel and well-organized emergency-response preparedness to deal swiftly and effectively with foreign animal disease. Subsequently, the benefits of creating the EP apparatus were made evident when EP staff effectively coordinated the elimination of sheep scabies in 1973, exotic Newcastle disease in 1974, classical swine fever in 1978, and an outbreak of highly pathogenic avian influenza from U.S. poultry flocks in the northeast in 1984.

Emergency Programs Section of APHIS

The EP section of Veterinary Services in APHIS carries out numerous functions relative to foreign animal disease control including surveillance, training, simulation exercises, diagnostic investigation, and coordinated response in the event of an actual foreign animal disease outbreak. Surveillance activities are aimed at rapid detection and diagnosis of outbreaks of exotic diseases in the United States. The EP staff is assisted in its efforts by federal and state field veterinarians, animal health technicians, and disease specialists. EP is also able to draw on the assistance of the national cadre of veterinarians in the private sector who have been federally accredited through the National Veterinary Accreditation Program, usually just after graduation from veterinary school. Currently, over 60,000 federally accredited veterinarians are in the national APHIS database.

EP provides training on foreign animal disease control to a wide range of prospective participants, including federal and state veterinarians, diagnosticians, animal health technicians, epidemiologists, port veterinarians, foreign veterinary medical officers, VS program specialists, and others who require knowledge of foreign animal disease diagnosis and identification. In the event of a foreign animal disease outbreak, these

Table 9-9   Some Significant Milestones and Accomplishments in Regulatory Veterinary Medicine in the United States Achieved by the Bureau of Animal Industry and its successor, Animal and Plant Health Inspection Services (APHIS)[a]

Date	Event
1833	Hog cholera first reported in southern Ohio and along the Wabash River in Indiana
1843	Contagious bovine pleuropneumonia (CBPP) first introduced into the United States
1870	First known outbreak of foot-and-mouth disease (FMD) in the United States
February 1879	British government places restrictions on U.S. cattle because of CBPP
1879–1881	European countries restrict U.S. pork imports because of trichinosis
May 29, 1884	Congress creates the Bureau of Animal Industry (BAI) to eradicate CBPP and other contagious animal diseases
1887	Congress gives BAI authority to purchase and destroy diseased animals
1888–1989	BAI scientists discover that ticks are the vectors of Texas cattle fever
August 30, 1890	Congress gives BAI quarantine authority over domestic ruminants and swine and imported animals
March 3, 1892	First tuberculin test made in United States on Jersey dairy herd in Pennsylvania
Sept. 26, 1892	CBPP eradicated after 8-year campaign using basic procedures of quarantine, slaughter, and disinfection
1906	BAI begins eradication efforts against cattle fever ticks and Texas cattle fever
1910	*Brucella abortus* first isolated from cattle in the United States
1916	First outbreak of vesicular stomatitis reported in Nebraska cattle shipped to Kansas City, MO
March 4, 1917	Congress appropriates $75,000 to begin bovine tuberculosis control effort; 5 % of U.S. cattle are infected
1924	First reported U.S. outbreak of fowl plague spreads to eight Eastern and Midwest states
1929	Fowl plague eradicated
1929	Last of nine U.S. outbreaks of FMD (1870, 1880, 1884, 1902, 1908, 1914, 1924, and 1929) is eradicated
June 17, 1930	Tariff Act prohibits imports of meat and animals from countries infected with foot-and-mouth disease
1934	Glanders, a horse disease, is eradicated
July 19, 1934	Efforts against bovine brucellosis begin as part of a "cattle reduction plan" caused by severe drought
1935	National Poultry Improvement Plan begins with major goal of eliminating pullorum disease
November 1, 1940	All states are Modified Accredited Bovine TB (cattle infection rate less than 0.5%)
1942	Dourine, a horse disease, is eradicated; suppression campaign began April 1, 1902
1943	Texas cattle fever eradicated after 37-year campaign; quarantine zone established in Texas
1947	First U.S. case of scrapie diagnosed in Michigan sheep flock
1952	Efforts begin to eradicate scrapie
1952	Presence of bluetongue confirmed in U.S. sheep; vaccination advised
1952-53	Vesicular exanthema spreads to 42 states and District of Columbia; most outbreaks are in garbage-fed swine
July 1, 1958	Screwworm eradication begins in the southeastern United States, using sterile insect technique; eradication achieved in 1959

(continued)

Table 9-9   Some Significant Milestones and Accomplishments in Regulatory Veterinary Medicine in the United States Achieved by the Bureau of Animal Industry and its successor, Animal and Plant Health Inspection Services (APHIS)[a] (Continued)

Date	Event
1959	Vesicular exanthema of swine declared eradicated
1961	Swine brucellosis program begins
September 6, 1961	Congress authorizes a hog cholera eradication program
June 1971	Outbreak of Venezuelan equine encephalitis (VEE) stopped in south Texas; task force sprays 13 million acres for mosquitoes and vaccinates 2.8 million horses for VEE
November 1971	Parrots from South America introduce exotic Newcastle disease into commercial poultry in southern California
March 14, 1972	Emergency declared to combat a spreading outbreak of exotic Newcastle disease in southern California; 117,000 km² quarantined
January 1973	Sheep scabies eradicated
July 3, 1974	Exotic Newcastle disease eradicated after the destruction of nearly 12 million chickens; cost, $56 million
Jan. 31, 1978	United States declared free of hog cholera; program costs $140 million versus $1.12 billion disease costs without a program
March 1978	Contagious equine metritis diagnosed in Thoroughbred horses in KY; by year's end, the outbreak was controlled
January 16, 1981	Emergency funds made available to APHIS to eradicate African swine fever from Haiti; eradicated by 1984
1983–1984	Outbreak of avian influenza eradicated from PA, VA, MD, and NJ; 17 million chickens destroyed; cost, $65 million
1984	USDA Beagle Brigade begins to detect prohibited agricultural items in the baggage of international travelers
January 16, 1986	First genetically engineered vaccine licensed by APHIS, for pseudorabies in swine
1989	APHIS adopts standards for state-federal-industry program to eradicate pseudorabies in swine
1991	Field trial successfully completed for first genetically engineered oral raccoon rabies vaccine
1991	Bovine TB recognized as serious problem in deer and elk
October 2, 1992	Scrapie Voluntary Flock Certification Program begins
Summer 1995	APHIS cooperates with southwestern states to combat serious outbreak of vesicular stomatitis
January 31, 2001	National brucellosis program achieves zero cattle herds under quarantine for first time

[a]A more complete list, from which this shorter list is derived, is available through the APHIS website on the internet at http://www.aphis.usda.gov/oa/history.html.

trained professionals would be involved in the disease control effort.

One key aspect of maintaining readiness through training is the implementation of test or simulation exercises. Each year, two regional task forces in the United States receive such emergency response training. Known as the Regional Emergency Animal Disease Eradication Organization (READEO), these task forces consist of APHIS-VS employees, state veterinarians, military support personnel, industry liaisons, and representatives from other units with VS, APHIS, and the USDA. EP also conducts foreign animal disease training courses at its headquarters in Riverdale, MD; at the National Veterinary Services Laboratories in Ames, IA; and at the Foreign Animal Disease Diagnostic Laboratory in Plum Island, NY. There are currently about 400 veterinarians in the United States, mostly in federal and state government, especially trained as foreign animal disease diagnosticians, who are called in to evaluate possible cases of foreign animal disease flagged by veterinary practitioners and reported to state or federal regulatory authorities as discussed in the section below.

Emergency Response to Foreign Animal Disease

Mounting an effective response to the incursion of a foreign animal disease in livestock or poultry in the United States is a team effort involving producers, private practitioners, numerous state and federal agencies, industry, and, increasingly, the general public. The general public must understand, and be willing to cooperate with, efforts to control disease outbreaks effectively, as such efforts may disrupt normal routines, as illustrated by the outbreak of FMD in the United Kingdom in 2001. As America becomes increasingly urbanized and more detached from agricultural life, the challenge of mustering public support for foreign animal disease control efforts becomes more difficult. Though it represents an extreme view, the statement in 2001 by an official of the People for Ethical Treatment of Animals that the introduction of FMD into the United States would be "good for animals, good for human health, and good for the environment" offers an insight into the challenge of garnering public cooperaton in a foreign animal disease outbreak and the obstacles that might be encountered in mounting effective disease control efforts.

Responsibilities of Practicing Veterinarians

The first line of defense in controlling foreign animal disease in the United States is the private veterinary practitioner. Proactively, veterinarians can work with farmers and producers to develop dependable biosecurity measures for livestock operations to ensure that infectious agents are not introduced onto the premises. They can educate farmers about the risks of various foreign animal diseases and encourage them to call a veterinarian whenever some unusual disease manifestation is observed on the farm and not to move any animals until a veterinarian has visited the premises. Federally accredited practitioners are also responsible for examination of animals destined for sales, auctions, and markets in interstate or international trade and preparation of health certificates for those shipments. For any veterinary reader who is not federally accredited, information about the National Veterinary Accreditation Program, including application forms, is available through the APHIS website at http://www.aphis.usda.gov/ vs/nvap/. Also, practitioners can work with producers to help eliminate diseases endemic to the United States that are considered foreign animal diseases in other countries and thus limit foreign trade opportunities for American livestock producers. Examples include bovine leukosis, caprine arthritis-encephalitis, and paratuberculosis in cattle, sheep, and goats.

The most critical function of the practitioner, especially now with the heightened risks of foreign animal disease occur-

rence, is to remain aware and vigilant concerning those risks. Many of the most contagious and economically costly foreign animal diseases are clinically similar to diseases that already occur in the United States. On any given day, in any busy practice, the reality exists that a sick animal which on first impression appears to have a well-known indigenous disease, may in fact be exhibiting signs of an exotic disease newly introduced into the country. This point was brought home most recently by the outbreak of West Nile virus infection in horses in New York in 1999, in which the neurological signs observed mimicked those of equine neurological disorders already occurring in the United States such as equine protozoal myeloencephalitis, eastern equine encephalomyelitis, and the neurological form of equine herpesvirus 1 infection (equine viral rhinopneumonitis). The clinical signs of some major foreign animal diseases are presented in Table 9-10, along with the indigenous diseases that resemble them. As these comparisons suggest, the diagnostic challenges involved in recognizing and controlling foreign animal disease are significant. Practitioners must be vigilant and remain alert to the fact that a foreign animal disease may be present. A complete list of animal diseases monitored by the OIE is provided in Table 9-2.

A detailed review of the clinical and diagnostic features of all the foreign animal diseases that potentially threaten livestock and poultry in the United States is well beyond the size constraints of this text. However, there are a number of very useful sources of information, both written and visual, on the identification of foreign animal diseases that veterinary students and practitioners can easily access to improve their diagnostic acumen (Table 9-11). In today's media-driven world, the veterinary practitioner can be sure to receive abundant media attention if a foreign animal disease occurs in his or her practice area. It is far better to be featured on the news as the astute clinician who promptly identified and reported the outbreak than as the careless one who misdiagnosed or overlooked it.

The Emergency Response Cascade

If a private practitioner suspects the occurrence of a foreign animal disease, that practitioner should immediately notify the state veterinarians office of the office of the APHIS area veterinarian in charge (AVIC). The telephone numbers for all state veterinarians and APHIS AVICs are listed in the "Government Agencies" section of the annual *Directory and Resource Manual of the American Veterinary Medical Association*. Contact information for APHIS AVICs is also available on the APHIS website at http://www.aphis.usda.gov/vs/area_offices.htm.

The state and/or federal veterinarian will consult with the referring veterinarian and respond as soon as possible with a visit to the suspect premises to do a preliminary evaluation of the disease situation. If the history and physical findings are consistent with a possible foreign animal disease, then a foreign animal disease diagnostician (FADD) will be called in, assuming that neither the state or federal veterinarian already on the premises is a certified FADD. The FADD will take appropriate diagnostic samples for the disease in question, includ-

Table 9-10   Differential Diagnosis for Selected OIE List A and List B Diseases Foreign to the United States

Disease and Causative Agent	Major Clinical Signs	Differential Diagnosis in the United States
Foot and mouth disease (hoof and mouth disease, aftosa) Causative agent: aphthovirus	Fever, vesicles on feet and vesicles and mucosal sloughing on structures of oral cavity, slobbering, lameness, abortion; high morbidity, low mortality	**Swine:** vesicular stomatitis, swine vesicular disease, vesicular exanthema, foot rot, chemical and thermal burns; **Cattle:** vesicular stomatitis, infectious bovine rhinotracheitis (IBR), bovine virus diarrhea (BVD), malignant catarrhal fever (MCF), bluetongue, rinderpest; **Sheep and goats:** bluetongue, contagious ecthyma, lip and leg ulceration (sheep), foot rot
Rinderpest (cattle plague) Causative agent: morbillivirus	Fever, ocular and nasal discharge, ulcerative lesions of the oral cavity, diarrhea, anorexia, depression, dehydration, prostration, and death	**Cattle:** BVD, IBR, MCF, foot and mouth disease, vesicular stomatitis, salmonellosis, paratuberculosis, arsenic poisoning
Contagious bovine pleuropneumonia Causative agent: *Mycoplasma mycoides* subsp. *mycoides*, small colony type	Fever, anorexia, depression, coughing, thoracic pain, dyspnea, respiratory distress, and in calves, occasionally polyarthritis	**Cattle:** bovine pasteurellosis, other pneumonic conditions
Heartwater (cowdriosis) Causative agent: *Cowdria ruminantium*	Peracute death, or acutely, fever, anorexia, hyperpnea, and neurological signs including chewing movements, eyelid twitching, circling, progressing to recumbency, convulsions, opisthotonus, coma, and death	**Cattle, sheep, and goats:** peracute- anthrax; acute-rabies, listeriosis, polioencephalomalacia, tetanus, meningitis, lead poisoning, strychnine poisoning, organophosphate toxicity
Peste des petits ruminants (Small ruminant plague) Causative agent: morbillivirus	Fever, anorexia, serous to catarrhal nasal discharge, sneezing, respiratory distress, conjunctivitis, necrotic stomatitis with focal erosions, severe diarrhea, dehydration, emaciation, and death	**Sheep and goats:** no other single disease produces this entire constellation of signs, but respiratory or GI signs may predominate; rule out pasteurellosis, contagious caprine pleuropneumonia, bluetongue, contagious ecthyma, foot and mouth disease, coccidiosis, some plant poisonings
African swine fever Causative agent: African swine fever-like virus	Sudden death possible, or fever, red-to-purple skin discoloration (esp. on ears, tail, and extremities), variable diarrhea, abortion; affected pigs retain reasonable body condition	**Swine:** classical swine fever, erysipelas, salmonellosis, and eperythrozoonosis
Classical swine fever (hog cholera) Causative agent: pestivirus	Fever, depression, lethargy, vomiting, constipation followed by or alternating with diarrhea, conjunctivitis, staggering gait, marked loss of body condition, purplish discoloration of the skin, terminally convulsions and death	**Swine:** African swine fever, erysipelas, salmonellosis, eperythrozoonosis, salt poisoning
Swine vesicular disease Causative agent: enterovirus	Fever; vesicles (in mouth, on snout, and on feet), lameness; also shivering, unsteady gait, and jerky leg movements	**Swine:** foot and mouth disease, vesicular stomatitis, vesicular exanthema of swine, and chemical and thermal burns

(continued)

Table 9-10 Differential Diagnosis for Selected OIE List A and List B Diseases Foreign to the United States[a] (Continued)

Disease and Causative Agent	Major Clinical Signs	Differential Diagnosis in the United States
Contagious caprine pleuropneumonia Causative agent: *Mycoplasma capricolum* subsp. *capripneumoniae*	Fever, coughing, lethargy, nasal discharge, dyspnea, awkward stance associated with thoracic pain	**Goats:** pasteurellosis, lungworms, other pneumonic conditions
Lumpy skin disease Causative agent: capripox virus	Fever, generalized nodular swellings of the skin, depression, anorexia, salivation, oculonasal discharge, agalactia, and emaciation	**Cattle:** bovine herpes mammillitis, streptothricosis, ringworm, ox warbles (*Hypoderma bovis*), photosensitization, bovine papular stomatitis, insect bites
Sheep pox and goat pox Causative agent: capripox virus	Fever, depression, conjunctivitis, lacrimation and rhinitis followed by generalized, raised circumscribed skin lesions that are vesicular at first and later scabbed	**Sheep and goat:** bluetongue, contagious ecthyma, photosensitization, insect bites, caseous lymphadenitis, streptothricosis, mange
Rift Valley fever Causative agent: phlebovirus	Fever, anorexia, weakness, depression, and death in young stock; adults have fever, anorexia weakness, excessive salivation, and a variable fetid diarrhea; abortion is the most prominent sign in pregnant animals	**Sheep and goats:** brucellosis, ovine enzootic abortion, enterotoxemia, bluetongue; **Cattle:** brucellosis, vibriosis, trichomoniasis, other causes of abortion
Bovine spongiform encephalopathy (mad cow disease) Causative agent: prion	A slowly progressing chronic neurological disease; signs include apprehension, nervousness, or aggression; incoordination; tremors; difficulty in rising; hyperaesthesia to sound and touch; also loss of body condition and milk production	**Cattle:** lead poisoning, listeriosis, brain abscess, hypomagnesemia, spinal trauma, and rabies (at least initially, since rabies has a much shorter clinical course)
African horse sickness Causative agent: orbivirus	Pulmonary form: fever, profound respiratory distress, tachypnea, sawhorse stance, profuse sweating, short, fatal course; Cardiac form: fever, edematous swelling of head and neck, petechiation on tongue and conjunctivae, prostration and death	**Equines:** equine viral arteritis, purpura hemorrhagica, equine infectious anemia, other causes of pneumonia
Dourine Causative agent: *Trypanosoma equiperdum*	Genital, perineal, and ventral edema in mares or stallions; genital vesicles; conjunctivitis and keratitis; later neurological signs, including restlessness, progressive weakness, incoordination, and paralysis, leading to recumbency and death	**Equines:** anthrax, equine viral arteritis, equine infectious anemia, coital exanthema, and in mares, purulent endometritis, including contagious equine metritis

(continued)

Table 9-10   Differential Diagnosis for Selected OIE List A and List B Diseases Foreign to the United States[a] (Continued)

Disease and Causative Agent	Major Clinical Signs	Differential Diagnosis in the United States
Glanders (farcy) Causative agent: *Pseudomonas mallei*	Chronic disease forms more common than acute; yellow-green nasal discharge, nodules and ulcers of nasal mucosa, multiple cutaneous nodules following lymph channels and nodes, possible lung involvement with coughing and dyspnea	**Equines:** strangles, ulcerative lymphangitis, sinusitis, gutteral pouch empyema, other causes of pneumonia
Highly pathogenic avian influenza (fowl plague) Causative agent: influenza virus	Severe depression, ruffled feathers, anorexia, marked thirst, swollen combs and wattles and edema around eyes, cessation of egg production, watery green to white diarrhea, hemorrhage (combs, conjunctivae, and legs), variable respiratory signs depending on extent of tracheal mucus	**Chickens, ducks, geese:** infectious laryngotracheitis, fowl cholera, infectious coryza, colibacillosis of poultry, Newcastle disease
Newcastle disease Causative agent: paramyxovirus	Sudden drop in egg production followed by high mortality 24-48 hours later or edema of the head, greenish diarrhea, respiratory distress and some neurological signs including drooping wings, torticollis, and ataxia	**Chickens, ducks and geese:** highly pathogenic avian influenza, infectious laryngotracheitis, fowl cholera, and infectious coryza

[a]The front line of defense against the introduction of foreign animals disease is the private veterinary practitioner, who must always keep in mind that exotic diseases may show clinical similarity to more familiar, indigenous diseases. The descriptions of clinical signs presented here focus primarily on the acute manifestations of each disease, though many of these conditions can assume peracute, subacute, and sometimes chronic forms. More descriptive details of these diseases is available from the United States Animal Health Association in their handbook Foreign Animal Diseases,[34] now also available on the internet at http://www.usaha.org/.

ing postmortem samples when necessary (Fig. 9-4), and those samples will be dispatched to either the Plum Island Foreign Animal Disease Laboratory in New York (Fig. 9-5) or the National Veterinary Services Laboratory in Ames, Iowa, depending on the disease in question. If the FADD considers that it is highly likely that the suspect cases are in fact a foreign animal disease, the samples are sent Priority 1, so that preliminary results are available within 24 hours. In such highly suspect cases, the state veterinarian will place a quarantine on the farm and establish an appropriate movement control zone around the premises. Local agricultural and emergency officials will be notified, and all contacts to the farm will be traced.

The laboratory diagnosis may be completed in two phases. In the first, more-rapid phase, a presumptive positive diagnosis can be made on the basis of antibody responses or detection of antigens. The second, confirmatory or definitive diagnosis requires actual isolation of the agent and, in the case of virus isolation, may take a week or longer to complete. An emergency response can be initiated on the basis of the presumptive positive diagnosis and then ratcheted up if and when the confirmatory diagnosis is made. In March 2001, APHIS issued a new set of guidelines outlining the national emergency

response to a highly contagious disease. Once a presumptive positive diagnosis is made from samples taken in the initial investigation, that case becomes the index case, and the following actions are taken according to the new national emergency response guidelines:

A conference call is conducted among the laboratory, the state veterinarian, the federal AVIC, the FADD, and the APHIS Emergency Management Leadership Team. This conference call will outline action steps specific to the disease under consideration. The framework of this action plan is as follows.

The state veterinarian will

- Quarantine the affected premises
- Consider stopping movement of animals within the state
- Consider active case finding based on suggestive clinical signs in the states using information from field veterinarians, the Food Safety and Inspection Service, extension agents, industry partners, and public awareness campaigns

Table 9-11   Useful Resources for Information on and Identification of Foreign Animal Diseases

1. **Foreign Animal Diseases.** This inexpensive handbook, referred to as "The Grey Book" is published by the Committee on Foreign Animal Diseases of the United States Animal Health Association. It was revised and updated most recently in 1998. The text provides informative and easy-to-read information on the natural history, diagnosis, and control of all the major foreign animal diseases of livestock and poultry as well as a section of color photographs of the major clinical signs and postmortem lesions for most of the diseases discussed. There are also useful appendices on laboratory submission of samples and procedures for cleaning and disinfection. Every practitioner should have a copy of this book in the office or practice vehicle. United States Animal Health Association. Foreign Animal Diseases. Richmond, VA: USAHA, 1998. Information on ordering this handbook is available on the internet at www.usaha.org/. Also, since November 2001, the full text of "The Grey Book" is available on-line at this same USAHA website.

2. **Keeping America Free from Foreign Animal Diseases.** This is a 7 volume set of slides with accompanying text and videotapes bound in loose-leaf notebooks. These materials provide excellent visual aids for the identification of major foreign animal diseases. It is produced by USDA APHIS and has been distributed to veterinary college libraries throughout the United States. The diseases covered include vol 1, African horse sickness; vol 2, African swine fever; vol 3, contagious bovine pleuropneumonia; vol 4, lumpy skin disease, sheep pox, and goat pox; vol 5, malignant catarrhal fever; vol 6, rinderpest and peste des petits ruminants; and vol 7, vesicular diseases, including foot and mouth disease, vesicular stomatitis, swine vesicular disease, and vesicular exanthema of swine. The slide and text portions of these materials are available for viewing on the APHIS Emergency Programs website at http://www.aphis.usda.gov/vs/ep/fad_training/bibpage.htm

3. **The Website of the Office International des Epizooties.** The OIE website is an essential source of information about foreign animal disease. While there are no visual aids for disease identification, there are descriptions of the OIE list A and B diseases including etiology, epidemiology, diagnosis, prevention, and control. There is also current information on the locations of recent disease outbreaks, lists of countries in which specific diseases are enzootic, standards for laboratory diagnosis, sources of diagnostic reagents, and contact information for world experts on the various diseases. The internet address is http://www.oie.int/.

4. **Outbreak! The Role of the Veterinary Community.** At the annual meeting of the American Veterinary Medical Association in 2000, a symposium was held to focus on the veterinary response to foreign animal disease outbreaks and other animal health emergencies. A number of very interesting presentations were made on related topics, including the threat of accidental foreign animal disease introduction, mapping of disease outbreaks using GIS, the role of vaccination in disease outbreaks, the role of private practitioners, the role of livestock industries, emergency animal disease response programs at the state and federal level, and building an animal disaster program. The full texts of these presentations are available at the APHIS Emergency Programs website, http://www.aphis.usda.gov/vs/ep/avma/avma-sym.html.

- Consider depopulation of affected herd(s) in consultation with USDA, industry, and other stakeholders

- Determine whether wild animals may be a risk factor in the dissemination or persistence of infection

- Notify appropriate contacts (such as the commissioner of agriculture, state emergency management director, and others deemed necessary) who would be needed to support a response

- Review the operational guidelines for the specific highly contagious disease at hand

- Designate incident commanders and an emergency operations center in consultation with local APHIS officials and state emergency managers

The Area Veterinarian in Charge (AVIC) will

- Notify appropriate contacts who would be needed to support a response (e.g., USDA State Emergency Board, field force, and others as predetermined during discussions with the state veterinarian)

- Prepare to participate in the Joint Incident Command as described in the state emergency plan. (Most state emergency management agencies follow protocols and procedures for emergency response as defined by the National Incident Command System)

The READEO director will

- Notify all AVICs in the region of the presence of the foreign animal disease and traceback findings

- Give the READEO team members notice to be prepared for deployment (see Fig. 9-6)

- Prepare to support the Joint Incident Command in their actions or become the incident commander in states unable or unwilling to take appropriate actions to control and eradicate the disease

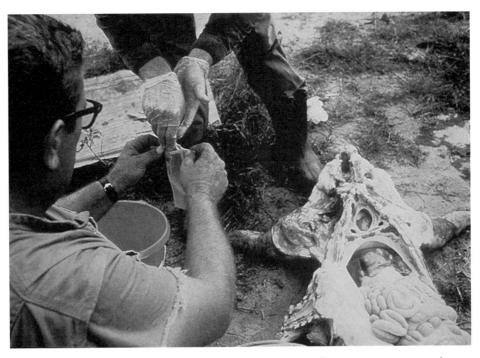

Figure 9-4. USDA/APHIS foreign animal disease diagnostician collecting postmortem samples on swine during a field investigation of possible foreign animal disease. Samples are dispatched to the Plum Island Animal Disease Center on Long Island Sound for analysis. Hundreds of such field investigations are carried out each year around the United States by foreign animal disease diagnosticians, at the request of state veterinary authorities in response to alerts from practitioners or producers. (Photo courtesy of Dr. Robert Brady, USDA/APHIS Veterinary Services)

The USDA/APHIS will

- Conduct isolation and typing of the highly contagious foreign animal disease agent
- Initiate national and North American communication plans
- Place national READEO leaders on high alert
- Alert USDA Crisis Management staff
- Activate the APHIS Emergency Operation Center
- Institute active case finding based on suggestive clinical signs in all states, to include the state veterinarians, extension agents, industry partners, and public awareness campaigns

Industry will

- Communicate with their constituencies
- Support state and national response efforts

Once the laboratory actually isolates and identifies the causative agent, the presumptive positive case becomes a confirmed case and triggers an additional set of responses as follows:

The state veterinarian, AVIC, or incident commanders will

- Initiate depopulation and disposal of the infected herd/flock if not yet accomplished under the presumptive positive diagnosis
- Initiate the process to request a governor's declaration of emergency, thus implementing the state emergency response plan
- Continue quarantine and movement restrictions
- Continue active case finding

The state emergency management director/Emergency Management System will

- Activate the state response plan
- Support local Emergency Management System efforts at the site of the outbreak
- Request a governor's declaration of emergency
- Enforce movement controls within the state
- Evaluate the need to request a presidential declaration of emergency, thus implementing the federal response plan

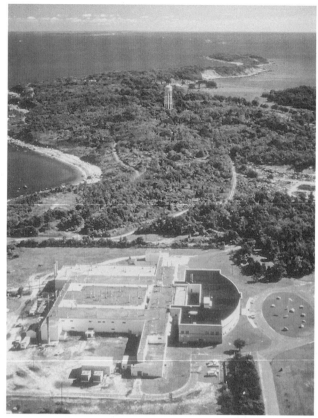

Figure 9-5. The Plum Island Animal Disease Center (PIADC) is American agriculture's "first line of defense" against foreign animal diseases such as FMD and African swine fever. The center is a self-contained facility located on Long Island Sound accessible by boat from Greenport, New York, and Old Saybrook, Connecticut. Two USDA agencies are active on the island. The Agricultural Research Service (ARS) carries out foreign animal disease research. The Animal and Plant Health Inspection Service (APHIS) operates the Foreign Animal Disease Diagnostic Laboratory and offers training courses in foreign animal diseases. Plum Island also is home to the North American Foot and Mouth Disease Vaccine Bank, which is financially supported and shared by the United States, Mexico, and Canada. (Photo and caption information from the USDA website http://www.ars.usda.gov/plum/index.html.)

The USDA will

- Notify appropriate federal agencies of the emergency declaration
- Consolidate and present the official daily situation report to the secretary of agriculture
- Coordinate the response activities of all USDA agencies to support APHIS and, until presidential emergency declaration, coordinate all requests for the support of other federal agencies
- Impose on the affected state a federal quarantine for interstate commerce and request enforcement by the affected state and adjoining states

- Identify a source and start evaluating a process of acquiring an effective vaccine when appropriate
- Coordinate national surveillance activities

The deputy administrator of Veterinary Services through the APHIS Emergency Management Operations Center will

- Provide international and national communication on the status of the situation
- Involve federal, state, and industry partners in the decision-making process with respect to the consequences of the disease on the United States
- Designate the associate deputy administrator of Veterinary Services the national incident coordinator

The secretary of agriculture will

- Declare an emergency or extraordinary emergency, if necessary, to release the funds to cover expenses for response activities, including funds for indemnity
- Call on other federal agencies to provide assistance
- Mobilize federal agricultural resources to assist the state

Industry will

- Communicate with their constituencies
- Support state and national response efforts
- Coordinate efforts with state, national, and international industry groups

In the case of highly contagious diseases, additional premises beyond that of the initial, index case, may be infected early in the outbreak. Therefore, early surveillance activities may identify additional presumptive positive cases, referred to as *secondary cases*. These secondary cases will be handled in the same manner as the index case, first as presumptive for the foreign animal disease and subsequently as confirmed cases. The response plan extends to those cases, and the process of quarantine, movement control, depopulation, and disinfection continues until the outbreak is officially declared to be under control.

This concise, orderly outline of stepwise response belies the logistical complexity, social disruption, economic cost, and human drama associated with a large-scale foreign animal disease control effort. Television images from the United Kingdom during the FMD outbreak of 2001 showing trenches full of dead cows and blackened skies over burning pyres of dead sheep offered a more graphic picture of the challenges associated with bringing a highly contagious epizootic disease under control (Fig. 9-7).

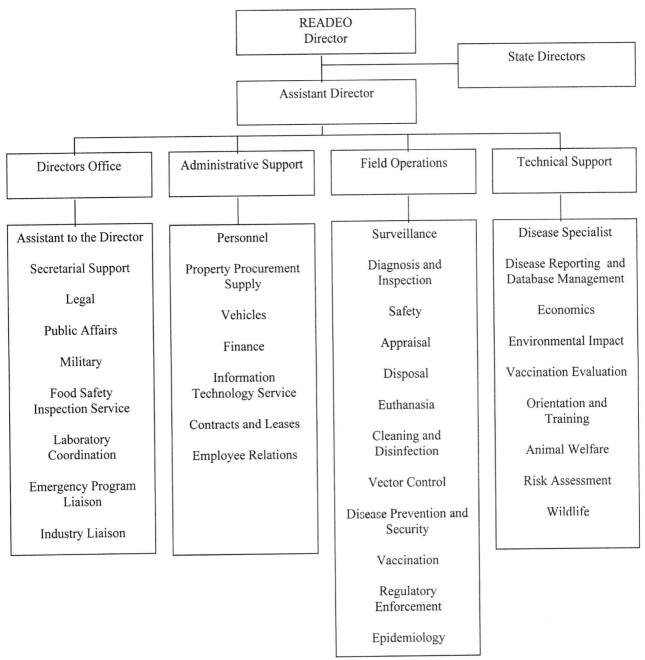

Figure 9-6.   The structure of the APHIS Regional Emergency Animal Disease Eradication Organization, READEO. This organizational chart is presented so that the reader can appreciate the array of administrative, technical, and logistical expertise that must be called into play in the event of a bona fide foreign animal disease emergency in the United States. The United States is divided into two regions, with the Eastern READEO responsible for coordination of emergency response in states essentially east of the Mississippi River and the Western READEO responsible for the states west of the river. The various responsibilities identified are assigned to various APHIS area veterinarians in charge and their staff within the region. These READEO resources are available to states experiencing a foreign animal disease outbreak.

Facing the Future

At the time of this writing, the FMD outbreak of 2001 in the United Kingdom was drawing to a close. Veterinary authorities in the United States, who had been on a heightened state of alert concerning the risk of introduction of FMD from Europe, were just beginning to feel that the immediate threat was subsiding, when the terrorist attack of September 11, 2001 occurred. Once again, the specter of foreign animal disease loomed, but this time not as the result of accidental introduction of contaminated animals or animal products, but rather through the malicious intent of bioterrorists. In the aftermath of September 11, a good deal of attention has focused on the preparedness of APHIS and other agencies to continue to successfully prevent incursions of foreign animal disease into the United States, especially in the context of

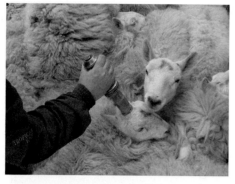
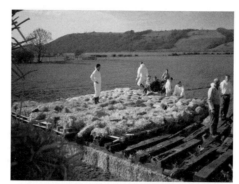
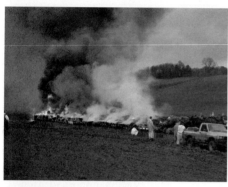
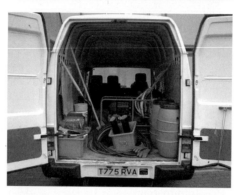
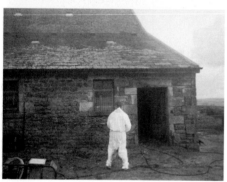
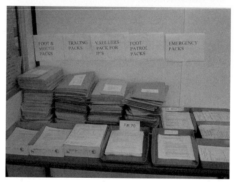

Figure 9-7.   Scenes from the FMD outbreak in the United Kingdom, March 2001. *Top left,* Killing sheep with a captive bolt. *Top right,* Preparing a pyre for disposal of carcasses by burning. *Middle left,* Monitoring a burning pyre. *Middle right,* A mobile cleaning and disinfection unit with equipment shown. *Bottom left,* Decontamination of infected premises by pressure spraying. *Bottom right,* Paperwork required for epidemiological investigation, animal appraisal, and other aspects of the control effort. (Photos courtesy of Dr. Donald E. Hoenig, Division of Veterinary Services, Maine Department of Agriculture and Mr. Richard Davies, Department of Environment, Farms and Rural Affairs, Preston, UK)

highly infectious disease agents being used as weapons of mass destruction.

APHIS entered the 21st century with a laudable record of achievement. In the case of FMD, for example, the agency has successfully kept the disease out of the country for 70 years, the last recorded outbreak having occurred in 1929. Nevertheless, genuine concerns have surfaced. Government downsizing and budgetary cutbacks have taken their toll. APHIS personnel has been reduced by approximately 500 positions over the course of the 1990s. While the APHIS budget remained essentially flat, the percentage of that budget allocated to the VS division was down from 37 to 27% over the same period. Thoughtful and conscientious observers have expressed real concern about the agency's ability to remain effective in the face of growing international trade and travel and the emerging threat of bioterrorism, citing inadequate manpower, insufficient training in foreign animal diseases among the nation's veterinarians, and outdated or inadequate laboratory diagnostic facilities.

Cognizant of the challenges facing Veterinary Services in safeguarding the health of the nation's livestock and people, VS commissioned an external review of its structure, function, and performance in 2000. The review was conducted by the National Association of State Departments of Agriculture (NASDA) and called upon the expertise of people in government, academia, and animal industry. The review was intended to identify existing strengths and weaknesses and recommend enhancements or new initiatives that would improve the overall safeguarding system. Four separate review committees were established to evaluate four main areas of concern:

- Exclusion activities-efforts designed to prevent the introduction of invasive species, pests, and diseases from entering the country

- International information-collection and analysis of data needed for timely decision making to analysis risk, to create regulations, to identify threats, and to facilitate trade

- Domestic surveillance and detection-activities that monitor for diseases/pests affecting the U.S. animal population, including efforts to identify diseases/pests exotic to this country

- Response-actions needed to prepare for and address adverse animal health events including the incursion of foreign animal disease

The safeguarding review was completed in October of 2001. The full text of the review is available on the internet at http://www.aphis.gov/vs/safeguarding.pdf. The primary recommendation of the review panel is that "Congress and the United States Department of Agriculture must provide funding and act to rebuild the state and national infrastructure for animal disease control, emergency disease preparedness, and response." In the meantime, in response to developments in Europe relative to FMD and BSE, Congress signed a bill into law in May 2001 to establish a federal interagency task force to coordinate actions to prevent the outbreak of BSE and FMD in the United States, and in October 2001, the U.S. secretary of agriculture announced that $1.8 million in grants will be distributed to 32 states to bolster emergency animal disease prevention, preparedness, response, and recovery systems.

Discussion Points

1. What were the principal equine disease problems of concern to Australian officials relative to the importation of horses for the Sydney Olympics in 2000? Review the regulatory procedures imposed and evaluate their appropriateness.

2. How will the production of organic livestock products affect herd health programs for different livestock operations, and what threats and opportunities does it present to the practice of veterinary medicine?

3. Select one of the diseases of concern to EMPRES as an important transboundary disease. What is the current global situation for this disease? What knowledge about the disease is lacking? What tools are needed to control it more effectively? Develop a plan to contain this disease in a country where it has a serious impact on production and trade.

4. If foot and mouth disease was introduced into the United States, would you support or oppose the use of vaccination to control an outbreak? What are the technical, social, political, and economic issues that must be considered in such a decision?

5. The debate on antibiotic resistance related to fluoroquinolone use in animals rages on. Some believe that the dissemination of drug resistant strains of bacteria is promoted by use of the drug in human medicine or by the introduction of resistant strains from overseas travelers and that the risk assessments linking use of fluoroquinolones in livestock to drug-resistant bacteria in humans are flawed. Opponents stand firm that the use of the antibiotics in livestock is the principal cause of antibiotic resistance in bacteria infecting humans. Review the debate and the data available and clarify your own position. What further research needs to be done to validate your position?

References

1. Bridges V, Cummings D. The potential for international travelers to transmit foreign animal diseases to U.S. livestock and poultry. Fort Collins, CO: USDA:APHIS:VS, 1998. (Available on the internet at www.aphis.usda.gov/vs/ceah/cei/health.htm#travelers)

2. Brown C, Bolin CA, eds. Emerging Diseases of Animals. Washington, DC: American Society for Microbiology, 2000.

3. Chivian E. Global environmental degradation and biodiversity loss: implications for human health. In: Grifo F, Rosenthal J, eds. Biodiversity and Human Health. Washington, DC: Island Press, 1997.

4. Diallo A. Peste des petits ruminants: a threat for developing countries. In: Gruner L, Chabert Y, eds. Proceedings of the 7th International Conference on Goats, Tours, France, vol 1. Paris: Institut de l'Elevage, 2000:278–279.

5. Dunlop RH, Williams DJ. Veterinary Medicine, An Illustrated History. St. Louis: Mosby-Yearbook, 1996.

6. Ekboir JM. Potential impact of foot and mouth disease in California. University of California, Davis, CA: Agricultural Issues Center, Division of Agriculture and Natural Resources, 1999. (Available on the internet at http://aic.ucdavis.edu/pub/fmd.html)

7. Epstein PR. Emerging diseases and ecosystem instability: new threats to public health. Am J Public Health 1995;85:168–172.

8. Epstein PR. Climate and health. Science 1999;285(5426):347–348.

9. Franz DR, Jahrling PB, Friedlander AM, et al. Clinical recognition and management of patients exposed to biological warfare agents. JAMA 1997;278(5):399–411.

10. Friedman TL. The Lexus and the Olive Tree. New York: Farrar, Strauss, & Giroux, 1999.

11. Gao F, Bailes E, Robertson DL, et al. Origin of HIV-1 in the chimpanzee *Pan troglodytes troglodytes*. Nature 1999;397(6718):385–386.

12. Hamir AN, Cutlip RC, Miller JM, et al. Preliminary findings on the experimental transmission of chronic wasting disease agent of mule deer to cattle. J Vet Diagn Invest 2001;13(1):91–96.

13. Headrick ML, Tollefson L. Food-borne disease summary by food commodity. Vet Clin North Am Food Anim Pract 1998;14:91–100.

14. Hodges J. The genetically modified food muddle. Livestock Prod Sci 1999;62:51–60.

15. Hollinger K, Wray C, Evans S, et al. *Salmonella typhimurium* DT104 in cattle in Great Britain. J Am Vet Med Assoc 1998;213:1732–1733.

16. Hogue AT, White PL, Heminover JA. Pathogen reduction and hazard analysis and critical control point (HACCP) systems for meat and poultry. Vet Clin North Am Food Anim Pract 1998;14:151–164.

17. Jongejan F, Goff W, Camus E, eds. Tropical Veterinary Medicine: Molecular Epidemiology, Hemoparasites and Their Vectors, and General Topics. Ann NY Acad Sci 1998;849:1–503.

18. Kla J, Tollefson L. Producer quality assurance programs. Vet Clin North Am Food Anim Pract 1999;15:197–208.

19. Leighton JK. Center for Veterinary Medicine's perspective on the beef hormone case. Vet Clin North Am Food Anim Pract 1999;15(1):167–180.

20. Linthicum KJ, Angamba A, Tucker CJ, et al. Climate and satellite indicators to forecast Rift Valley fever epidemics in Kenya. Science 1999;285(5426):397–4000.

21. Mariner JC, House JA, Sollod AE, et al. Comparison of the effect of various chemical stabilizers and lyophilization cycles on the thermostability of a Vero cell-adapted rinderpest vaccine. Vet Microbiol 1990;21:195–209.

22. Morris RS, Wilesmith JW, Stern MW, et al. Predictive spatial modelling of alternative control strategies for the foot-and-mouth disease epidemic in Great Britain, 2001. Vet Rec 2001;149(5):137–144.

23. Office International des Epizooties. The economics of animal disease control. Sci Tech Rev 1999;18(2).

24. Plowright W. Effects of rinderpest and rinderpest control on wildlife in Africa. Symp Zool Soc London 1982;50:1–27.

25. Rabsch W, Hargis BM, Tsolis RM, et al. Competitive exclusion of *Salmonella enteritidis* by *Salmonella gallinarum* in poultry. Emerging Infect Dis 2000;6(5):443–448. (Available on the internet at http://www.cdc.gov/ncidod/eid/vol6no5/rabsch.htm)

26. Roelke-Parker ME, Munson L, Packer C, et al. A canine distemper virus epidemic in Serengeti lions (*Panthera leo*). Nature 1996;379(6564):441–445.

27. Sagodira S, Buzoni-Gatel D, Iochmann S, et al. Protection of kids against *Cryptosporidium parvum* infection after immunization of dams with CP15-DNA. Vaccine 1999;17:2346–2355.

28. Schlosser E. Fast Food Nation: The Dark Side of the All-American Meal. Boston: Houghton Mifflin, 2001.

29. Singer P. Animal Liberation. A New Ethics for Our Treatment of Animals. New York: Avon Books, 1977.

30. Sundrum A. Organic livestock farming: a critical review. Livestock Prod Sci 2001;67(3):207–215.

31. Thompson SR. International harmonization issues. Vet Clin North Am Food Anim Pract 1999;15(1):181–195.

32. Thorns CJ. Bacterial food-borne zoonoses. Rev Sci Tech OIE 2000;19(1):226–239.

33. United Nations Environmental Programme. The Contamination of Food. UNEP/GEMS Environmental Library no. 5. Nairobi: UNEP, 1992.

34. United States Animal Health Association. Foreign Animal Diseases. Richmond, VA: USAHA, 1998.

35. Weiner DB, Kennedy RC. Genetic vaccines. Sci Am 1999;281(1):50–57

36. World Health Organization. Emerging and other Communicable Diseases. Strategic Plan 1996–2000. Document WHO/EMC/96.1. Geneva: World Health Organization, 1996.

Suggested Readings

For additional useful readings and resources on the subject of emerging diseases, see Table 9-6; on the subject of food safety, see Table 9-7; and on the subject of foreign animal disease diagnosis and control, see Table 9-11.

Chapter 10
Career Opportunities in International Veterinary Medicine

OBJECTIVES FOR THIS CHAPTER

After completing this chapter, the reader should be able to

- Undertake a self-evaluation to determine his or her own suitability for international work

- Better understand the employment landscape for veterinarians interested in adding an international dimension to their careers in veterinary medicine

- Develop preferences for the type of international employment and employer desired and begin to develop a personal plan to prepare for such work

Introduction

The accelerated rates of technological advance, economic growth, political transformation, and environmental change that have occurred over the last half of the 20th century have created a new professional landscape for veterinarians. This book has attempted to describe key features in that landscape and to identify emerging areas of professional activity for veterinarians tending to the needs of people and animals in the global village. A brief summary of emerging areas of professional opportunity in veterinary medicine is given in Table 10-1. While the varied, professional challenges of a global society are becoming increasingly clear, the career opportunities for veterinarians to address those challenges are less well defined and still somewhat difficult to identify. At present, relatively few formal positions for North American veterinarians to work

in the international arena are specifically advertised. There are several reasons for this.

One reason is that historically among the developed countries, America has not been as internationally active or globally connected as many of its European counterparts. For better or for worse, countries such as Britain, France, the Netherlands, Spain, Portugal, Belgium, and, to a lesser extent, Germany and Italy have strong colonial histories that resulted in distinct spheres of cultural and economic influence that persist to this day. In contemporary Ethiopia, for example, where Italian control ended in 1941, you can travel for hours over dusty unpaved roads to a small, remote town, walk into the only open restaurant and still be served a perfectly prepared al dente spaghetti bolognese and a delicious, fresh-brewed cappuccino, a truly jarring, but nonetheless pleasant, cultural juxtaposition that reflects the indelible mark that Italian influence has left on

Table 10-1	**Examples of Professional Activities for Veterinarians Interested in an International Dimension to Their Career**
Develop and strengthen veterinary service delivery systems for the underserved	
Assist in education and training of veterinarians and paraprofessionals	
Participate in zoonotic disease control and public health activities	
Develop regional and international animal disease surveillance and control programs	
Conduct research on disease resistance in indigenous breeds of animals	
Identify and verify the efficacy of local ethnoveterinary medicines and practices	
Promote poverty alleviation and empowerment of women through introduction of livestock	
Develop local capacity in human resources and strengthen community through livestock projects	
Promote food security in developing countries through improved animal health and production	
Promote sustainable, environmentally friendly, livestock production	
Promote food safety and quality assurance in national, regional, and world markets	
Facilitate expanded international trade in livestock and livestock products	
Harmonize international trade in livestock and livestock products	
Develop, test, and market new animal health products in world markets	
Identify, investigate, and help to solve global environmental health problems	
Participate in the protection and propagation of endangered species	
Participate in wildlife conservation efforts	
Promote the preservation of biodiversity	
Promote animal population control efforts and the humane care of dogs and cats in developing countries	
Provide assistance for improving the health and well-being of zoo animals in developing countries	
Practice clinical veterinary medicine	

the nation. More significant, however, is the persistence of economic ties. Italy remains an important trading partner for Ethiopia, purchasing animal hides and skins for shoe production and other fine, finished leather goods, and exporting many finished consumer goods back to Ethiopia. The trade connection is even stronger for neighboring Eritrea, which Italy first colonized in 1890 and occupied through 1941.

European governments with colonial pasts continue to cultivate cultural and economic relationships with former colonies in the postcolonial era by a number of mechanisms. The British Commonwealth, for example, is an organization based on voluntary membership that fosters ties among former members of the British Empire (i.e., colonies). Its 52 member states regularly consult and exchange views on a number of topics of common interest including economic affairs, international terrorism, drug trafficking, and technical assistance to less-developed states. Another example is the Communaute Financiere Africaine (CFA). From 1948 through 1994, via the CFA, the government of France pegged its currency, the French franc, to the currency of 14 French-speaking West African nations,

13 of which were former French colonies. This arrangement stabilized the CFA franc, the currency of the participating nations, and protected it from devaluation. In the commercial sector, many European companies have been maintaining and cultivating overseas markets for decades. European nationals may have family members who lived and worked in Africa, Asia, the Middle East, and Latin America. They are more aware of the culture and politics of these regions and exploit this knowledge and experience to cultivate and maintain business connections.

The United States, in general, does not have these historical linkages forged from a colonial past. On the one hand, it is a disadvantage in that Americans may lack familiarity with, and connections to, developing regions of the world. On the other hand, it offers an advantage in that Americans may deal with emerging nations in the political and economic sphere in an atmosphere relatively free of the resentment, suspicion, and grievance that is often directed towards former colonial powers. The challenge, of course, is to avoid generating new resentments, suspicions, and grievances aimed specifically at the United States. The terrorist attacks of September 11, 2001 in New York and Washington, D.C., and the ugly anti-American rhetoric that followed from some quarters suggests that the United States has been less than wholly successful in this regard.[5]

Another reason that international positions are not widely advertised for North American veterinarians is that most people outside the veterinary profession do not appreciate the breadth and depth of a veterinarian's training and the variety of functions that veterinarians are capable of carrying out. Frequently, international positions are described for which veterinarians would be admirably suited, even though a veterinary degree or veterinary experience is not specifically mentioned or sought in the advertisement. Such advertisements, for example, might be seeking public health specialists, individuals with experience in agribusiness, livestock production experts, or field researchers in wildlife conservation. There is little awareness within the general public that veterinarians receive training in biostatistics, research methodology, comparative medicine, public health, epidemiology, food safety, toxicology, and a variety of other useful, transferable, and relevant subjects that can serve a wide range of applications in the global marketplace. We have not done a good job collectively as a profession in promoting our own potential for working outside the sphere of domestic, private, clinical practice.

Thirdly, international employment opportunities for veterinarians are not easily categorized, and no single, centralized source exists where they are consistently advertised. Graduates seeking employment in small animal practice in the United States can reliably go to the *Journal of the American Veterinary Medical Association* every 2 weeks and find a robust list of potential job opportunities neatly broken down by state location. No parallel, comprehensive coverage currently exists for international jobs in veterinary medicine. No doubt the journal would be happy to run such advertisements for international employment, but prospective employees may not be aware of the journal as an advertising medium or, more significantly, may not recognize the sizable potential interest that exists among North American veterinarians to work internationally. At present, North American veterinarians interested in working abroad must be persistent and imaginative and cast a wide net to identify opportunities for international work. They may need to rely on word of mouth more than on classified ads. In fact, they may need to create their own positions through persuasion and personality and justify their continued employment through quality performance and output. All of us who are interested in international veterinary work must function as explorers, scouts, and beaters to track down and flush out the opportunities that exist and to create new ones where the potential remains untapped.

This is not to say that international opportunities do not exist. They just may be hard to find. In 1995, the results of a survey conducted at North Carolina State University were reported in the *Journal of Veterinary Medical Education*.[4] The survey was intended, in part, to identify opportunities for employment in international veterinary medicine. A questionnaire was mailed to various types of organizations involved in international work to determine how many had employed veterinarians in the past and how many would be likely to do so in the future. Of the 366 organizations receiving a mailed questionnaire, 177 (48%) responded. The respondents included both governmental and nongovernmental organizations (NGOs). Among these organizations, 50.3% had hired veterinarians prior to the survey, and 38% were currently employing veterinarians. In addition, 53.8% of the remaining organizations with no history of hiring veterinarians said they would consider hiring veterinarians in the future.

In another, albeit rough, indication of employment opportunities abroad for North American veterinarians, the 2001 *Membership Directory and Resource Manual* of the American Veterinary Medical Association[2] lists 374 AVMA members with foreign country addresses other than Canada, another 188 AVMA members living in United States territories, and 81 members listing military post offices, for a total of 643 AVMA members (some of whom may not be Americans or Canadians) who are potentially working internationally as veterinarians. This represents about 1% of the total active AVMA membership reported for the year.

This chapter is intended to provide practical information on career opportunities and job identification to veterinarians interested in adding an international dimension to their professional lives. The chapter begins with guidelines for conducting a self-assessment to determine the reader's own suitability for international work and the type of international work that might best reflect the reader's personality and interests. This is followed by a discussion of how the reader can acquire relevant skills, training and experience during different stages of his or her professsional development. Suggestions are provided for readers at the undergraduate, veterinary school, and post graduate level. Next, there is a presentation of the various types of organizations that might employ veterinarians for international work. The activities of various categories of agencies are described and examples of organizations in each category are provided. Finally, the chapter closes with a discussion of how to go about finding work that matches the reader's interests, skills and experience.

Defining International Work on Your Own Terms

If you have read this far in the book or even this far in the chapter, something is telling you that you are interested in international work. Where and what do you see yourself doing? Do you picture yourself

- Driving to Paris for the weekend in your BMW after a busy week working in international marketing at the Animal Health Business Group Headquarters of Bayer Corporation in Germany, where you have been assigned by Bayer's American subsidiary?

- Swooping over the African savanna in a helicopter, tranquilizer gun poised to dart a white rhino as part of a translocation and reintroduction program sponsored by an international conservation group?
- Traveling from village to village in a Land Rover through the mountains of Nepal to visit trainees in a community-based animal health care network that has been set up by an American (NGO) in cooperation with the Nepalese government?
- Helping to care for foundling orangutans at a rehabilitation center in Borneo, orphaned as a result of prolonged forest fires in their natural habitat?
- Organizing an international symposium on nontariff barriers to trade in animal products between Russia and the United States for the U.S. government?
- Providing emergency care for injured and stranded livestock following a severe hurricane in Central America?
- Helping dairy farmers and their veterinarians make the transition to privatization in former republics of the Soviet Union as part of a U.S. Agency for International Development (USAID) project?
- Working on the development of effective vaccines for the control of trypanosomiasis?
- Supervising the importation of a shipment of alpacas from Bolivia to the United States?
- Setting up a global program for monitoring the health of pelagic birds potentially at risk from endocrine-disrupting chemicals?
- Inspecting beef products in South America destined for the United States?
- Doing private small animal practice in Hong Kong?

All of these are realistic possibilities of international work for North American veterinarians. Despite the variety of interests and activities represented, all these experiences are valid examples of "international veterinary medicine," a field that demands to be broadly defined. It would be the rare individual however who would find all of these scenarios equally interesting or attractive or who could picture himself or herself pursuing each and every example. Even if that person existed, various circumstances of family ties, financial obligations, and other extenuating circumstances might eliminate some of the potential options.

The point, of course, is that opportunities in international veterinary medicine are defined to a great extent by the interests, attitudes, aptitudes, convictions, and commitments of individuals thinking about working internationally. International veterinary medicine is as diverse as the people who choose to pursue it.

The first step, therefore, in developing a plan and strategy to develop your career prospects in international veterinary medicine is to define what international veterinary medicine means to you in your own terms. To do this you have to honestly and carefully examine your motivations, your goals, your interests, and your capabilities. To do this, it will help to ask yourself, and answer thoughtfully, to your own satisfaction, the basic defining questions that journalists are taught to ask to clarify and characterize any new, unfamiliar situation—who, what, when, where, and why?

While your initial attempts to answer these questions will likely occur in private through personal reflection, list making, and conversations with colleagues and family members, it is also important to seek out people with first hand international experience and engage them in discussions of your evolving ideas.

If you are a veterinary student at a large university, it should not be too difficult to find a host of appropriate people to engage in conversation. Most likely, right within your own veterinary college there will be veterinary faculty and graduate students with first-hand international experience who will be happy to listen to you and share their opinions and perspectives. Yet even if you in practice in a small town somewhere, frequently you can still find people with international experience. They may be recent immigrants, former Peace Corps volunteers, veterans, or high school teachers who have worked or studied abroad during summers. Actively seek these people out. Such persistence in the pursuit of available resources itself demonstrates a desirable and necessary habit for successfully working internationally. If you cannot find appropriate people to talk to, books are available that guide readers through a self-assessment process when considering career path or career change. One title recommended by several sources is *What Color is your Parachute?* by Richard Nelson Bolles.[3] This book was first published in 1970, but a newly revised and updated edition is released regularly.

The "Who?" of International Work

It is important to have a sense of who you are as a person, both professionally and personally. We have all prepared job resumés that catalog our education, training, work experience, and professional accomplishments, thus defining ourselves chronologically according to our accumulated achievements for consideration by prospective employees. When thinking about international work, it can be useful, as a self-assessment, to prepare a parallel account of who you are using a more personal framework for evaluation. Try developing a resumé of the attitudes, habits, beliefs, personality traits, and other individual characteristics that define you as an individual. Think about how these various traits might enhance or hamper your effectiveness in international work. In other words, practice being self-aware. You may develop a better understanding of your own personality and gain some insight into your motivations for international work. It may help you understand how you are likely to respond to unfamiliar and unexpected situations or how well you may get along with people whose backgrounds and experience are very different from your own.

Also, when thinking about who you are, take into account the fact that you are an American, a citizen of perhaps the wealthiest and most powerful nation on Earth. You may not be accustomed to thinking about yourself in this context or feel that it has any major bearing on who you are as an individual, but rest assured, virtually everyone you meet abroad will consider you in terms of your citizenship. Their reactions may be positive or they may be negative, but they will very likely be colored by the fact that you are an American. When I first visited Kenya in 1969, I was asked by schoolchildren, whose image of the United States at that time was shaped primarily by old American cowboy movies shown in Nairobi cinemas, where my six guns were. They simply could not believe that I, an American, did not wear a gun belt and carry two loaded six-shooters. They also wanted to know when I, as an American, would be walking on the moon, a feat accomplished by American astronauts Neil Armstrong and Michael Collins just months before. Like it or not, when you travel abroad, you are an informal ambassador of the United States. How you behave will be assumed to represent how all Americans behave. Regardless of your own personal politics or convictions, local people will project their own perceptions of the United States upon you and may expect you to defend or disavow your country's policies and actions. Be aware of how America's policies and actions have affected a particular country or people both in historical terms and under present circumstances.

In addition, many Americans, until they work abroad, do not truly recognize or appreciate the incredibly high standard of living we enjoy and how sharply it contrasts with conditions in other places. The comfort, convenience, safety, and general efficiency that we experience in our everyday lives is unparalleled in much of the world. Even if, as an individual, you do not consider yourself wealthy, your mere arrival in some remote places confirms a degree of wealth, power, and control of resources that is unimaginable to many local people. The "walking around" money in your wallet may exceed a month's salary for average citizens in many places. Such disparities will inevitably influence your relationships with others, and you need to be aware of this.

Finally, when considering the "who?" question, think about the people you see yourself interacting with on a daily basis in your international work. Who will your coworkers and constituents be? Do you see yourself working with a team of research scientists? global marketing executives? government ministers and functionaries? trade negotiators? dairy farmers? game wardens? goat herders? church officials? soldiers? relief workers? other veterinarians? International veterinary work offers the potential to work with any or all of these different types as well as others. Obviously, your own temperament, interests, and professional skills will lead you toward some groups of coworkers and the kind of activities they represent and away from others. Also try to imagine what these people will be like. What will be the color of their skin? their gender? their level of education? What language will they speak? What religion will they practice? What foods will they eat? Be

open to the diversity of opportunity that international work offers, but be honest with yourself about your own biases and preferences. Be honest with yourself and with others about who you are and what you represent.

The "What?" of International Work

What is it you would like to do and what would you like to accomplish? As the introductory list of bulleted examples point out, the menu of opportunities in international work offers many options. What you choose, of course, depends largely on your personal and professional interests. Are you interested in wildlife conservation? food production? transboundary disease control? public health? socioeconomic development? the anthropology of animal keeping? pharmaceutical research and development? animal welfare? environmental health?

Do you see yourself working in an office? a laboratory? a classroom? a village? a ranger station? a clinic? a livestock market? a food-processing plant? a forest? When you close your eyes and think about your international career, are you sitting at a desk looking at a computer screen in air-conditioned comfort in the heart of a major European capital developing a technical service plan to support the marketing effort for a new anthelmintic? Perhaps you are standing on a narrow platform high in a tree in a rainforest in the middle of the night, drenched in sweat, waiting to capture a nocturnal mammal whose population is threatened by deforestation? Are you trying to convince a group of African cattle herders, armed with AK-47s, that it is in their best interest to pay their paraveterinarian for the drugs they use so that he will be able to resupply and serve them again in the future? Are you advising a group of investors and their technical staff on the installation and management of a large, intensive swine-production unit in Southeast Asia? Are you raising funds to set up a clinic for the care and treatment of donkeys in Pakistan?

As part of developing your international career strategy you should clearly define your interests and then match them up against your present skills and experience. Is your international career goal a natural extension of what you are already doing at home, or does it represent a new professional direction altogether? If you need new skills, how will you get them? If your skills are appropriate, but your international work experience is limited, how will you address that?

If you are still in veterinary school, your options for acquiring additional appropriate training and experience will be more varied and easily accessible than if, for example, you have already been in practice for several years. As a practitioner, on the other hand, you may already have, by virtue of experience, better management, organizational, communication, and hands-on technical veterinary skills than the student. Individual circumstances and the intensity of your motivation to do international work will dictate how much, and what kind of, additional training and experience you need and how easy or difficult it will be for you to obtain it. With some site-specific preparation through reading and discussions with informed individuals, a large-animal practitioner may capably serve as a privatization advisor to livestock veterinarians in the newly independent states of the former Soviet Union with a minimum of additional training, while an exotic animal practitioner might readily be able to provide useful training and clinical services to a wildlife rescue and rehabilitation center in Costa Rica on the basis of on existing skills and experience. However, if each practitioner decided he or she wanted to pursue the alternative opportunity, the need for additional training and experience becomes readily apparent.

The "When?" of International Work

The "when?" of international work refers both to the timing and the duration of your professional activity. First, at what stage of your career are you approaching the possibility of international work, and second, what time commitment do you wish to make to working abroad. Depending on to the stage of your career, the options for international work, and how easily you can make the transition, will change with your level of experience and type of training as well as with personal considerations of income, health, family responsibility, and financial obligation. Some newly minted veterinarians may already have significant international experience, special expertise, or advanced degrees as a result of activities or studies undertaken prior to veterinary school. Most recent veterinary graduates will not, and this may limit their options regarding available and appropriate international opportunities. Volunteer opportunities, advanced training programs, or military service in the veterinary corps may be the most likely opportunities at this stage.

Midcareer veterinarians thinking about international work may face a different set of challenges. Practitioners, regulatory veterinarians, or veterinary academicians, for example, may have a strong foundation of relevant technical know-how but limited understanding or experience in applying that knowledge in an international context. Sabbaticals or volunteer work abroad, transfers into industry positions with the potential for international assignment, or professional retooling through fellowships or advanced degrees with an international focus may facilitate midcareer international activities. Many veterinarians reaching retirement age may want to leave the pressures of daily practice but still wish to remain professionally active: Volunteer work again becomes an attractive option, as does private consulting for business and industry.

One also must decide, in the context of personal and professional considerations, what constitutes a comfortable and appropriate length of assignment. How much time do you have to spend abroad, if any, to fulfill your desire to be involved internationally. Will your circumstance allow you to work abroad continuously for years at a time? A position with the Food and Agriculture Organization of the United Nations (FAO) at its headquarters in Rome might be for you. Would you prefer a situation in which your base of professional activity is at home, but regular short-term international assignments are ensured? A teaching position at a veterinary faculty with an internationally based research program would serve well. Are you committed to a position in the United States but have a strong commitment to at least occasionally work

abroad? Short-term volunteer opportunities that can be carried out during vacation times are available. The Massachusetts Veterinary Medical Association, for instance, organizes an annual trip for interested practitioners to the Dominican Republic to provide clinical veterinary services to livestock in and around the town of Samana (Figure 10-1). Are you simply unable to get away at all but want to be involved? Then consider hosting a foreign veterinary student in your practice, working with your church or Rotary club to raise funds to buy books and journals for an overseas veterinary faculty, or helping to improve conditions at an urban zoo in a developing country. The possibilities are limited only by your imagination, interests, and sense of commitment.

The "Where?" of International Work

Think about where you would like to work and the reasons why. Personal reasons for selecting a location may be just as valid as professional ones. You may have developed a keen in-

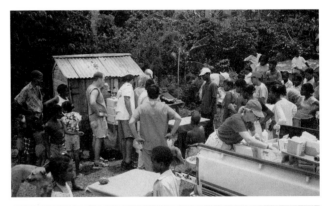

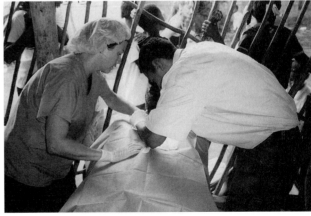

Figure 10-1.   Project Samana is an international outreach program of the Massachusetts Veterinary Medical Association and can serve as a useful model for similar programs by other state veterinary medical associations. The project focuses on animal population control, improving the health and productivity of draft animals, and provision of training to local veterinarians in Samana, Dominican Republic. Top, Massachusetts veterinarians set up a spay and neuter clinic in a schoolyard amidst a throng of curious local residents. Bottom, Massachusetts practitioner, Dr. Cindy Duerr, guides a Dominican veterinarian through a spay procedure. Dr. Duerr spent 2 years in the Peace Corps in Ghana before entering veterinary school. (Photos courtesy of Dr. Jay Merriam)

terest in, and knowledge of, a certain part of the world through the writings of a favorite author, interest in the art and music of a certain culture, or formal studies in college. You may have studied Spanish, French, or Russian for years in high school and university but always felt frustrated that you were never able to use your language skills on a regular basis. Perhaps you visited someplace as a tourist and thought you would like to come back some day in a professional capacity and make a contribution to the well-being of the people, the welfare of domestic animals, or the conservation of a beautiful, wild place and its denizens.

On the professional side, different interests may point you to different countries, regions, or ecosystems. You may, for example, recognize significant commercial livestock or aquaculture business opportunities for American agribusiness or pharmaceutical firms in a specific country with a growing economy somewhere in Asia, Africa, or Latin America. You may have a research interest in physiological adaptations of animals to water scarcity that could take you to any number of semiarid ecosystems around the world. A specific interest in mountain gorilla conservation would oblige you to work in Uganda, Rwanda, or the Democratic Republic of the Congo. Special expertise in the control of camel diseases may get you consulting invitations to various countries in the Middle East, while special expertise in swine medicine would pretty much guarantee that you never got invitations to those same countries, due to Islamic proscriptions against pigs as discussed in Chapter 3.

Keep in mind that no matter where you choose to go, you will be undertaking a cross-cultural experience. You must carefully consider how much cultural difference you can comfortably accommodate, both mentally and physically. People have different psychological thresholds for discomfort and unfamiliarity, and you need to have a sense of where yours is. Can you adapt to driving on the left-hand side of the road? Are you comfortable with having no access to high-quality emergency medical care? Can you tolerate losing your electrical power unpredictably for hours or days at a time? Are you prepared to have diarrhea for weeks at a time? How frustrated will you become if you have to dial a long distance call 30 times before getting connected? Would you be able to buy and consume meat from an open-air shop thick with flies? Can you live some place where alcoholic beverages are prohibited? How about living someplace where women are not permitted to drive? Would you be willing to eat insects if they are offered to you? How well do you sleep without air conditioning when the humidity is 90% and the temperature is even higher? Can you entertain yourself without access to television? Be honest with yourself about such issues. If you are not sure of your limits, then test yourself before you commit to the unknown. In your own city, are you willing to go walk in a neighborhood where you normally would never go and have dinner in a restaurant there? Would you go camping for a long weekend when the forecast calls for rain? How about taking a vacation in a developing country where no English is spoken? Do some experimenting, and try to establish the limits of your comfort zone. Do not, however, under any circumstances, practice driving on the left-hand side of the road while you remain in the United States!

The "Why?" of International Work

Examine your motivation for wanting to do international work. Why do you want to add a global dimension to your personal and professional life? Consider both personal and professional reasons. On the personal side, it may be, among other things, your spirit of adventure, a love of travel, the lure of unfamiliar places, or the opportunity to live in some place that has special meaning for you. These are somewhat generic impulses, but they are nonetheless, valid contributors to your decision to work abroad. Some other personal motivations may be less valid, for instance, the notion that international work is glamorous or that it makes you a more interesting person.

Perhaps you have other, personal motivations that are more focused, such as a strong personal philosophy, religious faith, or social conviction that can find expression through your work as a veterinarian. Examples might include helping people to feed themselves, encouraging peace through food security, promoting sustainable agriculture to protect natural resources and improve environmental health, securing a viable future for endangered species, improving the welfare of domestic animals in nations where animal welfare has not been a high priority, supporting the traditional lifestyles of nomadic peoples, or stimulating economic growth in developing countries.

Your motivations may be related to specific professional challenges and opportunities that are best realized in an international context. For example, you might be interested in the development of heat-stable vaccines against livestock diseases that occur in remote areas where it is difficult to deliver and maintain refrigerated inventories of vaccine. Other examples might be the identification, characterization, and evaluation of indigenous plants in Asia that have been used by local farmers as anthelmintics and insecticides; the collection of basic health data on a threatened animal species so as to help develop a realistic long-range conservation plan; the integration of appropriate microlivestock species into rural farming systems where human diets are low in protein; training and capacity building projects to improve mastitis control programs for the dairy industry in various countries of the former Soviet Union; or improving methods for ensuring that exotic animal diseases do not accidentally enter the Untied States.

Preparing Yourself for International Work

Once you have answered for yourself the general questions of who?, what?, when?, where?, and why? in relation to your interest in international work, it is time to tackle the most critical question in terms of realizing your international aspirations, namely, How do I go about preparing myself for the kind of international work I think I would like to do? To find out how, you must first gather information about the kinds of international employment opportunities available that reflect your interest and identify the types and extent of international experience and technical skills required for such jobs. Then you must begin to develop a plan for acquiring the appropriate experience and skills. In this section, some suggestions for networking and information gathering are offered as well as some guidance for gathering relevant international experience and strengthening your skill base.

Networking and Information Gathering

There is no simple, centralized, easily accessed source of information that focuses specifically on career opportunities in international veterinary medicine. Personal initiative through networking and information gathering remain critical aspects of identifying and/or creating international employment opportunities in veterinary medicine.

A number of guides are available at public libraries and bookstores that can help introduce newcomers to the general landscape of international jobs and career opportunities. Though they may contain little or no information specific to veterinary medicine, they are still useful introductions for veterinarians with little or no first-hand international experience or for students who have not yet been involved in any serious job hunting. One publisher, Impact Publications, has dozens of titles dealing with different aspects of international employment, including career planning, self-assessment, resumé writing, and job directories, among others. Another publisher, Intercultural Press, has many titles dealing with cross-cultural issues, including those related to working abroad. Few printed resources are specifically targeted to veterinarians interested in international work. One useful book in this area is Dr. Carin Smith's *Career Choices for Veterinarians: Beyond Private Practice*.[11] This recent volume has a chapter entitled "International, Volunteer, and Assistance Work" and also addresses international opportunities in chapters on working for the federal government, uniformed services jobs, consulting, and careers in industry. Another useful text, though written from a British perspective, is *Working with Animals: The UK, Europe and Worldwide*, by Victoria Pybus, which covers nonprofessional and some professional opportunities to work with animals in a variety of contexts involving livestock, companion animals, wildlife, and zoo animals.[9]

For veterinary-specific information about the nature and availability of international opportunities, it is important to network with veterinarians who have international experience or who are affiliated with specialties and organizations that have an international frame of reference. The annual AVMA meeting is a good place to begin. Many companies and organizations with international perspectives or activities have displays in the exhibition area staffed by informed people who are happy to answer questions and provide information. For instance, at the 1999 convention in New Orleans, I walked up to the booth of the American Association of Food Hygiene Veterinarians and had a very enjoyable and informative conversation with Dr. Joe Blair, the executive vice president of the association. It turned out that he himself had had numerous international assignments during his career, working as a consultant to USAID in

Latin America to ensure a high level of hygienic standards in local food-processing establishments. He showed me the newsletter of his association, which provides members with useful, current information about new developments, challenges, and opportunities in this important field, which is bound to expand as consumption of livestock products continues to expand. He also was able to refer me to others in the field with similar experience.

Many other public and professional organizations with an international perspective were present at the 1999 AVMA meeting, with representatives eager to talk and share information. These included (in alphabetical order), the American Academy of Public Health Veterinarians, the American Academy on Veterinary Disaster Medicine, the American Association of Zoo Veterinarians, the American Board of Veterinary Toxicology, Christian Veterinary Mission, the International Wildlife Rehabilitation Council, Livestock Conservation Institute (with information on foreign animal disease preparedness), Medical Books for China International, the Morris Animal Foundation (supporting gorilla conservation in East Africa), the U.S. Air Force Public Health Service, the U.S. Army, the United States Department of Agriculture (USDA) Food Safety and Inspection Service, the United States Public Health Service (which includes veterinarians posted at the Centers for Disease Control and Prevention (CDC), the Environmental Protection Agency (EPA), and the Food and Drug Administration (FDA)), and the World Veterinary Association (with information about the annual World Veterinary Congress).

In addition, a number of veterinary schools and colleges were represented that offered postgraduate training programs relevant to a career in International Veterinary Medicine, for example, the University of California at Davis, which offers a Masters in Preventive Veterinary Medicine. Commercial exhibitors also included a number of pharmaceutical and animal feed companies with international scope, including Bayer Corporation, Merck and Co., Merial Limited, Pasteur Merieux Connaught (now Aventis), Novartis Animal Health, Pfizer Animal Health, Ralston Purina Company, Schering-Plough Animal Health, and Waltham.

For those who cannot afford the time or expense to travel to the AVMA meeting, the *Membership Directory and Resource Manual* of the AVMA is a valuable reference.[2] An updated version is mailed annually to AVMA members at no cost and contains sections on organizations related to veterinary medicine. All the professional organizations and government agencies present at the 1999 AVMA meeting are included in the directory, as well as some relevant groups that were not present, for example, the Society for Tropical Veterinary Medicine. The directory provides relevant contact information for these organizations. In addition, all the world's veterinary schools are listed, with detailed contact information provided for North American schools. A separate list of international veterinary organizations includes contact information for the national veterinary associations of individual countries around the world, as well as international professional societies and organizations such as the World Association of Transport Animal Welfare and Studies, the

World Health Organization, and the World Association of Wildlife Veterinarians, to name but a few relevant examples.

Of course, in the age of global electronic communications, internet sites are also becoming a vital source of up-to-date information for veterinarians interested in international work. Again, as with print media, there is no single source that caters specifically to international interests. Several internet resources targeted at veterinarians have evolved in recent years and may contain relevant, useful information about international veterinary medicine, though in no case is that their primary function. NetVet and the Electronic Zoo, available at the same site, basically serve as a comprehensive clearing house with linkages to other pertinent web sites of interest to veterinarians. For example, if a veterinarian was interested in international issues related to primate conservation, he or she could go to the Electronic Zoo, click on "Primates" and receive an extensive list of related website links that deal with primate biology, primate medicine, primate conservation, primate rescue, and primate welfare, all a mouse click away from the Electronic Zoo page. It is available free to everyone at http://netvet.wustl.edu/.

Another useful electronic resource, VetPlus, is an interactive list for veterinarians, physicians, supporting technicians, and veterinary and medical students. It is available free to individual subscribers who must sign up electronically (see http://www.vetprof.com/ on the internet). Membership is worldwide, with over 37% of subscribers in 1998 coming from outside North America, including members in South America, Europe, Africa, Asia, and Australia. It is a good place to exchange technical and professional information with colleagues worldwide and begin to appreciate different cultural perspectives. In one discussion group, for example, veterinarians from the United States, the UK, Australia, and Sweden discussed the practice of declawing cats, the ethics of declawing, and the laws governing such practices in their respective countries. Declawing is illegal, by the way, in all of those countries except the United States.

Most of the potential employers listed below in sections of this chapter have web sites. Web sites usually provide a useful overview of the structure of an organization, its overall mission, the types and locations of international activities in which it is engaged, and frequently, even up-to-the-minute job postings that can help to give you an idea of the kinds of work available and the level of experience and training required to compete successfully for such positions.

For students, the university itself is often an excellent source of international information, if for no other reason than the size and scope of the library resources available there. In addition, however, large universities often have numerous international student groups that have meetings and sponsor cultural activities, lectures, or films on specific countries or regions. There may be whole departments focusing on various cultures or regions, such as a Middle Eastern Studies or African Studies Department, and of course there may be many faculty with field research projects overseas who can use student assistants on campus during the school year and, possibly, on site during the summer. Do not restrict yourself to veterinary medicine, as there may be important, useful opportunities with faculty in related areas of study such as conservation biology or agriculture, to name just two.

Experience Gathering

One of the frequently perceived obstacles in obtaining international work is the common requirement for prior international experience. This can be frustrating, especially for recent graduates. They don't qualify for advertised positions because they don't have experience, and they cannot gain experience because they do not qualify for advertised positions. So why do prospective employers place such a strong emphasis on prerequisite experience for international work? The reasons vary, depending on the type of position, the duration of the assignment, and the level of responsibility involved.

One function of the experience requirement is to enable employers to discourage frivolous applications from people simply not qualified to perform international work. Do not, however, be so easily deterred. If you were considering applying for a job that called for 5 years of international experience, but you had a strong, relevant skill base and 2 solid years of international experience instead of 5, it would be reasonable to apply for the position anyway. There is probably more flexibility in the decision-making process than is apparent simply from reading the advertisement. The worst that can happen is that they say no.

At another level, demonstration of some successful international experience on your resumé may be a shorthand method for potential employers to confirm that you are adaptable and flexible in unfamiliar situations and not likely to disrupt the work of foreign and expatriate colleagues in the field with personal complaints about unpaved roads, faulty plumbing, intermittent electricity, unreliable phone service, traveler's diarrhea, or any of the other routine inconveniences of international work that many Americans do not usually encounter in their daily lives.

In addition, a record of work experience abroad tells employers that you are able to apply your technical skills productively in a cross-cultural context. Veterinarians educated in North America are blessed with excellent clinical training and can draw on the most up-to-date information and technologies in the practice of veterinary medicine. In many parts of the world, advanced clinical and diagnostic services are not available, and veterinarians must perform their jobs drawing heavily on their physical diagnostic skills and their experience of what conditions are likely to occur locally. The successful expatriate veterinarian working abroad must be able to work effectively within the constraints of local conditions and be creative in maximizing accomplishments and minimizing complaints.

At the highest level, genuine, first-hand, long-term experience in a specific region or country can, in itself, be a critical asset, highly valued by potential employers. If, for example, you were going to be seconded to a government ministry for 3 years to help establish a national surveillance system for livestock diseases, it would be extremely important to know the politics, culture, geography, economic situation, livestock husbandry practices, and even the major language in that country. An individual with such background could hit the ground running, work effectively with a wide variety of personnel, capably evaluate problems, and develop solutions in an appropriate local context.

You must also recognize that prospective employers may assess short-term international experience differently than long-term experience. In other words, 12 1-month experiences in different locations represents a different profile of experience to a prospective employer than 1 12-month experience in a single place. Successful short-term professional experience may represent a capacity for efficiency, good organizational skills, and problem-solving ability, while long-term experience can represent a capacity for accommodation, staying power, and perhaps a deeper insight into the culture and commerce of a specific country or region. In developing a base of experience, it is best to have both short-term and long-term experiences in your portfolio. Bear in mind also that the type of experience is important. Active professional experiences are ranked more highly than passive, nonprofessional ones. A 3-week vacation in England, albeit an international experience of sorts, should not be included on a resumé. Attendance at an international scientific conference or professional meeting can be listed but is not likely to be considered very significant, unless you organized or chaired the event.

Before Veterinary School

The earlier in your life you recognize your interest in international work, the easier it will be to develop a marketable base of experience. Some fortunate individuals may have lived abroad as children with parents on international assignment or have grown up as citizens of other countries whose families later emigrated to the United States. For most people, however, opportunities to gain international experience relevant to career development usually become available during college. Such opportunities include, among others, an academic year abroad, summer in-country language study programs, summer research assistantships on overseas field projects, or a variety of volunteer opportunities. All such opportunities should be exploited.

The period following college can be a good time to gain useful international experience. College graduates who know they want to be veterinarians may find it a difficult personal decision to defer their attendance at veterinary college. However, college graduates who know with certainty that they want to do international veterinary medicine may be well served by gaining some long-term international experience prior to veterinary school. It will likely help them tailor their subsequent veterinary training, through elective course selection, externships, and summer work experiences, to match their international interests. The United States Peace Corps has been, since 1961, an important vehicle for many individuals to gain valu-

able, long-term experience on the path to international careers while doing useful, productive work in developing countries. Peace Corps service offers a special opportunity to gain hands-on, people-to-people field experience with full cross-cultural immersion. Future employers generally consider such experience highly relevant toward meeting their overall experience requirements.

Other long-term opportunities are also available. In recent years, for instance, numerous programs have arisen that place American students in foreign countries to teach English as a second language. While this activity per se may not be directly applicable to a future veterinary career, it offers a chance to acquire long-term experience in a country of interest to you, gives you the opportunity to learn or strengthen a foreign language skill, and gives you time to explore other connections and resources that may be useful in your future professional work. In addition, there are numerous volunteer, internship, and short-term work opportunities available overseas, some of which are potentially useful as preparatory experiences for future veterinarians. Once again, the public library and the internet are good places to begin to identify such opportunities, bearing in mind that the printed and electronic resources available through the library and the web must be used with patience and perseverance, as very few international opportunities are indexed or characterized specifically as opportunities for veterinarians, though they very well may be.

During Veterinary School

For veterinary students, the opportunity to gain international experience during veterinary school is increasing. Over the last 20 years, there has been a major shift in the veterinary curriculum to allow more elective time in the course schedule and to facilitate off-campus externship experiences during the period of clinical training. This means that students with an international focus may begin to build veterinary-specific international experience while still in veterinary school. Many individual students show admirable initiative in arranging their own externship opportunities. Some schools have structured international clinical externships. Texas A&M and UC-Davis, for example, have institutional arrangements with veterinary schools in Mexico to facilitate student externships there. Tufts University, in collaboration with the Massachusetts Society for the Prevention of Cruelty to Animals, offers a practice externship opportunity for its students in Morocco. The International Veterinary Student Association (IVSA) helps to coordinate international externship opportunities for students who wish to work as volunteers in foreign veterinary practices for periods of 2 weeks or longer. Each veterinary college in North America has its own student representative to the IVSA, coordinated through its local chapter of the Student American Veterinary Medical Association (SAVMA).

A variety of nonclinical externships or clerkships relevant to preparation for future international veterinary work are also available. A list of such positions, including opportunities in industry, corporate agriculture, government, and other categories has been compiled by the Center for Government and

Corporate Veterinary Medicine at the Virginia-Maryland Regional College of Veterinary Medicine. Listings can be viewed at their website, http://www.vetmed.umd.edu/cgcvm/.

An excellent opportunity for veterinary students at U.S. veterinary schools to gain valuable professional experience abroad emerged in 1996. This is the Frontiers in Veterinary Medicine Program created by the Geraldine R. Dodge Foundation. The program was created to encourage students to think outside the traditional confines of veterinary education and to develop new approaches to the humane treatment of animals through student-driven research. The program originally offered competitive grants of $5000 to approximately 35 students per year to promote student-conceived research projects in emerging areas of veterinary medicine such as conservation medicine, veterinary ethics, livestock in development, animal welfare, and other nontraditional areas in which the humane treatment of animals can be fostered. The program operated continuously from 1996 through 2000. After a 1-year hiatus in 2001 to conduct an external evaluation of their program, the Dodge Foundation has decided to continue with the Frontiers in Veterinary Medicine Program again in 2002, offering grants of up to $6000 each. Program information and application guidelines are available on the internet at http://www.grdodge.org/vet/index.html.

In the first 3 years of the Frontiers for Veterinary Medicine initiative, 1996 to 1998, a total of 109 projects was funded. Approximately 40% were focused on companion animals, 30% on large animals, and 30% on wildlife. Overall, a full one third of these funded projects had an international focus or cross-cultural perspective (Table 10-2). Students have shown remarkable creativity and imagination in developing research project initiatives that reflect a wide range of values and interests and clearly have demonstrated the variety of challenges and opportunities that can be identified in the field of international veterinary medicine. Students with the skills, resourcefulness, and determination to compete successfully for one of these grants, who can effectively implement field research projects in a cross-cultural context, bring home meaningful results, and leave a favorable impression with colleagues abroad, are students who are well on the road to establishing rewarding and productive international careers.

Some veterinary schools have been able to identify international opportunities for their own students through externally supported programs. For example, Washington State University, Texas A&M, Tufts University, and Purdue University formed a consortium that was able to procure federal funding in support of internationalization of veterinary education. In 1996, the group was awarded a grant by the National Security Education Program (NSEP) for its proposal "Enhancing International Veterinary Medical Education through University Curriculum Development." Implemented in partnership with eight host institutions in Latin America, the grant has provided opportunities for U.S. veterinary students to study Spanish while in veterinary school and to gain first-hand experience through student-defined externships and field projects in Latin America, with an emphasis on the countries of Argentina, Chile, Uruguay, and Mexico. These four countries together account for over 90% of the region's livestock trade with the United States.

In the changing landscape of veterinary education, it has now become possible for veterinary students interested in pursuing an international career to graduate from veterinary school with two full summers of field-based research experience, some foreign language skills, elective courses relevant to international veterinary medicine, and some clinical externship experience outside the United States (Fig. 10-2). The opportunities for students to maximize their international experience during veterinary school differ from institution to institution, as there is still considerable variation among schools in the extent to which they have committed to internationalizing the curriculum or encouraging and facilitating international student activities. Prospective veterinary students interested in international careers should ask very specific questions about international programs during the veterinary school application process. First of all, does the school actively promote and foster international activities? Is there a specific international program? Are there specific faculty members identified to support international activities by students? How many such faculty members are there and how much time do they allocate to that role? Are there relevant elective course offerings within the veterinary school or other colleges on campus? Are there any internal funds to support overseas clinical, research, and service opportunities for students? How many students from the school have been successful in obtaining grants in the Frontiers of Veterinary Medicine Program? These are all indicators of how well or poorly your interest in international veterinary medicine will be accommodated and supported during your time in veterinary school.

After Veterinary School

As just discussed, it is becoming easier for veterinary students to obtain professionally relevant, short-term, international experience while still in veterinary school. Nevertheless, new graduates may still lack the kind of long-term international experience that is attractive to many employers, especially for jobs with a high level of responsibility and commensurate pay. Their short-term experience and veterinary degree, however, will open some new doors for professional work, particularly if personal financial circumstances allow deferral of higher income for several more years.

Once again, as an option after veterinary school, the Peace Corps offers an excellent opportunity for appropriate long-term international experience. If you were not a Peace Corps volunteer before veterinary school, the value of the Peace Corps experience to you as a graduate veterinarian will be enhanced by your newly learned veterinary skills. You may also be able to make a more significant contribution in your host country. While most veterinarians in the Peace Corps recognized it as a positive, valuable experience, I have had one returning Peace Corps veterinarian tell me that the Peace Corps sees you as "a Peace Corps volunteer first, and a veterinarian second," implying that the organization did not make full use

Table 10-2 Student Projects with an International Perspective That Were Funded Through the Frontiers of Veterinary Medicine Program of the Geraldine R. Dodge Foundation in the First Three Years of the Program, 1996–1998

Award Year	Title of Project	Focus of Project	Project Location	Student's Veterinary School
1996	The Influence of Religion on the Humane Treatment of Animals	Dairy workers and dairy cattle	Israel	University of California-Davis
1996	Mongolian Livestock Management Systems	Mongolian herders and their goats	Mongolia	Michigan State University
1996	Impact of Veterinary Auxiliaries among the Twareg and Wodaabe of Niger	Pastoralist herders and their stock	Niger	Tufts University
1996	Rain Forest Biodiversity Conservation: Offsetting Hunting Pressures through Husbandry of Game Farmed Rats	Cane rats	Gabon	Tufts University
1996	Swiss Dairy Farmers in Quebec: Have the Swiss Brought with Them Management Practices Which Promote Animal Comfort and Demonstrate Respect for the Environment?	See title	Canada	University of Montreal
1996	The Fate of Unwanted Vietnamese Pot-Bellied Pigs: A Survey of Humane Organizations and Slaughter Houses	See title	United States	Ohio State University
1996	Application of Herd Health Principles to Yak in Western Nepal	See title	Nepal	Colorado State University
1996	Epidemiological Surveillance of Antibiotic Resistance as a Measurement of Disease Transmission from Humans to Wild Chimpanzees	See title	Uganda	Tufts University
1996	Improving the Welfare of African Chimpanzees through the Development of Local Solutions to Nutrition and Environmental Enrichment Constraints	See title	Uganda	Tufts University
1996	An Evaluation of the Value of Natural Forage for Captive Chimpanzees	See title	Kenya	Tufts University
1996	Conservation through Health Care and Molecular Biology: A Veterinary Role in Human-Wildlife Interactions	Chimpanzees and local fisherman	Tanzania	Tufts University
1997	Adaptation of Tufts Thermostable Rinderpest Vaccine for Aerosol Vaccination of Wildlife and Free Ranging Domestic Animals	See title	Kenya	Tufts University
1997	Survey of Pack Animal Health Care in Peten, Guatemala	Horses, donkeys, mules	Guatemala	Tufts University
1997	Survey and Support of the Nepali Paravet Program	Paraveterinarians and the livestock and villagers served	Nepal	Washington State University
1997	Chadian Manatee Conservation through Village-based Education and Genetic Analysis	Freshwater manatees	Chad	Tufts University

(continued)

Award Year	Title of Project	Focus of Project	Project Location	Student's Veterinary School
1997	Health, Fiber, and Welfare Survey of Goat Production in Namibia	See title	Namibia	Tufts University
1997	Comparison of the Sedative Effects of Different Preanesthetic Agents for Use in Field Clinics Performing Spay and Neuter Surgeries in Remote Areas	Dogs and cats	Guatemala	University of Tennessee
1998	The Introduction of Exotic Animals through Pet Shops: An Ecological and Ethical Issue Affecting the Native Fauna of Puerto Rico	See title	Puerto Rico	Kansas State University
1998	Situation Analysis for the Improvement of the Management and Veterinary Medical Treatment of the Working Buffalo in the Nile Delta Region of Egypt	See title	Egypt	Purdue University
1998	Epidemiological Study of Snakebite Mortality and Morbidity in Livestock and Humans in the Terai Region of Nepal	See title	Nepal	Washington State University
1998	Implications of the Forest Reserve Act of 1990 for the Health and Welfare of Retired Thai Logging Elephants	Asian elephants	Thailand	Tufts University
1998	Post-War Influences on Veterinary Education in Sarajevo: Impact on Meeting Animal Welfare Needs	University of Sarajevo, Faculty of Veterinary Medicine	Bosnia	University of California-Davis
1998	Cheetah Conservation on Namibian Livestock Ranches: Examining the Risk on Interspecies Disease Transmission	Cheetahs	Namibia	Tufts University
1998	Determination of the Prevalence of *Brucella abortus* in Equine Fistulous Withers in Remote Regions of Guatemala	Horses	Guatemala	University of Tennessee
1998	Assessing the Long-Term Viability of the Declining African Lion Population in Queen Elizabeth National Park, Uganda	Lions	Uganda	University of California-Davis and Tufts University
1998	Development of an Aerosol Rinderpest Vaccine for Use in Free Ranging Domestic Animals and Wildlife	See title	Kenya	Tufts University
1998	Field Assessment of Disease Status and Transmission of Malignant Catarrhal Fever in Wild and Domestic Hoofstock	Wildebeest and domestic livestock	Kenya and Tanzania	Colorado State University
1998	Environmental Mercury Contamination: A Role for Veterinarians in Turtle Rescue	Turtles	Venezuela	Tufts University

(continued)

Table 10-2	Student Projects with an International Perspective That Were Funded Through the Frontiers of Veterinary Medicine Program of the Geraldine R. Dodge Foundation in the First Three Years of the Program, 1996–1998 *(Continued)*			
Award Year	Title of Project	Focus of Project	Project Location	Student's Veterinary School
1998	A Survey of Leptospirosis in Stray and Companion Dogs in Puerto Rico	Dogs	Puerto Rico	Tuskegee University
1998	Canine Distemper Virus: Assessing Current Risks to Lions, Leopards, and Jackals in Botswana	Lions, leopards, and jackals	Botswana	University of California-Davis
1998	Clinical Ecology: Using Coral Disease as a Bio-Indicator of Reef Ecosystem Health	Coral Reefs	Philippines	Tufts University
1998	Assessment of Aviculture for Conservation: A Survey of the Pet Bird-Human Bond in Mexico	Parrots	Mexico	Tufts University
1998	Developing a Vaccine for a Significant Worldwide Disease of Cattle through International Scientific Collaboration	Cattle and anaplasmosis	United States	Washington State University
1998	Vocal Repertoires of Pack Ice Seals around the Antarctic Continent	Weddell seals	Antarctica	University of Georgia
1998	Using Prevalence of Parasite Infection to Predict Herbivore Overcrowding on Wildlife Reserves	Zebras	Kenya	Tufts University
1998	Identification of Common Intestinal Parasites and Prevalence of Equine Babesiosis in Guatemalan Work Horses	Horses	Guatemala	University of Tennessee

More-complete descriptions of these projects and others as well as information for applying for future grants can be found on the internet at http://www.grdodge.org/vet/index.html.

of that veterinarian's skills and training. As with any new position, be sure to clarify the job description, duties, and responsibilities before signing on. One potential problem with the Peace Corps for recent graduates of veterinary school, of course, may be finances. The Peace Corps is essentially a volunteer program that pays only a modest monthly stipend. If you have major student loans to pay off or a family to support, your circumstances may not allow you to exercise the Peace Corps option.

A more financially rewarding option may be military service. The uniformed veterinary services of the United States government actively recruit veterinary students and recent graduates and offer another potential opportunity to gain appropriate long-term field experience in international work. The Army and Air Force maintain approximately 40 permanent bases overseas, primarily in Asia and Europe, where veterinarians may be posted. The pay and benefits are significantly higher than in the Peace Corps, and there are opportunities for additional professional training and long-term career development as well. The minimum commitment is 3 years. The

likelihood of international assignments should be discussed during the recruitment process. In addition to the Army and Air Force, the Public Health Service actively recruits recent graduate veterinarians and also has opportunities for international assignments, at least intermittently.

Volunteer opportunities other than the Peace Corps also exist as ways to gain valuable field experience. A considerable number of environmental, wildlife conservation, rural development, and relief organizations have volunteer opportunities. Sometimes these positions are advertised as unpaid internships. Many volunteer and internship positions are appropriate for veterinarians, even though the organizations offering the opportunities may not identify veterinary skills as a prerequisite. When reviewing such opportunities, you may have to do the mental work of determining how the position might fit into your own long-term career plan. If you believe it would, then you will have to convince the organization that not only are you qualified, but that your veterinary background will bring a valuable fresh perspective to their mission. For example, in July 1999, the NGO coordination organization Inter-

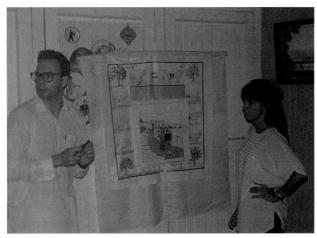

Figure 10-2. Dr. Diana Davis had the opportunity to work for a summer in Pakistan while a student at Tufts University School of Veterinary Medicine on developing training materials for a community-based animal health care program in Afghanistan. In this picture, Dr. Davis is discussing the layout of silk-screened flip charts for use in training with representatives of the International Rescue Committee who had the facilities for mass producing the silk-screened materials. The project on which Dr. Davis worked was funded by USAID and executed by Tufts University School of Veterinary Medicine in conjunction with the NGO Mercy Corps International. (Photo by Dr. David M. Sherman)

Action, based in Washington, DC, offered a 20-hour per week unpaid internship to work with its Disaster Response Committee. The position would give the intern an opportunity to work with professionals from a variety of NGOs, review and report on ongoing disaster intervention activities by NGOs, learn how international agencies respond to crises, and attend meetings related to humanitarian crises. Such a position would be an excellent learning experience for any veterinarian interested in pursuing a career in international veterinary disaster medicine. At the same time, a veterinarian in the intern position could raise awareness of the role of animals in helping people rebuild their lives following disasters and help to build animal rescue initiatives into future contingency plans for disaster mitigation.

Midcareer

The advantage of considering international work midcareer is that you have not only developed a strong professional grounding as a veterinarian, but also have gained additional, valuable skills. If you are a practitioner, you likely have developed strong skills in small business management. If you are on a veterinary school faculty, you have developed some valuable teaching skills. If you worked in the pharmaceutical industry, you likely know quite a lot about marketing, product testing and setting up field trials, quality control procedures, and/or dealing with government regulatory agencies.

The likely drawback of choosing to add an international dimension to your work midcareer is that your current situation

and responsibilities may not allow you the flexibility to acquire international experience, particularly long-term experience. However, some options are available. If you are committed to a full-time job and must continue in that job, there still may be opportunities to gain international experience during vacations, academic or corporate sabbaticals, or leaves of absence negotiated with employers, partners, or colleagues.

Midcareer veterinarians may still be able to undertake short-term overseas assignments with a variety of volunteer organizations who use veterinarians for abbreviated consultancies, such as Agricultural Cooperative Development International/Volunteers for Overseas Cooperative Assistance (ACDI/VOCA) or Christian Veterinary Mission, to name but two (Fig. 10-3). Another option is short-term participation in ongoing field research programs. Earthwatch is a nonprofit organization that arranges volunteer participation in such projects around the world. Volunteer stints average 2 weeks (9 to 16 days) duration. A wide variety of projects of potential interest to veterinarians are featured in the areas of animal behavior, biodiversity and ecology, endangered species protection, and wildlife management, among others, with field locations in virtually every continent.

Alternatively, working veterinarians might compete for paid fellowships aimed at midcareer professionals, which can provide opportunities to redirect their careers. The Congressional Science Fellowship of the AVMA is one such fellowship (on the internet, see http://www.avma.org/avmf/fellows.htm). The Science and Technology Fellowships offered by the American Academy for the Advancement of Science (AAAS) represent another example (on the internet, see http://fellowships.aaas.org/). A careful assessment of finances, family ties, professional responsibilities, community obligations, and personal motivation are required before pursuing such options. The guiding principle however, should be "Where there is a will there is a way."

Skill Gathering

The previous section emphasized the importance of experience gathering in international career development because the ability to function effectively in a cross-cultural context is a fundamental attribute of successful international work. In addition to experience, however, it is important to develop a professional skill base that is appropriate for the type of international work you wish to do. Once you have decided on a general area of international work, be it livestock production, wildlife conservation, commerce and trade policy, rural development, food safety, environmental health, zoonotic disease control, or any other of the many other exciting opportunities available to veterinarians in the global village, then it is necessary to develop a plan for gathering the skills relevant to that area of interest. When pursuing an international veterinary position, being a qualified veterinarian is only the general admission ticket. You need to develop a distinctive set of skills and experience that distinguishes you from other veterinarians interested in the same position.

There are two main categories of skills to be considered. The first are your professional skills. These are technical capabili-

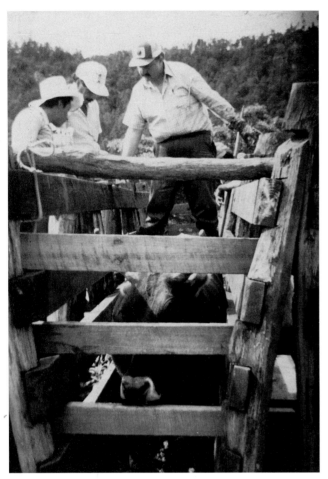

Figure 10-3. Dr. Roger Ellis, while a busy dairy practitioner in Vermont, organized his practice schedule to make time to volunteer for the Peace Corps' Farmer to Farmer Project sponsored by ACDI/VOCA in Honduras. In this photo, Dr. Ellis performs cattle pregnancy examinations for local farmers near San Marcos de Colon. He also provided training in animal health and husbandry to Peace Corps Volunteers working on cattle projects in Honduras. Those projects frequently received their cattle through Heifer Project International which partnered with the Peace Corps to provide follow-up support to farmers receiving cattle. Dr. Ellis is currently a state field veterinarian in New York and remains active in international veterinary medicine (Photo courtesy of Dr. Roger Ellis).

ties, advanced training, specialized expertise, or multidisciplinary knowledge that you have accumulated in your professional development. The second category are your life skills, which also may have evolved from your work as a veterinarian but, alternatively, may have arisen from different or separate facets of your life. Some examples of useful and marketable skills that are not veterinary specific but that may have derived from your work as a veterinarian include computer skills, bookkeeping, personnel management, public speaking, technical writing, grantsmanship, and project management. Avocational life skills with potential value in international work might include such things as artistic talent, language fluency, orienteering abilities, or certification as an airplane pilot.

Professional Skills

Just as with experience gathering, your approach to skill gathering will depend a great deal on your personal circumstances and the current stage of your veterinary career. It will also depend on the type of international work you wish to pursue. The traditional approach to accumulating additional and appropriate professional skills is to acquire formal education or training. This does not necessarily mean returning full time to school, as the range of options for additional education is expanding. Options may include formal Ph.D. programs taking 3 years or more, to participation in relevant short courses taking 3 weeks or less. Therefore, you should be able to find some educational opportunity that fits your situation. Numerous factors will influence what level of additional education you might be able to obtain. These factors include the stage of your career, your financial situation, academic qualification, geographical location, schedule constraints, and willingness to take on additional studies.

If you are still an undergraduate, you have the opportunity to pursue a major course of study that will enhance the value of your subsequent veterinary degree for international work. While you will be obliged to fulfill various preveterinary coursework requirements, there should be adequate opportunity to build knowledge in a complementary field. The selection will depend on your interests. A business major prior to veterinary school, for example, might make you more attractive to international pharmaceutical companies than a veterinarian with no business background. Similarly, a major in conservation biology or ecology would strengthen your appeal to international conservation organizations following graduation from veterinary school, while a major in rural sociology or agricultural economics might make you particularly attractive to rural development organizations working in developing countries.

For veterinary students, elective courses, externships, and summer breaks can be used to focus on subject areas and skills relevant to your evolving international interest. If the veterinary school permits coursework in other academic units of the university, appropriate course offerings should be investigated and pursued, as many useful ancillary subjects may not be offered within the veterinary curriculum. Similarly, appropriate off-campus externships should be found and followed up. For instance, if you are interested in rural development work, you might want to enhance your experience with animal species of importance abroad that may be underrepresented in your required clinical rotations, such as poultry, goats, or rabbits. If you are interested in wildlife, you might take additional exotic animal rotations in clinics and pursue externships at zoos, wildlife parks, or primate research centers. If you are interested in corporate work, you might want to arrange an externship in the research and development section of a pharmaceutical company or work as a research assistant for a faculty member in the pharmacology department or in the clinical sciences department evaluating a new product or treatment regimen. For many industry positions, experience with organizing and conducting properly executed research trials is an important skill.

The menu of choices for building additional professional skills is probably greatest immediately following graduation from veterinary school, as a wide array of internships, residencies, and graduate school programs are available that offer the potential to enhance your ability to find jobs and work effectively in international veterinary medicine. Once again, you need to be clear on your own goals and select carefully so that the advanced training you choose provides an appropriate extension of your skill base. Some programs may afford you the opportunity to enhance your skills and your international experience simultaneously, if you choose a graduate program that enables you to carry out your field research and thesis work abroad. For example, the International Livestock Research Institute, with campuses in Nairobi and Addis Ababa, has been the site of laboratory or field-based research for numerous graduate students enrolled in graduate programs in their home countries, including the United States. Areas of postgraduate study that might complement your veterinary training relative to different areas of international veterinary medicine are given in Table 10-3. Educational opportunities for veterinarians are routinely published in the classified section of the *Journal of the American Veterinary Medical Association*. Many are potentially valuable for graduates interested in international careers. When considering such programs, you must explore their flexibility during the inquiry phase. How likely is it that the training or study can be tailored to accommodate your special international interests? Clinical internship and residency programs, some of which are relevant to international work are published annually in the *Directory of Internships and Residencies* by the American Association of Veterinary Clinicians. Each veterinary school receives copies that are available to students for review.

If student debt or other obligations require that you begin to earn substantial income, then formal training or degree programs after veterinary school may not be a viable option, as such positions may provide only modest income, if any, and also may require additional tuition. Conditions vary from position to position, however, so do some investigating before writing off the idea of additional formal training altogether. There may be opportunities for advanced education associated with employment as well, since some employers with international activities are structured to provide additional training to selected individuals once employed. This is true of the U.S. Army Veterinary Corps as well as some other corporate and government employers, for example, the U.S. Public Health Service (USPHS) and Animal and Plant Inspection Service (APHIS). The author is aware of an Army veterinarian and an APHIS veterinarian, both with active international careers, who were able to pursue graduate programs in public health and epidemiology while employed by their respective

Table 10-3	Examples of Areas of Undergraduate or Postgraduate Study That Will Complement Your Training As a Veterinarian When Pursuing Different Categories of International Work
Focus of Employment Activity	**Relevant Areas of Formal Study**[a]
Livestock production	Agricultural economics, agriculture, animal science, agricultural engineering, preventive medicine, epidemiology
Rural development	Anthropology, sociology, agricultural extension, education, communication
Agribusiness	Business, marketing, management, international law, international relations
Disease control	Public health, epidemiology, computer science, medical geography, microbiology, immunology, molecular biology, pathology, statistics
Food safety	Public health, epidemiology, microbiology, molecular biology, pathology, toxicology
Pharmaceuticals	Pharmacology, physiology, pathology, molecular biology, botany, business, marketing, management, statistics
Trade and regulatory activities	International studies, international relations, international law, business, administration, mediation
Environmental health	Ecology, toxicology, environmental studies, marine biology, engineering, physical geography
Wildlife medicine and conservation	Zoology, ecology, conservation biology, forestry, reproductive physiology, zoo or exotic animal medicine, pathology

[a]These are examples, not prescriptions, for developing an appropriate mix of interdisciplinary knowledge and perspectives. Requirements for specific positions will vary, and in some cases, a strong record of practical relevant experience can substitute for additional training or specific coursework. These categories are somewhat arbitrary, and there may be overlap between categories. If agribusiness positions involve livestock activities, then subjects listed under Livestock production will also be relevant to Agribusiness.

institutions. Also, a commitment of 3+ years to a residency and/or Ph.D. program is not always necessary. A 1-year Masters Program in Public Health, for example, can be a very valuable credential for a wide range of international career opportunities.

Even when financial and personal situations allow it, many veterinary school graduates simply cannot embrace the prospect of additional, extended formal education or training right on the heels of veterinary school graduation, despite a clear interest in international careers. As there is no established career path for international work, no one is going to be penalized for going into practice for a period of time before choosing to seek additional training or education. In fact, practice itself can provide some important life and professional skills transferable to the international arena. If nothing else, practice will allow the recent graduate to apply the clinical training received in veterinary school and adapt it to a real-world setting. However, numerous short-term, nondegree educational opportunities exist that can be very valuable in furthering your international aspirations and that may be integrated into your work schedule. These may be short courses, intensive workshops or seminars, correspondence courses, or, increasingly, internet-based learning opportunities. Finding such opportunities can be facilitated by joining professional organizations working in your area of international interest. Newsletters or journals of organizations such as the Society for Tropical Veterinary Medicine or the American Association of Zoo Veterinarians frequently identify relevant learning opportunities, as will the internet. For example, the website EpiVetNet, based at Massey University in New Zealand, maintains a list of formal postgraduate programs as well as short courses and internet-based learning opportunities in epidemiology. The site is at http://epiweb.massey.ac.nz/.

Electronic learning opportunities on the internet are becoming increasingly available and offer an excellent opportunity for distance learning, allowing great flexibility for the working veterinarian. One current example of relevant internet study is the series of courses offered by the Federal Emergency Management Agency (FEMA) through their Emergency Management Institute, which cover various aspects of emergency management, including management of animals in disasters (see course descriptions and enrollment information at http://www.fema.gov/emi/crslist.htm). These courses would be relevant to individuals interested in international veterinary disaster medicine. Another example is the series of course offered by the Environmental Systems Research Institute (ESRI) on the theory and applications of global informational systems (GIS) using ARC/INFO software. The virtual campus of ESRI can be found on the web at http://campus.esri.com/. Familiarity with use of GIS would be an asset to veterinarians interested in international work involving disease surveillance, environmental toxicology, wildlife conservation, and other fields in which the spatial distribution of populations or events is important. The Global Health Network offers an informative, internet-based, public health course entitled "Epidemiology, the Internet and Global Health" at http://www.pitt.edu/~super1/index.htm.

Life Skills

As with professional skills, life skills may be acquired in a variety of ways. The ease with which they are accrued will depend again largely on personal circumstance and stage of career development. Veterinarians who own practices acquire by training and/or experience an important set of transferable skills related to business management, personnel management, accounting and finance, and interpersonal communication. They may also acquire computer skills using spreadsheets and database management software as well as computer-based farm management or herd health programs. Military veterinarians may acquire valuable skills in emergency management. Veterinary faculty frequently have well-developed writing, speaking, and teaching skills, while industry veterinarians may have developed strong skills in research design and evaluation.

If your work experience has not provided opportunities to develop specific skills needed for a particular sphere of international work, there may be numerous opportunities to do so within your community through adult education offerings at a local high school or public library, courses at community colleges, or opportunities to volunteer with local organizations. Do you need public speaking experience? Dr. Carin Smith highly recommends joining a Toastmasters group. Do you need to develop or document leadership skills? Offer to become an officer for a local community group or charitable organization or coach a youth sports team or scout troop. Do you want to establish credentials as a technical writer? Take a writing course at a community college and offer to write an animal health column for a local newspaper. Do you need teaching experience? Offer to teach a basic course in animal care through the community adult education program. Good oral, written, and interpersonal communication skills are valuable assets no matter what aspect of international work you pursue. Do not feel that locally acquired life skills are somehow less valuable than those received in more formal or structured settings. A record of active participation in the life of your community will be considered a very positive attribute by most private voluntary organizations involved in community development work in the developing world. Besides, maximizing your use of locally available resources is a fundamental characteristic of anyone destined to be successful in international work.

One life skill that merits specific discussion is language proficiency. The ability to read, speak, and write in a language other than English is a desirable skill, and anyone interested in international work should consider developing additional language skills. Speaking a local language will greatly enrich any personal or professional experience that you have abroad. The lack of language can make the simplest activities unduly complicated and obstruct the normal rhythm and flow of daily life. Speaking the local language unlocks doors. It facilitates the development of more complex and lasting interpersonal relationships with friends and colleagues. Many people are sincerely flattered by your willingness and ability to speak their language, and it raises your esteem in their eyes. Nevertheless, facility in a second or third language is not a consistent prerequisite for international work. Some jobs will always be available to speakers of English only, though more jobs may be available to multilingual applicants, at least on a regional basis.

There is no denying that English is rapidly becoming the predominant language of global commerce and communication. Nevertheless, distinct regional language spheres continue to exist, the obvious example being the Spanish-speaking countries of Latin America. French is still an important language in North and West Africa and southeast Asia, and it is humbling to remember that well over 1 billion people in Asia speak some form of Chinese. Clearly, knowledge of any of these languages will enhance your competitiveness for international positions in the respective regions where they are spoken. English, French, and Spanish remain the official languages of the United Nations, and many UN positions require fluency in at least two of the three tongues. A final reason to learn a language is to do your part to overcome the famous stereotype that Americans are unable or unwilling to learn additional languages. This perception is embodied in a painful joke, told to me by several, impressively multilingual Europeans. What do you call someone who can speak three languages? Trilingual. What do you call someone who can speak two languages? Bilingual. What do you call someone who can speak one language? An American!

The Attitude Factor

In 1958, William J. Lederer and Eugene Burdick published a novel entitled *The Ugly American*.[8] The book was organized as a series of individual profiles of a group of Americans working in the imaginary southeast Asian country of Sarkhan in the period preceding American involvement in the Vietnam war. The "ugly American" of the title is a retired engineer named Homer Atkins. His ugliness is literal, in that he is physically unattractive. Everything else about the man is meant by the authors to be seen as attractive and admirable. Homer Atkins is an American expatriate committed to the development of the Sarkhanese people. He spends his time in the countryside among the villagers, observes local customs and practices, learns the local language, works with the people to identify their needs, welcomes advice and criticism, applies his engineering skills in technologically appropriate ways using local resources to solve local problems, empowers local people to implement the technological advances they have created together, and draws his satisfactions from the success achieved by others.

In contrast, to Homer Atkins, the authors present a large cast of American officials and U.S. Embassy employees who work in various divisions of the Foreign Service in Sarkhan's capital city, Haidho. In contrast to Homer Atkins, the ugliness of these Americans is figurative. It is manifest not in their physical appearance, but in their attitudes and actions with respect to the country in which they live and work. The authors paint an un-

flattering portrait of these characters as arrogant, contemptuous, intolerant, insulated, self-serving, intellectually lazy, incompetent, corrupt, and shallow. These Americans mingle only with themselves, never leave the capital city, disdain contact with Sarkhanese people, fail to understand the condition of the country's ordinary citizens, misrepresent the local situation to superiors back in Washington to protect their own positions, and basically resent the intrusions of work on their carefully constructed social life, complete with its incessant round of cocktail parties and trips to the commissary to stock up on American goods.

Drawing from their own experiences in southeast Asia during the Eisenhower years, Lederer and Burdick intended their book as a wakeup call to the American public and policymakers about the ineffectiveness and misguided conduct of our foreign policy efforts. It came at a time when popular support for communism was spreading rapidly through the rural populations of Southeast Asian nations. The authors wanted to get the point across that the communists, regardless of the merit of their ideology, were effectively organizing peasants in southeast Asia at the grassroots level through a campaign of community education and participation, while the American foreign policy effort was essentially limited to expensive, large-scale, showy development projects carried out in partnership with national governments that drew little or no support from their own citizens. In the battle for "hearts and minds," the communists were clearly winning in the late 1950s when the book was written, and the authors were not shy about placing blame.

The Ugly American was a multi-million-copy bestseller. The book triggered a study commissioned by President Eisenhower to evaluate U.S. military aid programs, which led to much-needed reform. It is not surprising that within 3 years of the book's publication, President John F. Kennedy established the Peace Corps. Kennedy recognized the need to get Americans working overseas out of the cocktail and commissary circuit and into the countryside where they would be able to learn and teach simultaneously, to better understand and to be better understood, and to build partnerships in progress. The Peace Corps was an affirmation of the need for people-to-people contact in foreign relations, an approach grounded in a basic respect for the dignity of all human beings.

Clearly, attitudes are as important as aptitudes in successful international work. No matter how good you are technically, if you are arrogant, supercilious, impatient, rude, condescending, insensitive, disrespectful, disdainful, complaining, or constantly critical, the value of your technical contributions will be diminished or rendered wholly ineffective. In addition, your opportunities for future international work will be scarce. Personality and character influence professional performance, and experienced employers hiring for international positions recognize this. Obviously there is no official body that determines and sanctions correct behaviors, attitudes, and personality traits suitable for international work, nor should there be. However, there is surprising consistency in the characteristics that experienced professionals list as factors for successful international work. Some of these key attributes are discussed below.

Demonstrate respect for human dignity and the value of the individual. All people share similar hopes and aspirations for their own future and the future of their children. All individuals carry within themselves the inherent dignity of human life. What differs most about people is the circumstances under which they must live their lives and how such circumstances inhibit or encourage opportunities for fulfillment and happiness. It is critical in successful international work to maintain the conviction that people have the potential to grow and flourish when opportunities are created. If we find ourselves complaining about "those people" in foreign countries and their inadequacies or deficiencies, we have rendered ourselves ineffective for international work. Americans, living in the "land of opportunity," have become accustomed to an economic system that encourages and rewards individual initiative, a democratic government that provides the basic services necessary for a civil society, and a rule of law that protects the rights of individual citizens. We must not lose sight of the fact that until ordinary citizens in other nations also have access to such a framework for personal and social growth, people will continue to live in undignified circumstances. They must not, however, be considered to have lost their inherent dignity.

A basic lack of respect for people is not difficult to detect. I have observed foreigners working in the developing world who were rigidly hierarchical in their dealings with other people. Such individuals were polite and deferential to peers and superiors in the workplace, but rude and abusive to inferiors. This inconsistency was evident to all except themselves, and the behavior was costly in terms of diminished overall effectiveness and erosion of good will. One of the great strengths of the United States, admired around the world, is the inherent egalitarianism of our democratic society, our tendency to greet the doorman with the same respect and enthusiasm that we would greet the CEO with moments later. Projecting this egalitarian conviction is a fundamental asset in international work. It reflects a respect for the individual and his or her inherent dignity.

Demonstrate a respect for the environment. Much of the international work that veterinarians may become involved in is directed toward promoting economic development and social progress. While these are usually considered admirable objectives in themselves, it has become increasingly apparent that efforts to improve the quality of life for the world's people must be balanced with the need to conserve natural resources, protect ecological services, and maintain environmental health. Development agencies from small local NGOs to the World Bank are now including environmental impact assessments into the planning stages of their development projects in recognition of the fact that short-term economic advantages can be negated by unforeseen adverse environmental consequences. Increasingly in the future, those professionals who are successful and effective in international development work will be the ones who can demonstrate a commitment to sustainable develop-

ment in both word and deed. Suppose, for example, an American veterinarian representing an agribusiness company is invited to Africa to advise on the development of large-scale, intensive livestock production units near a large lake where numerous lakeshore communities derive their livelihood from fishing. It would be irresponsible for that veterinarian not to draw attention to the fact that animal-waste-handling issues are a critical aspect of the project's long-term success because water pollution, eutrophication, and fish kills could potentially occur if a careful waste management plan was not put in place. At the very least, that veterinarian should suggest making an environmental impact assessment and developing a waste management plan before a final decision is made on moving forward with the intensive-production units. No justifiable net gain would be realized if the production units went forward at the expense of lost livelihoods for local fisherman as well as serious disruption of the lake's ecology.

Be flexible. The ability to adapt to unexpected situations and to do so gracefully without loss of composure are critical attributes of successful international professionals. In the United States we have become accustomed to a high degree of material comfort and personal independence, and we have come to expect that our social institutions and technical infrastructure will function with a high degree of efficiency and reliability. You must always keep in mind that in a global context, this situation is largely the exception rather than the rule. One must be able to "roll with the punches" in the face of unexpected delays, changes in plans, malfunctioning equipment, washed-out roads, unavailable supplies, poorly trained technicians, skipped appointments, failed electrical supply, or any other of a variety of predictable obstacles to efficiency and productivity that inevitably crop up in international work. Not only is it necessary to accept these disruptions with good nature, one must also be creative and flexible in getting the job done anyway, in spite of these obstacles. In America, we have come to expect a great deal of personal control over the details of our daily lives and a minimum of inconvenience. If you are not prepared psychologically to relinquish some of that control and to accept a higher level of inconvenience and unfamiliarity, then international work decidedly is not for you.

In addition, flexibility in international work sometimes requires a fairly high tolerance for risk, discomfort, and even danger. In relief and development work, for example, societies that are largely dependent on animals are frequently caught up in military conflicts or natural catastrophes such as drought that affect animal health and disrupt veterinary service delivery. Somalia, Sudan, and Afghanistan are countries that come readily to mind in this context. Such situations provide opportunities for expatriate veterinarians to provide valuable services and support working with international agencies. However, working conditions are frequently difficult and threats to personal safety may be high. Though I do not wish to encourage reckless bravado among young veterinarians wishing to establish careers in international veterinary medicine, it cannot be denied that a willingness to work under conditions of increased risk offers opportunities for employment and valuable experience that, under more settled circumstances, would likely go instead to older individuals with considerably more experience already in their resumés.

Be a team player. International employment opportunities often derive from the fact that you have distinguished yourself through possession of a unique set of skills, specialized training, or established experience. In other words, you are, to some degree, recognized as an expert in your particular field. While such inherent acknowledgment of your professional accomplishments is gratifying, it is also fraught with psychological risks. One must not let "expert" status go to one's head. As soon as you believe you have "all the answers" or expect that others will automatically defer to your opinions by virtue of your expert status or your professional standing, your effectiveness in international work is diminished. While the technical aspects of a problem or project may appear similar from site to site, local culture, politics, geography, and a myriad of other variables must be taken into account to formulate appropriate assessments, recommendations, and plans of action. This requires active solicitation of input from others. In other words, it requires being a team player.

In international work, you are rarely, if ever, working alone. It is critical to the success of any project that the opinions and perspectives of all stakeholders be heard. Collecting the relevant information requires listening to others, be they expatriate or local scientists, officials, workers, or project beneficiaries. Truly listening is a skill. It requires an inherent respect for the opinions of others and a sense of humility that allows you to avoid defensiveness when others may not agree with you. In the international context, good listening requires a basic interest or curiosity about the unfamiliar and a willingness to learn about it. It also requires some cross-cultural awareness. When something seems self-evident to you in a given situation, it may not be self-evident to a local counterpart with different background, upbringing and experience. In fact, it may not be intrinsically self-evident at all. It may be plain wrong in the local context.

As a veterinarian working abroad, you may frequently be involved in an interdisciplinary team effort. For example, I had the opportunity to serve as team leader for an FAO team investigating a skin disease problem in sheep and goats in Ethiopia that was adversely affecting the quality of skins processed in the nation's tanneries for export to Europe. The drop in skin quality due to disease was costing the industry millions of dollars annually in lost export revenue. The FAO team included a veterinary diagnostician, a veterinary pathologist, a specialist in the technical aspects of the tanning industry, and an agricultural economist. In addition, each of these expatriate specialists had an Ethiopian counterpart on the team. Successful clarification of the problem and the development of appropriate corrective actions resulted from the experience and input of *all* team members-veterinarian and nonveterinarian alike, expatriate and Ethiopian alike (see sidebar in Chapter 8 "Ethnoveterinary Medicine: To Spray or Not to Spray? That is the Question").

Nowhere is the need for teamwork and cooperation more evident than in the area of wildlife conservation. This is a truly multidisciplinary field in which the inputs of a great many different types of natural scientists are required to understand and manage the forces that affect the viability of animal populations in a given ecosystem. Overlaid on the scientific issues are a complex set of social and economic factors that influence the amount of stress that human activity places on habitat and wildlife populations. In addition to the natural scientists already mentioned, various social scientists and policymakers may be involved in conservation efforts to address those social and economic issues. Veterinarians, as discussed in Chapter 7, have important roles to play in wildlife conservation. However, they must be prepared to work as part of a complex, multidisciplinary team to be effective. They must be willing to accept different points of view and assimilate different scientific perspectives. At a recent international zoological conference, veterinarians and nonveterinarians came together for a workshop entitled "Veterinarians in Conservation Biology," and the results of the workshop have been published.[10] At the workshop, nonveterinarians acknowledged the valuable role that veterinarians have played in wildlife conservation. However, they also voiced significant concerns about the attitudes of some veterinarians with whom they have worked. Some of the concerns expressed that veterinarians need to acknowledge and address are as follows:

- Some veterinarians present an arrogant or cavalier attitude. It seems that because they are trained in comparative medicine, some believe they know about all species, wild or domestic, and may act overconfidently when dealing with wild animals.

- In dealing with wild animals, some veterinarians have demonstrated a lack of accountability and a lack of awareness concerning the ethics and values issues concerning wildlife conservation.

- There seems to be a lack of appreciation by some veterinarians of what "wild" means. A zebra may be anatomically and physiologically similar to a horse, but its life, habits, and very essence as a wild animal are different in profound ways.

- Some veterinarians do not look beyond the application of their technical expertise to reflect upon the implications of their actions.

- Some veterinarians seem unprepared to be comfortable with, and react intelligently to, the ever-occurring question in wildlife medicine, "What do I do when I don't know what to do?"

- Some veterinarians appear not to be sensitized to knowing when not to intervene. They must be open to considering alternatives proposed by nonveterinary colleagues.

- All veterinarians must embrace an ethic of teamwork to participate effectively in wildlife conservation.

Be tactful and diplomatic. In international work, you are always someone's guest. Act accordingly. The well-mannered guest remains polite and courteous even when tested, and tested you will be when working abroad. When disagreements arise, remember that you don't change people's points of view by being angry or rude. That only tends to solidify their disagreement and encourages them to dig in their heels. Do not however, confuse being polite or diplomatic with being weak. You have a job to do and your position, if you believe in it, must be heard. Always be clear about the particular issue or point of view that is the subject of disagreement. In presenting your position, find the balance between being firm and being overbearing. Also, choose your battles carefully and save your reserves of good will for those issues that matter most. Finally, never forget the cardinal rule of international travel for Americans. If someone does not understand English, their comprehension is not improved by having you speak English to them more loudly.

Maintain a high standard of professionalism and personal integrity. Whether you are conscious of it or not, you always represent your country and your profession when you are working abroad. Much has been made about the extent of corruption that occurs in other countries, particularly in developing countries, though recent scandals in Europe involving the European Parliament indicate that the problem is by no means limited to developing countries. It is not unlikely that at some point during your work abroad, you will encounter some manifestation of corruption. Resist any temptation to participate, even if it seems expedient or appears to be commonplace. You must demand honesty, integrity, and fairness in all your dealings and lead by example, though it may cause you some discomfort and conflict in the process.

In summary, self-awareness is a critically important aspect of international work. Be conscious of how you behave, especially how you react to unfamiliar people and unexpected situations. If you are unsure of your reactions in an international context, test them out before you commit to an international career. At the very least, take a vacation abroad and do a self-evaluation. Were you irritated by minor inconveniences? Did you find yourself annoyed that local people did not speak English? Were you constantly comparing local conditions to those at home and finding them wanting? Be honest with yourself about your attitudes and responses. If your threshold for unfamiliarity was low when you simply had the task of relaxing and enjoying yourself, imagine how irritating this unfamiliarity would be if you were actually trying to get work done. International work may not be your cup of tea after all.

Potential Employers

Numerous types of organizations will potentially hire veterinarians for international work. The categories of potential employ-

ers and examples of organizations within each category are presented in Table 10-4 as a convenient overview of the information presented in this section. Within any organization, opportunities for employment will vary with your level of experience, training, and the possession of other unique or desirable life skills and professional skills. Some employers (e.g., the U.S. Army) are eager to recruit veterinarians right out of veterinary school. In fact, they may help pay for veterinary school if you enlist while a student. At the other end of the spectrum are United Nations organizations and private consulting and contracting firms, which usually require 5 or more years of experience specifically in an international setting before considering you for employment. When applicable, in the following discussion, some indication is given if a specific employer is likely to hire entry-level, midlevel, and/or advanced-level veterinarians.

United States Government Agencies

The U.S. government employs veterinarians in a broad range of capacities in a variety of agencies. While most of these veterinarians work within the United States, a number of opportunities for international veterinary work exist in the areas of food safety, international trade, public health, disease investigation and control, national defense, emergency response, and foreign aid and development.

Some federal positions, for instance, in food safety and inspection, specifically require veterinarians. However, positions for which veterinarians may qualify and indeed may be perfectly suited are often not listed as veterinary positions in federal job descriptions, so one must keep an open mind when perusing federal job listings. Positions advertised for biologists, zoologists, researchers, animal scientists, public health specialists, epidemiologists, food technologists, and others are often open to veterinarians even though a veterinary degree is not listed as a requirement.

Veterinarians working in government, when surveyed, generally express high job satisfaction Some of the positive factors cited are a good deal of independence, a high level of professionalism, a feeling that they are doing important work, a dynamic working environment, and being challenged in areas beyond their formal veterinary training. Some of the less favorable aspects of government work include a high degree of bureaucracy and paper work, and slow decision making. Veterinarians with families, especially school-aged children also site frequent relocation as a drawback of government work, at least in some positions. The mean salary for veterinarians working in government falls within the range of mean salaries for different types of private practice. Regular fixed working hours are the rule, and benefits for government employees are generally good.

Uniformed Services

The various agencies within the U.S. government that employ veterinarians, fall into two broad categories-the uniformed and the nonuniformed services. The uniformed services include the U.S. Army, the U.S. Air Force, and the United States Public Health Service Commissioned Corps.

Table 10-4	Summary of Potential Employers of Veterinarians for International Positions As Discussed in This Chapter by Employer Category
Type of Employer	**Examples of Employers**
United States government agencies	U.S. Army, U.S. Air Force, U.S. Public Health Service, Centers for Disease Control and Prevention, Animal and Plant Health Inspection Service, Food Safety and Inspection Service, Agricultural Research Service, Foreign Agricultural Service, U.S. Fish and Wildlife Service, National Wildlife Health Center, U.S. Peace Corps, U.S. Agency for International Development, Environmental Protection Agency, National Zoological Park
Academic institutions	Colleges of veterinary medicine, schools of public health, other related academic institutions, policy institutes
Private industry	Bayer, Hill's Pet Nutrition, Hoechst, Merial, Merck, Novartis, Pfizer, Ralston Purina, Schering-Plough, Waltham, other pharmaceutical, feed, and agribusiness firms
International donor institutions	World Bank, International Fund for Agricultural Development, African Development Bank, Asian Development Bank, Islamic Development Bank, Inter-American Development Bank, European Union
International technical institutions	Food and Agriculture Organization, World Health Organization, Pan American Health Organization, International Atomic Energy Agency, United Nations Environment Programme, United Nations Children's Fund, United Nations Development Programme, Office International des Epizooties
International research institutions	International Livestock Research Institute, International Center for Agricultural Research in Dry Areas, International Center for Living Aquatic Resources Management, International Center for Research in Agroforestry, International Centre of Insect Physiology and Ecology
Nongovernmental organizations	Veterinarians in Voluntary Assistance, Christian Veterinary Mission, VetAid, Vetwork, Veterinaires Sans Frontieres, Heifer Project International, FARM Africa, Agricultural Cooperative Development International/Volunteers for Overseas Cooperative Assistance, Mercy Corps International, Oxfam, Winrock International, World Concern, International Donkey Protection Trust, World Society for the Protection of Animals, World Wildlife Fund, Wildlife Trust, Morris Animal Foundation, African Wildlife Foundation, International Gorilla Conservation Programme, Wildlife Conservation Society (Bronx Zoo) and many other zoo-based international conservation programs
Private consulting firms	Land O' Lakes International Development Division, RDP Livestock Services, PAN Livestock Services, Development Alternatives Inc., Chemonics, Louis Berger International, Ronco Consulting Corporation
Independent consultant	Provide individual professional services as a contractor to many of the organizations listed above

United States Army Veterinary Corps The U.S. Army Veterinary Corps evolved over the 19th century in response to the growing need for proper care of cavalry horses. These services were first provided by farriers and then by civilian veterinarians. In 1862, during the Civil War, Congress authorized a position of military veterinary surgeon with the rank of regimental sergeant major. While the horse cavalry is largely ceremonial today, the Army still maintains an active Veterinary Corps, involved in a wide range of research and service activities at home and abroad. Currently, there are over 750 Army active and reserve component Veterinary Corps officers.

The principal function for most Army veterinarians is to ensure a safe food supply for military personnel. This function is carried out not only at U.S. bases, but also at the 35 or so permanent U.S. Army installations in Europe (Germany, England, Belgium, Italy, the Netherlands) and Asia (Japan and South Korea). They may also be assigned to bases of other military services as well as to embassies. Being involved in food procurement in foreign lands, Army veterinarians also serve as an advanced guard for identifying emerging foreign animal disease problems and communicate with USDA and other government agencies to alert them of possible importation hazards. Army veterinarians have also been directly involved in foreign animal disease control, for example, screwworm control in Panama.

Army veterinarians accompany Army units deployed overseas during military or peace-keeping operations, such as during the Gulf War in 1991 and more recently, in the Balkans. Overseas deployment of U.S. troops has been increasing. Under President Clinton, overseas major deployments occurred at the rate of four times per year, compared with an average of once per year in the years preceding the Clinton administration. This means more overseas opportunities for Army veterinarians. According to Lt. Col. Jeff Melander of the U.S. Army Veterinary Corps at Fort Bragg, in 1998, 11 veterinary teams were dispatched from Fort Bragg alone for international assignment, including 7 teams to Central America, 1 to Thailand, 1 to Egypt, and 2 to the Balkans (Fig. 10-4).

In addition to food procurement and safety issues, veterinarians at Army posts in the United States and elsewhere are also involved in caring for companion animals belonging to army personnel as well as for maintaining the health of working animals such as dogs used for guarding, rescue, police work, or bomb and mine detection. Furthermore, many Corps veterinarians actively participate in research and development activities, some with an international orientation. A main focus of research activity is to develop capabilities for protecting military personnel from biological and chemical weapons and improving quality of care for injured combat personnel. Many of

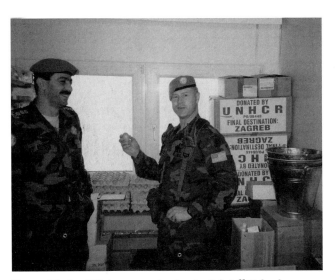

Figure 10–4. U.S. Army veterinarian Lt. Col. Jeff Melander, a graduate of the University of Minnesota College of Veterinary Medicine, visits with Jordanian United Nations peace keepers as they distribute food to Displaced Persons Camps in the former Yugoslavia. When not on assignment abroad, Dr. Melander is stationed at Fort Bragg in North Carolina. (Photo courtesy of Major Jeff Melander)

the biological agents under study are tropical disease agents. Army veterinary researchers, for example, have been involved in studying the pathogenesis of Ebola virus and the development of effective botulism antitoxins. While much of this work occurs in the United States, Army researchers have been posted to defense research laboratories in Asia and Africa as well.

In recent years, the Army has become increasingly involved in a new sphere of activity, namely, civil and humanitarian actions. For example, following the devastation of Hurricane Mitch in Central America in 1998, the U.S. Army was actively involved in emergency relief efforts. Thirty Army veterinary service officers and technicians actively participated in that effort. While such humanitarian responses have largely been ad hoc, there is increasing interest among social analysts and policymakers to formalize the role of the military in disaster relief and humanitarian aid. Such analysts and policymakers believe that in the future, threats to national security will derive more from environmental disruptions, climate change, water and food shortages, and emerging diseases and less from organized armed conflict. Based on this premise, governments are being urged to consider new goals and objectives for their military establishments and to rechannel some human and physical resources toward developing responses other than armed responses. This could mean greater opportunities in the future for veterinarians to pursue international careers in emergency preparedness, disaster medicine, disease control, and humanitarian aid as Army veterinarians.

Veterinarians enter the Army as officers at the rank of captain. The Army Veterinary Corps welcomes veterinary students and recent graduates and offers 3rd and 4th year scholarships to veterinary students. Once in the Army, there are also opportunities, available on a competitive basis, for furthering your education, including fully funded advanced degree programs in public health, laboratory animal medicine, veterinary microbiology, pathology, physiology, toxicology, pharmacology, and food technology. There are also residency training programs leading to eligibility for board certification in veterinary pathology and laboratory animal medicine. The Army represents a good entry-level opportunity for building an international career. More information can be obtained from an Army health care recruiter.

United States Air Force Biomedical Sciences Corps The U.S. Air Force does not have a Veterinary Corps, per se, but actively recruits veterinarians for its Biomedical Sciences Corps. In general, clinical services for working animals or companion animals owned by Air Force personnel are handled by veterinarians from the U.S. Army Veterinary Corps. Air Force veterinarians in the Biomedical Sciences Corps serve as public health officers (PHOs). As in the Army, Air Force veterinarians are responsible for issues of food safety for Air Force personnel. However, they may be involved in a wide range of other public health-related activities. In the words of the Air Force's own position description, PHOs

prevent disease, disability and premature death through effective population-based public health programs. They conduct epidemiologic surveillance and analyze communicable, environmental and occupational disease to establish and prioritize prevention and control strategies. They manage programs to reduce the effects of communicable disease, occupational illness, and disease carrying pest populations. They also manage food safety programs, preventive medicine programs and respond to disaster situations. They are consulted in infection control, health promotions and medical readiness programs. During contingencies, PHOs lead preventive actions to reduce the impact that endemic disease, dangerous plants, animals and climate have on personnel. They direct patient decontamination in the event of exposure to hazardous substances.

PHOs are assigned to a base clinic or hospital. The Air Force has about 16 permanent bases overseas in England, Germany, Italy, the Azores, Saudi Arabia, Turkey, Japan, and Korea. The Air Force is willing to discuss assignment locations during the recruitment process, but international postings are not likely to go to veterinarians fresh out of veterinary school unless they have some other special qualification or experience.

Veterinarians enter the Air Force as officers with the rank of first lieutenant or higher, depending on education or experience. As with the Army, the Air Force, depending on its needs, offers some opportunities for additional training, including pursuit of advanced degrees in epidemiology, public health, food technology, and toxicology, and will pay up to 75% of tuition and fees. More information can be obtained form Air Force health professions recruiters.

United States Public Health Service Commissioned Corps The USPHS was conceived and promoted by President John Adams in the 1790s. President Adams saw a role for the federal government in protecting and ensuring the health of its citizens. Veterinarians, working as civil servants, took on an active and visible role in the USPHS in the 1920s, helping to develop a national Grade-A milk sanitation program. In 1947, the Veterinary Medical Officers Corps of the USPHS Commissioned Corps was created. Currently, there are approximately 100 veterinary officers on active duty in the Corps.

The overall goal of the USPHS is to improve and advance the health of the nation's people. Toward that goal, the mission of the Commissioned Corps, according to its own descriptive literature, is to

> provide highly-trained and mobile health professionals who carry out programs to promote the health of the Nation, understand and prevent disease and injury, assure safe and effective drugs and medical devices, deliver health service to Federal beneficiaries, and furnish health expertise in time of war or other national or international emergencies.

The USPHS is part of the federal government's Department of Health and Human Services (DHHS). There are eight operational divisions within the DHHS to which USPHS Officers may be assigned. Veterinary Officers are most often used in four of these divisions, namely, the National Institutes of Health (NIH), the CDC, the FDA, and the EPA. The NIH, with headquarters in Bethesda, Maryland, employs the most Corps veterinarians, approximately 60, in its various branches. However, the CDC likely provides the most opportunities for USPHS veterinarians to work internationally. The CDC also hires veterinarians in nonuniformed positions.

The Centers for Disease Control and Prevention The CDC has its headquarters in Atlanta, Georgia, but also has branch activities around the country and abroad. For example, CDC supports a vector-borne disease programs in Fort Collins, Colorado, to which veterinarians are assigned. The mission of the CDC is "to promote health and quality of life by preventing and controlling disease, injury, and disability." Veterinary officers assigned to the CDC work in a wide range of disciplines including epidemiology, public health, toxicology, laboratory animal medicine, and pathology and may also assume managerial and administrative duties. Potential activities include, among others, investigations of communicable disease outbreaks, environmental health evaluations of hazardous waste sites, control of food-borne and water-borne diseases, tuberculosis eradication, research work with special pathogens such as Ebola virus, service as program officers in the National Immunization Program, and participation in international health programs.

CDC work demands mobility in many cases. Veterinary epidemiologists participate in public health teams responding to crises such as refugee movements, weather disasters, famines, and war-related emergencies. Such teams carry out rapid needs assessments through establishment of disease and injury surveillance systems, to help establish public health priorities. In addition to being willing to travel frequently, you must be able to accept a relatively increased degree of personal risk, as the situations just described tend to be risky.

There are definitely opportunities for CDC veterinarians to become involved in international work, particularly for those individuals who are willing and interested. Long-term and short-term assignments abroad are possible, as are research and policy activities within the United States with significant potential impact in the international arena. According to Dr. Richard Spiegel, a veterinarian working for CDC in the Division of Public Health Systems, he and his veterinary colleagues have been involved in a number of international activities in recent years. Since 1990, Dr. Spiegel himself was stationed for a total of 3 years in Nigeria working on issues of child health, while another colleague spent 3 years in Cameroon also working on epidemiological surveillance of child health and an additional 4 years in Niger working on Guinea worm eradication. Another colleague has a long-term assignment in China to work on polio eradication programs. Other CDC veterinarians have had recurrent short-term field visits abroad to work on parasitic disease issues, epidemiology of hemorrhagic virus diseases, and rabies control programs.

As mentioned, the CDC hires veterinarians as civil servants as well as obtaining veterinarians through the USPHS Commissioned Corps. Entry-level civil servant jobs are not easy to obtain at CDC. Most veterinarians working there have advanced degrees or extensive experience in a specialized area. However, the Commissioned Corps actively recruits DVMs with no additional training, and some are assigned to CDC.

The CDC also offers a 2-year work/training program for Epidemic Intelligence Service (EIS) officers who are assigned to various state health departments to deal with a wide range of issues including zoonoses, animal bites, rabies control, human disease investigations, community environmental hazards, and occupational safety and health. Though trainees are not assigned internationally for a full term, there may be opportunities for international travel and establishing mentorships with national and international health agencies. Veterinarians are eligible for this program, but they must have a Masters in Public Health or previous public health experience to apply. The program accepts 60 to 80 health professionals annually. Training as an EIS officer would be very useful fur subsequent international work. CDC also sponsors a number of internship programs, some of which are open to veterinary students, including 6- to 8-week epidemiology rotations for senior students-an excellent way to begin to network with CDC veterinarians and find out what kinds of international activities they are involved in. A complete list of internship opportunities can be viewed on the web (http://www.cdc.gov/hrmo/intshps4.htm).

Nonuniformed Services

A number of federal agencies employ veterinarians in a civilian, or nonuniformed, capacity, though international employment opportunities are more common in some agencies than others. A good overview of the landscape of federal employment for veterinarians and useful pointers on how to apply for such positions is provided by Smith.[11]

United States Department of Agriculture The USDA is the largest government employer of nonuniformed veterinarians and employs them in a number of its various agencies. At present, the greatest opportunity for veterinarians to add an international dimension to their work is through employment with the APHIS.

Animal and Plant Health Inspection Service (APHIS) APHIS is the agency responsible for protecting America's crops and livestock from the introduction of new diseases and the spread of existing diseases beyond their present range. It also is the agency responsible for ensuring compliance with the Animal Welfare Act wherever live animals are maintained for commercial or research purposes. There are five major program units at APHIS including Animal Care, Wildlife Services, Plant Production and Quarantine, Veterinary Services, and International Services. Their functions, as directly described at the APHIS website (http://www.aphis.usda.gov/) are as follows:

Animal Care (AC) conducts inspections to ensure the proper stewardship of animals used in research, exhibition, or other regulated industries.

Wildlife Services (WS) works to reduce wildlife damage to agriculture and natural resources, minimize potential wildlife threats to human health and safety, and protect threatened and endangered species. WS cooperates with foreign governments, international organizations, and other government and private organizations with respect to animal and bird damage and nuisance control.

Plant Protection and Quarantine (PPQ) protects the nation's agricultural resources from the international spread of plant and animal pests and diseases. PPQ inspectors at international airport terminals, seaports, and border stations check passengers and baggage for products that could harbor pests or diseases. PPQ also checks ship cargoes, rail and truck freight and mail from foreign countries; certifies U.S. agricultural products for export; and helps combat plant pests within the United States. PPQ's National Biological Control Institute provides leadership for biocontrol programs. PPQ also coordinates the development and execution of biotechnology regulatory policy for APHIS and other USDA agencies and issues permits for the movement and release of genetically engineered plants and organisms. Another part of PPQ is involved with environmental monitoring and residue analysis.

The Veterinary Services (VS) Branch of APHIS protects the health of the nation's livestock and poultry resources by regulating the entry of imported animals and animal products. VS is prepared to take emergency action against foreign diseases and, with the states, operates eradication programs for domestic animal diseases. VS provides health certification for exported animals and animal products. VS also conducts diagnostic tests and issues licenses for veterinary biological products and manufacturers.

International Services (IS) works outside the United States to protect U.S. agriculture and enhance agricultural trade. IS maintains a comprehensive information network, exchanges technical information, and provides expertise to foreign governments and international groups. IS also negotiates with foreign agricultural officials concerning entry requirements for U.S. agricultural products, conducts cooperative agricultural pest and disease programs in foreign locations, and manages preclearance programs for agricultural products shipped to the United States.

The IS unit of APHIS is the only federal government agency that hires veterinarians specifically for foreign service work. Currently, APHIS has 18 veterinarians on duty tours of 2 to 4 years in numerous foreign postings, including Austria, Australia, Belgium, the Caribbean, Chile, China, Colombia, Guatemala, Japan, Korea, Mexico, and Panama. IS veterinarians encounter a great variety of responsibilities and challenges in their work. Their professional activities might include implementation and administration of international animal sanitary monitoring programs, science and technology information exchange with foreign counterparts, administration of foreign disease eradication programs, supervision of technical and nontechnical personnel representing a diverse range of expertise, participation in trade negotiations, and interagency and intergovernmental collaboration on issues related to agricultural trade.

Dr. Karen Shank Sliter, an APHIS-IS veterinarian in Mexico, spoke on international career opportunities in the federal government at the 1999 AVMA convention in New Orleans, referring to such opportunities as "the best kept secret in veterinary medicine." She offered specific examples of the kinds of work that IS veterinarians have been involved with in recent years:

- Review of the equine encephalitis situation in Mexico

- Review of regionalization proposals to declare specific portions of foreign countries disease free for purpose of export of agricultural commodities to the United States

- Organization of trade symposiums in Russia and Mexico

- Participation in international disease conferences

- Attendance at livestock meetings

- Participation in the Gore-Mbecki Commission on Economic and Technological Cooperation between the United States and South Africa

- Clearance of ostrich egg importations to the United States from Namibia

- Clearance of cattle importations from Zimbabwe

- Inspection of foreign processing facilities that produce sausage casings for export

In the VS unit of APHIS, veterinarians may get temporary tours of duty abroad, usually from 1 to 3 months' duration to work on special assignments such as a specific animal importation or a country review. In addition, there are short-term travel opportunities for a variety of purposes including disease investigations, trade symposiums, attendance at scientific meetings, or participation in site visits, trade negotiations, or regionalization reviews. A number of VS veterinarians, as well as some state veterinarians from around the U.S., participated in the foot and mouth disease control effort in the United Kingdom in 2001 (Fig. 10-5). There are also limited career appointments in APHIS with special assignments to a single country for 3 to 5 years for a particular program or project.

Given the contemporary emphasis on globalization of trade and concern for food safety worldwide, it is surprising that so few veterinarians are employed by APHIS-IS. There is recognition within APHIS that more veterinarians will be needed in the future, but it is unrealistic for the prospective job applicant to expect that hundreds or even dozens of new job opportunities will become available in the near future. The main constraint on APHIS is budgetary, since the federal government has been in a general downsizing mode in recent years. With little budgetary opportunity to create new positions, APHIS hopes that through a process of employee attrition by retirement and reclassification of vacated positions, the number of APHIS-IS veterinarians working abroad will approach 30 within the next few years. In addition, APHIS will make increased use of veterinarians from the VS unit for short-term assignments abroad. Even with these constraints, APHIS still represents a good, though competitive opportunity for young veterinarians to add an international dimension to their careers. A good indication of the international perspective and activities of APHIS can be obtained by looking at the web page of the Center for Emerging Issues at http://www.aphis.usda.gov/vs/ceah/cei/index.htm.

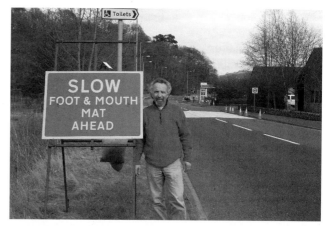

Figure 10-5. Dr. Don Hoenig, a graduate of the University of Pennsylvania School of Veterinary Medicine, is the state veterinarian of Maine. Dr. Hoenig went to the UK in 2001 to assist in the foot and mouth disease control effort when offered the opportunity through APHIS. This experience was valuable to Dr. Hoenig in developing a foot and mouth emergency response plan for the state of Maine upon his return. (Photo courtesy of Dr. Donald E. Hoenig)

Other USDA Agencies   Several other agencies within the USDA regularly hire veterinarians, but opportunities for international career development are less well defined in these agencies.

The Food Safety and Inspection Service (FSIS)   The FSIS regularly hires veterinarians primarily as supervising inspectors for meat and poultry slaughter and processing plants. It does have regular positions in the Commonwealth of Puerto Rico and the U.S. Virgin Islands. Beyond that, there are no longer any permanent FSIS postings for veterinarians abroad, though senior veterinary medical officers within the FSIS system may make periodic oversight visits to processing plants in foreign countries that export meat products to the United States. They may also travel abroad to participate in trade negotiations as advisors on issues concerning food safety. Entry level veterinary medical officers are unlikely to be assigned to these international positions.

The Agricultural Research Service (ARS)   The ARS identifies itself as "the principal scientific research agency of the U.S. Department of Agriculture," with the overall goal of ensuring an uninterrupted and adequate supply of high-quality food and fiber to meet the needs of the American people. With facilities at 114 locations across the United States, the ARS focuses on research to solve technical food and agricultural problems over a wide range of agricultural ecosystems. The agency has six specific research areas: soil, air and water conservation; plant productivity; animal productivity; food technology; human nutrition and wellness; and systems integration. Over 8000 people are employed by ARS on a full-time basis. One third of these employees are scientists and engineers.

Among the ARS research facilities are at least 18 focusing specifically on animal health. Notable among these, from the international veterinary perspective, is the Plum Island Animal

Disease Center, sharing its island venue with the APHIS Foreign Animal Disease Diagnostic Laboratory. Plum Island is in Long Island Sound, off the coast of Greenport, New York. These two laboratories focus primarily on the diagnosis of foreign animal diseases, performing thousands of tests each year to identify over 35 animal diseases exotic to the United States. Samples come from quarantine facilities, domestic regulatory veterinarians, and foreign veterinarians. These two laboratories also are involved in vaccine testing, production of diagnostic reagents, and development of new technologies for diagnosing and controlling foreign animal disease and are responsible for maintaining the North American Foot and Mouth Disease Vaccine Bank.

In addition to these technical functions, the Plum Island facility has an educational and training function. Research scientists, military veterinarians, veterinary students, APHIS veterinarians, and others may attend regularly scheduled training sessions in foreign animal disease. In addition, some graduate students are able to carry out laboratory research on foreign animal diseases as part of their degree programs in collaboration with their own degree-granting institutions. Employment as a veterinary research scientist at Plum Island would definitely add an international dimension to your veterinary career, though you may not necessarily work abroad. Research positions at Plum Island are not entry-level positions, as most veterinary scientists working there have advanced training and degrees in relevant specialty fields such as virology or immunology.

The Foreign Agricultural Service (FAS)   The FAS of USDA represents the interests of the U.S. food and agricultural sector abroad through improved market access for U.S. food and agricultural products, including livestock products. In addition, FAS carries out food aid and market-related technical assistance programs as well as legislatively mandated import and export programs. FAS also works with other government agencies and universities to enhance the global competitiveness of U.S. agriculture. It is also committed to increasing income and food availability in developing nations through stimulation of economic growth in the agricultural sector. FAS collects, analyzes, and disseminates information about global supply and demand, trade trends, and emerging market opportunities. Much of this trade information is available on the FAS website at http://www.fas.usda.gov/default.htm.

FAS operates worldwide, with staff located in over 75 posts covering more than 130 countries. Overseas personnel are supported by a team of analysts, negotiators, and marketing specialists in Washington, D.C. FAS does not routinely hire veterinarians. However, because of the growing importance of livestock products in U.S. agricultural exports, FAS may have international positions requiring livestock expertise for which veterinarians may be appropriate candidates, particularly if they have agribusiness experience.

United States Department of Health and Human Services   Three agencies within the USDHHS employ veterinarians. These are the FDA, the NIH, and the CDC. Of the three, the

CDC is most likely to engage veterinarians in international activities. These activities are described earlier in the chapter in the section on federal government jobs in the uniformed services, as veterinarians in the Commissioned Corps of the Public Health Service are regularly assigned to the CDC in addition to civilian veterinarians.

The FDA employs a good number of veterinarians, particularly through its Center for Veterinary Medicine (CVM). They are involved primarily in the regulation of new drugs and medical devices for use in veterinary medicine, with regard to safety and efficacy. International opportunities in the CVM are limited at present. CVM does have a summer intern program for veterinary students. More information is available on the internet at http://www.fda.gov/cvm/intern/student_intern.htm. Veterinarians also work at the NIH, primarily in the areas of laboratory animal care and as participating scientists in health research. Again, the opportunities for international veterinary work through NIH are currently limited.

United States Department of Interior   Two groups within the Department of Interior employ veterinarians in positions and offer good potential for international activity. These are the United States Fish and Wildlife Service (USFWS) and the National Wildlife Health Center (NWHC), administered through the United States Geological Survey.

United States Fish and Wildlife Service   The USFWS was established as a distinct entity within the Department of Interior in 1940, though precursor agencies and activities within the federal government can be traced back to 1871 when the U.S. Commission on Fish and Fisheries was created by Congress to study and recommend solutions to the obvious decline in marine food fish supplies. The USFWS has headquarters in Arlington, Virginia, and has numerous regional offices around the country, which it divides administratively into seven regions.

The mission of USFWS today is to work with citizens, other agencies, and organizations to conserve, protect, and enhance fish, wildlife, and plants and their habitats for the continuing benefit of the American people. While the focus of USFWS is on natural resources within the United States, it recognizes the global dimension of conservation efforts and the potential for forces outside U.S. borders to exert effects within those borders. As such, USFWS maintains an International Affairs Branch to facilitate interactions with other nations on the implementation of international treaties and conventions that help ensure the conservation of global commons and the species they support, for example, migratory birds that may traverse dozens of countries in their annual flights. The International Affairs Branch of USFWS has three Offices: the Office of International Affairs, the Office of Scientific Authority, and the Office of Management Authority.

The Office of International Affairs provides international leadership on conservation issues, ensures implementation of the service's international statutory and treaty responsibilities; and supports U.S. foreign policy initiatives to complement those responsibilities. The International Affairs Office focuses on three regional areas: the Western Hemisphere; Russia and China; and the Near East, South Asia, and South Africa. As an illustration of USFWS international activities, the goal of the Western Hemisphere Program is to develop and strengthen the capacity of Latin American and Caribbean nations to manage and conserve biological diversity for the benefit of local communities. Toward this goal, USFWS supports human resources development, information exchange, and environmental education projects throughout the hemisphere.

The Office of Scientific Authority (OSA) provides objective, biologically based advice to USFWS on implementation of the Convention on International Trade in Endangered Species of Wild Fauna and Flora (commonly referred to as CITES), the Endangered Species Act, and the Wild Bird Conservation Act. The Office of Management Authority implements domestic laws and international treaties to promote long-term conservation of global fish and wildlife resources.

The USFWS does employ a small number of veterinarians and also routinely advertises jobs for which veterinarians would potentially be qualified. There are not any specific veterinary positions within the International Affairs Branch, but once employed, the potential would exist for transfers to other branches.

National Wildlife Health Center   The NWHC is a science center of the Biological Resources Division of the United States Geological Survey of the Department of the Interior, located in Madison, Wisconsin (see http://www.nwhc.usgs.gov). The NWHC was established in 1975 as a biomedical laboratory to assess the impact of disease on wildlife and to identify the role of various pathogens in contributing to wildlife losses. It has approximately 40 employees and many of the professional staff are veterinarians. While most of the center's activities are focused on wildlife health and disease issues in the United States, there is a distinct international orientation as well. Several of the center's activities relating to international wildlife health include the following:

- Technical assistance on wildlife health issues through workshops and seminars both at the center and at other locations nationally and internationally.

- In-house training for senior veterinary students, wildlife biologists, and foreign scientists interested in wildlife diseases

- International collaborative scientific activities including projects with Russian counterparts for the study of wildlife diseases of mutual interest, with the Wildlife Institute of India in developing faculty expertise in wildlife disease, and with an Egyptian veterinarian who spent 1 1/2 years at the center training to assist development of wildlife health capabilities in Egypt

- Production of a videotape on lead poisoning in migratory birds that is widely used by the national and international conservation community

- Technical consultations with government scientists and officials in Australia, New Zealand, Japan, Denmark, France, Russia, and England regarding lead poisoning in wild birds

- Evaluation of wildlife disease risks associated with New Zealand's endangered species program

Independent Federal Agencies   Several federal agencies are independently administrated and do not fall under the authority of any of the major departments of the executive branch of the federal government, such as Agriculture, Interior, or Health and Human Services, as discussed above. Several of these independent federal agencies are of interest to veterinarians wishing to add an international dimension to their careers, as these agencies provide opportunities to garner international experience, pursue relevant training, or find international employment. These agencies include the Peace Corps, the Agency for International Development, the EPA, and the National Zoological Park of the Smithsonian Institution.

The United States Peace Corps   The Peace Corps, an independent federal agency established in 1961 by President John F. Kennedy, is America's international volunteer service corps. The Peace Corps sends American citizens overseas to participate in people-to-people development projects. Currently, 80 countries are served by the Peace Corps through the efforts of approximately 6700 volunteers. Peace Corps projects fall broadly into six main sectors-education, environment, health and nutrition, business, community development, and agriculture. In recent years, the Peace Corps has added country programs in Eastern Europe and newly independent states of the former Soviet Union to its existing programs in developing countries of Asia, Africa, Latin America, and the Pacific island nations.

The Peace Corps is an excellent entry-level opportunity for veterinarians to develop valuable international skills and experience. The Peace Corps will test your flexibility and adaptability while improving your cross-cultural sensitivity, your problem-solving skills, and your ability to work effectively in a team setting. Volunteers gain significant insights into the problems and challenges facing people in developing countries and garner new perspectives on the forces that constrain development in such places.

Volunteers commit to the Peace Corps for 27 months—3 months for training and 24 months in the field. No salary is provided. The Peace Corps pays for transportation to and from the volunteer's assigned country and provides a modest stipend to cover local living expenses. Dental and health care are provided, and there is a readjustment allowance of $6075 provided at the end of the full service period. There are also 2 days of vacation time earned for every month of service. Student loan payments for Stafford loans, Perkins loans, Federal

Consolidation loans and Direct loans can be deferred while the loan recipient is a Peace Corps volunteer.

Another opportunity of potential interest to veterinarians considering Peace Corps service is the Masters International Program. This allows qualified Peace Corps volunteers to enroll in graduate school in selected disciplines and earn academic credit toward their masters degree for the time spent in the field as a Peace Corps volunteer. Over 30 universities participate in the program, and a variety of disciplines of study are offered, some very relevant to veterinarians considering international careers. Such disciplines include public health, agriculture, business, agribusiness, environmental education, and NGO development/nonprofit management. Details of the Masters International Program including information about specific universities and degree programs are available at the Peace Corps web site at http://www.peacecorps.gov/gradschool/masters/index.cfm.

The United States Agency for International Development (USAID) The USAID is the independent agency of the federal government that provides economic development and humanitarian assistance to foreign nations to advance U.S. economic and political interests overseas. USAID was established in 1961 by President John F. Kennedy, the same year that he established the Peace Corps. USAID headquarters is in Washington, D.C., and a large staff is maintained there. In addition, however, USAID maintains staffed missions in countries where it funds foreign aid programs and may also have regional offices with coordination functions for aid programs of individual countries in the region, for example the Regional Economic Development Services Office for East and Southern Africa (REDSO/ESA) located in Nairobi, Kenya, but involved in activities throughout eastern and southern Africa.

There are a number of different ways to work for or with USAID. Full-time employees may be hired as Foreign Service or Civil Service employees. In addition, USAID recruits supplemental employees as needed for particular projects and organizational activities, under personal service contracts (PSCs). These contracts, which frequently involve overseas assignments, are usually for periods of 12 to 24 months. In some cases, PSCs may be renewed, but this does not equate with permanent employment. PSC opportunities, as well as other USAID employment vacancies, are posted on the internet with job descriptions and details for applying at http://www.info.usaid.gov/about/employment/.

Finally, USAID frequently requires outside consultants for short-term assignments to make site visits as technical advisors, program reviewers, or project evaluators, usually for periods of several weeks. These opportunities are not regularly advertised and effective networking is the best way to learn about, and be recruited for, such positions.

Regrettably, USAID rarely offers positions specifically for veterinarians. As with other government agencies, there may be positions advertised for which your skills and experience make you eminently qualified, but it is unlikely that you will be successfully recruited because you are a veterinarian. In fact you may be in the unfortunate positions of convincing your application reviewers that you are the right person in spite of being a veterinarian, taking pains in your application to emphasize those aspects of your professional life that USAID may be more interested in, such as your administrative skills, management skills, writing skills, international experience, or knowledge of development practices. One possible route of entry for veterinarians into a USAID career is through the New Entry Professional Program for Overseas Opportunities, formerly known as the International Development Intern (IDI) program. Information about this program is available at http://www.info.usaid.gov/about/employment/nepbro.htm.

While the terms "new entry" and "intern" suggest entry level positions, in fact, the programs favor applicants with some professional experience already in hand. In reality, most veterinarians who find employment through USAID end up doing so indirectly, by working for academic institutions, NGOs, or consulting firms that have received USAID funding to carry out contract projects abroad. Veterinarians working at such organizations may be directly involved in developing the project concept, preparing the project documents, and meeting with USAID officials to convince them that the project should be funded. Therefore, a knowledge of USAID perspectives and practices is very useful for veterinarians interested in international work.

There is a fellowship opportunity that offers interested veterinarians an excellent chance to learn about the organization, operation, and policies of USAID. This is the Diplomacy Fellowship offered by the American Academy for the Advancement of Science. Several veterinarians have competed successfully in the past for this fellowship and have earned valuable career experience in a wide range of areas. These veterinarians have served in the Office of Research in USAID's Bureau of Research and Development, in the Global Bureau of USAID's Human Capacity Development Center, and in the Bureau of Global Programs of USAID's Center for the Environment. Their various activities focused on subjects as diverse as technology transfer, agricultural program review, and preservation of biodiversity through sustainable development. The AAAS Diplomacy Fellowship is more of a midcareer opportunity than an entry-level opportunity. In addition to USAID, Diplomacy Fellows may apply to work at the USDA, the U.S. Department of State, or the Fogarty International Center of the NIH. More information is available on the internet at http://fellowships.aaas.org/diplomacy/index.html.

Environmental Protection Agency The EPA was established as an independent agency of the federal government in 1970, with headquarters in Washington, D.C. The mission of the EPA is to protect human health and to safeguard the natural environment, namely the air, water, and land upon which life depends. As such, the agency has evolved as the nation's principal regulatory agency for environmental health. It monitors and regulates a variety of national environmental concerns including reduction of air and water pollution, solid waste disposal, pesticide use, and radiation hazards, as well as other toxic substances. EPA is also involved in scientific inquiry and policy making in relation to environmental health. The EPA is committed to seeing that the United States plays a leadership role in working with other nations to protect the global environment. Toward that end, EPA maintains an active Office of International Activities and is involved in numerous international collaborations to address a variety of global environmental problems, many of which are discussed in Chapter 6. Some of the EPA's relevant international activities, as presented in the 1998 annual report of the Office of International Activities include:

- Collaborative agreements with Canada on improved water quality in the Great Lakes through reductions in sulfate and nitrate pollutants

- Technical and financial assistance to Russia for processing spent nuclear fuel from decommissioned nuclear submarines at Murmansk and other northern bases to reduce radiation pollution of terrestrial and aquatic Arctic environments

- Commitments secured from all eight Arctic (bordering) nations to phase out production and use of PCBs and to help Russia develop appropriate PCB disposal protocols

- Agreement between the United States and other Caribbean Basin States to establish wastewater effluent standards to be required under a legally binding regional agreement, promising significant potential benefit to coral reef ecosystems and the general public health

- Successful lobbying of the International Maritime Organization to implement a Mandatory Ship Reporting requirement for the protection of right whales

- Development of emissions trading agreements in China, Russia, and the Ukraine to reduce global greenhouse gas emissions

- Signing protocols with 50 countries of Europe, the former Soviet Union, and Canada to reduce the transboundary air movement and deposition of certain persistent organic pollutants (POPs), restrict the unintentional creation or release of dioxins and furans, reduce the content of mercury in medical and other products, and develop and exchange emission and source inventories

- Conducting workshops in Central America on proper pesticide use as part of an overall program of community-based environmental protection

At present, the EPA does not directly hire veterinarians for work at the agency, though veterinarians do work there. These individuals are usually assigned to EPA from the Commissioned Corps of the USPHS, described earlier in the section on uniformed services. As with other federal agencies, however, there may be positions advertised at EPA for which veterinarians are suited, even though a veterinary degree is not specifically solicited. Veterinary toxicologists, for example, would most certainly would be able to compete effectively for some EPA positions. EPA puts out an Environmental Career Resources Guide. It also offers a number of training programs including a Federal Environmental Internship Studies Program and the EPA Management Intern Program.

National Zoological Park The National Zoo, in Washington, D.C., is part of the Smithsonian Institution, an independent trust agency of the United States, established in 1846, which in addition to the zoo, is composed of 16 museums and galleries and numerous research facilities in the United States and abroad.

The National Zoo has an active Veterinary Services Program that involves clinical care, research, and training both nationally and internationally. On the international side, for example, veterinarians at the National Zoo's Center for Conservation and Research in Front Royal, Virginia, have been involved for many years in ongoing collaboration with colleagues in southern Africa. Activities include ongoing studies on the genetics and reproductive physiology of the cheetah in Namibia and continuing studies in Kruger National Park, South Africa, on a number of veterinary topics including anesthesia of giraffes; genetics of the sable antelope; basic studies of reproductive physiology in selected antelopes, elephants, and felids; and development of the Genome Resource Bank for preservation of frozen sperm from endangered animals of southern Africa.

In addition there are disease studies in Kruger National Park on the impact of feline immunodeficiency virus in free-ranging lions, leopards, and cheetahs as well as studies of bovine tuberculosis in African buffalo and its potential spread to lion, cheetah, elephants, and rhinoceros, which would adversely affect ongoing relocation programs.

Veterinary jobs at the National Zoo are not generally entry-level positions, as they usually require specialized clinical experience and/or advanced training or degrees in a specialized area, such as pathology or reproductive physiology. However, the National Zoo has a number of training opportunities for veterinarians and students interested in wildlife conservation and zoo animal medicine, including formal internships and residencies as well as summer and senior rotation externships and preceptorships in zoo animal medicine and veterinary pathology.

Academic Institutions

Employment in a faculty position at a veterinary college or other related academic institution represents an excellent opportunity for expanding one's professional activities into the international arena. Short-, medium-, and long-term activities abroad are all possible, and international activities may involve teaching, research, service delivery, or any combination of the three. While faculty positions are not likely to be entry-level opportunities, entry into academic medicine as a clinical resident or graduate student can in itself offer possible exposure to international activities and provide the necessary skills and experience to secure a faculty position as a later step in one's career.

Foreign Academic Institutions

There are close to 400 veterinary colleges in the world, all but 31 of them outside of the United States and Canada. A listing of these schools is provided in the AVMA *Membership Directory and Resource Manual*.[2] It would seem then, on first appearance, that the most direct and successful route to an international academic career would be to seek employment at a foreign veterinary college. In fact, this approach is not likely to be rewarding, as direct hire of foreigners is uncommon for a number of reasons.

Countries with veterinary schools, both in the developed and developing world, also have their own veterinary graduates, and these graduates represent an indigenous pool of talent and skill for the recruitment of new faculty. In many countries, immigration and job protection laws prohibit hiring foreign nationals or at least make such hiring very difficult. While a surprising number of veterinary schools use English as the language of instruction, many do not, and fluency in the local language of instruction, in addition to academic credentials, would be required. Even if faculty positions were available, many Americans, particularly those with families to support, would be deterred by faculty salaries abroad. While reasonably competitive in most industrialized countries, salaries can be startlingly low in many developing countries, as little as several hundred dollars per month! Despite these obstacles, it cannot be unequivocally stated that no direct-hire teaching positions are available abroad. Personal initiative, appropriate networking, and luck may pay off. If you know a particular place you would like to work and believe that you are qualified and have something to contribute, go ahead and contact the veterinary schools in that country or region. You may be able to arrange a special opportunity for yourself that might not be otherwise advertised or considered.

While direct hire is not a likely route for foreign academic employment, some possibilities do exist, though most of these opportunities require that you first be a faculty member at a North American university. From such a position, opportunities for sabbaticals, invited lectures, or teaching assignments, participation in faculty exchanges, or involvement in collaborative research activities with foreign universities offer the possibility for at least short- and medium-term opportunities abroad. Occasionally, at least in the past, long-term teaching contracts abroad were also available through development projects supported by foreign aid. For example, in the late 1960s and early 1970s, USAID provided funding for a number of American veterinary faculty to work in Kenya to help establish the new veterinary faculty of the University of Nairobi at Kabete and strengthen its institutional capacity. Managed through Colorado State University, the project recruited participating American faculty from a number of different universities. In the 1980s, faculty from the University of Minnesota were able to get short- and long-term assignments in Morocco as part of a USAID-funded program with the Institut Agronomique et Veterinaire Hassan II in Rabat for postgraduate training of Moroccan veterinary faculty. It is difficult to predict if such team teaching contracts will be available again in the future. Certainly the need exists to rebuild and strengthen the capacity for training veterinarians in countries where war and socioeconomic upheaval have undermined the ability of existing institutions to provide adequate training. Afghanistan, Vietnam, and the Central Asian Republics that emerged from the former Soviet Union all come to mind.

Domestic Academic Institutions

Faculty positions at North American veterinary colleges and related academic institutions, such as schools of public health, represent an excellent and growing opportunity to pursue international activities in the areas of education, research, outreach and extension, consultation, and provision of service. Don't be disappointed, however, if you do not find advertisements that specifically recruit faculty for positions in "International Veterinary Medicine." While such faculty positions may become more common in the future, at present, to the author's knowledge, only Tufts University School of Veterinary Medicine has faculty positions dedicated exclusively full-time to international veterinary medicine. This means that veterinarians seeking to add an international dimension to their academic careers must first qualify as faculty members for traditionally defined faculty appointments, usually by academic discipline and then either create or capitalize on opportunities to participate in international work. Such opportunities for adding a global dimension to faculty activity in this manner are likely to continue to increase, and at an accelerating rate, over the next few years.

Justification for this optimism comes in part from attendance at the 14th symposium on veterinary medical education of the American Association of Veterinary Medical Colleges (AAVMC) held at the University of Georgia in 1996. The symposium was entitled "The Internationalization of Veterinary Education: Strengths, Challenges, and Opportunities." It was clear that leaders in organized veterinary medical education were coming to the realization that globalization of communication and trade, environmental degradation, increasing world demand for food, and other major global trends presented new challenges for the education and preparation of future veterinarians able to respond effectively to a rapidly changing world. Internationalization of the curriculum was recognized as an important goal, and expanded opportunities for faculty and students to gain international experience were recognized as important elements in that internationalization process. The proceedings of this symposium, published in the *Journal of Veterinary Medical Education*, are useful reading for anyone interested in international veterinary medicine in general and the internationalization of veterinary education in particular.[1]

Internationalization of veterinary education is also discussed further in this text in Chapter 8.

Nevertheless, recognition of the need for change does not translate into immediate action in all cases, and it is clear that some veterinary schools are much more active in their support of internationalization than others. This is supported by a survey on internationalization of veterinary teaching facilities carried out by faculty at Washington State University, the results of which were presented at the AAVMC symposium in Georgia.[6] All but one veterinary school in the United States and Canada responded to the survey questionnaire. Virtually all veterinary schools recognized the need to internationalize their programs and institutions and offered appropriate and relevant rationales for doing so. Yet, only 26.7% indicated that their international activities and programs would increase greatly in the next 10 years. Three quarters of the responding schools indicated that they had an identifiable international position on the faculty or in the administrative staff, but the average time commitment of these individuals was small, averaging 20% of that persons' work load. In fact, many schools seem to have a designated international position in name only. In 1997, the author sent a questionnaire to the International Veterinary Student Association (IVSA) representative at each veterinary school in the United States and Canada asking that the IVSA representative identify a faculty person or administrator that students would look to for advice on international issues relating to their veterinary education. IVSA representatives from approximately one third of the veterinary schools had difficulty identifying an appropriate contact person within their faculties.

There are no established standards for determining how well a veterinary college is meeting the international expectations of its constituents, be they students, faculty, practitioners, or others. Dr. Carin Smith, in researching her book *Career Choices for Veterinarians*, identified several schools that offered visible opportunities for students interested in international careers. These include, in alphabetical order, the University of California at Davis, the University of Illinois, Purdue University, Texas A&M, Tufts University, and Washington State University. Table 10-2 provides a list of the international student projects funded by the Geraldine R. Dodge Foundation. The list also gives the schools where these students were enrolled, and that list serves as a reasonable guide for determining a school's interest in, and commitment to, internationalizing veterinary education. Appearance on the list implies that the school made an effort to distribute the announcement of the Dodge grant program to students; that students at that school had interesting ideas for international projects; that those students were able to find faculty mentors willing and interested in serving as advisors in the preparation, submission, and execution of the project; and, that the faculty member was able to find time to carry out this mentoring role. Taken together these factors suggest an institutional climate that supports international activities by students and faculty. Schools listed in Table 10-2 that are not already identified by Dr. Smith in her book include Colorado State University, University of Geor-

gia, Kansas State University, Ohio State University, Michigan State University, University of Montreal, University of Tennessee, and Tuskegee University. This list is not meant to be definitive or exhaustive, just illustrative. For example, Cornell University and University of Guelph are also well known to actively support student learning activities abroad and have faculty actively engaged in international activities.

The point is that different veterinary teaching institutions vary in their commitment to internationalization and their support for faculty to participate in international activities. If you pursue an academic career primarily as a way to become professionally involved in international work, then you need to thoroughly explore the potential for international work at any given institution. It is critical to determine if the university itself has a commitment to globalization and whether the administration at the veterinary school supports that commitment. If so, how does that translate into faculty opportunities for international work? Are international activities and time spent away from the home institution considered favorably toward promotion and tenure consideration, or are they seen as detractors? Has there been any effort to introduce international content into the curriculum? Has it been resisted or accepted? Do any faculty have ongoing research grants or service contracts that require time in the field overseas? Do department heads support this and help to facilitate appropriate coverage of teaching or clinical responsibilities during one's absence? Do other faculty support or resent international work? What is the college's policy on international consulting? Even though you may be applying for a faculty position in epidemiology, microbiology, pathology, large animal medicine, exotic animal medicine, or any other relevant academic discipline, these are some of the questions that must be asked and answered satisfactorily if you hope to use your faculty position successfully to further your interests in international veterinary medicine for your own personal satisfaction and for the advancement of the profession.

Private Industry

Opportunities for veterinarians in the corporate domain have long been available within in the United States, primarily with pharmaceutical companies but also within the pet food industry and in the corporate livestock production sector. For many veterinarians, employment in "industry" has represented an attractive alternative to private practice, offering regular hours, good pay and benefits, and considerable job satisfaction. Statistics of the AMVA identify 1562 veterinarians working in industry in 2000, and industry veterinarians have their own association, the American Association of Industrial Veterinarians, which encourages student membership as a means of becoming aware of the opportunities in industrial veterinary medicine and the best way to prepare for those opportunities.

The globalization of business, commerce, and trade that has been so evident in recent years has included industries that employ veterinarians, especially the manufacturers of pharmaceuticals and biologicals. Many such companies, through growth or extensive mergers and acquisitions, have become multinational firms, developing new markets and competing for market share around the globe. As a result, there are, and will continue to be, increased opportunities for veterinarians to have short-, medium-, and long-term international assignments within these multinational corporations. Examples of such companies include Bayer, Hills Pet Nutrition, Hoechst, Merial, Merck, Novartis, Pfizer, Ralston Purina, Schering-Plough, and Waltham.

Veterinarians are engaged in a variety of employment functions in industry. In the pharmaceutical industry, for instance, they may be involved in marketing and sales, technical services, new product research and development, and regulatory clearance. The latter is particularly important in the international context. Many companies wish to take existing products and introduce them into new and different markets around the world. As each country has its own regulatory policies, it is often necessary to develop new, site-specific safety and efficacy data for the drug. Industry veterinarians working with local counterparts play an important role in the design, implementation, evaluation, and presentation of new safety and efficacy data. Local regulators may also desire modifications of manufacturing, formulation, and packaging of existing drugs, and veterinarians may be involved in negotiations to avert or minimize potentially costly modifications of existing products. An emerging area that may offer more specialized employment opportunities in the future is ethnoveterinary medicine, discussed in Chapter 8. Many animal owners and traditional healers around the world use indigenous remedies derived from local plants. Without doubt, a good number of these traditional medicines contain effective compounds, but very little work has been done to identify active ingredients or evaluate their efficacy under controlled conditions. Veterinarians with good clinical skills and/or advanced training in pharmacology can contribute to the identification of effective traditional remedies worldwide and help bring derivative products to the marketplace.

Veterinary students can begin to explore industrial veterinary medicine while in school. Many companies recruit "student agents" to disseminate information about their products to fellow students. This represents an opportunity for the student agent to begin to network with veterinarians working for corporations that have veterinary opportunities abroad. There are also some clerkships in industry available to veterinary students to gain experience in corporate veterinary work. Some of these are listed at the web site of the Center for Government and Corporate Veterinary Medicine at the Virginia-Maryland Regional College of Veterinary Medicine (http://www.vetmed.umd.edu/cgcvm/). The American Association of Industrial Veterinarians also encourages student membership, which provides a regular newsletter of industry developments.

Specific international positions for veterinarians in industry are not likely to be entry-level positions. Some previous experience in practice or in industry would be expected, and some relevant international experience would be desired. If you are a recent graduate considering employment in indus-

try with an eye toward an international career, it would be wise to seek a domestic position with a multinational company and work within the company to position yourself for international appointments.

International/Intergovernmental Agencies

A number of international institutions offer potential employment to veterinarians. For the sake of discussion they can be roughly divided into three broad categories, though any individual organization may have multiple functions that overlap the categories designated here—funding institutions, technical institutions, and research institutions.

International Donor Institutions

A number of international donor institutions provide funding, usually to national governments, to support large- and small-scale development projects within the country. This funding may be in the form of loans or grants. Examples of international donor institutions include the World Bank and the International Fund for Agricultural Development (IFAD), which are United Nations agencies, as well as the Asia Development Bank, the African Development Bank, the Islamic Development Bank, the Inter-American Development Bank, and the European Union. Individual countries, through their specific foreign aid agencies, may also serve as donor agencies. Examples of such institutions are the USAID in the United States, the Canadian International Development Agency (CIDA) in Canada, Danish International Cooperation (DANIDA) in Denmark, Department for International Development (DFID) in the UK, and the Deutsche Gesellschaft fur Technische Zusammenarbeit (GTZ) in Germany. European government agencies, including the European Union are unlikely to hire American or Canadian nationals.

Projects supported by international donor institutions may be in a wide range of areas, including physical infrastructure development, health, education, environment, or agriculture, to name a few. Individual countries determine their internal needs, but development of the overall project, its budget, and plans for implementation are often finalized as a result of extensive consultation between the donor organization and the applying country. The final terms of some projects include provisions for a technical assistance package that includes a team of outside consultants with specified qualifications and experience. These consultants may be paired with local, professional counterparts working on the project to provide technical assistance and management support during project implementation. The technical assistance packages are often bid upon by private consulting firms who supply or recruit the technical experts required for the particular project. Private consulting firms as potential employers are discussed below in this section of the chapter.

Projects of potential interest to veterinarians are funded by international donor agencies. Such projects may involve livestock health and production, veterinary service delivery, public health, environmental health, and/or preservation of biodiversity. With regard to livestock, for example, the World Bank, between 1991 and 1999, approved at least 60 loans in 39 countries for agricultural projects that included an animal resource component in the overall project design. The size of individual loans for these various projects ranged from US$4.0 million to US$444.4 million, with the total amount lent exceeding US$3.83 billion.

There are several ways that veterinarians may find employment in association with donor institutions. Direct hiring by the institution as a full-time employee is possible, but such opportunities are infrequent. Donor institutions do require some in-house expertise on a variety of subjects to help make internal decisions about loan and grant priorities and strategies. The World Bank, for example, has an Agriculture and Natural Resources Department that employs several specialists familiar with different aspects of the livestock sector, including economics, marketing, production, and health. This team includes at least one veterinarian. Veterinarians qualifying for such positions would have to have a great deal of international experience and preferably some training or experience in business, finance, economics, administration, or project management.

In addition to full-time employers, donor institutions may use the services of consultants on a short-term basis. Consultants are likely to be retained for field visits to prepare feasibility reports on proposed projects, to conduct midterm progress and performance reviews on existing projects, or to conduct troubleshooting visits for projects encountering difficulties. Such consultants may be hired directly by the donor institution, or if a team of evaluators is required for the feasibility study or midterm review, the field mission may be put out for bid to private consulting firms. Finally, when the terms of the project loan require technical assistance teams, requests for proposals are usually advertised by the donor institution and/or the loan recipient country for competitive bids and proposals from private firms. Such firms may recruit outside consultants to fill specialized positions on the technical assistance team. Regardless of the route of employment, all these opportunities require the services of seasoned professionals.

International Technical Organizations

A number of international organizations, mostly agencies of the United Nations, provide programmatic and technical services to national governments. Different agencies have particular areas of specialization. These specializations are often directly evident from their names, for example, the Food and Agriculture Organizaton of the United Nations (FAO), the World Health Organization (WHO), the United Nations Environmental Programme (UNEP), the United Nations Development Program (UNDP), and the International Atomic Energy Agency (IAEA). Regardless of their area of focus, such organizations are involved in a variety of activities: education and training, data collection and analysis, policy advising, technical assistance on project development and implementation, and even regulatory and monitoring functions, when member nations sign treaties empowering the agency to perform such functions. The agencies just mentioned, as well as most other

UN agencies, have web sites that describe the agency's mission, organization, and activities. Most also have a web page for employment opportunities within the organization.

Of the agencies mentioned, the FAO, with headquarters in Rome; the WHO, with headquarters in Geneva; and the IAEA, with headquarters in Vienna, specifically hire veterinarians as regular staff members. UNEP and UNDP also hire veterinarians but more likely on an as-needed basis. All of these agencies, in addition to their headquarters facilities and staff, maintain regional offices or specific national offices in countries where they have active programs. Therefore employment opportunities may exist in a variety of locations. Be advised that national offices are usually staffed by citizens of the country in which the office is located. Nevertheless, expatriate project managers and technical experts may receive specific, project-related assignments to those offices, lasting from months to years.

Brief descriptions of those international technical institutions of potential interest to veterinarians as employers are given in the following paragraphs. As these agencies are so relevant to international veterinary medicine, their activities are discussed repeatedly in different chapters of this book. Refer to the index for more specific references to the organizations elsewhere in the text.

Food and Agriculture Organization of the United Nations The FAO was founded in October 1945, with a mission to raise levels of nutrition and standards of living, to improve agricultural productivity, and to better the condition of rural populations. Today, FAO is the largest autonomous agency within the UN system. It has 175 member nations and employs over 4300 staff members around the world. FAO deals with all aspects of agriculture and food production including crops, livestock, aquaculture, and fisheries. Within FAO there is an Animal Production and Health Division whose mission is the promotion of sustainable livestock production and improved food security. Its goal is to increase productivity of domestic animals by making better use of available resources (see http://www.fao.org/ag/aga/index_en.htm on the internet).

The division promotes the development of animal health and production technologies and provides strategy formulation and policy advice to member countries. It collects and disseminates information on animal health, feed resources, animal genetic resources, and livestock production systems and also provides an international forum where governments discuss policies and negotiate international agreements in the area of animal production and health. Technical support is offered in the areas of animal health; genetic resources; breeding and reproduction; feeds, nutrition and forage; husbandry and management; product handling and processing; specialized information systems; and, livestock development policy and planning. At the request of member nations, the division may initiate and fund a Technical Cooperation Programme, or TCP, to address a particular problem that is causing adverse economic or health effects. TCPs usually require recruiting expert consultants for site visits, field research, and training exercises to address the problem at hand. These expert consultancies offer potential opportunities for veterinarians when the problem involves livestock production and health (Fig. 10-6).

The Animal Health Service (AGAH) within the Animal Production and Health Division is responsible for assisting member countries to develop strategies for the economic control of animal diseases. The Infectious Disease Group and Parasitic Disease Group within AGAH work to promote international coordination of the prevention, diagnosis, and control of important diseases, such as foot and mouth disease, rinderpest, African swine fever, and various tick-borne diseases of economic importance.

World Health Organization Creation of an international health agency was first proposed at the United Nations in 1945, and the constitution of the WHO was ultimately ratified by member nations in 1948. Today the WHO has over 3800 employees worldwide working at its headquarters in Geneva, Switzerland, or through its six regional offices around the

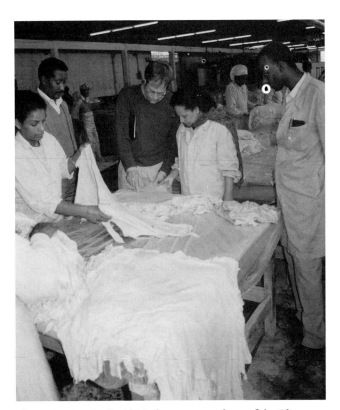

Figure 10-6. Dr. David M. Sherman, a graduate of the Ohio State University College of Veterinary Medicine, working as a private consultant in Ethiopia for the Food and Agricultural Organization of the United Nations. In the photo, Dr. Sherman (*center*) and his Ethiopian counterpart, Dr. Kassa Bayou (*left*), inspect sheep skins at a tannery on the outskirts of Addis Ababa to evaluate the impact of external parasites on skin quality. The visit was part of an FAO Technical Cooperation Programme requested by the Ethiopian government to find ways to improve the quality of sheep and goat skins from Ethiopia for the profitable export market. (Photo provided by Dr. David M. Sherman)

world. The Pan American Health Organization is the regional representative of the WHO in the Americas. The mission of the WHO is to promote the highest level of health and well-being for all the people of the world in a physical, mental, and social context.

WHO carries out a wide range of functions and activities in support of its broad mission. WHO acts as the directing and coordinating authority on international health work and promotes technical cooperation on international health issues; it assists governments in strengthening health services when requested to do so and furnishes, also on request, appropriate technical assistance and emergency aid; it encourages work on the prevention and control of epidemic, endemic, and other diseases; it promotes the improvement of nutrition, housing, sanitation, and other aspects of environmental hygiene; it supports and coordinates biomedical and health services research; it promotes improved standards of teaching and training in the health, medical, and related professions; it encourages the establishment of international standards for biological and pharmaceutical products and diagnostic procedures; it fosters activities in the field of mental health; and it advances standardization of international nomenclature of diseases, causes of death, and public health practices through conventions, agreements, regulations, and policy recommendations.

Through its Division of Communicable Disease Surveillance and Response (CSR), the WHO supports programs and activities related to zoonotic diseases (see http://www.who.int/emc/diseases/zoo/). The Zoonoses Unit is headed by a veterinarian. Areas of interest include a number of specific diseases such as anthrax, brucellosis, cestode infections, leptospirosis, Lyme borreliosis, Q fever, rabies, Rift Valley fever, toxoplasmosis, transmissible spongiform encephalopathies, and tuberculosis. In addition to specific disease concerns, there are general program interests in antimicrobial resistance, vector control, and disease risks associated with xenotransplantation. Veterinarians employed by the WHO generally have considerable experience or advanced training in relevant fields such as public health, immunology, or microbiology. Permanent or consulting opportunities may be available to qualified individuals.

International Atomic Energy Agency (IAEA) The IAEA is a specialized agency of the United Nations, established in 1957. IAEA headquarters are in Vienna, Austria. The roles of the IAEA are to foster the development of peaceful uses of atomic energy, set standards for nuclear safety and environmental protection, provide technical support to member countries, and foster exchange of information on nuclear issues. The IAEA also carries out monitoring and inspection functions for nuclear plant facilities in member countries and is involved in programs of preparedness and response to nuclear accidents, as discussed in Chapter 6 in relation to the nuclear accident at Chernobyl.

As part of its program to foster peaceful uses of nuclear technology, the IAEA is involved in developing medical and veterinary applications for radionuclides. As such, the agency supports work on radioimmunodiagnostics for veterinary diseases such as rinderpest through training and technical assistance. It also supports research and application of radiation-based sterilization techniques for insect pest control programs such as screwworm. The IAEA employs some veterinarians in support of these various activities.

United Nations Environment Programme (UNEP) A relatively young UN agency, UNEP was established in 1972 and maintains headquarters in Nairobi, Kenya. UNEP serves as the international forum for environmental matters of global concern. It coordinates international environmental conventions and accords, conducts monitoring and surveillance activities, engages in data collection and dissemination on various aspects of environmental change, and encourages and coordinates sound environmental practices and policies. Some examples of UNEP activities on specific topics of global environmental concern such as climate change, global warming, and the control of persistent organic pollutants are discussed in Chapter 6. UNEP also expresses programmatic interests in preservation of biodiversity, the relationship of livestock to environmental health, and the promotion of sustainable systems of animal agriculture. As such there is considerable potential for UNEP to require the services of veterinarians in the future.

Other United Nations Agencies Other agencies within the United Nations may sometimes become involved in projects or activities outside their primary missions, and such programs may require the services of veterinarians. For example, the UNDP was involved in providing support to rural Afghanistan during the protracted civil unrest there. UNDP activities included a variety of infrastructure support projects such as road construction, flood control, and reconstruction of agricultural irrigation systems. However, it became increasingly clear to UNDP staff that livestock health was a critical concern of the rural population and that healthy animals were vital for both work and agriculture. In response, UNDP established a paraveterinary program for rural Afghanistan and recruited expatriate veterinarians as technical advisors. Subsequently, the animal health program was transferred to the FAO in 1995, as livestock-related projects such as the paravet program are normally under their purview, and by that time, FAO had an active agricultural support program operating in Afghanistan as well.

Similarly, the United Nations Children's Fund (UNICEF) became involved in humanitarian relief efforts in the southern Sudan in the 1990s as the coordinating agency of the Operation Lifeline Sudan (OLS) program. A major goal of UNICEF was childhood immunization, but they found it difficult to organize vaccination campaigns in the war-torn region of traditional cattle pastoralists. It soon became evident that the health and welfare of children in the region was inextricably tied to the health and well-being of cattle, which served as the nutritional and economic basis of local society. UNICEF then began to support and coordinate paraveterinary programs focused on livestock vaccination in the region, which, coincidentally gave them better access to children as well as cattle, when herders assembled their herds and families for vaccination clinics. Many

veterinarians have participated in the OLS initiative, some through UNICEF, but most through the various NGOs and universities that have been involved in the regional effort. Tufts University has been very active in the OLS campaign, with several expatriate veterinarians becoming involved in the effort.

While very few jobs in United Nations agencies would be entry-level positions, there is an opportunity, albeit limited, to gain experience in the UN system as a UN intern. The UN internship program is open to students under 30 years of age enrolled in graduate programs and gives selected volunteers work at UN headquarters to gain first-hand insight into UN operations and practices. It is structured as three 2-month periods spread over a year. Participation for veterinary students in the internship program may be problematic, given the tight scheduling of veterinary school. Veterinarians pursuing Ph.D. programs after veterinary school would be more likely to be able to take advantage of the UN internship program. For veterinary students, it might require some very intensive negotiation with school administrators to possibly arrange a 1-year leave of absence and then return to school to finish with the class that followed your own. More detailed information about eligibility for the internship program, its goals, and the application procedure can be found on the internet at http://www.un.org/Depts/OHRM/examin/internsh/intern.htm.

The United Nations also runs a Volunteer Program (UNV) with eligibility requirements quite different than the internship program. Volunteers must be out of school and already have some experience or special expertise in a field desired by the UNV program. Assignments are in the field in countries other than the volunteer's home country. Volunteers actively participate in ongoing field projects and programs, along with regular UN employees. The main difference is the absence of pay. For those who can afford it and are selected, a UNV position represents a valuable and important means to develop credible international experience, gain better understanding of the operation of international agencies, and begin the critically important process of networking with other international professionals to identify future job opportunities. Information on the UNV program, including eligibility requirements and preferred areas of specialization are available on the internet at http://www.unv.org/.

Office International des Epizooties (OIE) The OIE or, in English, the International Office of Epizootics, is the principal world intergovernmental agency dealing with matters of animal health. It was established in 1924. The OIE is not a United Nations agency but frequently works jointly on projects with UN agencies, particularly WHO and FAO. The OIE currently has 158 member countries, each of which is represented at the OIE by national delegates. These delegates are frequently senior veterinary administrators in their respective federal governments. The current delegate for the United States, for example, is the deputy administrator of the Veterinary Services unit of USDA APHIS. Delegate positions are elected term positions that require intermittent attendance at OIE business meetings and assemblies and do not represent the delegate's primary employment.

The main objectives of the OIE, as defined by the organization, are to inform governments of the occurrence and course of animal diseases throughout the world and of ways to control these diseases; to coordinate studies devoted to the surveillance and control of animal diseases; and to harmonize regulations for trade in animals and animal products among member countries. These functions and the activities involved in executing them are discussed in more detail in Chapter 9.

The OIE has its headquarters in Paris, France, from where the Administrative Commission operates. The Central Bureau of the OIE consists of the director general's office, as well as four additional departments: administration and finance; information and international trade; publications; and science and technology, all with full-time staff. In recent years, an American veterinarian has been head of the Scientific and Technical Department. In addition to the Central Bureau, the Administrative Commission coordinates the four Specialist Commissions of the OIE, which address fish diseases, foot and mouth disease and other epizootics, the international animal health code, and standards. There are also five Regional Commissions dealing with matters related to Africa, the Americas, Asia/Oceania, Europe, and the Middle East. Employment opportunities for veterinarians potentially exist within the OIE system, but most jobs would require a high level of experience in regulatory affairs, administration, epidemiology, and/or disease diagnosis and control. More information about the OIE is available on their website, including job openings (http://www.oie.int/).

International Research Institutions

Veterinarians interested in international careers need to be aware of the existence of the Consultative Group on International Agricultural Research, commonly referred to as CGIAR. CGIAR's mission, as defined by the organization, is to contribute to food security and poverty eradication in developing countries through research, partnership, capacity building, and policy support.

The CGIAR was established in 1971. It is an informal association of 58 public and private sector members that supports a network of 16 international agricultural research centers. The CGIAR's budget for 1998 was fully funded at US$345 million with member contributions. Members include industrial and developing countries, foundations, and international and regional organizations. The World Bank, the FAO, the UNDP, and the UNEP are cosponsors of the CGIAR.

The 16 research institutions in the CGIAR network are distributed at locations around the world. Each research institution has a particular focus of research activity related to agriculture, often in the context of the local agroecology where the institution is located. A list of the CGIAR institutions and their locations is given in Table 10-5. These institutions have research, educational, and outreach functions. Graduate students enrolled in universities around the world may come to CGIAR centers as graduate fellows to carry out their thesis research, working with staff scientists to address important challenges in agricultural productivity and sustainability. Much CGIAR research is applied and practical, with an aim toward transferring new technologies to farmers, herders, veterinarians, and others who can use these new discoveries. Several of the CGIAR institutions should be of interest to veterinarians, as they deal with issues of livestock health and production and offer potential as sites for field research related to future graduate studies and also as potential future employers.

The main CGIAR institute dealing with animal health and production is the International Livestock Research Institute (ILRI). This institute actually represents the merger of two separate CGIAR institutions that functioned independently until 1995. These were the International Livestock Centre for Africa in Addis Ababa, Ethiopia, and the International Laboratory for Research on Animal Diseases (ILRAD) in Nairobi, Kenya. Historically, ILRAD activities were more laboratory oriented and focused on bioscience research, for example, the pathogenesis and control of vector-borne diseases in livestock, particularly trypanosomiasis and East Coast fever (*Theileria parva* infection). Projects at ILCA were more field oriented and focused on sustainable production systems, with an emphasis on technology transfer to farmers. Since the merger, there has been an effort to integrate these activities. ILRI's research and programmatic activities follow several defined themes including: tropical ruminant genetics, tropical ruminant diseases, feed resources for tropical ruminants, systems analysis and impact assessment, livestock policy analysis, livestock productivity and the environment, smallholder dairy systems, capacity development for National Agricultural Research Services, and systemwide support for CGIAR livestock program activities.

In addition to hosting graduate fellows, ILRI also has a student associate program open to qualified veterinary students committed to carrying out short-term research projects. It also welcomes research fellows, who are staff members at other institutions who, at the request of their home institute, come to ILRI for periods of up to 1 year to enhance their skill base or further their research endeavors. This could be a good opportunity for young university faculty interested in adding an international dimension to their careers. Information about these opportunities and ILRI in general is available on the internet at http://www.cgiar.org/ilri/training/training.cfm.

Several other CGIAR institutes may be involved in research activities of interest to veterinarians. The activities of the International Center for Agricultural Research in the Dry Areas (ICARDA) in Aleppo, Syria, includes research on the nutrition, health, and production of animals adapted to arid systems, especially sheep and goats. The International Center for Living Aquatic Resources Management (ICLARM) in the Philippines carries out studies on small-scale aquaculture and its integration into farming systems. The International Center for Research in Agroforestry (ICRAF) studies, among other things, the integration of livestock into forest and plantation agriculture systems. Information about these CGIAR institutions and all the other institutions in the CGIAR network can be accessed from the CGIAR homepage on the internet at http://www.cgiar.org/.

Table 10-5 International Research Centers in the Network of the Consultative Group on International Agricultural Research

Acronym	Full Name	Location
CIAT	Centro Internacional de Agricultura Tropical[a]	Cali, Colombia
CIFOR	Center for International Forestry Research	Bogor, Indonesia
CIMMYT	Centro Internacional de Mejoramiento de Maiz y Trigo[b]	Mexico City, Mexico
CIP	Centro Internacional de la Papa[c]	Lima, Peru
ICARDA	International Center for Agricultural Research in the Dry Areas	Aleppo, Syria
ICLARM	International Center for Living Aquatic Resources Management	Manila, Philippines
ICRAF	International Centre for Research in Agroforestry	Nairobi, Kenya
ICRISAT	International Crops Research Institute for the Semi-Arid Tropics	Patancheru, India
IFPRI	International Food Policy Research Institute	Washington, D.C.
IWMI	International Water Management Institute	Colombo, Sri Lanka
IITA	International Institute of Tropical Agriculture	Ibadan, Nigeria
ILRI	International Livestock Research Institute	Nairobi, Kenya, and Addis Ababa, Ethiopia
IPGRI	International Plant Genetic Resources Institute	Rome, Italy
IRRI	International Rice Research Institute	Los Baños, Philippines
ISNAR	International Service for National Agricultural Research	The Hague, Netherlands
WARDA	West Africa Rice Development Association	Bouake, Cote d'Ivoire[d]

Translations:

[a]The International Center for Tropical Agriculture.

[b]The International Center for Maize and Wheat Improvement.

[c]The International Potato Center.

[d]Ivory Coast.

The general mission of each research center is suggested by the name. Additional information for each of the 16 centers including their missions, current projects, publications, and employment opportunities is available on the internet from the CGIAR website at http://www.cgiar.org/research/index.html

One additional research institute, not in the CGIAR system but of definite interest to veterinarians, is the International Centre of Insect Physiology and Ecology (ICIPE) in Nairobi, Kenya, which carries out valuable research on animal disease vectors and integrated pest management in a developing country context. Information about ICIPE is available on their website at http://www.icipe.org/.

Beyond the training opportunities available at CGIAR and other international research institutions, entry-level employment is not likely. Veterinarians hired by such institutions are almost certain to require advanced degrees and research experience.

Nongovernmental Organizations (NGOs)

NGOs are also referred to as private voluntary organizations, or PVOs. These are nonprofit organizations in the private sec-

tor that rely largely on charitable donations to support their staff and programs. Donations may come from private individuals, church groups, foundations, corporations, or other sources. In addition, NGOs may enter into contractual relationship with government agencies, for example, USAID, and thereby receive funding to carry out specific projects or services as subcontractors of the government agency. NGOs receiving funds from federal agencies have to be registered and approved by the agency.

Traditionally, NGOs have focused on charitable, humanitarian work, particularly in times of emergency when they mobilize to provide relief services to victims of natural disasters or wars. CARE and the Red Cross are examples of NGOs well known for emergency relief work around the world in times of crisis. Many such humanitarian agencies are now actively involved not only in short-term relief work, but also in sustained development activities. The role of NGOs in development work and the continuum between relief and development are discussed in more detail in Chapter 5.

Today, in the United States alone, there are well over 150 private humanitarian agencies carrying out relief and development work around the world. A good source of information about such NGOs is the organization known as InterAction, based in Washington, D.C. InterAction is an umbrella coalition of 159 humanitarian agencies that represents the interests of its members to government and the general public and supports and coordinates a variety of training and organizational activities for its members. InterAction produces a regular newsletter, *Monday Developments*, which reports on domestic and international issues relevant to its members and also lists available internships and jobs with member agencies, many of which are international. InterAction has a web site, located at http://www.interaction.org. A more-extensive, international list of humanitarian aid agencies, with contact information, is available on the internet at ReliefWeb, a site managed by the United Nations Office for the Coordination of Humanitarian Affairs. The home page for ReliefWeb, from which the Directory of Humanitarian Organizations can be accessed is http://www.reliefweb.int/.

Individual relief and development NGOs differ in their missions, expertise, strengths, and foci of activity, and not surprisingly, the likelihood of them employing or using veterinarians varies accordingly. A number of NGOs reliably require veterinary expertise. There are actually veterinary-specific NGOs that employ veterinarians or use them as consultants or volunteers in projects related to animal health and productivity around the world. Examples include Christian Veterinary Mission, a faith-based NGO, and Volunteers in International Veterinary Assistance (VIVA) in the United States; Vet Aid in the UK; and the various chapters of Veterinaires Sans Frontieres in France, Belgium, and Switzerland. Then there are NGOs that focus on agricultural development and emphasize livestock production as an effective tool for improving the quality of life for the rural, and even the urban, poor. Such agencies include Heifer Project International in the United States and FARM Africa in the UK. These groups also employ veterinarians as well as using them as paid consultants or volunteers. There are also NGOs, such as CARE, that emphasize natural resources management in relation to agriculture and food production as part of their overall development approach.

A number of other NGOs emphasize rural development and agricultural productivity in their work and may also promote livestock production activities as part of their overall program, though they may not identify livestock as a primary focus. Examples of such organizations include Agricultural Cooperative Development International/Volunteers for Overseas Cooperative Assistance (ACDI/VOCA), Mercy Corps International, Oxfam, Winrock International, and World Concern. In addition, there are NGOs that focus on international animal welfare issues, such as the International Donkey Protection Trust in the UK, which provides veterinary services, resources, and

training to improve the welfare of beasts of burden in developing countries, and the World Society for the Protection of Animals, which, among its other animal conservation and welfare activities, fields technical teams to rescue livestock and pets following natural disasters around the world.

Along with an increase in the number of NGOs focusing on humanitarian relief and development, there has also been a considerable expansion in the number of NGOs concerned with environmental issues in recent years. Within this community of environmental NGOs, a number focus on wildlife conservation matters and use the services of veterinarians in support of their programmatic activities and field projects, either as employees, consultants, or volunteers. Some examples include the World Wildlife Fund, Wildlife Trust, Morris Animal Foundation, National Wildlife Federation, African Wildlife Foundation, and the International Gorilla Conservation Programme. In addition, zoos, which are mostly nonprofit organizations, are increasingly involved in field-based international wildlife conservation activities in addition to their zoo-based conservation and education efforts. The Wildlife Conservation Society of the New York Zoological Society (Bronx Zoo) and the San Diego Zoo are but two examples of such zoos. The role of zoos in international conservation efforts is discussed further in Chapter 7. The American Zoo and Aquarium Association publishes an annual *Directory of Zoological Parks and Aquariums in the Americas*, which can help identify international wildlife conservation opportunities for veterinarians. A good general source of information about environmental and wildlife NGOs as well as other agencies and organization concerned with conservation of natural resources is the *Conservation Directory*, published annually by the National Wildlife Federation. For veterinarians interested in environmental work of any kind, not necessarily focused specifically on wildlife issues, the Alliance of Veterinarians for the Environment is an excellent resource. The organization maintains a website that includes a section entitled "The Career Changing Tool Kit," which advises veterinarians on how to prepare for careers in the environmental sector (see http://www.aveweb.org/). The section includes links to valuable information resources, related organizations, and directories of resources.

Regardless of the programmatic focus of the NGO, be it livestock oriented or wildlife oriented, veterinarians working with such NGOs may use their professional and life skills in a wide variety of tasks. Activities in which veterinarians are likely to be involved, based on actual NGO employment experiences, include administration, fund raising, project development and management, project evaluation, policy formulation, technical assistance and advising, education and training, community development, field-based research, and clinical service delivery. Veterinarians working with NGOs must have excellent "people skills," as on any given day in the field, they may be working side by side with pastoralists, professional colleagues, prime ministers, or any combination thereof. As many NGOs welcome volunteers, this group of potential employers offers abundant international experience-building opportunities for recent graduates or practitioners seeking to try their hands at international work. Paid employment as consultants or full-time employees will usually require some existing international experience or specialized skills.

Private Consulting Firms

Earlier in this discussion of potential employers, private industry was identified as a sector offering opportunities for international employment of veterinarians. A characteristic of the private industry sector is that companies in the sector have material products to sell, such as drugs, vaccines, or equipment for intensive livestock production. There is another category of private sector business that also potentially hires veterinarians, the private consulting firms. These firms do not sell physical products per se, but rather technical and management expertise. In that way they are similar to NGOs. However, while NGOs are structured as nonprofit organizations that depend extensively on organized fund raising and donations to fund their activities, private consulting firms are for-profit companies that bid on contracts to provide services for development projects. These projects are usually funded through national government or multilateral agencies such as USAID, the European Community, or the World Bank. The operating costs and profit margins of private consulting firms are built into their budgets.

Many private consulting firms offer their services in support of development assistance in the international arena over a wide range of technical areas including agriculture, engineering, education, environment, small business enterprise, and governance, to name but a few. Many of these companies maintain offices in or near Washington, D.C., as familiarity with governmental agencies and procedures and the ability to maintain personal contacts within government agencies are important aspects of doing business in this sector. Up-to-date information on programmatic agendas, regional priorities, and funding preferences within particular agencies that issue requests for proposals (RFPs) is critical for private consulting firms so that they can develop corporate strategies, plan and manage their resources effectively, prepare top-quality bidding proposals, and remain successful in a competitive environment

Like NGOs, different private firms promote different areas of expertise. There are, for example, private consulting firms that emphasize expertise in livestock health and production and related activities such as food processing and marketing. Some examples are the International Development Division of the farmer's cooperative Land O' Lakes in the United States, RDP Livestock Services in the Netherlands, and PAN Livestock Services and Livestock in Development in the UK. Other companies are more broadly involved in agricultural development but may still have livestock health and production components in their project activities. Examples of such firms include Development Alternatives Incorporated (DAI) and Chemonics in the United States. Some firms may participate in large, integrated development activities that include agriculture as one part of a larger project or national presence, for example, the engineering firm Louis Berger International. Some firms are highly specialized in their services, but these services may include animal-related activities and the poten-

tial use of veterinarians. For example, Ronco Consulting Corporation provides technical assistance in land mine clearance operations throughout the world, including the training and use of mine-sniffing dogs.

Firms with livestock-specific activities may employ veterinarians for their permanent organizational staff in positions in administration, management, project development, and project preparation and marketing. In most cases, veterinarians working for private consulting firms are temporary hires recruited specifically for specific projects and assignments abroad. In many cases, project proposals are submitted with potential field staff already identified. For the proposal to be competitive, listed staff must have convincing credentials in terms of international experience, relevant technical expertise, and appropriate training. Therefore, entry-level positions are unlikely in consulting firms, though some companies, for example, Land O' Lakes, sometimes have volunteer positions that may be appropriate.

Many private consulting firms maintain rosters of qualified individuals whom they can contact for inclusion in upcoming relevant proposals. Interested, experienced veterinarians can submit resumés to the human resources offices of these firms to be placed on the roster if the company deems the individual's credentials adequate and relevant. Many private consulting firms seeking individual specialists or looking to update their professional rosters will advertise in the *International Career Employment Weekly*, available as a newspaper or on the web by subscription (see http://www.internationaljobs.org/). Many firms have their own individual web sites where you can learn more about the organization and its activities as well as regularly review job openings at that company.

Self-Employment

For veterinarians with a great deal of professional experience or special expertise, private consulting may be a professionally and financially rewarding avenue for international work. While any number of specializations may be marketable for veterinary consulting, several skill areas have been traditionally associated with enhanced opportunities for international assignments. These include epidemiology, public health, agricultural economics, experience in agribusiness, and experience with intensive livestock-production systems. Currently and in the future, as new problems and challenges arise and program priorities are redefined by policymakers and funding agencies, new areas of expertise valuable to consultants are emerging. Such areas of expertise include environmental toxicology, conservation biology, wildlife management, experience in privatization of state-run enterprises, community development, sustainable agriculture, and delivery of veterinary services.

Independent consultants may work for a number of organizations including funding agencies, NGOs, consulting firms, and private industry. The length of assignments may vary from days to months, and a wide variety of work may be undertaken. The content of professional activities will of course vary with the employer, your area of expertise, and the nature of the project for which you are hired. Whatever the subject matter, likely activities of consultants include project feasibility assessments, project design, project evaluation, project implementation and management, technical consultation and advising, troubleshooting, or organizing and conducting workshops, training sessions, and scientific meetings.

Self-employed consultants face a special set of challenges related to the nature of their business. They must be willing to face the budgetary and scheduling uncertainties associated with intermittent work on irregularly occurring assignments. They must be extremely flexible and highly adaptable and have excellent people skills. Effective networking is a critical requirement for successful consultants, as they must ensure that prospective employers remember them, their skills, and their availability for future assignments. Dr. Carin Smith offers a good discussion of the pros and cons of veterinary consulting in her book *Career Choices for Veterinarians*.[11]

Private Practice

Private clinical practice is the activity for which North American veterinary education best prepares its graduates. However, it is, at present, the least marketable skill we have in the international arena. There are a number of reasons for this as discussed in more detail in Chapter 8 on delivery of animal health care services worldwide, but the main reason is one of eligibility. Practice acts and licensing regulations in other countries, as in our own, often present significant barriers for foreign veterinarians wishing to enter private practice. In some cases there are outright prohibitions, in others there may be complex requirements that effectively bar all but the most determined foreigner.

The situation is not completely without promise, however. A dramatic increase in pet ownership in Asia over the last decade has fueled a demand for small animal clinical expertise in many Asian countries. In 1998, for example, the Veterinary Surgeons Board of Hong Kong amended their rules so that graduates of AVMA-accredited schools with current licenses in the United States and Canada can register to practice veterinary medicine in Hong Kong without additional testing or training. In November 2000, the AVMA signed an agreement with the Royal College of Veterinary Surgeons (RCVS) so that graduates of AVMA-accredited veterinary colleges in the United States and Canada will be eligible for licensure in Great Britain. Applicants must have passed the National Board Examination and Clinical Competency Test or the North American Veterinary Licensing Examination. Details for application can be found at http://www.rcvs.org.uk/vet_surgeons/members/us_canada. html on the RCVS website. Similarly, in November 2000, an agreement was reached between the AVMA and the Australasian Veterinary Boards Council (AVBC) that will allow graduates of AVMA-accredited veterinary colleges in the United States and Canada to apply for licensure in Australia and New Zealand, though some states in Australia and New Zealand have existing legislation that must be changed to accommodate this new ruling. For further information, the AVBC can be contacted by email at avbc@ozemail.com.au.

Veterinarians interested in other private practice opportunities abroad should make a short list of countries in which they are particularly keen on practicing and then contact the veterinary association in each country to obtain specific information about eligibility and licensing requirements. Contact information for veterinary associations in different countries is available in the AVMA *Membership Directory and Resource Manual* in the section "International Veterinary Organizations."[2] While the veterinary association is not the rule-making body within a country, they are likely to have access to the desired information or at least be able to refer you to the proper authorities. Once you determine your eligibility, you might want to subscribe to a veterinary journal from that country or view it at a veterinary library to stay apprised of jobs. You may also want to notify the veterinary association of your interest in practice opportunities, especially in short-term relief work, which may be a way to get some experience in the country, make additional contacts, and set about the task of finding more-permanent work.

Finding a Job

If you have confirmed your commitment to international work and your suitability for such work, assessed your level of skill and experience, and identified a potential type of employer, then it is time to move forward with the process of finding a job. This may mean finding a specific international position or seeking domestic employment with an organization where the future likelihood of international opportunities is high.

A great many of the general suggestions offered earlier in the chapter for determining your interest and suitability for international work also apply during the process of job identification, though the process will now be more focused. You still need to gather information, attend meetings, canvas the internet, and network with colleagues and potential employers, but you may now narrow the process to your specific area of interest or type of employer.

For example, if you are interested in working for the pharmaceutical industry or in agribusiness, you should probably join the American Association of Industrial Veterinarians, attend their breakfast meetings at the North American Veterinary Conference, Central States Veterinary Conference, or Western States Veterinary Conference, or their annual meeting at the AVMA convention. You should read their newsletter, which comes out three times a year, and you should regularly check the magazine *Feedstuffs*, which runs classified employment advertisements with frequent job listings for technical services veterinarians, some of which are international positions. Also register with the AVMA Placement Service to be apprised of potential industrial job opportunities. Identify a list of prospective employers in your field of interest and visit their web sites regularly, as most industrial employers have web sites and regularly list job opportunities there. If you have former classmates or colleagues who work in industry you should visit with them by phone or in person about their positions, the work environment in their company, and the potential for employment. The importance of personal, professional contacts within a company cannot be overemphasized. Dr. Carin Smith points out that in preparing the chapter on industry opportunities for her book *Career Choices for Veterinarians*, she did not have a single person in a human resources or personnel position return her calls to discuss employment opportunities at their respective companies. All the information she got was from veterinarians working in different capacities within those same companies.

Likewise, if you are interested in rural development work in the NGO sector, check in regularly at the website of InterAction to identify upcoming meetings and conferences about relief and development topics. Attend some meetings and meet people working for different NGOs. Subscribe to the InterAction newsletter, *Monday Developments*, to keep abreast of issues facing the NGO community and to check for job possibilities. Visit the web sites of individual NGOs to find out what kind of work they do and the likelihood that they might hire veterinarians. Also identify the NGOs that use volunteers and/or maintain rosters of potential volunteers and/or consultants and send your resumé along with the requisite application forms, often available directly from the web. Determine if any NGOs have offices near you and visit those offices to get acquainted. You might be able to provide some volunteer services, become known to the organization, and parlay the relationship into a paying position. NGOs are headquartered in a variety of locations. For example, Heifer Project International is in Little Rock, Arkansas; Mercy Corps International in Portland, Oregon; Oxfam USA in Boston, Massachusetts; ACDI/VOCA in Washington, D.C.; and Christian Veterinary Mission in Seattle, Washington.

Similar approaches can be taken for wildlife conservation positions, federal government positions, international agency positions, private consulting firms, or any other sector that you might pursue for international employment opportunities. The key is to know the terrain for that specialized field or sector, become associated with the relevant organizations, communicate regularly and widely with people in your field of interest, take advantage of the power of the internet to define and identify opportunities, and keep your eyes and ears open at all times (Fig. 10-7). At the same time, whenever possible in the progression of your career, be sure to keep adding appropriate skills and experiences that will enhance your desirability to employers in the sector in which you are interested. These will not necessarily be additional technical veterinary skills, but may instead be management, leadership, communication, language, cross-cultural, or any other type of life skills.

You must remember that international veterinary medicine is not a recognized or acknowledged field, and therefore, jobs for veterinarians interested in international work are not easily categorized or compiled. Always bear in mind that jobs may be advertised for which you are qualified as a veterinarian even though the employers do not recognize that a veterinarian is eminently qualified to fill the position. For some nontradi-

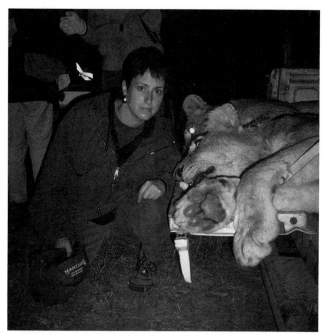

Figure 10-7. Following graduation from Tufts University School of Veterinary Medicine, Dr. Ellen Messner Rogers gained valuable experience in wildlife capture through a volunteer fellowship in South Africa. Upon completing the fellowship, she worked in conjunction with South African veterinarians and parks boards on wildlife translocations. Currently, Dr. Rogers coordinates wildlife field courses for American veterinary students in South Africa. The two lions in this picture have been immobilized for tuberculosis testing. Lions in and around Kruger National Park have a high incidence of tuberculosis. (Photo courtesy of Dr. Ellen Messner Rogers)

tional positions, one of your biggest challenges may be to convince employers that your veterinary qualifications and experience are an advantage and not an impediment to your employability! Be patient and thorough in your search, and don't pigeonhole yourself.

In the search for employment, your resumé can be a very important document. Know what characteristics and abilities potential employers are looking for and make sure your resumé reflects the desired characteristics. A resumé submitted for an academic position can and should look different than a resumé submitted for a position with a pharmaceutical company or an NGO. For example, the American Association of Industrial Veterinarians in its informational brochure, identifies some of the qualifications sought by industrial employers. In addition to veterinary qualifications and a good scholastic record, employers look for evidence of business skills and knowledge, good written and verbal communication skills, and excellent interpersonal skills to participate successfully in the many cooperative team efforts that occur in the industrial environment. Your resumé should be user friendly and make it easy for a prospective employer in industry to identify such skills. In demonstrating your qualifications do not feel compelled to confine your resumé to professional activities. For example, if you are a scout leader in your community or a member of the school board, such activities demonstrate leadership and teamwork skills and should be clearly presented as reflecting such skills in your resumé.

When searching for international career opportunities be prepared to accept the fact that the ideal international position you envision may not be available at the moment. In fact, it may not be available at all. One of the potential frustrations of international veterinary medicine is that many institutions and organizations do not yet recognize the valuable contribution that veterinarians can make in a global context. In that sense, veterinarians seeking to work internationally are essentially pioneers and sometime proselytizers, who must "preach the gospel" of globalization. Therefore, it may be necessary, when constructing an international career to accept positions in organizations where the potential for international activity is high but as yet unrealized. The challenge then, once inside the system, is to understand the goals and objectives of the organization and identify constructive opportunities to internationalize their mission and activities. Effective pioneers, particularly in government, academics, and industry, should be able to define global opportunities and get themselves placed in positions of their own suggestion or creation.

Finally, there are many individual veterinarians who are interested in international issues but whose circumstances will not allow them to follow an international career track. Such individuals have the opportunity to "think globally and act locally" within their daily professional work. It may mean putting up posters in a waiting room that promote an agency involved in improving agricultural production in Africa or having promotional literature on the illegal exotic pet trade and its impact on biodiversity in Latin America. It can mean writing a column on international issues in a local newspaper, hosting a foreign veterinarian in an externship in your practice, or organizing a textbook, journal, and equipment donation to a foreign veterinary school or veterinary association.[7] The possibilities for becoming involved are only limited by your interest, imagination, and commitment.

Discussion Points

1. Identify the former colonies of Britain, France, the Netherlands, Spain, Portugal, Germany, and Italy. How does a colonial past manifest itself in the life of currently independent nations that were former colonies? Was the United States ever a "mother country"? If so, where and how?

2. Some critics contend that the activities of contemporary, western-based multinational companies in developing countries represent a form of "neocolonialism." What does this mean? What is the basis for the charge? If you worked overseas for an American-based pharmaceutical or agribusiness firm, how would you defend against such charges?

3. Think of some examples of anti-American activity that have occurred in recent years. What was the basis for these actions? If you were in a country where anti-American activity had occurred and a foreign colleague criticized the United States for certain practices or situations, how would you respond?

4. Identify a useful role for a veterinarian in an international position of interest to you personally and professionally. Develop an appropriate project or activity based on that role and develop a presentation or proposal to convince your employer that it would benefit the organization or institution to have you pursue that role.

5. Even if you never work abroad, what can you do in your practice or other professional activity to support the notion of thinking globally and acting locally on a topic of interest to you?

References

1. American Association of Veterinary Medical Colleges. The Internationalization of Veterinary Education: Strengths, Challenges, and Opportunities. Proceedings of the 14th symposium on veterinary medical education. J Vet Med Educ 1996;23(Special Issue).

2. American Veterinary Medical Association. Membership Directory and Resource Manual. 50th Ed. Schaumburg, IL: AVMA, 2001.

3. Bolles RN. What Color is Your Parachute? 2002 Edition: A Practical Manual for Job-Hunters & Career Changers. Berkeley, CA: Ten Speed Press, 2002.

4. Correa MT, Anderson KL, Stevens JB, et al. Employment in international veterinary medicine: a survey of requirements and opportunities. J Vet Med Educ 1995;22(1):25–29.

5. Ford P. Why do they hate us? Christian Science Monitor, Sept. 27, 2001:1,5–10.

6. Noel JC, Henson JB, Memon MA, et al. The internationalization of United States and Canadian colleges of veterinary medicine. J Vet Med Educ 1996;23:12–21.

7. Nolen RS. Veterinarians donate supplies to Albania. JAVMA 2001;218(9):1406.

8. Lederer WJ, Burdick E. The Ugly American. New York: Norton, 1958.

9. Pybus V. Working with Animals: The UK, Europe, and Worldwide. Oxford, UK: Vacation Work, 1999.

10. Sherman DM, Pokras M, English AW. Preparing veterinarians for meaningful participation in wildlife conservation. J Vet Med Educ 1999;26(1):26–29.

11. Smith CA. Career Choices for Veterinarians: Beyond Private Practice. Leavenworth, WA: Smith Veterinary Services, 1998.

Suggested Readings and Resources

Centers for Disease Control and Prevention. Health Information for the International Traveler 2001–2002. Atlanta, GA: U.S. Department of Health and Human Services, Public Health Service, 2001.

Central Intelligence Agency. World Factbook, 2001. An up-to-date summary of pertinent information on the world's nations available on the internet at http://www.odci.gov/cia/publications/factbook/index.html.

Godden R. Coromandel Sea Change. New York: William Morrow, 1991.

Hess JD. Whole World Guide to Culture Learning. Yarmouth, ME: Intercultural Press, 1994.

Kingsolver B. The Poisonwood Bible. New York: Harper Flamingo, 1998.

Marshall T. Whole World Guide to Language Learning. Yarmouth, ME: Intercultural Press, 1990.

Micou P. The Music Programme. Secaucus NJ: Carol Publishing Co., 1989.

Rose SR. International Travel Health Guide. 12th Ed. Northampton, MA: Travel Medicine, 2001.

Storti C. Figuring Foreigners Out: A Practical Guide. Yarmouth, ME: Intercultural Press, 1999.

Thomas, M. Come to Africa and Save Your Marriage. New York: Soho Press, 1987.

Travel Medicine Incorporated. A private company providing useful products and information related to safe and healthful international travel. Informative website at http://www.travmed.com/.

U.S. Department of State. Travel warnings and consular information sheets. Updated, country by country information on travel risks, on the internet at http://www.travel.state.gov/travel_warnings.html#a.

World Health Organization. International Travel and Health: Vaccination Requirements and Health Advice. Geneva: WHO, 2001. Available on the internet at http://www.who.int/ith/english/index.htm

Appendix

Contact Information for Agencies and Organizations Relevant to International Veterinary Medicine

The landscape of international veterinary medicine remains, to some extent, uncharted. Throughout this text, various organizations, agencies, and institutions have been identified that serve as useful guideposts for readers interested in pursuing information, training, volunteer opportunities, or employment relative to the various aspects of international veterinary medicine discussed in the book. Contact information for key entities mentioned in the text is provided in this appendix. They are grouped in alphabetical order under the various categories listed as follows:

Biodiversity, Wildlife and Environmental Groups
Donor and Lending Institutions
International Government Development and Aid Agencies
International Technical Organizations
NGOs—General Relief and Development
NGOs—Veterinary Relief and Development

Pharmaceutical and Animal Nutrition Firms
Private Consulting Firms
Professional Veterinary and Related Organizations
Research and Policy Institutions
Training, Fellowship, and Grant Opportunities
United States Government Agencies

Readers with access to the internet are encouraged to first visit the websites for those entities that are of interest to them. At the very least, the website usually provides an overview of the organization's mission, structure, and activities. In some cases, the website offers a wealth of additional resource information in the form of statistical databases, useful links to related organizations, lists of relevant publications, current news of international veterinary interest, and sometimes, full text versions of useful publications. In the lists that follow, URL addresses preceded by an asterisk (*) indicate websites that are particularly rich in information and resources and that should definitely be explored in detail.

Please recognize that organizations may change their names, cease to exist, or merge with other entities. This latter phenomenon is particularly prevalent in the pharmaceutical industry of late. Organizations may also change officers, addresses, email addresses, website locations, and telephone numbers. Also note that international telephone numbers may not have the seven digit configuration so familiar in North America. Every effort was made to provide current information at the time of publication, but undoubtedly, some information will become out of date. For organizations specifically related to veterinary medicine, the *Annual Directory and Resource Manual* of the American Veterinary Medical Association can serve as a useful backup source to find updated contact information when the trail followed in this appendix runs cold.

BIODIVERSITY AND WILDLIFE AND ENVIRONMENTAL ORGANIZATIONS

African Wildlife Foundation
1400 Sixteenth Street, NW, Suite 120
Washington, DC 20036 USA
Phone: 1-202-939-3333
Fax: 1-202-939-3332
Email: africanwildlife@awf.org
URL: www.awf.org

American Zoo and Aquarium Association
8403 Colesville Road, Suite 710
Silver Spring, MD 20910-3314 USA
Phone: 1-301-562-0777
Fax: 1-301-562-0888
URL: www.aza.org

Birdlife International
Wellbrook Court
Girton Road
Cambridge CB3 0NA UK

Phone: 44 1 223 277 318
Fax: 44 1 223 277 200
Email: birdlife@birdlife.org.uk
URL: http://www.birdlife.net/

Center for Biodiversity and Conservation
American Museum of Natural History
Central Park West at 79th Street
New York, NY 10024 USA
Phone: 1-212-769-5742
Fax: 1-212-769-5292
Email: biodiversity@amnh.org
URL: http://research.amnh.org/biodiversity

Center for Marine Conservation
1725 De Sales Street, NW, Suite 600
Washington, DC 20036 USA
Phone: 1-202-429-5609
Fax: 1-202-872-0619
Email: cmc@dccmc.org
URL: www.cmc-ocean.org

Center for Plant Conservation and Missouri Botanical Garden
PO Box 299
St. Louis, MO 63166-0299 USA
Phone: 1-314-577-5100
Email: cpc@mobot.org
URL: www.mobot.org

Charles Darwin Foundation Inc.
407 North Washington Street, Suite 105
Falls Church, VA 22046 USA
Phone: 1-703-538-6833
Fax: 1-703-538-6835
Email: darwin@galapagos.org
URL: www.darwinfoundation.org

CITES Secretariat, UNEP
International Environment House
15 Chemin de Anemones,
CH-1219 Chatelaine, Switzerland
Phone: 41-22-917-8139
Fax: 41-22-797-3417
Email: cites@unep.ch
*URL: www.cites.org

Conservation International
1919 M Street, NW, Suite 600
Washington, DC 20036 USA
Phone: 1-202-912-1000
URL: www.conservation.org

Greenpeace, USA
702 H Street, NW
Washington, DC 20001 USA
Phone: 1-800-326-0959
URL: www.greenpeaceusa.org

International Wildlife Rehabilitation Council
4437 Central Place, Suite B-4
Suisan City, CA 94585-1633 USA
Phone: 1 707 864 1761
Fax: 1-707-864-3106
Email: iwrc@inreach.com
*URL: www.iwrc-online.org

IUCN—The World Conservation Union
Rue Mauverney 28
1196 Gland, Switzerland
Phone: 41-22-999-0001
*URL: http://www.iucn.org/

Morris Animal Foundation
Mountain Gorilla Veterinary Project
45 Inverness Drive East
Englewood, CO 80112-5480 USA
Phone: 1-800-243-2345
Fax: 1-303-790-4066
URL: www.morrisanimalfoundation.org

National Audubon Society
700 Broadway
New York, NY 10003 USA
Phone: 1-212-979-3000
Fax: 1-212-979-3188
Email: education@audubon.org
URL: www.audubon.org

National Wildlife Federation
11100 Wildlife Center Drive
Reston, VA 20190-5362 USA
Phone: 1-703-438-6000
URL: www.nwf.org

Rainforest Action Network
221 Pine Street, Suite 500
San Francisco, CA 94104 USA
Phone: 1-415-398-4404

Fax: 1-415-398-2732
Email: rainforest@ran.org
URL: www.ran.org/ran/

Sierra Club
85 Second Street, 2nd Floor
San Francisco, CA 94105-3441 USA
Phone: 1-415-977-5500
Fax: 1-415-977-5799
Email: information@sierraclub.org
URL: www.sierraclub.org

Society for Conservation Biology
4245 N. Fairfax Drive
Arlington, VA, 22203 USA
Phone: 703-276-2384
Fax: 703-525-8024
Email: information@conservationbiology.org
URL: conbio.net/scb

The Nature Conservancy
4245 North Fairfax Drive, Suite 100
Arlington, VA 22203-1606 USA
Phone: 1-703-841-5300
Email: comment@tnc.org
URL: http://nature.org/

Wildlife Conservation Society
2300 Southern Boulevard
Bronx, NY 10460-1099 USA
Phone: 1-718-220-5100
Email: feedback@wcs.org
URL: www.wcs.org

Wildlife Trust
61 Route 9W
Palisades, NY 10964-8000 USA
Phone: 845-365-8337
Fax: 845- 365-8177
URL: www.wpti.org

World Wildlife Fund
1250 Twenty Fourth Street, NW
Washington, DC 20077-180 USA
Phone: 1-202-861-0350
URL: www.worldwildlife.org

Zoological Society of London
Regents Park
London, NW1 4RY UK
Phone: 44- 20-7449 6293
URL: www.zsl.org

Zoological Society of San Diego
PO Box 120551
San Diego, CA 92112-0551 USA
Phone: 1-619-231-1515
URL: www.sandiegozoo.org

DONOR AND LENDING INSTITUTIONS

African Development Bank
Rue Joseph Anoma, 01 BP 1387
Abidjan, 01 Cote d'Ivoire
Phone: 225-20-20-44-44
Fax: 225-20-21-77-53
Email: recruit@afdb.org
URL: www.aafdb.org

Asian Development Bank
PO Box 789
Manila, 0980 Philippines
Phone: 63-2-636-2550
Fax: 63-2-636-2444
Email: adb@adb.org
URL: www.adb.org

Grameen Bank
Mirpur Two
Dhaka 1216, Bangladesh
Phone: 880-2-803 559
Email: grameen.bank@grameen.net
URL: www.grameen-info.org/index.html

Inter-American Development Bank
1300 New York Avenue, NW
Washington, DC 20577 USA
Phone: 1-202- 623-1000
URL: www.iadb.org

International Fund for Agricultural Development
107 Via del Serafico
Rome, 00142 Italy
Phone: 39-6-54591
Fax: 39-6-5043463
Email: ifad@ifad.org
URL: www.ifad.org

Islamic Development Bank
PO Box 5925
Jeddah, 21432 Saudi Arabia
Phone: 966-2-646-7373
Fax: 966-2-637-2069
Email: ypp@isdb.org.sa
URL: www.isdb.org

World Bank
1818 H Street, NW
Washington, DC 20433 USA
Phone: 1-202-477-1234
*URL: www.worldbank.org

INTERNATIONAL GOVERNMENT DEVELOPMENT AND AID AGENCIES

Canadian International Development Agency
200 Promenade du Portage
Hull, Quebec KIA 064 Canada
Phone: 1-819- 997-5456
URL: www.acdi-cida.gc.ca/index.htm

Danish International Development Assistance
Asiatisk Plads 2
DK-1448
Copenhagen, Denmark
Phone: 45-33 92 00 00
Fax: 45-32 54 05 33
Email: um@um.dk

Department for International Development
Abercrombie House, Eaglesham Road, East Kilbridge
Glasgow, G75 BEA UK
Phone: 44-1-355-84-31-32
Fax: 44-1-355-84-36-32
Email: enquiry@dfid.gtnet.gov.uk
URL: www.dfid.gov.uk

Deutsche Gesellschaft fur Technische Zusammenarbeit
Dag-Mammarskjold-Weg 1-5
Eschborn, 65760 Germany
Phone: 49-6196-79-0
Fax: 49-6196-79-115
Email: personal@gtz.de
URL: www.gtz.de/home/english/index.html

Norwegian Agency for Development Cooperation
Ruselokkveien 26, PO Box 8034
Oslo, 0030 Norway
Phone: 22-24-2060
Fax: 22-24-2066
Email: informasjoyssenteret@norad.no
URL: www.norad.no

Swedish International Development Cooperation Agency
Stockholm, 105 25 Sweden
Phone: 46-8-698-5000
Fax: 46-8-20-8864
Email: info@sida.se
URL: http://www.sida.se/Sida/jsp/Crosslink.jsp?d=107

INTERNATIONAL TECHNICAL ORGANIZATIONS

Animal Production and Health Division, Animal Health Service
Food and Agriculture Organization of the United Nations
Viale delle Terme di Caracalla
Rome, 00100 Italy
Phone: 39-6-57051
Fax: 39-6-5705312
Email: samuel.jutzi@fao.org
*URL: www.fao.org/ag/AGA/default.htm

Division of Communicable Disease Surveillance and Response, Zoonosis Unit
World Health Organization
Avenue Appia 20
Geneva 27, 1211 Switzerland
Phone: 41-22-791-21-11
Fax: 41-22-701-21-11
Email: csr@who.ch
URL: www.who.int/emc/index.html

Food and Agriculture Organization
Viale delle Terme di Caracalla
Rome, 00100 Italy
Phone: 39-06-570 54243
Fax: 39-06-570 53152
Email: FAO-HQ@fao.org
*URL: www.fao.org

International Atomic Energy Agency
PO Box 100, Wagramer Strasse 5
Vienna, A-1400 Austria
Phone: 43-1-2600-0
Fax: 43-1-2600-7
Email: official.mail@iaea.org
URL: www.iaea.org/worldatom

Office International des Epizooties
12 rue de Prony
Paris, 75017 France
Phone: 33-1-44-15-1888
Fax: 33-1-44-15-1888
Email: oie@oie.int
*URL: www.oie.int

Ozone Secretariat of the UNEP
PO Box 30552
Nairobi, Kenya
Phone: 254-2-62-1234
Fax: 254-2-62-3601
URL: www.unep.ch/ozone/home.htm

United Nations Children's Fund
3 United Nations Plaza
New York, NY 10017 USA
Phone: 1-212-326-7000
Fax: 1-212-887-7465
Email: netmaster@unicef.org
*URL: www.unicef.org

United Nations Development Programme
One United Nations Plaza
New York, NY 10017 USA
Phone: 1-212-906-5315
Fax: 1-212-903-5364
Email: hq@undp.org
*URL: www.undp.org

United Nations Environmental Programme
PO Box 30552
Nairobi, Kenya
Phone: 254-2-62-1234
Fax: 254-2-62-3927
Email: ipainfo@unep.org
*URL: www.unep.org

World Meteorological Organization of the UN
7 bis Avenue de la Paix
Geneva, CP 2300-1211 Switzerland
(Includes the Intergovernmental Panel on Climate Change)
Phone: 41 22 730 8111
Fax: 41 22 730 8181
Email: ipa@www.wmo.ch
*URL: www.wmo.ch

World Trade Organization
Centre William Rappard, Rue de Lausanne 154
Geneva 21, CH-1211 Switzerland
Phone: 41-22-739-5111
Fax: 41-22-731-4206
Email: enquiries@wto.org
*URL: www.wto.org

NGOS—GENERAL RELIEF AND DEVELOPMENT

ACDI/VOCA
Agricultural Cooperative Development International/
Volunteers for Overseas Cooperation Assistance
50 F Street, NW, Suite 1100
Washington, DC 20001 USA
Phone: 1-202-383-4961
Fax: 1-202-783-7204
URL: www.acdivoca.org

Catholic Relief Services
209 West Fayette Street
Baltimore, MD 21201-3343 USA
Phone: 1-410-625-2220
Fax: 1-410-685-1635
Email: webmaster@catholicrelief.org
URL: www.catholicrelief.org

InterAction
1717 Massachusetts Avenue NW, Suite 701
Washington, DC 20036 USA
Phone: 1-202-667-8227
Fax: 1 202 667 8236
Email: ia@interaction.org
URL: www.interaction.org

Intermediate Technology Development Group
Bourton Hall
Bourton-on-Dunsmore
Rugby CV23 9QZ UK
Phone: 44-1926-634-440
Fax: 44-1926-634-441
Email: itdg@itdg.org.uk
*URL: www.itdg.org/

International Rescue Committee
122 East 42nd Street
New York, NY 10168-1289 USA
Phone: 1-212-551-3000
Fax: 1-212-551-3180
Email: irc@theIRC.org
URL: www.intrescom.org

Mercy Corps International
3030 SW First Avenue
Portland, OR 97201 USA
Phone: 1-800-292-3355
Email: info@mercycorps.org
URL: www.mercycorps.org

Oxfam America
26 West Street
Boston, MA 02111-1206 USA
Phone: 1 800 776 9326
Fax: 1-617-728 2594
Email: info@oxfamamerica.org
URL: www.oxfamamerica.org

World Concern
19303 Fremont Avenue North
Seattle, WA 98133 USA
Phone: 1-800-755-5022
Fax: 1-206-546-7269
Email: wconcern@crista.org
URL: www.worldconcern.org

NGOS—VETERINARY RELIEF AND DEVELOPMENT

Christian Veterinary Mission
19303 Fremont Avenue North
Seattle, WA 98133 USA
Phone: 1-206-546-7569
Email: rkf@crista.org
URL: www.vetmission.org

FARM Africa UK
9–10 Southampton Place
Bloomsbury, London, WC1A 2EA UK
Phone: 44-20-7430-0440
Fax: 44-20-7430-0460
Email: farmafrica@farmafrica.org.uk
URL: www.farmafrica.org.uk

Heifer Project International
PO Box 808
1015 South Louisiana
Little Rock, AR 72203 USA
Phone: 1-800-422-1311
Fax: 1-501-376-7631
Email: info@heifer.org
URL: www.heifer.org

International Donkey Protection Trust
The Donkey Sanctuary
Sidmouth, Devon EX10 0NU UK
Phone: 44-1395-578-222
Fax: 44-1395-579-266
Email: thedonkeysanctuary@compuserve.com
URL: www.thedonkeysanctuary.org.uk/

Massachusetts Society for the Prevention of Cruelty to Animals
350 South Huntington Avenue
Boston, MA 02130 USA
Phone: 1-617-522-7400
URL: www.mspca.org/world/world_main.html

VetAid
Pentlands Science Park
Bush Loan
Penicuik, Scotland EH26 OP2 UK
Phone: 44-131-445-6241
Fax: 44-131-445-6242
Email: mail@vetaid.org
URL: www.vetaid.org

Veterinaires San Frontieres
14 Avenue Berthelot 69361
Lyon, Cedex 07 France
Phone: 33-4-78-69-79-59
Fax: 33-4-78-69-79-56
Email: vsf@vsf-france.org
URL: www.vsf-france.org/

Vetwork UK
35D Beach Lane

Musselburgh, EH21 6JX UK
Phone: 44-131-665-2417
Email: stephen@vetwork.org.uk
*URL: www.vetwork.org.uk

Volunteers in International Veterinary Assistance
Dr. Robert Pelant
1015 Louisiana Street
Little Rock, AR 72202-3815 USA
Email: robert.pelant@heifer.org

World Society for the Protection of Animals
United States Office
34 Deloss Street
Framingham, MA 01702 USA
Phone: 1-508-879-8350
Fax: 1-508-620-0786
Email: wspa@wspausa.com
URL: www.wspa-international.org/

PHARMACEUTICAL AND ANIMAL NUTRITION FIRMS

Bayer Corporation
100 Bayer Road
Pittsburgh, PA 15205-9741 USA
Phone: 1-412-777-2000
Fax: 1-412-777-2034
URL: www.bayerus.com

Intervet International BV
PO Box 31
5830 AA Boxmeer The Netherlands
Phone: 31 485 587 600
Fax: 31 485 577 333
Email: info@intervet.com
URL: www.intervet.com

Merck & Co. Inc.
One Merck Drive, PO Box 1000
Whitehouse Station, NJ 08889-0100 USA
Phone: 1-908-423-1000
Fax: 1-908-423-2592
URL: www.merck.com

Merial Limited
2100 Ronson Road
Iselin, NJ 08830 USA
Phone: 1-888-637-4251
Fax: 1-732-855-9366
URL: www.merial.com

Novartis Animal Health Inc.
3200 Northline Avenue, Suite 300
Greensboro, NC 27408 USA
Phone: 1-336-387-1000
URL: www.us.novartis.com/who_we_are/
    desc_animal_health.html

Pfizer Animal Health
235 E. 42nd St
New York, NY 10017 USA
Phone: 1-212-573-2323
Fax: 1-212-573-7851
URL: www.pfizer.com/ah

Ralston Purina Co.
Checkerboard Square
St. Louis, MO 63164-0001 USA
Phone: 1-314-982-1000
Fax: 1-314-982-2134
Email: hrfeedback@ralston.com
URL: www.ralston.com

Schering-Plough Animal Health
One Giralda Farms
Madison, NJ 07940-1010 USA

Phone: 1-973-822-7000
Fax: 1-973-822-7048
URL: http://usa.spah.com/home.cfm

PRIVATE CONSULTING FIRMS

Associates in Rural Development
159 Bank Street, 3rd Floor
Burlington, VT 05401 USA
Phone: 1-802-658-3890
Fax: 1-802-658-4247
Email: ard@ardinc.com
URL: www.ardinc.com

Chemonics International Inc.
1133 20th Street, NW
Washington, DC 20036 USA
Phone: 1-202-955-3300
Fax: 1-202-955-3400
Email: info@chemonics.com
URL: www.chemonics.com

Development Alternative Incorporated
7250 Woodmont Avenue, Suite 200
Bethesda, MD 20814 USA
Phone: 1-301-718-8699
Fax: 1-301-718-7968
Email: info@dai.com
URL: www.dai.com

Land O'Lakes International Development
PO Box 64406
St. Paul, MN 55164-0406 USA
Phone: 1- 800-851-8810
URL: www.landolakesidd.com/

PAN Livestock Services
PO Box 236
Reading, RG6 6AT UK
URL: www.veeru.reading.ac.uk/veeru2001/partners/PAN.htm

RDP Livestock Services
PO Box 523
3700 AM Zeist, The Netherlands
Phone: 31-30-6921-566
Fax: 31-30-6919-830
Email: Office@rdp.net
URL: www.rdp.net

Ronco Consulting Corporation
2301 M Street, NW, Suite 400
Washington, DC 20037 USA
Phone: 1-202-785-2791
Fax: 1-202-785-2078
Email: administration@roncowash.com
URL: www.roncoconsulting.com

Winrock International
38 Winrock Drive
Morrilton, AR 72110 USA
Phone: 1-501-727-5435
Fax: 1-501-727-5242
Email: conference@winrock.org
URL: www.winrock.org

PROFESSIONAL VETERINARY AND RELATED ORGANIZATIONS

Alliance of Veterinarians for the Environment
Gwen Griffith, 4801 Belmont Park Terrace
Nashville, TN 37215 USA
Phone: 1-615-297-8925
Fax: 1-615-297-8743
Email: avegwen@aol.com
*URL: www.aveweb.org

American Academy of Veterinary Disaster Medicine
Dr. Joanne Howl
4304 Tenthouse Court
West River, MO 20778 USA
Phone: 1-301-261-9940
Fax: 1-410-867-8406
Email: jovet@aol.com
URL: www.cvmbs.colostate.edu/clinsci/wing/aavdm/
    aavdm.htm

American Association of Food Hygiene Veterinarians
4910 Magdalene Court
Annandale, VA 22003-4363 USA
Phone and Fax: 1-703-323-9327
Email: joeblair@erols.com
URL: www.avma.org/aafhv

American Association of Industrial Veterinarians
PO Box 488
Oskaloosa, KS 66066-0488 USA
Phone: 1-785-863-2389
Fax: 1-785-863-3141
Email: aaiv@ruralnet1.com

American Association of Public Health Veterinarians
Dr. Fred Angulo
National Centers for Infectious Disease
Centers for Disease Control and Prevention
MS-A-38
Atlanta, GA 30333 USA
Phone: 1-404-639-2206
Fax: 1-404-639-2205
Email: fja0@cdc.gov
URL: www.avma.org/aaphv/default.htm

American Association of Zoo Veterinarians
Dr. Wilbur Amand
6 N. Pennell Road
Media, PA 19063 USA
Phone: 1-610-892-4812
Fax: 1-610-892-4813
Email: aazv@aol.com
URL: www.aazv.org

American Veterinary Medical Association
1931 North Meacham Road, Suite 100
Schaumburg, IL 60173 USA
Phone: 1-847-925-8070
Fax: 1-847-925-1329
Email: avmainfo@avma.org
URL: www.avma.org

International Veterinary Student Association
KVL, DSR
Dyrlaegevej 9
DK-1870 Frederiksberg DENMARK
Fax: 45 3528 2152
Email: info@ivsa.org
URL: www.ivsa.org

National Institute of Animal Agriculture
1910 Lyda Avenue
Bowling Green, KY 42104 USA
Phone: 1-270-782-9798
Fax: 1-270-782-0188
EmailNIAA@animalagriculture.org
URL: www.animalagriculture.org

Society for Range Management
445 Union Boulevard, Suite 230
Lakewood, CO 80228 USA
Phone: 1-303-986-3309
Fax: 1-303-986-3892
Email: srmden@ix.netcom.com
URL: http://srm.org

Society for Tropical Veterinary Medicine
Dr. Edmour F. Blouin
Dept. Veterinary Pathobiology
College of Veterinary Medicine
Oklahoma State University
Stillwater, OK 74078 USA
Phone: 1-405-744-6726
Fax: 1-405-744-5275 (fax)
Email: blouin@okstate.edu
URL: www.soctropvetmed.org

Student Chapter of the American Veterinary Medical
    Association
1931 North Meacham Road, Suite 100
Schaumburg, IL 60173 USA
Phone: 1-847-925-8070
Fax: 1-847-925-1329
Email: avmainfo@avma.org
URL: www.avma.org/savma/default.htm

United States Animal Health Association
P.O. Box K227
Richmond, VA 23288
Phone: 1-804-285-3210
Fax 1-804-285-3367
URL: www.usaha.org

World Association of Wildlife Veterinarians
Dr. A. W. English,
University of Sydney, Department of Animal Health,
Private Mailbag 3
Camden, NSW 270 Australia
Email: anthonye@camden.usyd.edu.au
URL: http://wildvet.home.netcom.com/home.html

World Veterinary Association
Rosenlunds Alle 8
DK-2720 Vanlose, Denmark
Phone: 45-387-10156
Fax: 45-387-10322
Email: wva@ddd.dk
URL: www.worldvet.org

RESEARCH AND POLICY INSTITUTIONS

Center for Health and The Global Environment
Harvard Medical School
333 Longwood Ave. Suite 640
Boston, MA 02115
Phone: 1-617-432-0493
Fax: 1-617-432-2595
Email: 1chg@hmg.harvard.edu
*URL: www.med.harvard.edu/chge/

Consultative Group on International Agricultural
    Research
The World Bank
MSN G6-601
1818 H Street, NW
Washington, DC 20433 USA
Phone: 1-202-473-8951
Fax: 1-202-473-8110
Email: cgiar@cgiar.org
*URL: www.cgiar.org

Cities Feeding People
PO Box 8500
Ottawa, Ontario KIG 3H9 Canada
Phone: 1-613-236-6163
Fax: 1-613-238-7230
Email: blwilson@idrc.ca
*URL: www.idrc.ca/cfp

Institute for Development Studies
University of Sussex
Brighton, BN1 9RE UK
Phone: 44-1273-606-261
Fax: 44-1273-621-202
Email: ids@ids.ac.uk
*URL: www.ids.ac.uk

International Centre of Insect Physiology and Ecology
PO Box 30772
Nairobi, Kenya
Phone: 254-2-861680
Fax: 254-2-860110
Email: icipe@icipe.org
*URL: www.icipe.org/cgi-bin/WebObjects/ICIPE

International Development Research Centre
250 Albert Street
PO Box 8500
Ottawa, Ontario K1G 3H9 Canada
Phone: 1-613-236-6163
Fax: 1-613-238-7230
Email: info@idrc.ca
URL: www.idrc.ca

International Food Policy Institute
2033 K St. NW
Washington, DC 20006-1002 USA
Phone: 1-202-862-5600
Fax: 1-202-467-4439
Email: ifpri@cgiar.org
*URL: www.ifpri.org

International Livestock Research Institute—Nairobi
P.O. Box 30709
Nairobi, Kenya
Phone: 254 2 630 743
Fax: 254 2 631 499
Email:ILRI-Kenya@cgiar.org
*URL: www.cgiar.org/ilri/ilri.cfm

International Livestock Research Institute—Addis Ababa
P.O. Box 5689
Addis Ababa, Ethiopia
Phone: 251 1 463 215
Fax: 251 1 461 252
Email:ILRI-Ethiopia@cgiar.org
*URL: www.cgiar.org/ilri/ilri.cfm

Land Tenure Center
University of Wisconsin—Madison
1357 University Avenue
Madison, WI 53715 USA
Phone: 1-608-262-3657
Fax: 1-608-262-2141
Email: ltc-uw@facstaff.wisc.edu
URL: www.wisc.edu/ltc

Organization for Tropical Studies
PO Box 90630
Durham, NC 27708-0630 USA
Phone: 1-919-684-5774
Fax: 1-919-684-5661
Email: nao@acpub.duke.edu
*URL: www.ots.duke.edu

Overseas Development Institute
111 Westminster Bridge Road
London SE1 7JD UK
Phone: 44 20 7922 0300
Fax: 44 20 7922 0399
Email: odi@odi.org.uk
*URL: www.odi.org.uk/

Pastoral Development Network
(Managed by the Overseas Development Institute)
111 Westminster Bridge Road
London SE1 7JD UK
Phone: 44 20 7922 0300
Fax: 44 20 7922 0399
Email: pdn @odi.org.uk
*URL: www.odi.org.uk/pdn/index.html

Transparency International
Otto-Suhr-Allee 97/99
Berlin, 10585 Germany
Phone: 49-30-343-8200
Fax: 49-30-3470-3912
Email: ti@transparency.org
*URL: www.transparency.org

World Conservation Monitoring Centre
219 Huntingdon Road
Cambridge, CB3 0DL UK
Phone: 44-1223-277-314
Fax: 44-1223-277-136
Email: info@unep-wcmc.org
*URL: http://www.unep-wcmc.org

World Resources Institute
10 G Street, NE, Suite 800
Washington, DC 20002 USA
Phone: 1-202-729-7600
Fax: 1-202-729-7610
Email: front@wri.org
*URL: www.wri.org

WorldWatch Institute
1776 Massachusetts Avenue, NW
Washington, DC 20036-1904 USA
Phone: 1-202-452-1999
Fax: 1-202-296-7365
Email: worldwatch@worldwatch.org
URL: www.worldwatch.org/

TRAINING, FELLOWSHIP AND GRANT OPPORTUNITIES

American Academy for the Advancement of Science
Science and Diplomacy Fellowship
1200 New York Avenue, NW
Washington, DC 20005 USA
Phone: 1-202-326-6700
Fax: 1-202-289-4950
Email: science_policy@aaas.org
URL: fellowships.aaas.org

AVMA Congressional Science Fellowship
101 Vermont Avenue, Suite 710
Washington, DC 20005 USA
Phone: 1-800-321-1473 ext 625
URL: www.avma.org/avmf/fellows.htm

Earthwatch
3 Clocktower Place, Suite 100
Box 75
Maynard, MA 01754 USA
Phone: 1-800-776-0188
Fax: 1-978-461-2332
Email: info@earthwatch.org
URL: www.earthwatch.org

Environmental Systems Research Institute
380 New York Street
Redlands, CA 92373-8100 USA
Phone: 1-909-793-2853
Fax: 1-909-793-5953
Email: info@esri.com
URL: www.esri.com

Federal Emergency Management Agency
Emergency Management Institute
16825 South Seton Avenue
Emmitsburg, MD 21727 USA
Phone: 800-238-3358
Fax: 301-447-1658
Email: emi@fema.gov
URL: www.fema.gov/emi/

EpiVet Net
Epi Centre
Private Bag 11222
Massey University
Palmerston North, New Zealand
Phone: 64-6-350-5270
Fax: 64-6-350-5716
Email: EpiCentre@massey.ac.nz
*URL: http://epiweb.massey.ac.nz

Geraldine R. Dodge Foundation
Frontiers in Veterinary Medicine
163 Madison Avenue
Morristown, NJ 07962-1239 USA
Phone: 1-973-540-8442
Fax: 1-973-540-1211
Email: vetinfo@grdodge.org
URL: http://www.grdodge.org/vet/index.html

United Nations Internship
Coordinator of the Internship Programme, Room S-2590D,
    United Nations
New York, NY 10017 USA
Phone: 1-212-963-7522
Fax: 1-212-963-3683
URL: http://www.un.org/Depts/OHRM/examin/internsh/
    intern.htm

United Nations Volunteer Program
PO Box 260111
Bonn, D-53153 Germany
Phone: 49-228-815-2000
Fax: 49-228-815-2001
Email: information@unvolunteers.org
URL: www.unv.org

University of California, Davis
Master of Preventative Veterinary Medicine, School of
    Veterinary Medicine
One Shields Avenue, University of California
Davis, CA 95616 USA
Phone: 1-530-752-1383
Fax: 1-530-752-2801
URL: www.vetmed.ucdavis.edu/mpvm/mpvm.htm

Veterinary Economics and Epidemiology Research Unit
University of Reading
PO Box 236
Reading, RG6 6AT UK
Phone: 44-118-931-8478
Fax: 44-118-926-2431
Email: veeru@reading.ac.uk
URL: www.veeru.reading.ac.uk

Virginia Maryland Regional College of Veterinary Medicine,
Center for Government and Corporate Veterinary Medicine
8075 Greenmead Drive
College Park, MD 20742-3711 USA
Phone: 301-314-6830
Fax: 301-314-6855
Email: cgcvm@vetmed.umd.edu
URL: www.vetmed.umd.edu/cgcvm/

Wageningen University
Postbus 9101, 6700

Wageningen, 6700 HB The Netherlands
Phone: 31-317-484-472
Fax: 31-317-484-884
Email: info@www.wag-ur.nl
URL: www.wau.nl

Wildlife Capture Course
Parawild Safaris
PO Box 4101
Nelspuit, 1200 South Africa
Phone: 27-82-468-7001
Email: safari@parawild.co.za
URL: www.parawild.co.za

Wildlife Veterinary Medicine Course
PO Box 90
Karino, 1204 South Africa
Phone: 27-13-747-2224
Email: jpraath@iafrica.com
URL: www.wildlifevets.com

UNITED STATES GOVERNMENT AGENCIES

**Animal and Plant Health Inspection Services—Veterinary
    Services**
United States Department of Agriculture
Washington, DC 20250 USA
URL: www.aphis.usda.gov/vs

Center for Veterinary Medicine
Food and Drug Administration
7519 Standish Place,
Rockville, Maryland 20855
301-827-3800
http://www.fda.gov/cvm/

Centers for Disease Control and Prevention
1600 Clifton Road, NE
Atlanta, GA 30333
Phone: 1-404-639-3311
URL: www.cdc.gov

Environmental Protection Agency
Ariel Rios Building
1200 Pennsylvania Avenue, NW
Washington, DC 20460 USA
Phone: 1-202-260-2090
URL: www.epa.gov

Food Safety and Inspection Service
1400 Independence Avenue, SW, Room 2932-S
Washington, DC 20250-3700 USA
Phone: 1-202-720-8601
URL: www.fsis.usda.gov

National Wildlife Health Center
6006 Schroeder Road
Madison, WI 53711 USA
Phone: 1-608-270-2400
Fax: 1-608-270-2415
URL: www.nwhc.usgs.gov/

National Zoological Park
3001 Connecticut Avenue, NW
Washington, DC 20008-2598 USA
Phone: 1-202-673-4721
Fax: 1-202-673-4607
Email: natzoo@nzp.si.edu
URL: http://natzoo.si.edu

Peace Corps
111 20th Street, NW
Washington, DC 20526 USA
Phone: 1-800-424-8580
Email: volunteer@peacecorps.gov
URL: www.peacecorps.gov/home.html

Plum Island Animal Disease Center
Foreign Animal Disease Diagnostic Laboratory
PO Box 848
Greenport, Long Island, NY 11944-0848 USA
Phone: 1-515-323-2500
URL: www.ars.usda.gov/plum/

United States Agency for International Development
Ronald Reagan Building
Washington, DC 20523-1000
Phone: 1-202-712-4810
Fax: 1-202-216-3524
URL: www.usaid.gov

U.S. Army Veterinary Corps
2250 Stanley Road
Fort Sam Houston, TX 78234-6100 USA
Phone: 1- 210-221-8149

Email: briannoland@ln.amedd.army.mil
URL: http://vets.amedd.army.mil/dodvsa/

US Fish and Wildlife Service
Main Interior, 301 MIB, 1849 C Street, NW
Washington, DC 20240-0002 USA
Phone: 1-202-208-4717
Fax: 1-202-208-6965
Email: contact@fws.gov
URL: www.fws.gov

US Public Health Service Commissioned Corps
Veterinary Medical Officers Corps
Recruitment/ODB, 5600 Fishers Lane, Room 4A-18
Rockville, MD 20857-001 USA
Phone: 1-301-594-3360
Email: phs@psc.gov
URL: www.usphs.gov/

Index

Pages numbers in *italics* denote figures; those followed by a t denote tables.

Franklin Pierce College Library

00139023

00139023